CONTRIBUTORS

V. JANE BLISS-HOLTZ, M.S.N., R.N.

Instructor, Nursing of Children, University of Pennsylvania
School of Nursing, Philadelphia, Pennsylvania

MEREDITH J. COWAN, R.N., B.S.N.

Assistant Head Nurse, Labor and Delivery,
Hermann Hospital, Houston, Texas

MADONNA CRONIN, R.N., M.S.

Staff Nurse, Neonatal Intensive Care,
George Washington University Hospital, Washington, D.C.

CORNELIA B. DEWEES, C.N.M., M.N.

Associate Professor, Nurse-Midwifery College of Nursing;
Nurse-Midwifery Staff, Medical University Hospital,
Medical University of South Carolina, Charleston, South Carolina

ELISSA A. EMERSON, C.F.N.P., M.S.

Assistant Professor of Community Health, School of Nursing
University of Texas Health Science Center
at Houston, Houston; Consultant, Gerontology,
Harris County Health
Department, Houston, Texas

SHERRY A. GILLESPIE, R.N., M.S.N.

Assistant Director, Obstetrics and Gynecology
Medical University of South Carolina
Charleston, South Carolina

KATHY ANNE HAUSMAN, R.N., M.S., C.N.R.N.

Neuroscience Consultant
Louisville, Kentucky

ALICE F. ILLIAN, R.N., B.S.N.

Assistant Clinical Lecturer, University of Texas School of Nursing;
Head Nurse, Turner Neonatal Intensive Care Unit and Neonatal
Transport Team, Hermann Hospital, Houston, Texas

M. LYNN LITCHFIELD, R.N., C.N.M., M.S.N.

Instructor, Neonatology, College of Nurse-Midwifery,
Medical University of South Carolina, Charleston;
Director, Maternal-Child Health, Spartanburg, General
Hospital, Spartanburg, South Carolina

CAROLE ANN MILLER McKENZIE, C.N.M., Ph.D.

Associate Professor and Chairperson,
Graduate Maternal Newborn Nursing
Medical University of South Carolina, Charleston, South Carolina

CAROLE ANN MILLER McKENZIE, C.N.M., Ph.D.

Professor and Dean, Division of
Nursing, Sumter Area Technical
College, Sumter, South Carolina; formerly
Associate Professor and Chairperson,
Graduate Maternal/Newborn Nursing Program, Medical
University of South Carolina, Charleston, South Carolina

ELAINE M. MOORE, C.N.M., M.S.N.

Staff Nurse-Midwife, Grady Memorial Hospital
Nurse-Midwifery Service, Atlanta, Georgia

JOY HINSON PENTICUFF, R.N., Ph.D.

Assistant Professor, School of Nursing,
University of Texas at Austin, Austin, Texas

JANE POHODICH, R.N., M.S.

Clinical Coordinator, Maternal and Child Health Nursing,
St. Joseph Hospital, Houston, Texas

PAMELA RODGERS, R.P.H., B.S.

Instructor, College of Pharmacy; Decentralized
Pharmacist/Supervisor, Medical University of
South Carolina, Charleston, South Carolina

ADITA LYNN ROOT, R.N., Ph.D.

Clinical Services Administrator,
Memorial Hospital, Houston, Texas

SHEILA SOUTHWELL

Perinatal Clinical Specialist, Moffett Hospital,
University of California, San Francisco, California

KAY STEPHENSON, R.N., M.S.N.

Director of Nursing, Maternal and Child Health Services,
Methodist Hospital of Dallas, Dallas; formerly Assistant Professor,
Graduate Program in Perinatal Nursing, Houston Baptist University
and University of Texas at Houston, Houston, Texas

HIGH RISK PERINATAL NURSING

by

The American Association of Critical-Care Nurses

Editors

KATHERINE W. VESTAL, R.N., Ph.D.

Associate Executive Director, Hermann Hospital, Houston;
Formerly Director of Pediatric Nursing, Hermann Hospital, Houston;
Assistant Professor of Pediatrics, The University of Texas
Medical School at Houston, Houston, Texas

CAROLE ANN MILLER McKENZIE, C.N.M., Ph.D.

Professor and Dean, Division of Nursing, Sumter Area Technical
College, Sumter, South Carolina; Formerly Associate Professor
and Chairperson, Graduate Maternal/Newborn Nursing Program,
Medical University of South Carolina, Charleston, South Carolina

1983

W. B. Saunders Company

Philadelphia • London • Toronto • Mexico City • Rio de Janeiro • Sydney • Tokyo

W.B. Saunders Company: West Washington Square
Philadelphia, PA 19105

1 St. Anne's Road
Eastbourne, East Sussex BN21 3UN, England

1 Goldthorne Avenue
Toronto, Ontario M8Z 5T9, Canada

Apartado 26370 – Cedro 512
Mexico 4, D.F., Mexico

Rua Coronel Cabrita, 8
Sao Cristovao Caixa Postal 21176
Rio de Janeiro, Brazil

9 Waltham Street
Artarmon, N.S.W. 2064, Australia

Ichibancho, Central Bldg., 22-1 Ichibancho
Chiyoda-Ku, Tokyo 102, Japan

Library of Congress Cataloging in Publication Data

Main entry under title:

High risk perinatal nursing.

1. Obstetrical nursing. 2. Pregnancy, Complications of—
Nursing. 3. Infants (Newborn)—Diseases—Nursing.

I. Vestal, Katherine W. II. McKenzie, Carole Ann.
III. American Association of Critical-Care Nurses.
[DNLM: 1. Obstetrical Nursing. 2. Perinatology—
Nursing texts. WY 157 H638]

RG951.H54 1983 610.73'678 82-24075

ISBN 0-7216-1005-6

Front and back cover illustrations are modified from illustrations appearing in *Victorian Stained Glass Pattern Book,* by Ed Sibbett, Jr., published by Dover Publications, Inc., New York, 1979

High Risk Perinatal Nursing   ISBN 0-7216-1005-6

Last digit is the print number: 9   8   7   6   5   4   3   2   1

TO RICHARD AND RICKY
TO ROGER AND RYAN

KATHERINE W. VESTAL, R.N., Ph.D.
Associate Executive Director,
Hermann Hospital,
formerly Director of Pediatric Nursing,
Hermann Hospital, Houston; Assistant
Professor of Pediatrics, The University
of Texas Medical School at
Houston, Houston, Texas

SHELLEY WALLISCH, R.N., M.S.
Nurse Clinician, Coney Island Hospital, Brooklyn, New York

FOREWORD

In recent years, technological advances have greatly improved the efficiency of living and coping with high risk situations. Technology has influenced health care services in many ways. However, health care providers and consumers must remain alert to the misuses and dangers related to technologically based health services, for misuses can lead to unfavorable consequences and other problems. Moreover, a preoccupation with or excessive dependency on technology could lead to problems in understanding and appropriately helping people. Hence technology has benefits and limitations in serving humans.

This comprehensive book reflects thoughtful attention to the role of technology in caring for high risk families and individuals. Technological assessment and procedures are carefully blended with different nursing caring activities. The blending of technological and nontechnological caring activities is important to provide highly skilled perinatal nursing care. Indeed, high risk perinatal nursing care has become a recognized specialty in nursing that necessitates care modalities to accommodate a variety of emotional, physical, social, and cultural health needs of clients.

Today, perinatal nurses are challenged to consider the health care needs of clients within a broad community frame of reference with diverse conditions and life stresses affecting people. This book provides such a community focus through discussions of ways to help clients and to detect life stresses that can affect perinatal families and individuals. Most importantly, suggestions for care of mothers and neonates from different geographic regions and communities are included. This community focus for high risk perinatal care provides the essential context to help nurses learn from clients ways to promote health or to prevent illnesses.

It is encouraging to see the book's emphasis on helping families prevent risk producing situations that limit favorable outcomes for the infant and mother during prenatal, natal and postnatal experiences. It is encouraging to see the ways in which the perinatal nurse can take an active leadership role as an advocate of healthy families and to prevent unnecessary illness conditions when other positive choices can be made for families. Today, the prevention of illness and the maintenance of health reflect the dominant and future directions for perinatal nursing care. The perinatal nurse is in a key position to demonstrate this trend.

The perinatal nurse must be well prepared and sensitive to the client's needs to be effective and successful in the professional role. The perinatal nurse must know how to help families and individuals whose cultural and economic lifeways are different from the normal expectations of professional nurses. Helping families maintain care outside, as well as inside, the hospital is most important. Technological and clinical learning and caring knowledge and skills are essential for nurses to function in human health care situations. Therefore, it is reassuring to find caring concepts and principles to guide nursing actions for high risk families and individuals included in this text. This caring emphasis reflects what I hold to be the central, unique, and distinct nature of nursing as a profession and discipline. It is essential to help nurses provide sensitive, skilled, and responsible care to high risk families and individuals. Thus I believe the nurse and all nurses are challenged to provide caring services rather than medical services as a major role activity of nursing. Caring is a humanistic and scientific domain to explain and know nursing activities, and this book points to several aspects of caring for perinatal clients and families. Caring can and does make a difference in the quality of human health services to people. But caring is also dynamic and requires the nurse to incorporate changes in techniques and method when clients indicate such a need.

In the future, we can anticipate that perinatal nurses will use research and theory to provide all health and nursing care services to families at high or low risk. Accordingly, the nurse must learn the principles, content, and methods presented so conscientiously in this book. The nurse must also study role activities and their therapeutic effect on clients and families.

In general, this book provides the reader with rich content and practice skills in high risk perinatal care, reflecting the authors' and editors' knowledge and skills. It is a book that can help to advance clinical nursing skills to high risk mothers and infants. Several examples are offered to help the reader grasp the nature and role expectations of the perinatal nurse in helping families with potential high risk conditions or problems. Sensitivity to life stresses affecting potential high risk families and individuals is an outstanding feature of this book. The readers will also recognize that a body of perinatal knowledge and clinical skills are growing in this subfield in nursing. Such knowledge and skills must be transmitted and incorporated in teaching, research, and practice in nursing. In achieving this goal, we will be able to say perinatal nurses can make a difference in the provision of humane health care to people.

MADELEINE M. LEININGER, R.N., Ph.D., F.A.A.N.
Professor of Nursing and Anthropology
Director, Center for Health Research
Wayne State University
Detroit, Michigan

PREFACE

The field of perinatology is developing at a rapid pace. The expansion of perinatal knowledge provides direct benefit to high risk perinatal patients who require sophisticated care directed toward ensuring the safety of the mother, fetus, and neonate, while at the same time promoting the welfare of the family unit. Such care does not happen without considerable planning and preparation of facilities, personnel, and resources. The need to continue to facilitate this planning and preparation is paramount to all health care workers in the perinatal arena, including nurses who assume major responsibilities in the management of the care of the high risk maternal fetal unit and the neonate. Obviously, not all high risk patients have rapid access to a sophisticated perinatal unit in a tertiary care center. This necessitates that all perinatal care facilities be capable of providing quality care for the high risk patient in an emergency. Nurses practicing in these settings must be able rapidly to assess and implement appropriate care based on valid knowledge.

High risk perinatal nursing focuses on a family centered approach to the needs of the mother and infant at risk, their families, and their friends. The nurse must utilize a basic knowledge of physiological and psychological concepts, pregnancy, and childbirth to formulate a plan of care for the patient at risk. The interdependency of all body systems and the superimposed pregnancy must be understood in order to assess the changing clinical picture adequately.

It is important for nurses practicing in the perinatal field to view the maternal-fetal-neonatal unit as a whole. All must be aware of the implications of risk in every aspect of the childbearing cycle. It is not adequate to segregate the care of the mother from the care of the baby. Indeed, such a view negates the basic premise of family centered care, which is a fundamental tenet of all perinatal nursing.

This book is designed to provide nurses who care for mothers, fetuses, and neonates with a concise guide to high risk perinatal nursing management. There is an element of risk with all pregnancy and childbirth, and rapid assessment and action can promote effective treatment. While it is helpful to have a basic understanding of maternal-neonatal nursing, this text will serve as a reference to any nurse faced with providing high risk perinatal care. Additional references and resources are included for the reader who desires further information.

An outline format is utilized as a means of providing a concise systematic presentation of material. Ready reference guides and charts are intended to consolidate critical information into a concise form. Instructors and students will also find this text useful as an orientation guide, study outline, or review course.

Section I addresses the concept of high risk perinatal care. The history and progression of this specialty reflect the rapid advances made in this field. The factors that produce the high risk condition are discussed, as well as potential outcomes. The important areas of regionalization of care and transport of both high risk mothers and high risk neonates are also explored, and the nursing care needed during transport is outlined.

Section II focuses on the psychosocial care of the high risk family unit. Family theory is utilized as a basis for exploring the strengths and deficits the high risk family bring to the health care setting. The concept of maternal-paternal-infant bonding is emphasized, in both assessment and implementation of nursing care. Techniques for the management of stress as it relates to the patient, family, and nursing staff in a perinatal crisis situation will be explored. Suggestions and resources for assisting the family during and following the crises are given.

Section III concentrates on maternal-fetal high risk care. Beginning with consideration of risk factors and assessment of the patient and family, the section emphasizes support for childbearing families at risk during the antepartal, intrapartal, and postpartal periods. Emergency procedures are outlined, and common instrumentation resources are described. The common critical medical conditions that might occur during the three partal periods—and nursing management of them—are discussed.

Section IV is devoted to neonatal high risk care. Beginning with discussion of risk factors and consideration of the neonate and his family, this section emphasizes support for the neonate at risk during the first 30 days of life. Emergency procedures, including resuscitation, are presented, and common instrumentation utilized in neonatal care is outlined. Common critical medical conditions that might be present during the neonatal period and general support areas, such as fluids and nutrition, thermoregulation, and stabilization, are also discussed.

Section V takes a futuristic look at high risk perinatal care and discusses ways to review and plan to meet regional high risk perinatal needs.

In addition, the appendices were developed to contain ready reference information for maternal and neonatal high risk procedures and drugs. These procedures and drugs are limited to common high risk entities and are not meant to be all inclusive. Other references may be helpful in providing additional material in these areas.

K.W.V.

C.M.McK.

ACKNOWLEDGMENTS

Special thanks go to Kathy Pitcoff of W.B. Saunders Company, whose support during this process was greatly appreciated, and to Bina Woodham, who spent many hours in the typing and preparation of this manuscript.

K.W.V.

C.M.McK.

CONTENTS

SECTION I   CONCEPTS IN HIGH RISK PERINATAL CARE

Chapter 1

THE NATURE OF HIGH RISK PERINATAL NURSING CARE 2

    Katherine W. Vestal, R.N., Ph.D., and Carole Ann Miller McKenzie,
    C.N.M., Ph.D.

Chapter 2

RISK FACTORS IN PERINATOLOGY 7

    Carole Ann Miller McKenzie, C.N.M., Ph.D.

Chapter 3

REGIONALIZATION OF HIGH RISK PERINATAL CARE 13

    Katherine W. Vestal, R.N., Ph.D.

Chapter 4

NEONATAL AND MATERNAL TRANSPORT 22

    Kay Stephenson, R.N., M.S.

SECTION II   PSYCHOSOCIAL CARE OF THE HIGH RISK
               FAMILY UNIT

Chapter 5

FAMILY-INFANT BONDING 64

    M. Lynn Litchfield, C.N.M., M.S.N.

Chapter 6

NURSING ASSESSMENT AND MANAGEMENT OF THE
CHILDBEARING FAMILY IN CRISIS 80

    Joy Hinson Penticuff, R.N., Ph.D.

Chapter 7

STRESS: THE INFANT, FAMILY, AND NURSE 97

    Shelley Wallisch, R.N., M.S.

SECTION III   MATERNAL/FETAL HIGH RISK CARE

Chapter 8

ASSESSMENT AND CLASSIFICATION OF THE HIGH RISK
MATERNAL-FETAL UNIT 120
  Elissa A. Emerson, M.S., C.F.N.P.

Chapter 9

OBSTETRICAL EMERGENCIES 137
  *Carole Ann Miller McKenzie, C.N.M., Ph.D., and
  Sherry A. Gillespie, R.N., M.S.N.*

Chapter 10

ANTEPARTAL CRISES 153
  Elaine M. Moore, C.N.M., M.S.N.

Chapter 11

INTRAPARTUM CRISES 191
  Sherry A. Gillespie, R.N., M.S.N.

Chapter 12

POSTPARTAL CRISES 258
  Carole Ann Miller McKenzie, C.N.M., Ph.D.

SECTION IV   HIGH RISK NEONATAL CARE

Chapter 13

ASSESSMENT AND CLASSIFICATION OF THE HIGH RISK
NEONATE 278
  Cornelia B. Dewees, C.N.M., M.N.

Chapter 14

NEONATAL EMERGENCIES 294
  Alice F. Illian, R.N., B.S.N.

Chapter 15

RESPIRATORY CRISES 325
  Adita Lynn Root, R.N., Ph.D.

Chapter 16

CARDIOVASCULAR AND HEMATOLOGICAL CRISES
IN NEONATES 353
  Sheila Southwell, R.N., M.S.

Chapter 17

NEUROLOGICAL CRISES 399
  Kathy A. Hausman, R.N., M.S., C.C.R.N.

Chapter 18
RENAL AND METABOLIC CRISES 429
Jane Bliss-Holtz, R.N., M.S.N.

Chapter 19
GASTROINTESTINAL CRISES AND NUTRITIONAL SUPPORT 452
Jane Pohodich, R.N., M.S.

Chapter 20
NEONATAL INFECTIONS 514
Madonna Cronin, R.N., M.S.

SECTION V   THE FUTURE OF HIGH RISK PERINATAL CARE
Chapter 21
PREDICTIONS, IMPLICATIONS, AND PLANNING FOR
HIGH RISK PERINATAL CARE 540
*Carole Ann Miller McKenzie, C.N.M., Ph.D., and
Katherine W. Vestal, R.N., Ph.D.*

APPENDIX A: MATERNAL PROCEDURES AND DRUGS 548

APPENDIX B: NEONATAL PROCEDURES AND DRUGS 596

INDEX 649

CONCEPTS IN HIGH RISK PERINATAL CARE

CHAPTER 1

THE NATURE OF HIGH RISK PERINATAL NURSING CARE

Katherine W. Vestal, R.N., Ph.D.
and
Carole Ann Miller McKenzie, C.N.M., Ph.D.

OBJECTIVES

Upon completion of this chapter the reader will be able to accomplish the following:

1. Identify the perinatal patient(s) at risk
2. Recognize the impact of perinatal crises on the family
3. Describe the high risk perinatal care-giver team
4. State the issues related to nurses' stress in those who function in the perinatal arena
5. Recognize the need for supporting nursing research in the high risk perinatal field.

High risk perinatal nursing care encompasses care of the childbearing family at risk from conception through the neonatal period. As a new specialty area in nursing the need to acquire knowledge and skills is essential. High risk perinatal families have always existed, but now the responsibility for meeting their special needs has become a part of nursing.

Statistics related to maternal/fetal and neonatal complications vary according to the source. Perinatal mortality (stillbirths and neonatal deaths) in 1977 was 1.6 per 1000 live births. Currently there are about 180 perinatal deaths for every maternal death.[5] Maternal mortality was reported to be 9.9 per 100,000 live births in 1978.[5] The number of deaths during the first 24 hours of life exceeds the number in the period from the second month to the first year of life, and the number of neonatal deaths is fewer than the number of fetal deaths.

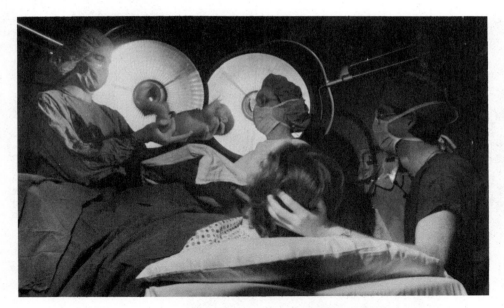

Figure 1-1. Family centered care is possible even in the high risk delivery setting. (Courtesy of Don Shaeffer, Hermann Hospital, Houston, Texas.)

These statistics indicate the need to improve care to the maternal/fetal unit and to better diagnose early fetal complications, which will occur as maternal transport systems are further developed to tap the resources of the regionalized center.

THE PERINATAL PATIENT

The perinatal patient may be the mother, the fetus, or the neonate. Risk to any one of these units may precipitate risk to another. While the father may not experience physiological risk, he is at risk with the mother and baby for psychological complications. The nurse who cares for the family must be aware of all the factors that influence risk and must be willing to include the total family in the development of care.

Obstetrical care is usually a normal positive environment for patients. It is difficult for staff to make the adjustment from the usual mode of care to that of high risk. Unfortunately it is the patient and family who suffer. At the time of crisis it is difficult to provide support that is not essential to physiological care. Staff members operate in a reactive mode to the crisis and are seldom able to provide a deliberative approach to the total patient.

Thus the need for planned comprehensive high risk care models is essential. These models should include biopsychosocial approaches to the family in a crisis situation and emphasize both short term and long term intervention.

The perinatal patient may include two patients if one considers the maternal/fetal unit. The fact that the nurse is caring for two patients, one of whom is unseen, complicates care. In a crisis this fact intensifies the need for a positive outcome. In addition, the adaptation required by the neonate to accommodate extrauterine life is paramount to survival. Thus complications of care increase logarithmically as crises evolve.

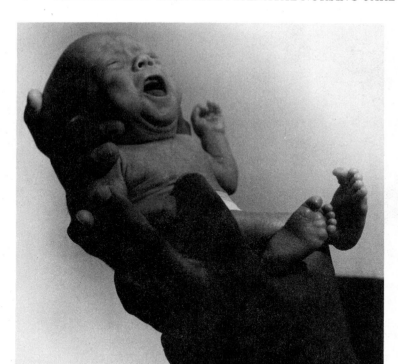

Figure 1-2. Outcomes for high risk neonate have significantly improved since the institution of perinatal care. (Courtesy of Don Shaeffer, Hermann Hospital, Houston, Texas.)

THE FAMILY

The impact of the high risk perinate has a tremendous effect on the family. These effects can indeed be catastrophic if one considers the potentially poor outcomes that may result. The crisis of the event as it affects the nuclear family cannot be underestimated. In addition to dealing with the usual aspects of birth, the nuclear family is forced to contend with a frightening crisis over which it has little control.

The extended family may not be geographically close enough to lend support or assist with events as they arise. Dependent on information derived from distraught family members, their anxiety may only lend further stress to the perinatal family. In a situation in which long term care is needed, absence of the extended family may induce greater economic and emotional strain on an already stressed family unit.

Nurses who work with the childbearing family at risk are in a position to help alleviate some of the stress. The nurse controls information about the event, is a constant source of support, and has limited ability to manage the environment. Control over such issues as visiting can make the difference in whether the crisis has a positive or negative result with the parents. The nurse is also instrumental in guiding the parents to develop coping mechanisms that are adequate to meet the crisis. This can be done by not overwhelming the parents with expertise but rather providing a competent and supportive environment in which they can relate to one another and their fetus or neonate.

THE STAFF

The perinatal team is generally composed of physicians, nurses, respiratory therapists, laboratory technicians, social workers, child life workers, chaplains, and transport team members. Often there are even more health care professionals who interact with the patient and family. This group of professionals has elected to provide care for high risk perinatal families, and their competence is evident as they respond to crisis. This competence is the result of experience, education, and the intangible desire to help families in crises on a day to day basis.

It is this constant stress that also places the team members at risk for their own crises. Because they are continually providing emotional support to others, they need adequate support systems provided for them. This can be accomplished through regular staff meetings, support groups, and counseling.

It is imperative that the administration of the institution recognize these risk factors of the staff. Failure to do so results in rapid turnover and disillusionment with the role. When this happens, the quality of care suffers, and the morale of the care providers is compromised. Administrative support can also be reflected in the provision of adequate staffing, educational resources, and reasonable equipment.

RESEARCH

There is a dearth of nursing research in the areas of perinatology. The existing studies tend to focus on psychosocial issues rather than physiological care, thus limiting the new information that is available to clinicians. It is imperative that nurses at all levels become active in seeking solutions to day to day problems that exist in perinatal care.

Perinatal interest groups in nursing must sponsor support for these studies through financial support and as resource centers. They can also provide a vehicle for reporting the findings at professional meetings and through professional journals.

CONCLUSIONS

The field of perinatology continues to develop at a rapid pace. The nurse's place in that development is critical. As the primary care giver for families in perinatal crises, the nurse is the constant stabilizing individual who remains with the patient on a 24 hour basis. The nurse is also the team member who can consider the patient from the total viewpoint, linking the physiological concerns with the psychological concerns. Coordination of the care giver, from crisis through transport to final resolution can provide the optimal outcome for the family. Challenges in the provision of this care are numerous. The nurse is in the role to meet these challenges.

_____ REFERENCES _____

1. Babson, S.G., Pernoll, M.L., and Benda, G.I.: Diagnosis and Management of the Fetus and Neonate at Risk: A Guide for Team Care, 4th ed. St. Louis, C.V. Mosby Co., 1980.
2. Butnarescu, G.F., Tillotson, D.M., and Villarreal, P.P.: Perinatal Nursing. Vol. 2: Reproductive Risk. New York, John Wiley and Sons, 1980.
3. Johnson, S.H.: High Risk Parenting. Philadelphia, J.B. Lippincott Co., 1979.
4. McKenzie, C.A.M., and Vestal, K.W.: Perinatal crises. _In_ Kinney, M., et al. (eds.): AACN's Clinical Reference for Critical Care Nurses. New York, McGraw-Hill Book Co., 1981.
5. Pritchard, J.A., and MacDonald, P.C.: Williams' Obstetrics, 16th ed. New York, Appleton-Century-Crofts, 1980.

CHAPTER 2

RISK FACTORS IN PERINATOLOGY

Carole Ann Miller McKenzie, C.N.M., Ph.D.

OBJECTIVES

Upon completion of this chapter, the reader will be able to accomplish the following:

1. Discuss the importance of risk assessment
2. List the sources that influence pregnancy and its outcome
3. List the criteria necessary for assessment of pregnancy as high risk
4. List the methods that are available to assess maternal and fetal well-being
5. Discuss the traditional methods of fetal assessment

Accurate and complete assessment is the most effective way to determine risk in the perinatal period. By assessing the childbearing family continuously throughout the childbirth experience, risks are identified early and can be managed. Early identification of risk is essential in providing positive perinatal outcomes. In an emergency situation, assessment must be quick and accurate to determine the thrust of intervention necessary. It is the nurse who usually must begin this process. The nurse may even, in some instances, complete the assessment and call the physician with the findings. Whatever the situation, the nurse must be ready with the information and skills necessary to provide the most accurate assessment.

This chapter will include a general overview of the influences affecting pregnancy and its outcome, the criteria for identification of high risk pregnancy, and the procedures utilized in risk screening during pregnancy. More specific information on assessment of the maternity patient is available in Chapter 8 and assessment of the neonate is available in Chapter 13. In addition, specific procedures are discussed in the appropriate chapters and in Appendix A, Maternal Procedures and Drugs.

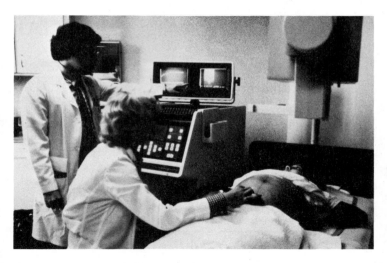

Figure 2-1. Accurate assessment of risk is essential in ensuring positive perinatal outcome. (Courtesy of Don Shaeffer, Hermann Hospital, Houston, Texas.)

It is important for the nurse to realize that regardless of the patient being cared for—mother, fetus, neonate, or father—the history of each influences the other. If the neonatal nurse is assessing risk in the baby, the history of the parents provide information about the neonate's outcome. If the neonate is having difficulty of some sort, the mother's postpartum course will be influenced. And if the father has any problems, they will influence the course of the pregnancy and neonatal outcome.

INFLUENCES ON PREGNANCY AND ITS OUTCOME

Table 2-1 lists the potential influences on pregnancy and its outcome. As one can see from the table, the factors that influence pregnancy and the neonate come from a variety of sources. Many of these factors come from the prepregnancy situation and can be assessed as part of prepregnancy counseling. With genetic problems this counseling is essential for favorable outcome. In time, it will probably be an essential component of care for the childbearing family.

CRITERIA FOR IDENTIFICATION OF HIGH RISK PREGNANCY

Table 2-2 provides a list of criteria that assist in identification of the high risk pregnancy. These criteria can be utilized to provide a check list of problems that contribute to the high risk situation. The criteria come from a variety of sources.

**TABLE 2-1. POTENTIAL INFLUENCES ON PREGNANCY
AND ITS OUTCOME**

Obstetric/ Gynecologic History	Medical/Surgical History	Paternal Influences	Biologic Factors
Grand multiparity	Chronic disease	Family history	Hormonal insufficiency
Previous surgical delivery	Hereditary disorders	Age	Weight
Previous prolonged labor	Psychiatric disease	Blood group	Height
Previous fetal loss or complication	Infectious disease	Chronic disease	Abnormal laboratory findings
Blood factor immunization	Family history	Hereditary disease	Age
Previous pregnancy			
Recent delivery			
Infertility			
Gynecologic complication			

Emotional Factors	Environmental Factors	Psychologic, Social, and Economic Factors	Present Pregnancy Factors
Family relationships	Stressors	Accidental pregnancy (unwanted)	Nutrition
Problems with other children	Smoking	Culture and race	Complications present
Any stress-producing factor	Drugs	Occupation/ education	Indifference to health needs
	Alcohol	Financial status	Lack of progression
	Genetic influences	Marital status	Gestation
	High altitude	Housing and environment	Surgery during pregnancy
	Infection	Support systems	Irradiation
	Exposure to environmental hazards	Age	

Reprinted with permission from McKenzie, C.M., and Vestal, K.: Perinatal Crises. *In* Kinney M., et al. (eds.): AACN's Clinical Reference for Critical Care Nurses. New York, McGraw-Hill Book Co., 1981.

TABLE 2-2. CRITERIA FOR IDENTIFICATION OF HIGH RISK PREGNANCY

Characteristics of the Patient
Age
 Teenage: under 18 at conception
 Elderly: 35 years and over at conception
Weight:
 Underweight: 100 lb or less
 Overweight: more than 20% over
  standard weight
 Gain: over 30 and under 15 lb

Height
 Short stature: 60 in or less

Race (specific problems affecting specific
 races, i.e., Tay-Sachs, sickle-cell anemia,
 cystic fibrosis)

Marital status
 Single
 Separated/divorced
 Widowed

Culture (specific cultural practice affecting
 pregnancy, i.e., pica)

Education/occupation
 Less than high school diploma
 Other than skilled or professional
  workers

Economics (lack of money for pregnancy
 care, housing and environment)

Available emotional supports (if none,
 may have emotional and other additional
 stressors)

Drug addiction or ingestion

Alcoholism

Smoking (two packs plus per day)

Emotionally stressed
 Fear
 Anger
 Hostility
 Anxiety and tension
 Lack of support
 Ambivalence
 Family problems
 Patient perceptions ("I know something
  is wrong")

Characteristics of the Father
Age
 Elderly: age 40 and over (increased
  incidence stillborn)
 Teenage: under 18 (lack of support
  and/or responsibility)

Blood group
 Rh positive with Rh negative mother
 ABO incompatibilities

Family history
 Genetically transferred conditions
 Genetically predisposed conditions

Chronic disease
 Drug addiction
 Alcoholism
 Diabetes mellitus

Previous Pregnancy History
Parity
 Grand multipara (seven or more
  pregnancies over 20 weeks or 500 gm)
 Primigravida

Previous surgical delivery
 Cesarean section
 Version
 Vacuum extraction
 Mid to high forceps
 Breech extraction

Previous outcomes
 "Early" fetal loss (two pregnancies
  terminated under 28 weeks)
 "Late" fetal loss (one or more at 28
  weeks plus)
 Live prematures (two or more under
  2500 gm)
 "Early" neonatal death (one or more
  under 7 days)
 "Early" fetal loss and live premature
  (one fetal loss under 28 weeks in last
  two pregnancies plus one live premature
  [any pregnancy])
 "Large" infant (one or more greater than
  4000 gm)
 "Damaged" or traumatized infant (one
  or more living or not)
 Infants small for gestational age

Pregnancy occurrence
 Less than 3 months after last delivery
 More than 5 years after last delivery

Labor length
 Prolonged or dystocia
 Precipitate

Medical/Surgical History (during
 nonpregnancy period, previous
 pregnancy, or present pregnancy)
Hypertensive disease
Renal disease
Diabetes
Cancer in past 5 years
Thyroid disease
Hereditary disorders
Cardiovascular disease
Respiratory disease

Table continues on following page.

TABLE 2-2 *(Continued)*

Blood factor sensitization
Severe malnutrition
Psychiatric disorder
Neurologic disease
Drug addiction or ingestion
Alcohol addiction or ingestion
Mental retardation
Lupus erythematosus
Infectious disease
Infertility
Gynecologic complication

Additional Medical Complications
  (during previous or present pregnancy)
Toxemia

Bleeding

Rubella

Anemia
  Hemoglobin 8 gm or less
  Hematocrit 30% or less
  Sickle-cell anemia
  Cooley's anemia

Multiple pregnancy

Abnormal positional problems

Abnormal presentation
Abnormal lie
Abnormal position

Indifference to health needs
  Missed appointments (three or more)
  Failure to follow recommendations
    consistently

Nutrition
  Weight loss and/or crash dieting, fasting
  Weight gain (less than 15 lb or more than
    30 lb)

Progression
  Incompatible fundal height with gestation
  Small for gestational age fetus
  Large for gestational age fetus
  Multiple pregnancy
  Incorrect calculation of dates
  Hydramnios or oligohydramnios

Other
  General anesthesia or surgery
  Abdominal x-rays
  High altitude
  Stressors
  Decreased fetal movement

Reprinted with permission from McKenzie, C.M., and Vestal, K.: Perinatal Crises. *In* Kinney, M., et al. (eds.): AACN's Clinical Reference for Critical Care Nurses. New York, McGraw-Hill Book Co., 1981.

The childbearing family must be assessed biologically, psychologically, environmentally, and socially, including economically. All of these areas provide information about the high risk situation. In addition, both the mother and father provide helpful information for accurate assessment.

METHODS TO ASSIST FETAL AND MATERNAL WELL-BEING

There are a variety of methods utilized in assessing maternal and fetal well-being. Table 2-3 lists these methods. Each of these methods is discussed in more detail in Chapters 8, 10, 11, and 13 and in Appendix A.

The more traditional methods of fetal assessment—estimation of fetal age, measurement of uterine size, estimation of fetal weight, detection and measurement of fetal heart rate, and detection and history of fetal movements—can all be viable methods of assessment when none of the other tools is available. However, a more complete picture of maternal and fetal well-being is obtained by utilizing the more sophisticated methods. Table 2-3 lists some of the more futuristic tools that are being utilized in some areas at this time. These certainly will have a place in the assessment process of tomorrow.

TABLE 2-3.   METHODS OF ASSESSMENT OF FETAL AND MATERNAL WELL-BEING

Traditional Methods	Laboratory Parameters	Serial Measurements of Fetal Growth
Estimation of fetal age	Antenatal genetic diagnosis	Radiography
Measurement of uterine size	Amniocentesis	Ultrasound
Estimation of fetal weight	Physiological maturity— amniotic fluid	
Detection and measurement of fetal heart rate	surfactant L/S ratio Creatinine	
Detection and history of fetal movements	Biochemical testing— Human chorionic gonadotropin Estriols	
Stress testing	*Future methods (utilized now in limited areas)*	
Oxytocin challenge tests	Amnioscopy	
Non-stress tests	Amniography	

CONCLUSIONS

The accuracy of diagnosis of an obstetrical or neonatal emergency or crisis is dependent upon the accuracy of the assessment of either patient. Since the nurse will usually be beginning and possibly completing this assessment, a working knowledge of the components of total assessment is essential. Thus the patient will be assured more complete and quality care in the childbearing period.

REFERENCES

1.   Babson, S.G., Pernoll, M.L., and Benda, G.I.: Diagnosis and Management of the Fetus and Neonate at Risk: A Guide for Team Care, 4th ed. St. Louis, C.V. Mosby Co., 1980.

2.   Butnarescu, G.F., Tillotson, D.M., and Villarreal, P.P.: Perinatal Nursing. Vol. 2: Reproductive Risk. New York, John Wiley & Sons, 1980.

3.   Jenson, M.D., Benson, R.C., and Bobak, I.M.: Maternity Care: The Nurse and the Family, 2nd ed. St. Louis, C.V. Mosby Co., 1979.

4.   McKenzie, C.A.M., and Vestal, K.W.: Perinatal crises. *In* Kinney, M., et al. (eds.): AACN's Clinical Reference for Critical Care Nurses. New York, McGraw-Hill Book Co., 1981.

5.   Pritchard, J.A., and MacDonald, P.C.: Williams' Obstetrics, 16th ed., New York, Appleton-Century-Crofts, 1980.

6.   Spellacy, W.N.: Management of the High-Risk Pregnancy. Baltimore, University Park Press, 1976.

7.   Varney, H.: Nurse-Midwifery. Boston, Blackwell Scientific Publications, 1980.

CHAPTER 3

REGIONALIZATION OF HIGH RISK PERINATAL CARE

Katherine W. Vestal, R.N., Ph.D.

OBJECTIVES

Upon completion of this chapter the reader will be able to accomplish the following:

1. List the common features of successful regionalized perinatal programs
2. Define regionalized high risk perinatal care
3. Describe the three levels of obstetrical and neonatal services
4. Identify the basic purposes of regional perinatal centers
5. Discuss the issues in regionalized perinatal care related to personnel, financial considerations, family centered concept, transport systems, and coordination with community hospitals
6. Describe planning and evaluation models for regionalized high risk perinatal care

Perinatology has been successful in implementing systems for the regionalization of high risk care. Regional networks have been designed to reduce perinatal mortality through referral to sophisticated centers equipped to provide high risk medical and nursing care. Despite this, the United States still has a relatively poor standing in perinatal outcome, as compared with other Western industrialized nations. Factors that may contribute to this poor standing include the ethnic and social heterogeneity of the population, the country's geographic vastness, and gaps in the general availability and delivery of perinatal care.[13]

In the mid 1960s increased attention to the outcomes of high risk maternal and infant care stimulated development of a new pattern of care delivery. The availability of sophisticated technology, transport equipment, and combined obstetrical and pediatric care led to development of a comprehensive regional plan for perinatal care.

This required the provision of centralized obstetrical and newborn intensive care services that provided the communications and referral systems to ensure that all at risk might have entry into the system. This system also addressed the costs of medical care by consolidating expensive resources, both technical and human, in centers, rather than having widespread duplication of services in many hospitals.

THE NATURE OF THE REGIONALIZATION PROCESS

Although the guidelines for regionalization of perinatal services have been well defined, the social and political process has been less well delineated. Viable regionalized programs share common features.[1]

1. Problems are defined by a broad spectrum of health care professionals in various settings—practice, academic, and public health—and representatives in geographical-demographical perspective.
2. Plans and programs involve all people responsible for the delivery of the primary care.
3. Programs build on the existing strengths of an area and are sensitive to local perspectives.
4. Programming reflects understanding and involvement of the general community.
5. A balancing of individual and institutional priorities must exist.
6. The needs of the service recipients are clearly in focus and central to the process.
7. Continual evaluation and improvement must be made in the program.

Underlying the development of perinatal centers is the constant realization that the service must meet the cultural needs of those it was designed to serve. This culture, its values, structures, and biases, may differ from those of the innovators and must be considered in all activities. The cultures of both the innovators and the recipients may change, and the fluid nature of the population must be considered when formulating new ideas, techniques, and policies.

DEFINITIONS

Regionalized high risk perinatal care can be defined as a service providing facilities capable of delivering care of varying degrees of complexity in a given geographical area. All facilities work in close coordination to provide efficient, high quality, cost effective care with a minimum of duplication and waste.[7] The most important aspect of this approach is to provide care, as close to their homes as possible, to women with high risk pregnancies and to minimize the number of sick infants who must be transported following delivery.

In general, hospitals with obstetrical and neonatal services can be classified as primary, secondary, or tertiary perinatal care centers according to the level of care they are prepared to provide.

Level I Facilities. Primary, or level I, facilities are designed to provide care to obstetrical and newborn patients who have no complications. Because the number of deliveries at these facilities is often low, it is not economically feasible to provide high risk perinatal care. Facilities offering primary care must, however, be prepared to identify complications of pregnancy or of the neonate when they arise and make a referral to a high risk center for treatment. Obviously they must also be prepared to handle emergency situations and initiate methods of stabilization prior to transport.

Level II Facilities. Secondary, or level II, facilities are designed both to provide normal obstetrical and newborn care and to handle most of the complications of pregnancy and the neonatal period. While not equipped with as extensive an intensive care environment as a level III facility, the secondary setting can provide care to both the mother needing continuous fetal monitoring and the baby requiring basic cardiorespiratory monitoring or general support. Major obstetrical or neonatal problems will require transport to a level III facility. Twenty-four hour laboratory facilities must be available.

Level III Facilities. Tertiary, or level III, facilities are able to provide sustained and complete care for the most complex obstetrical and neonatal problems. This type of facility should have a high delivery rate and serve a large population area. Densely populated urban areas may support several level III facilities, while in sparsely populated geographical regions a facility may of necessity be some distance from the community hospital.

The level III facility is usually associated with a medical school and has affiliation agreements with level I and II facilities to provide care for their complex cases. There must be provisions for expert transport and continuous back-up services for the facility. Extensive and ongoing education must be available for personnel.

The basic purposes of regional perinatal centers can be summarized as follows:[13]

1. To identify and treat high risk pregnancies early in the perinatal period
2. To further identify and treat high risk factors within the intrapartum and neonatal periods
3. To develop interhospital agreements on criteria for transfer of mothers and infants within the network
4. To develop support systems of consultation, laboratory services, education, and transportation within a region
5. To develop a record keeping system to allow evolution of the entire program

A conceptual model of a regional system is seen in Figure 3–1. This model indicates that all pregnant women are systematically monitored for risk factors. A criterion of risk may indicate treatment in the community hospital or in a higher level care center. Such a network will also provide the same support for neonates when problems arise. The unique roles of both community and university hospitals must be respected for regionalization to work and to improve access of the high risk mother or infant to the appropriate level of care.

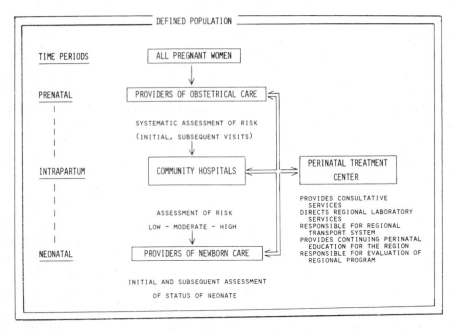

Figure 3-1. Conceptual model of a regional perinatal system within a defined geographic area. (Reprinted with permission from Merkatz, I., and Johnson, K.: Regionalization of perinatal care for the United States. Clin. Perinatol., *3*:272, 1976.)

PERSONNEL

Regionalization requires availability and proper distribution of medical and nursing personnel. Tertiary care centers are generally in constant need of neonatologists and neonatal intensive care nurses. This same shortage is often seen at the secondary level. In addition to physicians and nurses, there is an equally increasing demand for respiratory therapists, physical therapists, perinatal social workers, and other support personnel.

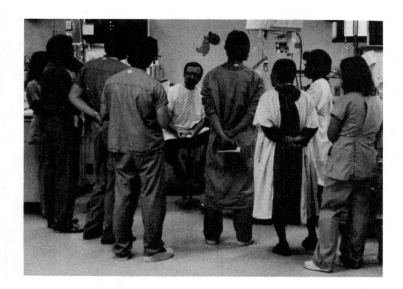

Figure 3-2. Education of high risk care givers is an important aspect of regionalized centers. (Courtesy of Hermann Hospital, Houston, Texas.)

The highly complex nature of the high risk perinatal setting demands knowledgeable as well as empathetic care givers. The resources for educating and supporting such personnel must be provided. This is usually done through university sponsored outreach educational programs for level I and II facilities. Regular, planned in-services can be provided as well as exchange facilities for clinical training.

FINANCIAL CONSIDERATIONS

The cost of regionalization cannot be underestimated. Financially the development of regional medical facilities is usually borne by individuals utilizing the services, i.e., patients, or the taxpayers. When one considers the costs of maintaining such facilities, combined with rising inflation, the financial picture is ominous. A high risk hospitalization can be financially devastating to a family or create considerable unpaid services for the facility. Despite this, the demand for high risk beds continues to increase. With less capital available for expansion and fewer dollars available for services, current overcrowding of facilities is not likely to diminish in the near future.

MAINTAINING THE FAMILY CENTERED CONCEPT

Family centered perinatal care helps the family to reach the goals of physiological well-being and strong positive emotional interaction with the newborn child.[19] It recognizes the impact of family attitudes and behaviors on the ultimate well-being of the child. With increased emphasis on the use of regionalized perinatal centers, the question arises how such settings can coexist with family centered care.

Superspecialization of perinatal care could lead to sacrifice of individualized attention to the family if it is not safeguarded. Perinatal practices must reflect careful attention to individual family variations and needs. For the high risk perinatal families there must be emphasis on their emotional needs as well as the technological. Regional high risk centers should attempt to offer the commonly sought family services, i.e., fathers welcome in the delivery room even for a high risk birth, rooming-in arrangements if possible, overnight accommodations for the husbands, liberal visiting hours, sibling visitations, and childbirth/parenting classes.

Transfer of mother, neonate, or both physically removes the family from their common support systems, so familiar people and physicians are helpful. The community physician needs access to the mother and baby if only for informational purposes. If the parents are separated from their sick infant, frequent communication between the doctor/nurse and family is imperative. Pictures of the baby are helpful, and visitation should be arranged as soon as the mother can travel. Nurses should be concerned about the family that initiates no contact with the regional center and should work diligently to establish rapport. Forced separation between the parents and infant may lead to poor bonding and increasing depression. There may be cases when it is best also to transfer the postpartum mother to the same facility as the infant to enhance their contact. When feasible, reverse transport returning the baby who has improved to the closest appropriate community hospital, is always helpful to the commuting family.

Regionalized quality high risk perinatal care can be reconciled with family centered maternal and neonatal care. It depends, however, on strenuous efforts by the primary care givers, both physicians and nurses, to develop close working relationships with the community hospitals.[11] Regional centers must be responsive to their referral sources and to the needs of the parents who wish not only medical excellence but also an active role in their newborn's care.

REGIONALIZED TRANSPORT SYSTEMS

Sophisticated and reliable means for transport of mothers and neonates was the development that insured the success of regionalization. As knowledge of stabilization and support techniques needed for moving critical patients became known, the basic impediment to centralized care diminished. Currently there are many systems available for both antepartum and neonatal transport.

While the technical aspects of transport are discussed in Chapter 4, the philosophical issues of transport are important in the concept of regionalization. The network of community hospitals that refers to a level II or III facility should devise a system that is effective and efficient for identifying and moving perinatal patients judged to be at high risk. The diversity of transport schemes that have developed reflects the striking regional differences in geography, political structures, professional personnel, facilities, and socioeconomic patterns.[18]

Most transport systems, both air and ground, are sponsored by the regional center and are designed to respond to requests from outlying hospitals. A transport team is sent to stabilize the condition of and move the mother or baby back to the center. Such a system is both costly and time consuming. Recently systems utilizing a "community based" transport process made up of well trained non-physician teams to escort the mother or baby to the regional center have proven effective.[18] This provides a reasonable alternative to the traditional method of transfers.

Maternal transport is also receiving increased attention as risk factors are being identified earlier in pregnancy. A high risk maternal transport system developed subsequent to a newborn transport system broadens the scope of intensive care and further reduces neonatal mortality and morbidity.[10] It seems logical that even greater reductions in neonatal crises could be achieved if the identified high risk mother were to be transported to a perinatal center for special management of prenatal or intrapartum complications known to affect neonatal outcome. A high risk maternal transport system should be expected to complement or supplement a well established newborn transport system and not replace it. Unfortunately, development of maternal transport systems has yet to attain the level of neonatal transport systems.

Regional Dispatch Systems. Contemporary issues related to high risk perinatal regionalization are now surfacing as the concept matures. One issue is related to the difficulty in locating available neonatal intensive care beds. Because of funding cutbacks, personnel shortages, and greater demand for beds, there are an increasing number of incidents in which critically ill newborns have been turned away from financially strained, overcrowded hospitals. This critical bed shortage exists in many regions, and there is no resolution in sight. Several perinatal centers have instituted a regional dispatch center to expedite location of beds in neonatal intensive care units.[22]

A regional dispatch system improves the efficiency of locating available high risk beds, reduces staff time required to locate beds, and helps provide a data retrieval system for future reference. Such systems utilize dispatchers and back-up physicians and nurses for a 24 hour a day, 7 day a week referral service. Neonatal centers are contacted once each shift to determine the number of intensive and intermediate care beds available. General guidelines for use when locating beds include (1) infant's condition, (2) closest appropriate center with an available bed, (3) physician's preference, and (4) location of the infant's home.[22] Nurses and physicians provide perinatal consultation to the dispatcher or referring physician. This link to a central source can be the key in providing timely and highly skilled assistance to a mother or a baby at risk.

COORDINATION WITH COMMUNITY HOSPITALS

The community hospital is an integral and important part of a regionalized perinatal program. The American Hospital Association considers a community hospital to be nonfederal, short term, general or otherwise specialized. Approximately 5900 of the 7100 hospitals in the United States meet that definition.[2] These hospitals have a high status in their communities and are important resources for the population. In 1972, over 25 per cent of these hospitals had fewer than 50 beds, and under 4 per cent had more than 500 beds.[2]

The community hospital is viewed as providing the comprehensive treatment that used to be provided by the family physician. The town babies are born there, children are treated, and the elderly die there. Some hospitals are reluctant to consolidate high risk services, either for reasons of pride or fear of loss of service, because they feel they would not be fulfilling their *community* obligation to provide family health care. Thus it is not difficult to see why the community hospital is an important entry point into the concept of regionalized perinatal care.

Over 60 per cent of the deliveries in the United States occur in hospitals with less than 500 deliveries per year, and the number of hospitals offering obstetrical services has increased each year since 1973.[14] Thus the ability to transfer patients at high risk from a community hospital to a perinatal center provides an option for care by highly expert professionals.

Paradoxically, the increased availability of regionalized centers has provided more efficient maternal and neonatal transport and better outreach educational support to the community. Hence their ability to care for the unexpected has been enhanced. The regional system should capitalize on the specific strengths of individual hospitals in addition to correcting weaknesses and provide teaching components that focus on the practical needs of the hospital at its own level of care.[5]

PLANNING AND EVALUATION OF
————— REGIONALIZED HIGH RISK PERINATAL CARE —————

Perinatal care is undergoing rapid change, predominantly because of innovations brought about by regionalization. Planning involves both evaluation and decision making. The well known processes of designing, gathering data, identifying goals, and determining resources apply to the perinatal regionalization process as well. Future changes will have to be evaluated with the current social and economic climate to establish priorities.

New clinical practices will emerge that will improve pregnancy outcome. Regional perinatal centers will need to show that they are looking critically at the processes by which their programs attempt to effect changes in health outcomes.[16] Perinatal mortality and birthweight have been commonly utilized as measures of program effectiveness, but additional measures are clearly needed. The potential for regionalization to produce more accurate data must be utilized to provide reliable means for conducting program evaluation.

There are three main strategies for evaluation:[16]

1. Description of program activities
2. Measurement of goal fulfillment
3. Measurement of cause and effect using vital statistics as they relate to the regionalized perinatal program

Regional perinatal programs must be committed to evaluation of their programs, and this should be planned for at the onset. Planning and evaluation provide a frame of reference for these programs and as well as evidence of the cost at which their efforts yield the benefits that they seek to attain.[16]

————————————— CONCLUSIONS —————————————

Regionalization of high risk perinatal services is intended to deliver comprehensive care to high risk mothers and neonates. In addition it educates parents and personnel and assumes the responsibility for follow-up using community resources. As a result the regional center is not just a repository for sick patients, but rather it is an institution in which education, current and comprehensive medical and nursing care, and ongoing evaluations of all facets of perinatal health care are coordinated and carried out for a designated region.[5]

_____ REFERENCES _____

1. Belton, H., and Meyer, P.: Regional care for mothers and their infants. Clin. Perinatol., 7:218, 1980.
2. Brown, I.: The management of high-risk obstetric transfer patients. Obstet. Gynecol., 51:198, 1978.
3. Brown, J.L.: The role of the community hospital in a regional program of obstetrics and neonatal care. Clin. Perinatol., 7:197–203, 1980.
4. Butterfield, L.J.: Organization of regional perinatal programs. Semin. Perinatol., 1:217–233, 1977.
5. Curet, L.B.: Perinatal centers and regionalization of perinatal care. 18:343, 1977.
6. Ellenberger, D., Kennedy, A.H., and Chase, C.: An educational program for nurses from referring hospitals in a perinatal regionalization system. J.O.G.N. Nurs., 8: 158–161, 1979.
7. Evans, H., and Glass, L.: Regionalization of perinatal care. Pediatr. Ann., 7:18, 1978.
8. Ferrara, A.: Evaluation of efficacy of regional perinatal programs. Semin. Perinatol., 1:303–308, 1977.
9. Florida perinatal program a mixed success. Am. Med. News, 24:12–14, 1981.
10. Harris, T.R., Isaman, J., and Giles, H.R.: Improved neonatal survival through maternal transport. Obstet. Gynecol., 52:294, 1978.
11. Klein, M.C., and Papageorgiou, A.N.: Can perinatal regionalization be reconciled with family-centered maternal care? J. Fam. Pract., 5:974, 1977.
12. Modanlou, H.D., Dorchester, W., Freeman, R.K., and Romnal, C.: Perinatal transport to a regional perinatal center in a metropolitan area: Maternal versus neonatal transport. Am. J. Obstet. Gynecol., 138:1157–1164, 1980.
13. Merkatz, I., and Johnson, K.: Regionalization of perinatal care for the United States. Clin. Perinatol., 3:272–274, 1976.
14. Ryan, G.M.: Regional planning for maternal and perinatal health services. Semin. Perinatol., 1:255–266, 1977.
15. Shott, R.J.: Regionalization: A time for new solutions. Pediatr. Clin. North Am., 24:651–657, 1977.
16. Siegal, E., Gillings, P., and Nugent, R.: Planning and evaluation of regionalized perinatal care: A general example. Semin. Perinatol., 1:284, 1977.
17. Sinclair, J.C., Torrance, G.W., Boyle, M.H., Horwood, S.P., Saigal, S., and Sackett, D.L.: Evaluation of neonatal–intensive care programs. N. Engl. J. Med., 305:489–494, 1981.
18. Sumner, J., Harris, H.B., Jones, B.J., Cassady, G., and Wirtschafter, D.A.: Regional neonatal transport: Impact of an integrated community center system. Pediatrics, 65:910, 1980.
19. Swartz, W.H., and Swartz, J.V.: Family centered maternity care. Its relationship to perinatal regionalization and neonatal intensive care. Clin. Perinatol., 3:433, 1976.
20. The regionalization of perinatal care. Am. J. Public Health, 71:571–572, 1981.
21. Usher, R.: Changing mortality rates with perinatal intensive care and regionalization. Semin. Perinatol., 1:309–319, 1977.
22. Vogt, J.F., Chan, L.S., Wu, P.Y., and Hawes, W.E.: Impact of a regional infant dispatch center on neonatal mortality. Am. J. Public Health, 71:577, 1981.
23. Watteville, H.: The future structure of perinatology. J. Perinat. Med., 3:8–10, 1975.

CHAPTER 4

NEONATAL AND MATERNAL TRANSPORT

Kay Stephenson, R.N., M.S.*

OBJECTIVES

Upon completion of this chapter the reader will be able to accomplish the following:

1. Define perinatal transport

2. Understand the rationale for the development of perinatal transport services

3. Differentiate between the types of perinatal transport services based on client focus, institutional responsibility/control and mode of transportation

4. Identify four elements of team selection, composition and/or roles that are paramount to the most successful functioning of the transport system

5. List the factors that are given consideration in selection of the best transport vehicle for a perinatal health care region

6. Outline the basic types of equipment required for maternal-fetal and neonatal transport

7. State the basic premise in determining the need for any transport of perinatal clients

8. List the most common indications for maternal-fetal and neonatal transport

9. Identify the four phases of the transport process. Describe the importance of each phase in the achievement of an optional outcome for the transport process

10. Describe a nursing role for perinatal transport

Transportation of patients to facilities designed to provide appropriate attention to their health care needs is not a new concept in the delivery of care. Unfortunately, an all too common scene in daily life is a speeding ambulance transporting an individual for emergency treatment of a life threatening condition. Military health care personnel have been involved in ground or air evacuation and transport of civilians and military service personnel probably since major wars began. Transporting patients from one

---

*The author wishes to thank the following perinatal transport nurses for their assistance: Sharon Bloom, R.N., M.S.N., Alice R. Gomez, R.N., C.N.P., and Julie Wood, R.N., B.S.N.

health care institution to another, however, has evolved largely as a result of specialization within the health care field. With the advancements currently available in the scientific base of medical practice as well as the sophistication of technological support, it is impossible for each health care professional and institution to provide all the services available for the patient with certain health care needs. Thus, transport can be an invaluable resource for perinatal health care providers.

PERINATAL TRANSPORT – THE CONCEPT AND RATIONALE

The disciplines of obstetrics and pediatrics combined efforts to provide comprehensive care for the high risk perinatal patient. Services have been developed that provide highly sophisticated diagnostic, monitoring, and therapeutic technology managed by advanced educational practitioners of more narrow specialization. These services are too costly to be provided at every institution offering care for perinatal patients, so the regionalization of these services has been an important concept to ensure availability, accessibility, and affordability. Referral of patients requiring specialized high risk services is inherent in the regionalization concept. Often such referral warrants the use of transport services.

There are inconsistencies in the literature that defines perinatal transport. The terms referral, transfer, and transport appear to be used interchangeably. For the purposes of this chapter, perinatal transport will be defined as the *supervised movement of one or more perinatal patients from one health care institution to another*. Supervision implies *the accompaniment of the patient by a professional or paraprofessional* member of the health care system. Health care institution is defined broadly as *any facility providing care to the patient for the purposes of meeting recognized health care needs*. Such institutions may include, but are not limited to, hospitals, clinics and private physicians' offices.

Although referral is a component of the transport of perinatal clients, transport is viewed as a more involved issue in the delivery of perinatal health care services. Transport dictates the need for a vehicle for transfer, designation of member(s) of health care professions for accompaniment, controlled physical movement of the patient, and provision of care during the process. Referral of the high risk maternal/fetal patient, at some designated point in the antepartum period, may result in a degree of freedom for the patient in planning and implementing her own method of travel, accommodations, and, to some extent, length of stay to receive care in the specialized center.

THE SYSTEM FOR TRANSPORT

There are many ways to organize and implement a transport system for the high risk maternal/fetal unit or newborn. In consideration of any transport system, attention must be given to the type of system, the team, the vehicle, the equipment, and the indications, as well as the process of the transport episode itself.

TYPE

There are three broad areas to be examined in discussing the types of transport systems employed for high risk perinatal patients. These are delineated by (1) patient focus—maternal/fetal or neonatal transport, (2) institutional responsibility and control—one-way or two-way transport, and (3) mode of transportation—ground or air. A type of transport system can be described by combining one of the two choices for each of the three areas, for example, two-way maternal air transport. There are at least as many types of transport systems presently employed for perinatal patients as there are permutations from the two choices in the three broad areas.

Regional areas often develop and utilize more than one type of system. This may occur concurrently, as the institutions in the region attempt to meet different needs, or progressively, as those involved in developing and utilizing the system recognize which type of system best suits their patient population, institutional philosophy, financial resources, and geographical locale. No one type of transport system automatically precludes the need for another type. The strengths and pertinent considerations of various types of transport systems can best be described within the framework of the three broad areas previously outlined.

Patient Focus—Maternal/Fetal and Neonatal Transport

Maternal/fetal transport, more simply referred to as maternal transport, is directed at supervised transfer of the pregnant woman and her developing fetus prior to delivery for the purpose of providing specialized high risk perinatal care. The nature of the care can be diagnostic, monitoring, or treatment, or it may be a combination. The need for specialized care can be determined or anticipated for the maternal patient, the fetus, or the newborn. The timing for transport can occur during the antepartum period, early in the intrapartum period, or in the postpartum period. The philosophy of maternal/fetal transport services is not to transport if delivery is imminent. There is a risk that delivery may occur en route and require emergency care for both maternal and neonatal patients.

Neonatal transport is directed at supervised transfer of the newborn who has demonstrated substantial risk or documented symptomatology that indicates the need for specialized high risk care. The timing of transport of the newborn is determined by assessment of the newborn's status by the referring health care personnel and recognition of the need for specialized services beyond the capabilities of their own institution.

The paramount consideration in developing any transport system is the patient. Patient focus determines vehicle, equipment, and team selection. To a lesser degree, patient focus influences decisions regarding air versus ground and one-way versus two-way types of transport systems. Certainly many aspects of preparation, organization, and communication at both the referring institution and specialized center are determined by the patient population targeted to receive the benefits of the service.

The paucity of literature on maternal/fetal transport as compared to the literature regarding neonatal transport might suggest that the "art and science" of maternal/fetal transport is, as yet, not as developed. Among the factors contributing to less development or utilization of maternal/fetal transport services in high risk perinatal care are:

1. The advent of neonatology as a specialty as compared to perinatology
2. The degree to which high risk pregnancy complications may be addressed via referral or consultation modes [3-5]
3. Controversy regarding the benefits of maternal transport in situations in which neonatal factors are the indication for transport
4. Different viewpoints of referring pediatricians (neonatal transports) and obstetricians (maternal/fetal transports) in the areas of monetary compensation and patient-physician relationship

Historically, organized neonatal transport appears to have had its advent in the late 1960s and early 1970s, parallel with the development and utilization of neonatal intensive care services. Significant improvement in infant mortality as a result of specialized care for the small, immature, sick newborn spurred the rapid development of advanced technology, the emergence of neonatology as a recognized subspecialty of pediatrics, and an increase in utilization of neonatal intensive care services.

Effort was made toward the goals of regionalization of neonatal services, and neonatal transport systems were a necessary component of implementation. Transport services improved as their impact on the overall mortality and morbidity was documented.[7]

With few exceptions, organization of maternal/fetal transport evolved a full decade later. Exceptions included military obstetrical health care services and services in the state of Arizona, the latter reporting the beginning of an organized system as early as 1973.[19]

Theoretically, risk identification in the maternal patient can be made prior to conception as it relates to personal health habits, preexisting disease, past obstetrical history, family history and psychosocial risk indices for the individual and family. During early and regular prenatal care there is the opportunity for risk identification as it relates to the development of maternal or fetal disease or both. Early consultation or referral may reduce the necessity for transport of the maternal/fetal patient. While a substantial percentage of risk to the perinatal patient cannot be identified in the antenatal period, intrapartum risk scores have been demonstrated to be most predictive of perinatal morbidity and mortality.[9,30,40,41]

The largest percentage of maternal/fetal transport has been for neonatal indications. The reasons mothers are transported most often are not that their personal health is at risk but rather that the newborn's health is at risk and intervention of a specialized nature might be required. In such situations the general feeling is that maternal/fetal transport would be preferable. It is intuitively felt that the uterine environment is the ideal transport vehicle for the neonate at risk.[6]

There are four distinct advantages of maternal/fetal transport over new-born transport:

1. A high level of obstetrical expertise and technology available for the mother at risk
2. Immediate intensive pediatric evaluation and support for the newborn
3. Reduced equipment needs, which increases the speed and efficiency of the system
4. Enhancement of mother/infant bonding by providing care for both perinatal patients in the same institution.[18]

Questions have been raised whether the advantages for the family and newborn in situations in which maternal/fetal transport is for neonatal indications "compensate for the hardships imposed by moving the mother outside her community to deliver."[38] Although limited and still somewhat controversial at this point, research has been undertaken to substantiate the advantage in relation to neonatal outcome.[27,28,34,38,39,47] This research appears particularly relevant in view of the following considerations:

1. The impact of neonatal intensive care on neonatal outcome has been well established. The role of neonatal transport in improved outcome has been examined.[12-15]
2. The majority of maternal/fetal transports are for neonatal indications.
3. Neonatal transport systems are necessary to meet the needs of those neonates for whom risk cannot be predicted in the antepartal period regardless of whether maternal/fetal transport services are available.

Much of the research examining neonatal outcome in maternal/fetal versus neonatal transport has been challenged because of methodology. Recent results, however, do indicate that premature newborns transported in utero have a lower incidence of respiratory distress syndrome, a lower than predicted mortality, and a shorter hospital stay than similar premature newborns transported in the neonatal period.[27,28,38,39,47]

Until such documentation is conclusive, obstetricians may be reluctant to transfer maternal/fetal patients who are not experiencing any problems that present immediate risk to the health of one or the other. In addition to the feeling by obstetricians that care of these maternal/fetal patients is well within their level of medical expertise, the establishment of rapport, trust, and commitment that often ensues between obstetrician and patient during the course of frequent antenatal visits may be a deterrent to transport of the maternal/fetal patient. The loss of input into the care of the patient as well as the loss of monetary compensation may also be factors in the obstetrician's reluctance to transport the maternal/fetal patient.[50]

Institutional Responsibility and Control—
One-way or Two-way Transport

Transport systems are also distinguished by the types of organization of services, most often from the perspective of institutional control and respon-

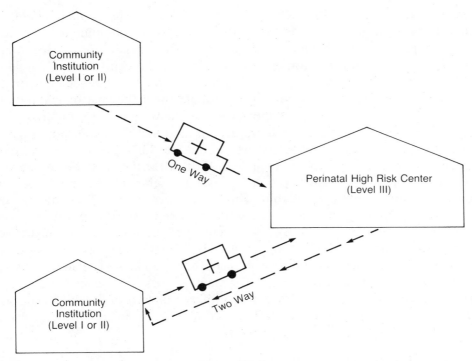

Figure 4-1. One-way versus two-way transport of perinatal high risk patients. (Courtesy of Terri Ingalls.)

sibilities in providing the service. Two such types of transport services are described in the literature.

One-way transport service is basically regarded as the responsibility of the referring institution for providing a mechanism and the appropriate personnel for supervision of transfer of the patient to the specialized high risk perinatal center. In two-way transport, the high risk center dispatches a transport service to the referring institution and provides supervised transfer for the client back to the center. The two types are depicted in Figure 4–1.

In the recommendations for the regional development of maternal and perinatal health services made by the Committee on Perinatal Health, transport of high risk perinatal patients was outlined as a responsibility of the level III (high risk perinatal specialty) center. Support for two-way transport was made in the committee's statement that "optimal management before and during transport will be possible if the transport team goes to the referring hospital with all necessary supplies and equipment." It was also suggested that the type of two-way service would allow the specialty center an opportunity to meet more fully its responsibility in providing education to the outlying referring institutions in its region by practical demonstration of stabilization techniques.[12] Support for the educational aspect of a two-way neonatal transport system is outlined in the report of a study by Skelton and associates at Vanderbilt University Medical Center in Tennessee.[49]

Theoretically, just by virtue of the assessed need to transport, it seems appropriate for the service to be provided by the organization most capable of providing specialized care for the perinatal patient. Evaluation of early systems of neonatal one-way transports showed that there were significant problems associated with such an approach. These problems included inadequately trained staff, inappropriate types and use of equipment (especially for temperature maintenance), lack of complete resuscitation facilities, and inappropriate administration and monitoring of oxygen therapy.[7] Support for two-way transport of critically ill newborns and its influence on neonatal morbidity and mortality is readily found, although the cost of maintaining such a service as well as the manpower requirement must be considered.

Conversely, in the limited literature on maternal/fetal transport there is a suggestion that one-way transport is more readily accepted in maternal/fetal transport situations. Boehm and Haire describe a highly organized, evolving one-way transport system for maternal/fetal patients in middle Tennessee affiliated with Vanderbilt University Hospital.[4] In view of the economic load for the regional center in maintaining both a two-way maternal and a two-way neonatal transport system, further consideration might well be given to the development and evaluation of maternal/fetal one-way transport systems when indications for transport are neonatal. The advisability of a one-way maternal/fetal transport system is questionable in situations in which maternal or fetal health is the primary concern or in which transport is being carried out in the intrapartum period.

Mode of Transportation—Ground or Air

Although not a sole consideration, a significant determinant in selection between air and ground transportation is the distance to be traveled by the high risk perinatal patient. The factor of distance, as utilized for decision making regarding the mode of transportation, is viewed from the aspects of both time and cost. For example, in air travel for intermediate distances, e.g., between 50 and 100 miles, the time involved in coordinating and transporting the team and the patient to and from the airport or heliport may outweigh the advantage provided by the speed of air travel.[16]

Other factors requiring careful consideration in deciding between air and ground modes of transportation are the client population; geographical terrain; climate; population density; traffic congestion; weather conditions; road conditions; the nature of the client's condition; urgency of the transport situation; and the cost, availability and organization of the system itself. These factors take precedence in making the decision about the type of system to be developed by a regional center, as well as in deciding, for each individual transport, which mode of transportation is advisable at the time for the specific situation.

TEAM

The team is a vital part of the transport system and may well be the most important component of any transport process.[26] In an expanded sense, the transport team is composed of numerous persons of many disciplines in all the institutions or agencies involved in any way with transport of the high risk perinatal client. Specifically, the transport team is most often considered

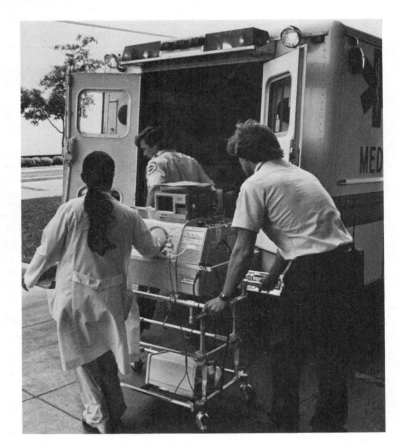

Figure 4-2. Ground transport of the neonatal patient. (Courtesy of Craig Stotts, Hermann Hospital, Houston, Texas.)

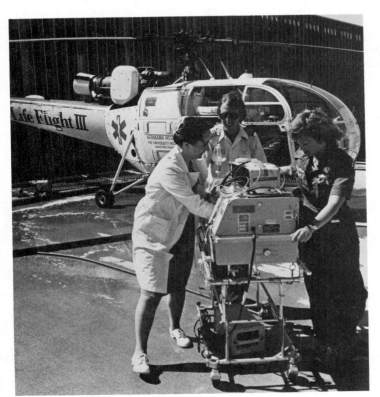

Figure 4-3. Air transport of the neonatal patient. (Courtesy of Craig Stotts, Hermann Hospital, Houston, Texas.)

TABLE 4-1. THE ADVANTAGES AND DISADVANTAGES OF GROUND AND AIR TRANSPORT SYSTEMS

Advantages	Disadvantages
Ground	

Point to point capability of patient transfer
  Less environmental exposure for the patient
  Fewer numbers of transfers from one transport conveyance to another
  Less chance for error in communication and coordination of services
 	
Accessibility to the patient during transport
 	
Ability to stop, thereby eliminating vehicle motion as a disadvantage, when the patient requires emergency intervention
 	
Use of audible monitoring equipment in surveillance of the patient's condition
	Restricted in situations of traffic congestion or hazardous road conditions
	
	Prolonged travel time as it relates to
	  Changes in the patient's condition without the availability of a full repertoire of perinatal care services
	  Utilization of limited supplies, particularly energy (battery) sources and oxygen
	  Need for stops for the purposes of refueling and personal needs of the team members
	  Fatigue of team members
	  Physiological and psychological stress of the patient
	  Unavailability of the service for transports of other patients

Air	

Rotary-winged
 	
Point to point capability of patient transfer in many situations
 	
Employment in situations in which distances are short and traffic congestion is a serious limitation to ground transport
 	
Fixed-winged
 	
Speed of travel for long distances
 	
Ease of travel, thereby increasing safety and speed, in areas where geographical terrain and climate make ground transport more hazardous
	Rotary- and Fixed-winged
	
	The necessity for some mechanism of ground transport for the team and patient in arriving and returning from the heliport or airstrip
	Numerous occasions for environmental exposure
	Numerous transfers as a result of multiple transport vehicles
	Increased complexity of organization and communications in coordinating all aspects of transport
	
	Limited accessibility to the patient as a result of
	  Poor lighting
	  Noise
	  Limited space
	  Turbulence
	
	Restrictions on choice of equipment due to
	  Poor lighting
	  Noise
	  Turbulence
	  Dynamics of altitude
	
	Physiological alterations as a result of
	  Change in atmospheric pressure
	  Acceleration and deceleration
	  Motion
	  Noise
	
	Necessity for additional training of team members specific to influences of flight and aerodynamics on their care giving abilities as well as on the condition of the patient
	
	Additional stress for patient and family when their experience with flying has been limited

to consist of those persons who are designated for and directly involved in supervised movement of the patient, which is the definition that is applied to the concept as it is used in this chapter.

Composition of the transport team varies from region to region throughout the country and has been reported to include usually two or three members from the health care disciplines—medicine, nursing, respiratory therapy, emergency care technical services, anesthesiology, and social work. The pilot of the aircraft or the ambulance driver must be considered as part of the team also. Total team membership, therefore, is usually no more than four.

Although team composition and organization reflects "the specific needs of the region [and the client] to be served and may be dictated by financial and personnel limitations," there are some elements felt to be paramount to the most successful functioning of any transport system.[15] The incorporation of these elements of composition and organization is also crucial in promoting an optimal outcome of the transport process. First, the team should be composed of personnel specifically determined by the health care organization to have responsibility and availability for perinatal transport services. The team should not be randomly selected from among any personnel present at the time of the request or documentation of the need for transport services. It is also important that prior arrangements be made for coverage during the entire transport process of any other duties that designated transport team members may have in the institutional setting.

In addition to team designation and selection, team size affects the functioning of the transport system and therefore may influence outcome. The team should be composed of as few members as possible to accomplish the transport process with an optimal outcome for the patient and family. A small team will reduce the probability of error by avoiding overcrowding of the transport vehicle, by facilitating communication, and by lessening the intricacies of coordinating the entire transport system.

Preparation of the team for transport is interrelated directly with specific designation of team members and indirectly with team size; it may well be the most crucial of all the elements in achieving optimal outcome of the transport process. The team should be specifically educated for the transport process. Members can be educated as a team, or the educational process be handled within the individual health care disciplines with content concentration according to role descriptions and role expectations among team members.

Regardless of the approach, the team should achieve "collective expertise"[32] in the following areas:

1. Assessment of the perinatal patient—historical, physical, and appropriate laboratory diagnostic work-up
2. Knowledge of the pathophysiology of conditions specific to the patient focus
3. Knowledge of the indication, administration, and effects of various treatment regimens for stabilization in these conditions
4. Clinical decision making based on nos. 1, 2, and 3.
5. Technical skills necessary in the performance of diagnostic work-up or treatment regimens

6.   Skills in crisis intervention

7.   Using and troubleshooting the equipment

8.   Recognition and management of variations in patient status as a result of specific effects of transport

9.   Insuring safety for themselves and the patient during transport

The last element influencing transport to be highlighted is inherent in the concept of team—functioning of the individual members as a cohesive unit is necessary for the success of any transport system. Role responsibilities should be clearly delineated according to expertise, yet where there is overlap in areas of knowledge and expertise, role flexibility must exist. Either a physician or nurse should serve as team leader in clinical decisions about the care regimen for the patient.[32] As expanded nursing roles have evolved in perinatal nursing, many transport teams are utilizing nurses as team leaders with physician consultation available by radio or telephone. The pilot or ambulance driver should assume a leadership role as it relates to the safety, advisability, and logistics of vehicle movement. Other team members may have primary or shared responsibility in providing patient care in coordinating activities and family support, and in operating equipment.

VEHICLE

Selection of a vehicle for transport of the high risk perinatal patient is a complex issue. The decision must take into consideration the specific region to be served and the institution that will maintain the service. The complexity stems from many interrelated factors that have a bearing on the choice of the "best" vehicle. These factors include cost, utilization, availability, patient focus, and the philosophy of patient care. The weight assigned to each one of these factors contributes to the individuality seen in vehicle selection and defines "best" for the region and the institution involved.

There are several choices of vehicles within the realm of either air or ground transport. Fixed wing aircraft include jet and single and twin engine propeller planes. Helicopters, rotary wing aircraft, are also available. Ground conveyance vehicles range from hearse-type, traditional van, ambulances built on an extended automobile chassis to custom designed coaches built on a motor home chassis.[16] Some type of ground transport vehicle may be necessary even with the consistent employment of an air transport system.

The financial resources of the institution providing the service balanced in some manner with vehicle utilization in the region are two factors that play a major role in vehicle selection. A small community hospital providing infrequent one-way transport services to the specialty center will have a different perspective from the high risk perinatal specialty center averaging 30 transports per month with adequate funding for regional services.

Availability is another factor and may absolutely dictate the vehicle to be utilized if purchase is not an option. The frustration of ensuring 24 hour availability with minimal response time can be incentive enough to purchase the vehicle. Contractual agreements necessary to ensure vehicle availability can often be more expensive than the purchase and maintenance costs for an ambulance. Consistent availability of a vehicle and pilot or driver is a related issue. The efficiency of the transport system is enhanced if the health care team members are familiar with the vehicular layout and operation of its standard equipment. Even minor changes that can be permanently incorporated into the vehicle to facilitate transport of the perinatal patient, as well as pilot or driver familiarity with the specific needs of the perinatal patient, can be important to the success of transport systems.

Patient focus contributes to the decision regarding the best vehicle for transport. Exterior design and interior compartment size and layout requirements are determined by the need to load and accommodate a stretcher and minimal equipment (maternal/fetal transport) versus the need for an incubator and equipment to outfit a mobile intensive care unit (neonatal transport). In some maternal/fetal transport systems or in individual situations in which total preparedness for the possibility of delivery en route is valued, all of the equipment necessary for both perinatal patients may need to be accommodated by the vehicle selected.

A factor closely interrelated with patient focus is the philosophy of care during transport adopted by the region or institution. Currently the predominant philosophy of care in two-way neonatal transport is to stabilize prior to departure from the referring hospital and to monitor the newborn whose condition has been stabilized with intensive care methods as needed. The return trip can then be made at safe recommended speeds, rather than "running hot" or "coding." There seems to be less attention to stabilization in the maternal/fetal patient, and in some situations (premature labor) a "speedy" return, although not at the expense of safety, may be desirable. Speed may also be a predominant factor in the philosophy of one-way transports since the objective is to get the patient, either maternal/fetal or neonatal, to the center as soon as possible for the required specialized care.

Regardless of how these various factors interplay in determining vehicle selection, the overriding consideration must be that the vehicle facilitate and not inhibit the delivery of care.[31] Extensive guidelines for selection of neonatal transport vehicles are available in the literature.[11,16] Many regional centers in reports of their transport services have provided pictorial descriptions of custom designed or specially adapted ambulances or aircraft that facilitate neonatal transport.[16,21,49] Similar information is not available in the literature reporting on maternal/fetal transport services. No doubt this is due to a limited need for special adaptation of the vehicle for transport of an adult patient. The following list highlights some general recommendations for perinatal transport vehicles regardless of patient focus. The vehicle should:

1. Meet safety requirements of the appropriate regulatory agency
2. Provide ample space for accessibility to the patient for the purpose of observation and provision of care
3. Have mechanisms for environmental control—temperature regulation and pressurization
4. Insure adequate lighting for monitoring the patient's condition and providing safe, accurate care
5. Provide ample storage space for equipment

6. Provide adequate seating for all team members

7. Have a power supply independent of the battery supply provided on the equipment

8. Carry additional oxygen and air supplies beyond those provided on portable equipment

9. Have a communication system between hospital and vehicle

10. Be available 24 hours with minimal response time

EQUIPMENT

The portable equipment selected for accompaniment with the transport team, as well as any equipment incorporated into the transport vehicle itself, is directly dependent on the specific patient focus for the perinatal transport services. The comprehensiveness of the equipment selected will be determined by the philosophy of care adopted by the institution responsible for the service. The greater the degree to which a transport service is functioning like a mobile hospital unit, the more extensive the equipment selection. In two-way transport, as the high risk perinatal center attempts to bring its specialization to the patient, there will be increased emphasis on the technological sophistication of the equipment.

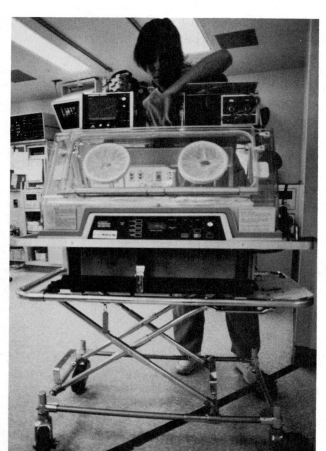

Figure 4-4. Neonatal transport equipment. (Courtesy of Hermann Hospital, Houston, Texas.)

Some of the equipment for transport must be portable. Basically the portable equipment should include a patient transfer conveyance, such as a stretcher or Isolette, ongoing life support equipment, and equipment for emergency resuscitation. The portable equipment should be compact and light enough in weight to permit maneuvering and loading by the team members without extra assistance. All portable equipment should be selected and evaluated with regard to the effects of vibration and environmental exposure on its accuracy in functioning (Fig. 4-4).

Although selection of additional equipment is based on the function it will serve, consideration should be given to safety, compactness, and versatility. Attention to these factors in selecting specific types of equipment will increase the efficiency of the transport system. There are limits with each type of transport vehicle on the type of equipment that may be used. This is particularly true of air transport in which noise, lack of electrical power, poor lighting, excessive motion or vibration, acceleration, deceleration, and changes in air pressure may create problems with the equipment's function.

The transport service should have its own equipment reserved for specific use in transporting high risk perinatal patients. Provision and maintenance by the transport service of the necessary equipment for monitoring and stabilizing the condition of the patient insures availability, familiarity, and reliability, thereby avoiding critical delays and problems in patient management.

Maternal/Fetal Transport

One major advantage of maternal/fetal transport in contrast to neonatal transport is the reduced equipment needs.[18] This is true, however, only for services that adhere to a policy of careful screening of the maternal patient and transport only when it is virtually assured that delivery will not ensue en route. Otherwise the service would need to equip the vehicle with items to provide care for both mother and newborn.

The basic equipment necessary for stabilization and for in-transit care of the maternal/fetal patient includes that for emergency resuscitation, oxygen administration, suction, intravenous therapy including infusion of blood or blood products, drug administration, manual pelvic examination, and monitoring of vital signs of both mother and fetus. A list of the equipment used to outfit one maternal/fetal transport service is presented in Table 4-2.

When desirable, equipment for providing routine delivery care can be carried and is compact enough to be contained within a large scrub basin. Such equipment includes items for preparing the perineum, performing and repairing an episiotomy, clamping the umbilical cord, and clearing the newborn's airway.[45] Obstetrical instruments such as forceps may be included if desired by the obstetrician. The equipment necessary to care for a potentially high risk newborn is extensive and is described in the following section.

Neonatal Transport

Equipment requirements for neonatal transport are extensive because of the intensive care provided for the high risk newborn. The one item that has

TABLE 4–2.   ARIZONA REGIONAL PERINATAL PROGRAM MATERNAL TRANSPORT EQUIPMENT LIST

Medications	Amount
Pitocin 10 U/L ml	4 ampules
Methergine 0.2 mg/1 ml	2 ampules
Ephedrine sulfate 0.05 gm	2 ampules
Epinephrine 1:1000 1 ml	2 ampules
Sodium Luminal grains 2/1 ml	2 ampules
Sodium Amytal 250 mg	2 ampules
Apresoline 20 mg/1 ml	2 ampules
Diazepam 10 mg	2 syringes
Sodium bicarb 50 mEq	4 syringes
Magnesium sulfate 50% 5 gm/10 ml	4 syringes
Magnesium sulfate 10% 2 gm/20 ml	4 ampules
Calcium gluconate 10 ml	2 ampules
Compazine 10 mg/2 ml	2 ampules
Benedryl 50 mg/1 ml	2 Tubexes
Naloxone (Narcan) 0.4 mg/1 ml	2 ampules
Xylocaine 1%	1 vial (20 ml)
Dramamine 50 mg	6 tablets
Aromatic ammonia	2 Vaporoles
Sterile H_2O for injection 10 ml	2 ampules

Equipment and Supplies: IV Solutions and Tubing	Amount
Dextrose 5% lactated Ringer's	500 ml
Dextrose 5% water	500 ml
Plasma	250 ml
IV tubing—Y type blood	1
IV tubing—standard	1

Miscellaneous Supplies	Amount
Angiocaths 18G, 16G, 14G	3
Tourniquet—elastic	2
Syringes—plastic	
3 ml	4
6 ml	4
12 ml	2
20 ml	2
60 ml	2
Tubex syringes	1
Needles 18G, 20G, 22G	4
Alcohol sponges	10
Adhesive tape ½, 1, and 2 in	1
Band-Aids	6
Doptone stethoscope	1
Ultrasound gel	1
B/P cuff with stethoscope	1
Reflex hammer	1
Padded tongue blade	2
Rubber airway	2
Ambu bag—adult size	1
Grocery bags with plastic liner	2
Chix wipes (box)	1

Reproduced with permission from Giles, H.: Maternal transport. Clin. Obstet. Gynecol., 6:203–214, 1979.

received the greatest attention in the literature on neonatal transport is the transport Isolette or incubator. The increased attention to environmental control for the newborn is related specifically to the dramatic impact temperature stabilization has been demonstrated to have on neonatal mortality. It is generally accepted that an incubator that maintains temperature by some means of warmed air convection and radiant heat is best for neonatal transport. A combination of both types of heat supply reduces heat loss during performance of procedures requiring the opening of the Isolette, and on exposure to a colder environment during transfer into the transport vehicle or failure of heat supply in the interior of the vehicle itself. There are many incubators available for newborns that are specifically designed for transport.[10,16,21,26]

In addition to maintenance of temperature, the transport Isolette functions in environmental control by providing humidity, maintaining increased oxygen concentration in the inspired air, and, to a degree, protecting from environmental contaminants.

Many transport Isolettes are designed as miniature intensive care units on wheels. With the exception of supplies, the equipment necessary for transport has been built into the overall system, making it basically a self-contained unit. Some transport teams prefer to use the more basic neonatal transport incubator and adapt their own support equipment onto the frame or onto a larger gurney carrying the Isolette. Regardless of design, other equipment that should be portable includes a ventilatory assistance device (usually with a capacity for continuous positive airway pressure [CPAP] and intermittent positive pressure ventilation [IPPV]), oxygen/air sources, a blender apparatus, suction apparatus, infusion pump, and a monitoring device. A complete resuscitation kit should accompany the newborn in all phases of the transport process as well.

Table 4–3 is a list of additional supplies that may be included to facilitate the care provided by the team during neonatal transport. Supplies include items for intravenous therapy, drug administration, diagnostic or monitoring procedures, specific treatment regimens, and respiratory support. The extensiveness of the supplies will be determined by the degree of stabilization the team wishes to achieve prior to arrival at the high risk perinatal center. Unless methods of stabilization are carried out in the transport vehicle, these supplies will need to be stored in a portable container.

THE INDICATIONS

The underlying purpose of transport of any perinatal patient is to achieve optimal outcome of the pregnancy for the family. Joint decisions for transport must be made by physicians at the referring institution and at the specialized high risk perinatal center, based on knowledge about the capabilities for care at both institutions; the patient's needs must be matched with the services available. As pointed out by the Committee on Perinatal Health in their 1976 report, "It is realized that expertise and services will vary at all levels within and among regional systems." Guidelines have been established by the committee and are presented in the report to be utilized by physi-

TABLE 4-3.   UNIVERSITY HOSPITAL, SAN DIEGO,
NEONATAL TRANSPORT EQUIPMENT LIST

LID
  1st Row
  O₂ tubing and mask (2)
  Cord clamp (1)
  Thermometer (1)
  Culture tubes (2)
  Kling
  Tourniquet (adult)
  2nd Row
  O₂ connecting tube (2)
  Redux cream
  5-in-1 Adaptor
  Q-tips—2/pkg (3)
  Arm board (1)
  Tongue blades (2)
  4 × 4s (4)
  Toppers (2)
  3rd Row
  1″ Adhesive
  ½″ Adhesive
  1″ Micropore
  ½″ Micropore
  1″ Blenderm
  ½″ Blenderm
  1″ Elastoplast

TOP SHELF
  Left Section
  IV scalp vein needles—
    25 ga long and
    short (2 ea)
    23 ga (2)
  Alcohol swabs
  Knife blades
    #10, 11 (2 ea)
  Lancets (4)
  Band-Aid (4)
  Gummed labels (4)
  Rubberbands (4)
  Needles
    Blunt #18, 20,
    23 (2 ea)
    Sharp #22, 25 (4 ea)
  Back Section
  Blood tubes
    Red (2)
    Blue (1)
    Gray (1)
    Lavender (2)
  Capillary tubes
  Tape measure (2)
  Dextrostix
  Critoseal
  Silk sutures—
    4-0, 5-0 (2 ea)
  50% Dextrose solu (1)

Right Section
Syringes
  T.B. (6)
  3 cc (2)
  6 cc (2)
  12 cc (3)
  20 cc (3)
Center Section
Meds
  S.P. Albumin
  Phenobarb. inj.
  Neosporin oint (2)
  Bacteriostatic H₂O (1)
  Nonpreservative H₂O
    (1)
  Decadron
  Bacteriostatic NaCl
  Na penicillin
  Glucagon
  Isoproterenol (2)
  Na bicarbonate (2)
  Epinephrine 1:10,000
    (2)
  Silver nitrate (2)
  Aqua Mephyton (2)
  Lasix (1)
  Lanoxin (2)
  Atropine (2)
  Dilantin (1)
  Valium (1)
  Dopamine (1)
  Ca gluconate (2)
  Gentamicin
  Oxacillin
  Kanamycin
  Ampicillin 125 mcg (2)
  Heparin
  Ca chloride
FIRST DRAWER
  1st Section
  Laryngoscope handle
  Laryngoscope blade (2)
  Guide wire
  Endotracheal tubes
    3.0 mm (2)
    3.5 mm (1)
    4.0 mm (1)
  Nasotracheal tubes—
    3.0 mm (2), 3.5 mm
      and 4.0 mm (1 ea)
  3 mm Adaptor
  Back Section
  Tr. benzoin
  Betadine
  Battery fuses
  Battery size AA (2)

Bulbs (2)
Surgilube
O₂ masks (3 sizes)
O₂ analyzer
Sterile instruments
  Scissors (2)—sharp,
    blunt
  Kelly (2)—curved,
    straight
  Forceps (1)
  Scalpel (1)

SECOND DRAWER
  Gloves—
    size 6 (1), 6½ (2),
      7 (2), 7½ (2), 8 (1)
  Bulb Syringe
  Mapleson bag
  EKG audio monitor
  DeLee suction (2)
  Umbilical catheter—
    3.5, 5 Fr. argyle
    (2 ea)
  Umbilical tape (2)
  Suction catheter—5,
    8 Fr (2 ea)
  Feeding tube—5, 8 Fr
    (2 ea)
  Trocar catheters—10, 12,
    16 Fr.
  Heimlich chest drain
    valve (2)

THIRD DRAWER
  D5W 250 cc.
  D10W 500 cc. (1)
  D5 & .2 N.S. 500 cc (1)
  D5 & .45 N.S. 250 cc (1)
  Normal saline
  THAM
  Pediatric IV set (2)
  Blood set (1)
  Metriset (1)
  3-Way stopcock (3)
  IV Extension tubing (2)
  Masking tape
  Coban
  Ambulance battery adaptor
  B.P. cuff
  Clipboard
  COA sheets (4)
  OR permits (6)
  Check list (4)
  Order sheets (4)
  Progress notes (4)
  ICU nursery notes (4)
  Medication sheets (4)

Reprinted with permission from Feldman, B.H., and Sauve, R.S.: The infant transport system. Clin.
Perinatol., *3*:469-478, 1976.

cians for determining the need for consultation and possible referral, transport, or both. These guidelines, established for both maternal/fetal and neonatal patients, were based on the differentiation among levels of care (levels I, II, and III) within the region according to specifications in the report.[12]

Maternal/Fetal Transport

The majority of maternal/fetal transports are for neonatal indications. Maternal patients have most often been transported because of some prediction of neonatal risk that might require immediate neonatal intensive care services. The neonatal risk most often influencing maternal/fetal transport is premature birth. Premature labor and premature rupture of membranes are the conditions cited almost consistently as the first and second ranked indications for transport of maternal/fetal patients. Premature labor alone accounts for almost 50 per cent of all indications for maternal/fetal transport reported. In combination with premature rupture of membranes without documented labor, premature labor accounts for as many as 80 per cent of the indications for transport reported by some maternal/fetal services.

Table 4–4 depicts in order of decreasing frequency the indications for maternal/fetal transport reported in the literature.[4,6,19,34,37,50] Associated with a number of the indications is a risk of premature delivery.

Preeclampsia was the second most frequent indication in a number of studies (although not in Table 4–4), its percentage in the total number of transports being always very close to that of premature rupture of membranes. All other conditions made up a small percentage of the overall indications for transport. Diabetes and hypertension were the maternal diseases most often cited as indications for transport. It is common for maternal/fetal patients to have more than one indication for transport.

TABLE 4–4. INDICATIONS FOR MATERNAL/FETAL TRANSPORT*

Premature labor

Premature rupture of membranes

Preeclampsia

Antepartum bleeding (third trimester)

Maternal disease
  Diabetes
  Hypertension
  Rh sensitization
  Venereal disease
  Sickle cell disease
  Pulmonary disease
  Drug abuse
  Amnionitis
  Hepatitis

Multiple pregnancies

Abnormal obstetrical history

*Referral, transport, and transfer were not consistently differentiated in the literature.

Neonatal Transport

Prematurity in the newborn is a dominant indication for neonatal transport. In many cases the documentation of the state of prematurity itself is the primary reason for transport, based on the knowledge that the premature infant is at risk for development of many disease states and conditions that complicate the neonatal course. Recognition of one or more of these disease states results in the majority of transports for neonates.

Because of more variation in categorization of diagnoses, indications for neonatal transport are not easily ranked in frequency of occurrence. Table 4–5 depicts the most common indications for neonatal transport in relative order of frequency.[1,2,3,7,13,48,51]

It is important to note that categories of diagnosis that contribute to a substantial portion of neonatal transports are those requiring expertise from other subspecialties within the division of pediatric medicine. Examples include congenital heart disease, neurological conditions, and conditions requiring surgical intervention.

THE PROCESS OF TRANSPORT

The process necessary to achieve the goal of perinatal transport consists of four phases: pre-transport communication, stabilization of the patient's condition, transport (movement), and post-transport communication.

Pre-transport Communication

The groundwork supporting an optimal outcome for the transport process is established long before the actual phone call requesting transport from the referral health care institution to the high risk perinatal center. Development of rapport among health care providers within the region served by the transport services, meticulous attention to the organization

TABLE 4–5. INDICATIONS FOR NEONATAL TRANSPORT

Prematurity

Respiratory distress
 Hyaline membrane disease
 Transient tachypnea
 Meconium aspiration
 Pneumonia

Perinatal asphyxia

Congenital malformations
 Congenital heart disease
 Surgical problems

Neurological problems
 Intraventricular hemorrhage (IVC)
 Seizure activity

Infections

and coordination of the logistics of transport, and the education of all involved personnel about the logistics as well as the patient care necessary for transport are critical factors in a successful transport process. Months of preparatory work are necessary to establish these factors for effective, efficient transport service. An approach by the high risk perinatal center as the deliverer of "all things wise and necessary" is not conducive to the establishment of such a solid base for the transport process. Rather, open communication is facilitated by an understanding of the role and its value of each individual and institution involved in the transport process.

Once communication lines have been established within the region, specific pre-transport communication can be put into operation. The success of this first phase will affect the outcome for the entire transport process. There is a component of pre-transport communication that occurs within each separate health care institution and between two institutions. The following outline highlights the nature of pre-transport communication that must occur in each component for optimal outcome of the transport process.

Pre-transport communication *within the referring hospital* must occur:

- Among health care personnel regarding assessment and documentation of the need for transport.
- Between health care personnel and patient or patient's family regarding advisability and specifics of transport for the purpose of obtaining informed consent
- Among health care personnel in coordinating and providing care for optimal stabilization of the patient prior to transport
- Among transport team leader, other team members and transport vehicle service personnel to mobilize the team and vehicle (one-way transport)
- Among various departmental personnel to obtain duplication of pertinent records, roentgenograms, and required blood samples to accompany the patient
- Among various departmental personnel, family and health care personnel to discharge the patient from the referring institution
- Between health care personnel and patient or patient's family for support and information throughout the pre-transport phase of the transport process.

Pre-transport communication *between the referring institution and high risk perinatal center* must occur:

- Between referring and consulting physicians to confirm the need and advisability of transport
- Between referring and consulting physicians regarding additional diagnostic work-up and care required for maximum stabilization
- Between transport team leader and a designated primary care provider for the patient to confirm approval for transport, to obtain additional detailed and updated information on patient's status for maximum preparedness, and to coordinate times of departure, transit, and arrival (direction of communication determined by one-way versus two-way transport)
- At predetermined intervals between designated personnel for the purposes of updating all aspects of the transport process

NEWBORN TRANSPORT WORKSHEET

To be completed by accepting physician

Date_____ Time_____ DOB _____ Time _____

Infant's Name: _____

Mother's Name: _____

Referring MD: _____

Problem List:	Premie/Gest. Age	☐	Birth Trauma	☐
	Resp. Dist.	☐	G.I.	☐
	Asphyxia	☐	Cardiovascular	☐
	R/O Sepsis	☐	Cong. Anom.	☐

Status: VS:	Temp ____	ABGS:	pH _____	Site:	Artery	☐
	HR ____		PO₂ _____		Vein	☐

Status: VS: Temp ____   ABGS: pH _____   Site: Artery ☐
             HR ____   PO$_2$ _____   Vein ☐
             RR ____   PCO$_2$ _____   Capillary ☐
             BP ____   HCO$_3$ _____   TCO$_2$ ☐
             Dstix ____   BE _____
             Hct ____   Blood cultures done? Yes No

Meds Given:

Antibiotics   — Please list name(s) _____

Aquamephyton — Amt: _____

Eye Prophy.   — Name _____

Maternal:

Total Pregnancies _____

Total Abortions _____ Spontaneous _____ Elective _____

Total Live Children _____

Labor: Spontaneous   Onset of Labor: Amniotic Fluid:
          Induced   Date _____   Clear
                          Time _____   Mec. Stained
                                                  Foul Smell
                                                  Bloody

Financial
Information:

Figure 4–5. Neonatal transport forms for documentation. (Courtesy of Hermann Hospital, Houston, Texas.)

Illustration continues on following page.

Newborn Transport Record

Part A

Person Receiving Call_____

Date Call Received_____ Time_____

Infant's Name_____

Age_____ Sex_____ Wt. _____ Gest. Age _____

Hospital of Origin_____

City_____ County_____ State _____

Referring MD_____ Accepting MD_____

Reason for Call: Premie ☐   Asphyxia ☐   Birth Trauma ☐   Cardiovasuclar ☐
Resp. Dist. ☐   R/O Sepsis ☐   G.I. ☐   Cong. Anom. ☐

Receiving Hospital:	HH ☐ TCH ☐ JDH ☐ JSH ☐ MEM ☐ Other ☐	Receiving Unit:	NICU ☐ NSCU ☐ IICU ☐ PICU ☐ Other ☐

Reported Status: Apgars 1_____/5_____

VS: Temp _____
HR _____ ABGS pH____ PO_2 _____
RR _____
BP _____ PCO_2____ HCO_3 ____BE____
Dstix _____

Site: Art ☐
Assist: Vein ☐
FiO_2 _____   Mask ☐   Cap. ☐
Spont._____   ETT ☐ TCO_2 ☐

Fluid Lines: UAC ☐   IVF:_____
UVC ☐   Meds Given: Antibiotics ☐
PIV ☐   Resuscitation ☐
CVL ☐   Aquamephyton ☐
Other ☐   Eye Prophy. ☐

Resuscitation at Birth:
Bulb Sx ☐
Cath Sx ☐
Mask ☐
Bag Ett ☐
Cardiac Mass. ☐

X-Rays Taken: CXR ☐   KUB ☐   FINDINGS_____

Type of Transport: Primary   Return to Hospital_____

Mode: Ground ☐   Transporting   Pediat. Res. ☐
Helicopter ☐   Personnel: Fellow ☐
Fixed-Wing ☐   NTN ☐
Other ☐   NICU Nurse ☐
Flight Nurse ☐
R. T. ☐

Time Log:	Time	Date
Birth	_____	_____
Call Recd.	_____	_____
Depart	_____	_____
Arrive Ref. Hosp.	_____	_____
Depart Ref. Hosp.	_____	_____
Arrive Rec. Hosp.	_____	_____

Mobilization Delay:
None ☐   Weather ☐
Elective ☐   Equipment ☐
Personnel ☐   Traffic ☐
Ambulance ☐   Communication ☐
Disposition ☐   Other_____

Figure 4–5 *(Continued)*

Part B

Maternal Age _____
   Total No. Pregnancies _____

   No. Abortions _____ { Therapeutic _____
                              Spontaneous _____
                              Elective _____
   No. Stillbirths _____
   No. Infants < 38 Wk. Live Born _____
   No. Infants > 42 Wk. Live Born _____ No. Live Borns Who Died Before 1 Mo. of Age ___
   No. Infants < 5 lb. 6 oz. (2500 gm.)   No. Infants > 9 lb. 14 oz. (4000 gm.)
                        Live Born _____   Live Born _____
   Pregnancy Problems (P = Previous Pregnancies; T = This Pregnancy)

Marked Emotional Tension	_____	Urine/kidney Infection	_____
Hyperemesis Gravidarum	_____	Other Infection 1st Trimester	_____
Accidents/Trauma	_____	Other Infection 2nd Trimester	_____
Bleeding 1st Trimester	_____	Other Infection 3rd Trimester	_____
Bleeding 2nd Trimester	_____	X-Rays During Pregnancy	_____
Bleeding 3rd Trimester	_____	Surgery During Pregnancy	_____
Preeclampsia/Eclampsia	_____	Premature Onset Labor	_____
Chronic Hypertension	_____	Premature R.O.M.	_____
Hepatitis or Exposure	_____	Oligohydramnios/Polyhydramnios	_____
Multiple Birth(s)	_____	Precipitous Delivery	_____
Nonvertex Delivery(ies)	_____	Rh Problems	_____
Placenta Previa	_____	Cong. anomalies	_____
Placental Disruption	_____	Diabetes mellitus	_____ Class ____
Alcohol/Drug Habituation	_____	Other _____	

Present Pregnancy and Delivery
   Date/Time Onset of Labor _____
   Labor: Spontaneous   Induced
   Indications for Induction: _____
   Membranes Ruptured: Artificially   Spontaneously   Hrs. Prior to Del. _____
   Abnormalities of Labor: _____
   Amniotic Fluid: Amount—Copious   Scant
                    Nature—Mec. Stained   Foul Odor   Other _____
   Type of Delivery: Vag.   C/S
   Meds During Pregnancy: _____
   Mother's Blood Type _____ Rh _____ Previous RhoGam   Yes   No
   Indications of Fetal Distress
      Bradycardia   Tachycardia

Figure 4–5 Continued.

Part C

Stabilization: H-Hosp;   T-Transport Team

H	T	
☐	☐	Intubated ETT Size_____
☐	☐	Sepsis Work-up
☐	☐	Blood Culture
☐	☐	Lumbar Puncture
☐	☐	U.A.C. Insertion Catheter Size _____ Placement X-Ray_____
☐	☐	N.G. Tube Inserted
☐	☐	Thoracentesis L _____ R _____
☐	☐	Pericardial Aspiration
☐	☐	Cardiac Massage Time Started_____

Medications:

Medication	Time	Route	Dosage	Signature

AMB T° / INC T°	T	P	R	Color	Tone	Dex	BP	FiO_2	pH	PO_2	PCO_2	HCO_3	BE	I:E	PIP	PEEP/ CPAP	Rate	Time

Psychosocial:

Spoke with Mother	Yes	No
Mother Saw Baby	Yes	No
Mother Touched Baby	Yes	No
Spoke with Father	Yes	No
Father Saw Baby	Yes	No
Father Touched Baby	Yes	No
Family Member to Admit Baby	Yes	No

Responsible Physician _____

Instructions to Referring Hospitals:
1. Written Order for Transfer
2. 10 cc. Clot Maternal Blood—Labeled
3. 10 cc. Clot Infant Cord Blood—Labeled
4. Copies of Maternal and Infant Charts
5. Copies of All X-Rays and Lab Results
6. Record Infant's Length in cm.

Transport Nurse _____

Source: Hermann Hospital, Houston, Texas.

Figure 4–5 Concluded

Pre-transport communication *within the high risk perinatal center* must occur:

- Among designated health care personnel in newborn intensive care and obstetrical services to determine the bed availability and adequate personnel coverage necessary for approval of transport
- Among specific transport team members of the health care personnel and personnel of the transport vehicle services to mobilize the team and vehicle for transport (two-way transport)
- Between personnel in communication with referring institution and receiving unit personnel to facilitate maximum preparedness for admission
- Among receiving unit personnel and emergency room personnel, personnel in the admission department and in various departments providing ancillary patient services in preparation for new patient admission
- Between perinatologist/neonatologist and other specialists when the need for immediate consultation is anticipated

Factors that have been demonstrated to enhance the efficiency of the pre-transport communication process include a special "hot line" telephone number for contact with the high risk perinatal center, designation of one person, free from direct patient care, to coordinate activities surrounding the transport process, the established algorithms for all personnel to follow in carrying out the numerous steps in any one area of the required communication outlined above.

Stabilization

Patient care during perinatal transport requires detailed attention to all aspects of care that contribute to optimal stabilization prior to movement. In one-way transport the care provided for the patient to stabilize his condition is performed by the health care personnel at the referring institution with the resources available there. Telephone consultation with the high risk perinatal center may be obtained to achieve as great a degree of stabilization as possible prior to transport. In situations in which two-way transport is employed, there are two phases to the stabilization process. Based on input from the specialists at the high risk perinatal center, the personnel at the referring institution provide care to achieve stabilization prior to the transport team's arrival. On arrival, after further assessment of the patient's condition, the transport team may intervene with additional measures to attempt to achieve greater stability.

Careful assessment and skill in clinical decision making are the precursors to the appropriate interventions to achieve stabilization of the patient's condition. Lengthy assessment is not inherent in the concept of careful assessment; time is often a critical factor in the stabilization process. A sound knowledge base is paramount to the team members' effectiveness and efficiency during the transport process.

Based on the indications previously reported for transport (Tables 4–1 and 4–2), the following areas are often the major concerns in stabilization of the condition of the maternal/fetal patient:

1. Cessation/control of labor
2. Control of blood pressure

3. Control of bleeding
4. Correction of metabolic imbalances

The areas below are often the major concerns in stabilization of the condition of the neonatal patient:

1. Establishment of respiratory efficiency
2. Correction of thermal instability
3. Establishment of cardiac efficiency
4. Correction of metabolic imbalances
5. Control of infection
6. Control of seizure activity

When transport of the perinatal patient is to be accomplished by air, interventions a step beyond those necessary for stabilization may be performed. Elective procedures, that is, procedures not required by the patient's condition at that point in time, may be performed as preventives of the effects of the flight, especially in unpressurized aircraft. They may also be performed because of the hazards of accomplishing them during flight if they are necessitated by a change in the patient's condition. The most common example of such a procedure is intubation and ventilation of the newborn to insure oxygenation and adequate ventilation.[21,22]

A component of stabilization often given cursory attention is the need of the perinatal patient or patient's family for psychological support. Few transport teams include a social worker or mental health nurse specialist, so the nurse must coordinate this aspect of care.

Transport

Movement of the perinatal patient is only one phase of the process of transport. However, it is the hallmark of the entire process. The movement of the patient is transport. Movement occurs in transferring the patient from any one bed to conveyance and vice versa, in traversing corridors, in loading and unloading the patient and conveyance on and off the transport vehicle, and in traveling the distance between the referring institution and the high risk perinatal center.

During movement of the client, the ability to provide direct care taking measures is compromised. It is for this reason that the stabilization phase is so vital in the entire transport process. The primary function of the transport team members during movement is insuring patient safety. Monitoring should include observation to confirm the maintenance of adequate stabilization and to detect any changes in condition.

Some changes in condition may be a result of the movement itself. Increased metabolic demands can result from activity and anxiety. In patients with little metabolic reserve or balance, changes in condition can be dramatic. Sensory and motor stimulation from motion and vibration can also affect the condition. Although not recognized in newborns, motion sickness in maternal/fetal patient is common. In unpressurized aircraft dramatic effects on the patient's condition can result from hypoxia and expansion of trapped gases. When intervention is indicated by a change in condition, movement can be stopped, except, of course, in air transport, and the necessary care provided.

In addition to the patient's condition, the functioning of all equipment should be monitored closely during movement. Common problems in equipment during movement include dislodgment and kinking of lines and tubing, leaks in respiratory equipment, loss of pressure, and inaccuracy in the readings.

Post-transport Communication

Once the perinatal patient has been transferred to the designated bed space in the receiving unit of the high risk perinatal center, the transport (movement) phase of the process is complete. The last phase in the entire process of transport is post-transport communication. As with pre-transport communication a component of post-transport communication occurs within each separate health care institution and between the two institutions. Overall the goals of the post-transport communication phase are education and support. The following outline highlights the nature of post-transport communication necessary within each component to achieve these goals.

Post-transport communication within the high risk perinatal center must occur:

- Between transport team members and receiving health care personnel in sharing data necessary to admit the client into the institution (two-way)
- Among health care personnel in the institution for the purposes of admission and stabilization of the condition of the patient
- Between health care personnel and the patient or patient's family in orientation to the new unit and new personnel, in updating the patient's condition, and for psychological support in coping with this phase of the process

Post-transport communication between the referring institution and the high risk perinatal center must occur:

- Between transport team members and receiving health care personnel in sharing data necessary to admit the patient into the institution (one-way)
- Between consulting and referring physicians in follow-up of transport to share information regarding accomplishment of transport, the patient's status/diagnosis, further care anticipated, and to give constructive feedback about the role and care provided prior to transport
- Between receiving and referring nursing staff in follow-up of transport to share updated information on the patient's status and the family's coping

— Between transport nurse and referring primary nurse in follow-up of transport to share updated information on the patient's status and the family's coping and to give two-way constructive feedback about the role and care provided during transport (two-way). (In one-way transport this feedback would have to be accomplished between transport nurse and receiving primary nurse.)

— Between receiving health care personnel (physician and nurse) and the newborn's family to share updated information on the patient's condition and to facilitate visitation/continued communication (neonatal)

Post-transport communication within the referring institution must occur:

— Between transport team members and other health care personnel regarding the outcome of the transport process (one-way)

— Among health care personnel in sharing information communicated back from receiving health care personnel

— Between health care personnel (physician and nurses) and the newborn's family in reinforcing/clarifying information communicated to them by the receiving institution personnel and in providing support throughout the mother's hospital stay (neonatal)

THE NURSING ROLE FOR PERINATAL TRANSPORT

Nursing interventions are specific to the major maternal/fetal and neonatal conditions that necessitate transport. Limits may be placed on the extent of care because of lack of available services or equipment during certain phases of the transport process. Decisions for intervention may be necessary without a full repertoire of diagnostic data. In such cases, decision making needs to be approached more from a perspective of assessment and treatment of acute clinical signs and symptoms to achieve stability of the condition and to maintain optimal homeostasis. Certain procedures for diagnostic purposes or for long term, more comprehensive care may need to be postponed until arrival and admission to the specialized unit within the high risk perinatal center.

A ready reference guide provides an overview of the nursing actions necessary to accomplish the transport process (Table 4–6). These actions, listed in sequence, are general in nature. Although more specific information is highlighted to differentiate between maternal/fetal and neonatal transport, the nursing actions specific to any one maternal/fetal or neonatal condition are not included here. Comments are provided to reemphasize and summarize certain aspects of one-way and two-way air and ground transport systems.

Table 4–6 follows.

TABLE 4-6. THE NURSING ROLE FOR PERINATAL TRANSPORT

Nursing Action	Rationale	Maternal/Fetal	Neonatal	One-Way	Two-Way	Air	Ground
Transfer ongoing responsibilities to other personnel upon confirmation of need for transport.	Certain responsibilities specific to transport need to be assumed as soon as notification is received.			Rarely employed exclusively for transport role; often primary care giver for patient to be transported.	A team member may be employed for transport role only.		
Communicate directly with designated primary care nurse at other health care institution.	Nurse to nurse communication facilitates exchange of information valuable to nursing care of patient and establishes rapport helpful in later contact during transport situation; primary care nurse usually has most updated information on patient's condition.	Exchange succinct information related to: name, age, prenatal obstetrical history, gravidity, parity, gestation, prenatal history, diagnosis, clinical course since admission, current status, family members/support person, coping status	Exchange succinct information related to: name, age, sex, gestation, history, prenatal labor and delivery history, diagnosis, clinical course since admission, current status, family situation, mother's condition	Nurse transporting patient calls nurse who will be admitting patient.	Nurse who will be arriving to transport patient back calls nurse currently caring for patient.		
Check transport equipment; stock additional equipment if warranted by information	Regardless of daily checks of equipment, a check prior to departure reduces chance of missing or	See section on equipment.	See section on equipment.	Equipment may need to be assembled for each transport; a list to facilitate collecting the equipment	Equipment should be reserved just for transport situation.	Equipment may vary somewhat depending on ground or air transport.	

Nursing action	Rationale			
on patient's condition.	nonfunctional items; personnel who use equipment should check equipment.	needed for transport should be available.		Include ambulance driver's and attendants' responsibilities.
Meet with other team members to clarify role responsibilities and share information about patient.	Team coordination is essential to efficiency of system and optimal outcome of process.	Particularly important since often no specifically designated team members.	Important when team composition varies according to patient's needs.	Include pilot's responsibilities.
Establish contact with patient's family as early as possible before departure; introduce self as member of transport team; provide information about transport process.	Early contact even if one is not yet involved directly in patient's care will allow more opportunity to establish rapport and trust in transport nurse. Family can begin to incorporate information earlier, which will allow more time to ask questions, state concerns, and make arrangements prior to departure; family can identify transport nurse as support person.	Encourage husband/significant other to make arrangements for stay in city where center is located and to have family member or friend accompany him as support person.	Encourage father to notify other family members or friends help as his support person and to stay with hospitalized mother if he is going to proceed to speciality center. If overnight stay is anticipated because of distance encourage him to make arrangements prior to departure.	Listing of possible accommodations near center plus directions and direct phone number for center should be available for family at referring institution. / May not be feasible at this point in process.
	Discourage family members from following directly behind ambulance.			

Table 4–6 continues on following page.

TABLE 4-6. THE NURSING ROLE FOR PERINATAL TRANSPORT (Continued)

Nursing Action	Rationale	Maternal/Fetal	Neonatal	One-Way	Two-Way	Air	Ground
Assess patient's status by reviewing or collecting data from history, physical examination, and diagnostic testing.	Establish baseline for interpreting changes in condition, making clinical decisions for intervention, and communicating information about the patient to other health care personnel.	Include past obstetrical, family, and prenatal history; progression of clinical course since p admission, including drug administration and response. Physical exam maternal vital signs, reflexes, fundal height, Leopold maneuvers, vaginal examination (if advisable), quality and timing of contractions, heart sounds, breath sounds, ophthalmic examination (if indicated), fetal heart tones. Diagnostic testing: complete blood count, urinalysis, electrolytes, fetal monitor strip, nonstress test (NST) (Additional assessment specific to symptomatology/condition/diagnosis and available services in referring institution)	Include history—maternal, labor and delivery progression of clinical course p admission including drug administration and response. Physical exam vital signs, heart sounds, breath sounds, respiratory effort, pulses, neurological examination, abdominal examination, general examination for color, edema, perfusion, trauma and anomalies Diagnostic testing: hematocrit, glucose, arterial blood gases	Important prior to departure even if stabilization has already been accomplished by other health care personnel.	Immediately upon arrival in referring institution (may be necessary to begin some intervention before complete assessment due to extreme unstable condition)	In situations in which referring personnel transport client to air strip to meet arriving two-way team, further assessment will be limited.	

52

					May be accomplished in extensively equipped vehicle for legal purposes and insuring sophisticated equipment (two-way).
		Beginning and completion of legal responsibility for patient should be carefully understood and documented.	One phase of stabilization prior to transport.	Two phases of stabilization prior to transport.	A greater degree of stabilization may be warranted because of limited access to patient. Some interventions prior to transport may be warranted in consideration of effects of flight on patient's condition.
Begin record keeping process; include pertinent data and documentation of nursing care specific to transport process.	Careful documentation is necessary for legal purposes, communicating information, and later evaluation of transport system and process.	In general: establish IV line, correct fluid/volume/electrolyte imbalances, correct metabolic imbalances, provide comfort (psychological and physiological), measures and medication for pain relief, position left lateral, administer O$_2$ as needed, achieve and maintain normotensive state, closely monitor and control labor, administer drug therapy as indicated, monitor maternal and	In general: maintain airway, insure respiratory adequacy, achieve and maintain thermal homeostasis, achieve and maintain normotensive state, establish IV line, correct fluid/volume electrolyte imbalances, correct metabolic imbalances, decompress abdomen, place on portable monitoring equipment to insure close surveillance.		
Assist in interventions necessary for stabilization prior to transport. Assure degree of stabilization felt to be necessary prior to transport.	Detailed attention to stabilization prior to movement reduces risk to patient, and it is hoped, minimizes need for intervention during movement.				

Table continues on following page.

TABLE 4-6. THE NURSING ROLE FOR PERINATAL TRANSPORT *(Continued)*

Nursing Action	Rationale	Maternal/Fetal	Neonatal	One-Way	Two-Way	Air	Ground
		fetal signs closely, especially when loading/titrating drugs.					
		(Additional intervention dependent on symptomatology condition/diagnosis)					
Communicate with family to share information and provide psychological support. Facilitate family in spending time with patient prior to departure.	Family is experiencing situational crises. Timely, appropriate intervention can be crucial to their coping abilities.		Facilitate parent-newborn interaction that will enhance attachment; encourage touching, talking, holding (if possible), naming newborn, picture taking. Transport Isolette can be taken into mother's room. Snapshot can be provided for mother to keep.		May be first opportunity to meet patient's family since arrival; will need to establish some degree of rapport quickly, assess their level of knowledge, correct misunderstandings, and obtain informed consent for center for transport and assume total responsibility for care. Excellent interpersonal skills are necessary to accomplish this and establish a sense of trust and support prior to departure.	Additional anxiety may be present if limited experience with air travel.	

With assistance, transfer patient to transport conveyance and move into transport vehicle.	Increased safety needs and certain effects on patient are inherent in movement.	Attention to continuous observation of patient, psychological support, safety (side rails, straps), positioning, comfort measures, personal integrity (clothing, draping), protection from environmental exposure (extra blankets, waterproof covering), patency of lines, monitoring at intervals (IV flow, contractions, vital signs)	Attention to positioning to allow continuous observation of newborn in Isolette plus equipment function, patency of lines, data on newborn's condition via monitor devices, additional heat control upon exposure to extreme cold, limited opening of Isolette portholes	Numerous transfers may be required; more exposure to environment can be anticipated.	Encourage husband/father to accompany team until patient is safely "settled" in transport vehicle.
Alert clerical personnel to notify receiving institution of time of departure.	Careful coordination for timing of arrival insures maximum preparedness.				
Position oneself in transport vehicle to allow for continuation of monitoring and to facilitate delivery of care during transport.	There is greater safety for team member if movement in vehicle can be minimized.	Position to side of patient close enough for hands-on monitoring of labor and vital signs and to facilitate communication to support patient.	Position to allow for continuous observation of newborn and visualization of data from monitoring equipment.	May be necessary to arrange for ground transportation at airstrip	Restrictive to certain types of observation and monitoring

Table 4-6 continues on following page.

TABLE 4-6. THE NURSING ROLE FOR PERINATAL TRANSPORT (Continued)

Nursing Action	Rationale	Maternal/Fetal	Neonatal	One-Way	Two-Way	Air	Ground
Monitor patient's condition and the functioning of equipment closely during transport; intervene with specific care measures only as indicated by change in condition.	Early intervention in response to slight changes in condition may decrease need for more involved intervention. Extensive intervention is limited during transport; problems with accuracy and safety are more probable. Some effects on patient's condition may result from the nature of transport itself.	Monitor vital signs, labor, IV fluid infusion, blood loss, urine output, fetal heart tones, degree of comfort (both physiological and psychological), equipment function, signs of motion sickness.	Monitor vital signs, patency of airway, respiratory effort/efficiency, IV fluid infusion, O_2 concentration, output (urine and G.I.), Isolette, temperature, equipment functioning.			Restrictive to use of certain types of monitoring equipment. Impossible in some aircraft to perform certain procedures. In unpressurized aircraft monitor closely for hypoxia and expansion of trapped gases	Noise may restrict use of stethoscope for pulse and BP. Motion/vibration may require need to stop vehicle.
Keep accurate records of patient's conditions and specifics of interventions during entire transport process.	Careful documentation is necessary for legal purposes, communicating information, and later evaluation of transport system and process.						

Intervention	Rationale	Potential complications
Maintain contact with appropriate personnel in receiving institution to update information on patient's condition and arrival time.	Updated information facilitates maximum preparation for admission at receiving institution.	May be necessary to change prior arrangements for coordinating availability of ground transport at airstrip
With assistance, move patient from vehicle to receiving unit and transfer to bed in unit.	Same considerations during movement as outlined earlier	
Participate in the care necessary to admit patient to the unit; relate transport information to receiving nurse and physician.	More continuity in care is insured; greater opportunity to share detailed information about patient is provided; patient is provided with advocate/liaison in new system. Often two nurses are required to meet newborn's needs and accomplish necessary admission procedures.	Legally, may not be advisable to participate in certain aspects of care at receiving institution. Availability to participate in care may be compromised by need for another transport
Complete ongoing documentation of transport process by including specifics of patient's condition on admission to receiving unit.	Complete documentation is important for legal purposes and later evaluation of outcome of transport process. Include vital signs, fetal monitor data, progression of labor, intake/output, general condition. Include vital signs, oxygenation status, acid base balance, intake/output, glucose level, neurological status.	Return to referring institution after completion of documentation; leave information to facilitate further contact prior to departure.

Table 4-6 continues on following page.

57

TABLE 4-6. THE NURSING ROLE FOR PERINATAL TRANSPORT *(Continued)*

Nursing Action	Rationale	Maternal/Fetal	Neonatal	One-Way	Two-Way	Air	Ground
Contact family to share information concerning arrival, changes in patient's condition, and more specific information regarding how to contact patient or primary care giver. Serve as family's advocate/liaison with new system.	A great deal of "energy" is necessary to cope with new system and possibly new city. Supportive intervention at this point may help family reserve energies for coping with other aspects of the crisis.			In most one-way neonatal transport situations, contact can be made with mother on return to referring institution.	Ideally, should be available to meet family member at center for introduction to new health care personnel		
Contact referring staff (physicians and nurses) for update on transport process and patient's condition. Encourage referring staff to follow up on patient's condition.	Beyond meeting the need for professional courtesy, notification serves important functions in ongoing public relations and education with referring institutions.			Update staff on return. Provide name and number of contact person at center.	Should be accomplished prior to resuming othre responsibilities for transport		
Restock equipment used for transport; alert clerical personnel to arrange for cleaning and maintenance of equipment used.	Immediate readiness for next transport situation is assured.			May be limited availability of certain equipment	May have "back-up" stock of equipment		

Initiate referrals
for patient or
patient's family
with appro-
priate profes-
sional agencies
or layman's
groups.

Appropriate refer-
rals will increase
resource/support
persons for
patient and
family and
contribute to
achievement of
comprehensive
care.

Transporting
nurse to
receiving
personnel

Transporting
nurse to
referring
personnel

Continue peri-
odical follow-
up with family,
and referring/
receiving health
care personnel.

Continued liaison
role with family
is supportive for
family. Follow-
up may increase
job satisfaction for
an episodic type of
nursing role.
Maintaining open
lines of commu-
nication between
institutions facili-
tates subsequent
transports.

59

————————————— REFERENCES —————————————

1. Blackburn, G., et al.: Experiences with transportation of the high-risk newborn. Med. Ann. D.C., 43:349–351, 1874.
2. Blake, A.M., Pollitzer, M.J., and Reynolds, E.O.R.: Referral of mothers and infants for intensive care. Br. Med. J., 2:414–416, 1979.
3. Blake, A.M., et al.: Transport of newborn infants for intensive care. Br. Med. J., 4:13–17, 1975.
4. Boehm, F.H., and Haire, M.F.: One-way maternal transport: An evolving concept. Am. J. Obstet. Gynecol., 134:484–491, 1979.
5. Boehm, F.H., et al.: Maternal-fetal transport: Inpatient and outpatient care. J. Tenn. Med. Assoc., 72:829–833, 1979.
6. Brown, F.B.: The management of high-risk obstetric transfer patients. Obstet. Gynecol., 51:674–767, 1978.
7. Chance, G.W., O'Brien, J.J., and Swyer, P.R.: Transportation of sick neonates, 1972: An unsatisfactory aspect of medical care. Can. Med. Assoc. J., 109:847–851, 1973.
8. Chance, G.W., et al.: Neonatal transport: A controlled study of skilled assistance. J. Pediatr., 93:662–666, 1978.
9. Chase, H.C.: Perinatal mortality. Clin. Perinatol., 1:3–17, 1974.
10. Colton, J.S., Pickering, D.E., and Colton, C.A.: Evaluation of a life support module used for air transport of critically ill infants. Aviat. Space Environ. Med., 50:177–181, 1979.
11. Committee on Fetus and Newborn: Hospital Care of Newborn Infants. Evanston, Ill.: American Academy of Pediatrics, 1977.
12. Committee on Perinatal Health: Toward Improving the Outcome of Pregnancy. White Plains, N.Y., The National Foundation–March of Dimes, 1976.
13. Cunningham, M.D., and Smith, F.R.: Stabilization and transport of severaly ill infants. Pediatr. Clin. North Am., 20:359–366, 1973.
14. Ellis, W.C., Bharara, J., and Snyder, R.: The regional newborn center–Effect on neonatal mortality of referring hospitals (Abstract). Pediatr. Res., 6:409, 1972.
15. Feldman, B.H., and Sauve, R.S.: The infant transport service. Clin. Perinatol., 3:469–478, 1976.
16. Ferrara, A., and Harin, A.: Emergency Transfer of the High Risk Neonate. St. Louis, C.V. Mosby Co., 1980.
17. Gibbons, H.L., and Fromhayen, C.: Aeromedical transportation and general aviation. Aerospace Med., 142:773–779, 1971.
18. Giles, H.R.: Maternal transport. Clin. Obstet. Gynecol., 6:203–214, 1979.
19. Giles, H.R., et al.: The Arizona high-risk maternal transport system: An initial view. Am. J. Obstet. Gynecol., 128:400–406, 1977.
20. Goldman, H.I., Lanzkowsky, P., and Sun, S.: Regionalized neonatal intensive care. N.Y. State J. Med.. 74:1835–1840. 1974.
21. Graven, S.N. (Chairman): Newborn Air Transport Conference. Denver, Mead Johnson Nutritional Division, 1978.
22. Graven, S.N. (Chairman): Maternal Air Transport Conference. Denver: Mead Johnson Nutritional Division, 1979.
23. Greene, W.T.: Organization of neonatal transport services in support of a regional referral center. Clin. Perinatol., 7:187–195, 1980.
24. Gunn, T., and Outerbridge, E.W.: Effectiveness of neonatal transport. Can. Med. Assoc. J., 118:646-649, 1978.
25. Guy, M.: Neonatal transport. Nurs. Clin. North Am., 13:3–11, 1978.
26. Hackel, A.: A medical transport system for the neonate. Anesthesiology, 43:258–267, 1975.
27. Harris, T.R.: Neonatal versus maternal transport: An analysis of dollar costs and mortality rates (Abstract). Clin. Res., 23:149A, 1975.
28. Harris, T.R., Isaman, J., and Giles, H.R.: Improved neonatal survival through maternal transport. Obstet. Gynecol., 52:294–300, 1978.

29. Henry, J.N., Krenis, L.J., and Cutting, R.T.: Hypoxemia during aeromedical evacuation. Surg. Gynecol. Obstet., *136*:49–53, 1973.
30. Hobel, C.J., et al.: Prenatal and intrapartum high-risk screening. I. Prediction of the high-risk neonate. Am. J. Obstet. Gynecol., *117*:1–8, 1973.
31. Honeyfield, P.R.: General condition of air transport. *In* Graven, S.N. (Chairman): Newborn Air Transport Conference. Denver, Mead Johnson Nutritional Division, 1978.
32. Honeyfield, P.R.: Staffing for Newborn Transport: Team Composition. *In* Graven, S.N. (Chairman): Newborn Air Transport Conference. Denver, Mead Johnson Nutritional Division, 1978.
33. Johnson, M.A., Owens, J., and Horwood, S.P.: Air transport of infants in Newfoundland and Labrador. Can. Med. Assoc. J., *119*:127–134, 1978.
34. Levy, D.L., Noelke, K., and Goldsmith, J.P.: Maternal and infant transport program in Louisiana. Obstet. Gynecol., *57*:500–504, 1981.
35. Makowski, E.L., et al.: Effect of maternal exposure to high altitude upon fetal oxygenation. Am. J. Obstet. Gynecol., *100*:852–861, 1968.
36. McCaffree, M.A.: Neonatal transport, 1976. J. Okla. State Med. Assoc., *71*:10–14, 1978.
37. Merenstein, G.B., et al.: An analysis of air transport results in the sick newborn. II. Antenatal and neonatal referrals. Am. J. Obstet. Gynecol., *128*:520–525, 1977.
38. Modanlou, H.D., et al.: Antenatal versus neonatal transport to a regional perinatal center. A comparison between matched pairs. Obstet. Gynecol., *53*:725–729, 1979.
39. Modanlou, H.D., et al.: Perinatal transport to a regional perinatal center in a metropolitan area: Maternal versus neonatal transport. Am. J. Obstet. Gynecol., *138*: 1157–1164, 1980.
40. Naeye, R.H., and Blanc, W.A.: Influences of pregnancy risk factors on fetal and newborn disorders. Clin. Perinatol., *1*:187–195, 1974.
41. Nesbitt, R.E.L., Jr.: Prenatal identification of the fetus at risk. Clin. Perinatol., *1*: 213–228, 1974.
42. Oetgen, W.J., and Landes, R.D.: Aeromedical evacuation of high risk infants: Experience at a military medical center. Milit. Med., *143*:712–713, 1978.
43. Oxer, H.F.: Aeromedical evacuation of the seriously ill. Br. Med. J., *3*:692–694, 1975.
44. Perez, R.C., and Burks, R.: Transporting high risk infants. J. Emerg. Nurs., *4*:14–18, 1978.
45. Perkins, R.P.: Air transport of mothers: Equipment. *In* Graven, S.N. (Chairman): Maternal Air Transport Conference. Denver, Mead Johnson Nutritional Division, 1979.
46. Pettett, G.P., et al.: An analysis of air transport results in the sick newborn infant. I. The transport team. Pediatrics, *55*:774–782, 1975.
47. Rapoport, P.J., et al.: In utero versus postpartum transportation of high-risk infants (Abstract). Pediatr. Res., *2*:541, 1977.
48. Roy, R.N.D., and Kitchen, W.H.: Nets: A new system for neonatal transport. Med. J. Aust., *2*:855–858, 1977.
49. Skeleton, M.A., et al.: Transport of the neonate. South. Med. J., *72*:144–148, 1979.
50. Souma, M.L.: Maternal transport: Behind the drama. Am. J. Obstet. Gynecol., *134*: 904–908, 1979.
51. Storrs, C.N., and Taylor, M.R.H.: Transport of sick newborn babies. Br. Med. J., *3*:328–332, 1970.
52. Sumners, J., et al.: Regional neonatal transport: Impact of an integrated community/center system. Pediatrics, *65*:910–916, 1980.

PSYCHOSOCIAL CARE OF THE HIGH RISK FAMILY UNIT

CHAPTER 5

FAMILY-INFANT BONDING

M. Lynn Litchfield, C.N.M., M.S.N.

OBJECTIVES

Upon the completion of this chapter, the reader will be able to accomplish the following:

1. Discuss the basic principles of parental-infant bonding.
2. List four differences between the concepts of bonding and attachment.
3. State changeable factors in the bonding process in which the nurse may have impact.
4. Discuss positive and negative clues concerning the bonding process that should be assessed in the delivery room.
5. Discuss the adaptive tasks of pregnancy and ways in which the unsuccessful meeting of those tasks may interfere with parental-infant bonding.
6. List 11 factors that may make parents at high risk for bonding problems.
7. Discuss nursing interventions designed to facilitate bonding with high risk parents.
8. Describe normal touch progression post partum.
9. Discuss nursing interventions designed to facilitate bonding in the postpartum period.
10. Describe differences between the "taking-in" and "taking-hold" phases and ways to facilitate bonding in these phases.
11. Discuss nursing interventions designed to facilitate bonding with premature or acutely ill newborns.
12. Discuss ways to facilitate bonding when the infant remains in the hospital after the mother has been discharged.
13. Discuss ways to facilitate bonding when the infant has been transferred to another hospital.
14. Discuss nursing interventions aimed at facilitating bonding with congenitally deformed infants.
15. Discuss bonding in situations in which the newborn dies or death is imminent.

Perhaps at no other point in the history of an individual family unit does the nurse have such an impact on the maternal-paternal-infant relationship as during the perinatal period. The attitudes developed during this period of individual and family crisis may have profound and lasting effects on the future family relationship. Much research, both with animals and humans, has been focused on this parent-infant bonding and attachment, and efforts

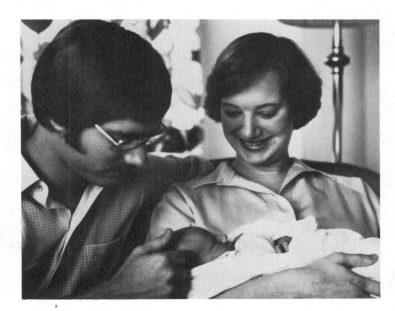

Figure 5-1. The attitudes developed during the perinatal period have profound affects on lasting family relationships. (Courtesy of Don Shaeffer, Hermann Hospital, Houston, Texas.)

have been made to relate such dysfunctions as child abuse, conditions involving failure to thrive, and childhood emotional disturbances with problems in these early processes.

PRINCIPLES OF BONDING

What is bonding? Klaus and Kennell hypothesized that a sensitive period exists in humans immediately following birth during which the mother is most likely to develop strong emotional ties to her infant. "This original mother-infant bond is the wellspring for all the infant's subsequent attachments and is the formative relationship in the course of which the child develops a sense of himself."[3] This hypothesis was based on animal studies that supported the theory that there exists in nature a sensitive period during which attachment of the animal mother and infant occurs. Species-specific behaviors of the animal infant appear to evoke maternal behaviors necessary for optimal mothering at a period in which the mother is most sensitive to these stimuli. Without these infant behaviors and the reciprocal maternal responses, survival of the species would be jeopardized.[8] For each species there exists a specific sensitive period; if this period is altered these normal behaviors do not occur.

Klaus and Kennell, after years of review of animal studies and their own research, postulated seven principles regulating human bonding:

1. A sensitive period exists immediately following birth during which the parents should have contact with the infant for optimal future parent-infant relationships to develop.

2. The mother and father exhibit species-specific responses when they are first introduced to their infant.

3. The mother and father can bond optimally to only one infant at a time. This principle has special impact for twins and other multiple gestational infants.

4. For optimal bonding to occur, the infant must respond in some manner (eye contact or body movement).

5. Persons observing the birth of an infant become strongly attached to the child.

6. It is difficult for parents to bond to their newborn and mourn the real or threatened loss of that newborn or another significant person at the same time. This principle has special impact for premature or acutely ill newborns.

7. Early events may have long-lasting effects. Fears concerning the prognosis of a newborn with temporary problems may adversely affect the long-term parent-infant relationship.[3]

DIFFERENCES BETWEEN BONDING AND ATTACHMENT

Although Klaus and Kennell used the terms bonding and attachment interchangeably, other researchers have made a distinction between them (Table 5-1). Attachment, according to Bowlby, is a more generalized term dealing with the affectional relationship between parents and infants developing during the first year of life.[1] She proposed that behaviors of the infant such as crying, smiling, sucking, and clinging serve the purpose of bringing the mother to the infant and keeping her there so that attachment can occur. Maternal responsiveness to her infant's needs and acceptance of that infant have been associated with securely attached infants at 1 year of age.[9]

Whether or not less than optimal bonding does have long-lasting effects on parental attachment and family relationships is still being researched. Studies support but do not conclusively prove the existence of a postpartum sensitive period for human maternal-infant bonding. Possibly the development of a strong maternal-infant bond would facilitate the gradual attachment process during the infant's first year by making the mother aware of her infant's behavioral cues. Ideally this would enhance the reciprocity of the mother-infant interaction and lead to infants securely attached to their parents.[9]

TABLE 5-1. DISTINCTION BETWEEN BONDING AND ATTACHMENT

	Bonding	Attachment
Directional	Parent → infant	Parent ⇆ infant
Timing	At birth	During first year of life
Infant response	Eye contact	Crying
	Body movement	Smiling
		Sucking
		Clinging
		Following
Influencing factors	High risk factors of parent or infant	Quality and timing of parent-infant experiences

Adapted from Taylor, P.M. (ed.): Parent-Infant Relationships. New York, Grune & Stratton, 1980.

_____ THE NURSE AND THE BONDING PROCESS _____

Does the nurse have an impact on the bonding process? Certainly there are factors that have an impact on the bonding process that are relatively unchangeable. The mother brings to the bonding process her own personal history of care taking by her mother, her relationship with family and significant persons in her life, her past obstetrical history, her cultural beliefs, and the events of the current pregnancy leading to delivery. Changeable aspects superimposed on these factors are such events as the type and manner of labor and delivery, the type and degree of emotional support provided by hospital personnel, the attitudes of medical and nursing personnel, the amount and timing of separation of the mother and infant, and hospital policies regulating the perinatal experience.[3] It is within this framework of changeable and unchangeable factors that the nurse must work to promote optimal maternal-paternal-infant bonding.

The first step for the nurse in dealing with the bonding process is to assess the maternal-paternal-infant interactions that are occurring (Table 5–2). The following case study highlights the signs that maternal-infant bonding is occurring.

TABLE 5–2.   OBSERVATIONS IN THE DELIVERY ROOM
TO ASSESS BONDING PROCESS

	Positive	Negative
How does the mother/father look?	Excited	Dejected
	Satisfied	Apathetic
	Relieved	Ambivalent
What does the mother/father say?		
Initial comments re: infant	Positive	Negative
Initial comments re: gender	Satisfied	Disappointed
General comments	Newborn-centered	Self-centered
Points out family resemblances in infant	Yes	No
Calls infant by name	Yes	No
Talks to support person	Yes	No
Requests infant to be taken away	No	Yes
What is emotional message in verbalizations to each other and to infant?	Excited	Apathetic
	Satisfied	Dejected
		Ambivalent
What does the mother/father do?	Views infant	Turns away from infant
	Reaches for/touches infant	Withdraws from infant
	Involves partner in exploration of infant	Does not involve partner
If breast-feeding:	Attempts to breast-feed in delivery room	Does not attempt to breast-feed in delivery room

Adapted from Rising, S.S.: The fourth stage of labor: Family integration. Am. J. Nurs., 74:870–874, 1974.

> Mrs. M., a 27 year old primigravida, delivered a female infant after an uneventful 12 hour labor. During the laboring process, her husband was extremely supportive of her. This pregnancy was planned, and both were excited over the prospect of an addition to their family. The delivery was a normal vaginal delivery with local anesthesia. Immediately following the birth the infant was placed on her mother's abdomen by the physician. The newborn was alert with her eyes open and looking around. The father supported the infant's head so that the mother and he could view her face. Both had little regard for other events happening around them. The mother exclaimed, *"She's so beautiful! She has your [husband's] mouth!"* The mother continued to view the infant, lightly stroking her head and body with her fingertips, examining the newborn's fingers and toes, and murmuring, *"Our own daughter!"* The father also explored his daughter, although more tentatively. Much time was spent on his part observing the interaction between his wife and his daughter. When the infant was taken to the nursery, the mother asked when she could see and hold her again.

Using Table 5–2, it can be seen that this case study is a good illustration of both maternal-infant and paternal-infant bonding.

The following case study reveals a different set of clues.

> Ms. M., an 18 year old unmarried primigravida, was admitted to labor and delivery in active labor. She related to the nurse that this was not a planned pregnancy; by the time she realized she was pregnant, her gestational age was too advanced for an abortion. Her boyfriend since that time had sporadically continued to see her but had refused to assume any responsibility for the baby or to be present during labor and delivery. The labor was a difficult one for Ms. M. Because of her prolonged labor and her inability to push effectively, Ms. M.'s physician performed a forceps delivery. A slightly depressed male infant was delivered. Ms. M. expressed relief that it was finally over and began crying. She resisted efforts by the nurse to look at or touch her baby. She said to the nurse, *"Take the baby away so I can get some sleep."* Her last comment about the newborn as he was being taken to the nursery was, *"Why is he crying?"*

Assessment using Table 5–2 indicates risk of poor maternal-infant bonding. The nurse, working within the framework of her own philosophy and that of the organization in which she works, can act to promote optimal

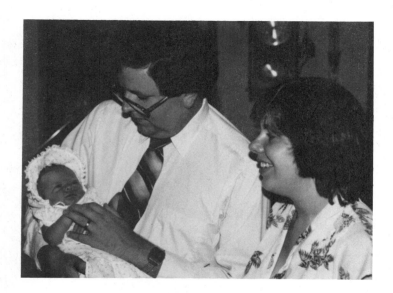

Figure 5–2. Throughout a normal pregnancy, parents anticipate the day when they will bring their new baby home. (Courtesy of L.W. Miller.)

bonding for this mother-infant unit. There are several statements made by the mother in the second case study that need clarification for the nurse to make an accurate assessment.

> When the nurse returned to the delivery room she commented to Ms. M., *"It's been a long and hard labor and delivery for you. You did a wonderful job. I'm sure that you must feel relief. Why are you crying?"*
>
> *"I wanted a girl. I didn't want a boy. He'll just remind me of Ned"* (her boyfriend).
>
> *"Is that the reason you didn't look at your baby?"* the nurse asked.
>
> *"Who does he look like?"* Ms. M. questioned.
>
> *"His face looks like yours. He has the same shaped mouth as yours and his hair is light like yours. I'm sure when you look at your baby you'll see resemblances to you and your family. A lot of times we think babies look like persons we want them to look like."*
>
> *"Why was he crying so much?"*
>
> *"Crying is the way babies communicate. After a few days you'll know which cry is for hunger or wet diapers or just being lonely. When babies are born, they're exposed to light and new noises and other new experiences. Sometimes babies cry a lot in the delivery room because it's a strange place for them. It's perfectly normal."*
>
> *"Is he a cute baby?"*
>
> *"Would you like to see him yourself? When you leave here to go to your room, I'll take you to the nursery first. Then you can see your baby for yourself and hold him if you wish,"*
>
> *"Yes, I would like that. Please stay with me."*

Based on what she had assessed, the nurse wrote a maternal-infant bonding assessment for the postpartum nurses who would be caring for Ms. M.:

Maternal-Infant Bonding Assessment—Ms. M.

At risk for M-I bonding:

1. Unplanned, unwanted pregnancy—questionable acceptance of pregnancy
2. No emotional support from infant's father
3. Desired female child, delivered male
4. Adolescent pregnancy
5. Did not view or hold infant in delivery room
6. Seems unknowledgeable concerning basic infant needs—crying

Plan to facilitate bonding:

1. Provide emotional support and acceptance of Ms. M.
2. Gradually encourage Ms. M. to hold and explore her baby.
3. Nurse present during M-I interactions for support and to provide information.
4. Encourage frequent M-I interactions.
5. Assess support systems—Bring in any support system available.
6. Social services consultation—Schedule home visit by nurse after discharge.
7. Point out positive factors of having male infant.
8. Provide information concerning infant's status and individual personality (how he soothes himself, prefers sleeping on stomach, and so on).

In making this assessment, the nurse utilized her knowledge of the adaptive tasks of pregnancy that must be met for successful bonding to occur.[2]

TABLE 5-3. ADAPTIVE TASKS OF PREGNANCY
FOR SUCCESSFUL BONDING

Adaptive Task	Ms. M.
Planning pregnancy	Unplanned
Confirming pregnancy	Unwanted—attempted abortion
Accepting pregnancy	Questionable acceptance
Perception of fetal movement	No data
Beginning perception of fetus as individual	No data
Delivery	Difficult delivery
Viewing the newborn	Refused
Seeing/touching newborn	Refused
Providing care for newborn	At risk

The nurse caring for the woman prenatally is in an ideal situation to begin promoting maternal-infant bonding by helping the woman and her partner meet these adaptive tasks. Unfortunately this is not always the case. The nurse caring for the patient during labor and delivery and the postpartum period must remain cognizant of these adaptive tasks and discover ways to facilitate their attainment for each individual family unit. If the mother has not successfully met the adaptive task of perceiving the fetus as a separate entity from herself, she may have difficulty in incorporating the birth process into her psyche, thereby limiting the energy available to her to begin exploring, identifying, and providing love and care for her newborn. Failure to have accepted the pregnancy by the time of birth may have grave implications for future mother-infant relationships.

Much has been written about problems in maternal-paternal-infant bonding with high risk newborns. The nurse must keep in mind, however, that certain parents with normal newborns may also be at risk for bonding problems. Ms. M. is a good example of a high risk parent (Table 5-4).

Parents with unplanned or unwanted pregnancies may have difficulty meeting the adaptive tasks of confirming and accepting their pregnancy. Women carrying fetuses conceived by traumatic means (rape, incest) are at grave risk for being able to fully accept, claim, and attach to the infant.

TABLE 5-4. FACTORS THAT MAY INHIBIT PARENTAL-INFANT BONDING

Unplanned pregnancy

Unwanted pregnancy by one or both partners

Adolescent parents

Emotionally immature parents

Parents with previous obstetrical or neonatal loss (stillborn, inevitable abortion, etc.)

Parents with real or threatened loss of loved one

Parents with poor emotional support systems, including dysfunctional family relationships, marital conflicts

Traumatic pregnancy: rape, incest

History of poor parenting by own parents: child abuse, child neglect

Chronic illness/pregnancy-induced illness

Parents with few life experiences, including sexual relationships, childbearing, child rearing

Adolescent parents or emotionally immature persons may lack the necessary ego functions to postpone gratifications and to self-sacrifice for the sake of the infant's well-being. Individuals lacking emotional support systems from significant others may be unable to continue investing the great amount of emotional energy necessary to meet the infant's basic needs of trust and dependency. Parents who have experienced previous obstetrical or neonatal losses may still have unresolved grief feelings from that loss that may inhibit the present bonding process. A nurse involved in this type of situation may have to assist the parents in grieving the loss of a past pregnancy or neonate before she can assist them in bonding with their infant. These parents may be unwilling to attach to their infant because of their fear, valid or invalid, of another loss and the associated pain they remember so vividly.

_____ NURSING INTERVENTIONS TO FACILITATE BONDING _____

Nurses are in an excellent position to help these high risk parents. Because it is the parents and not the infant who are at risk, the infant is usually healthy and available for increased amounts of exposure to the parents. The nurse must assess the situation carefully, however, since the parents must be ready for their infant. Forcing the parents and infant together without this readiness on the parents' part may do more harm than good. In cases of unwanted, unplanned, or traumatic pregnancies, this may exaggerate the feeling of the parents that their infant was forced on them. See Table 5–2 for readiness clues.

It is important to emphasize here that interventions must be focused on both parents rather than only on the mother. In an early study on attach-

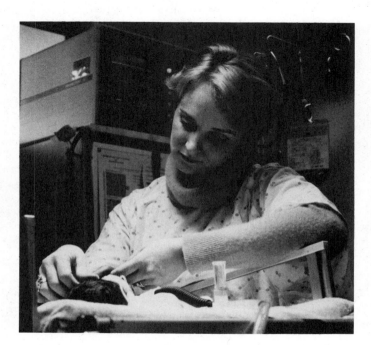

Figure 5-3. The hospitalized high risk infant needs the opportunity for close contact with the parents to facilitate bonding. (Courtesy of Don Shaeffer, Hermann Hospital, Houston, Texas.)

ment, the father was the primary attachment figure in 27 per cent of the sample studied, even though the mother was the primary care giver.[7] Frequently, in situations in which the infant is transferred to a regional center for neonatal care, the father necessarily becomes the bonding figure while the mother is confined to her postpartum bed. In fact, in situations with dysfunctional maternal-infant relationships, the father's attachment to the infant may prevent later emotional or psychological disturbances in the child.

What about the cues of readiness post partum? Perhaps one of the most obvious cues concerning bonding is in the progression of infant touching by the parents. Rubin purported the idea of maternal touch progression postpartum in early studies of maternal attachment. She discovered that the mother initially explores her infant from the periphery inward and begins by utilizing her fingertips, then her palms, and later, her whole arms in the touching process.[5] The infant's face and head take predominance in these early discoveries. The rate of progression is dependent on several factors— how the mother perceives herself in this role of mother, how the infant reciprocates her explorations, and the quality of the mother-infant relationship at any given time. Studies have shown that the rate of progression is increased when the infant is unclothed.[3] Paternal touch progression also follows this pattern.

The nurse must ensure quality time for the parent-infant interactions. The atmosphere must be one of unhurried concern and support on the part of the nurse. The nurse should not leave the mother alone with her new infant but provide guidance and information in the care giving tasks the mother is learning. The nurse should remember that the newborn is a stranger to the mother and father, even though they may have wanted a child desperately. They need time and patience in learning to know and love their infant, and they need respect for their own individuality. The nurse should allow the mother to progress with care giving at her own pace. Before answering questions the nurse should make sure that the question voiced is the real concern. The importance of this can be realized in the following case study:

> Ms. R. delivered a premature infant at 35 weeks' gestation. In the delivery room she overheard the pediatrician discussing possible hypoxia and the potential of brain damage to a group of new medical students on the service. The next day she asked the nurse if her baby was breathing properly and getting enough "air" in his lungs. The nurse replied that her baby was breathing fine *now*. Ms. R. took that statement by the nurse to mean that brain damage had been suffered. When she took her infant home, Ms. R. treated him as a brain damaged child. The child, as a result of the lack of stimulation, was slow developmentally and socially retarded. When he was 5 years old, Ms. R. took her son to a psychologist. She was amazed to learn that her son possessed a normal intelligence level.

It is important also not to confuse normal postpartal emotional and physical adjustments with dysfunctional bonding. During labor the mother progressively withdraws from her environment as she continues in active labor until all her energies are invested within herself. Postpartally the reverse occurs. The mother moves from an introverted state into a progressively extroverted one that once again encompasses persons and events not immediately present in her environment. Rubin divided this postpartal process into the phases of "taking in" and "taking hold."[5]

During the "taking-in" phase, which lasts 2 or 3 days, the mother is in a passive, restorative state. She cannot seem to get enough sleep, food, or information about the labor and delivery process. Concomitantly, she is also extremely interested in her infant's oral intake. The mother should be assisted in assimilating information concerning her labor and delivery so that she can free the energy invested in this process of reconstruction. She can then begin to identify the uniqueness of her birth experience and of her infant and can thus meet the adaptive task of realizing her infant as an entity separate from herself.

The "taking-hold" phase typically begins on the third postpartum day. The mother moves from a passive to an active state in which control of bodily functions becomes important and urgent. Within this framework of immediacy she becomes supersensitive and unduly critical of herself and her ability to care for her infant. Small upsets such as an infant that will not feed become exaggerated crises. The nurse must help the mother and father understand that these phases are normal processes. She must remain cognizant of these phases so that she does not label a mother as being at risk for bonding problems when on the third postpartum day she seems more concerned with her bowel habits than with her infant. Equilibrium occurs approximately 2 weeks postpartum. Unfortunately the nurse providing care in the hospital rarely sees this equilibrium.

HIGH RISK INFANT

What can the nurse do to facilitate parental-infant bonding when the infant is high risk? Typically, the parents experience guilt, anxiety, fear, grief, and frustration at the birth of a premature or ill newborn. They need special compassion and emotional support to accept their own ambivalent feelings and to deal with the prognosis of their infant. In situations in which the mother is hospitalized prior to the birth, the nursing staff can anticipate potential bonding problems and begin to intervene appropriately. The mother and father should be introduced to personnel who will be caring for their infant after birth. If at all possible, the parents should be taken to the nursery where the infant will be admitted and introduced to the equipment and apparatus that likely will be used. If the baby will be transferred to a regional center for intensive care nursery capabilities, the parents should be informed of the usual procedure and shown the equipment that will be utilized.

In the delivery room, if at all possible, the parents should be given an opportunity for bonding to occur. The mother should be allowed to see and touch her infant, if only for a few seconds. This gives her an image of her baby to relate to future communications concerning prognosis. In many situations in which the mother was not allowed to see her infant, her image of him was worse than reality warranted.

Information concerning the infant's status should be given as soon as possible and be optimistically realistic. Nursing and medical personnel must be careful to provide information at a level the parents can understand and be receptive to questions the parents may be hesitant to ask. Whenever possible, information should be relayed to both parents at the same time to prevent feelings of one or the other partner feeling "left out" or "not being told the whole truth." They should be reassured that the premature birth was not due to any wrongdoing on their part. This must be emphasized over and over again as the parents continue to look for an answer to the question, Why?

Parents of premature or ill newborns frequently begin a grieving process in anticipation of the death of the infant or at the loss of their imagined and expected normal, healthy, full term infant. As stated earlier, it is difficult for parents to attach and detach to an infant at the same time. As soon as the prognosis appears optimistic, the nurses should facilitate the termination of the grieving process and encourage attachment behaviors. This is not always easy to do. At times, the grief process has progressed to the point where it is difficult for the parents to believe their infant will survive or recover fully. The early guarded prognosis may have long term effects on the parent-infant relationship. Consider the following case study:

> Ms. L. delivered a 34 week female with respiratory distress syndrome. Initially the infant's prognosis was guarded, and she had several episodes of respiratory arrest. Ms. L. was convinced, even after her infant began improving, that the baby would not survive. Even at the age of 4 years, any respiratory problem of the child triggered Ms. L.'s fear of her child dying. She refused to let the child leave her house in inclement weather and gave her prophylactic cold and sinus medicines.

If the infant is admitted to the nursery in the hospital where the delivery occurred, nursery personnel should visit the mother and father at the earliest possible time to relay information about the infant's condition. The father should be taken to the nursery and introduced to the environment and equipment being utilized. A nurse should be assigned as the primary care giver so that the parents have someone they know to call on for information. The nursery personnel should visit the mother several times daily to keep her abreast of her infant's condition. The nursery telephone number should be given to her so that she may call the nursery at any time. As soon as possible, she should be taken to the nursery to view her infant. Ideally, her husband or partner should be with her; a nurse should also accompany the parental unit initially to provide support and to assess the bonding situation. In situations in which the infant is connected to many wires and tubes, the parents must be coaxed to see beyond the apparatus to their infant. Premature infants appear different from typical full term, healthy infants. Attempts should be made by nursing personnel to point out specific physical characteristics of the infant to dispel the perception of him as a "scrawny animal" or as a "little old man."

The infant in a closed Isolette poses additional problems for bonding. The parents are unable to use their olfactory and tactile senses for data gathering about their infant. The Isolette walls distort their view of their baby, and it is difficult for them to attain eye to eye contact with him or her. Because of the great amounts of energy being utilized by the premature infant for basic metabolic needs, the baby lies still in the Isolette and does not respond to the parents' efforts at communication with body movements as normal infants do. Any response to noise or stimulation, if it does occur, is usually a startle response, which frequently frightens the parents with its severity. When such an infant is startled, it is often difficult to soothe it, and the parents wonder to themselves how they will ever manage such an irritable baby.

As soon as the infant's condition stabilizes, the parents should be encouraged to provide as much care as possible. In some situations this may mean only touching the infant through the Isolette sieves. Breast feeding is an excellent way to maintain a mother-infant bond. The mother, by pumping her breasts for the infant's feedings, feels she is contributing something unique to the care of her infant—something that no one else can. The parents must be warned that the infant will not respond initially in the usual manner to being held or cuddled. Since the infant's reflexes are immature, it is a weak grasp reflex at best. Since the infant is neurologically deficient, the body movements are jerky and stiff. The parents may be looking forward to the first thme they can hold their infant, only to realize that the child is stiff in their arms and unresponsive. They must be informed that this will correct itself as the infant matures and becomes accustomed to handling.

The nurses should do all they can to emphasize the uniqueness of the infant. The parents should be encouraged to name their infant, and the infant should be called by that name by all involved with its care. When the condition permits the infant should be dressed in clothes brought from home or available in the nursery. Weekly or monthly birthdays and holidays should be remembered, and appropriate decorations made for the nursery. Milestones such as weight gain or the first oral feeding should be celebrated. Special items such as a stuffed animal brought by the parents should be placed on or in the Isolette. The nurses should relay information to the parents concerning unique aspects of the infant's care. Such items of information as how the infant soothes himself or herself, the best position for sleeping, and the best position for feeding all serve to involve the parents in the infant's care and enhance their perception of the infant as their own unqiue child.

If the infant remains in the hospital after the mother is discharged, a system should be set up to provide ongoing information to the parents and to encourage their continued involvement in the care given. The nurses should call the parents frequently to keep them abreast of the infant's condition. Frequent, liberal visiting privileges to the nursery should be encouraged.

TRANSPORTED INFANTS

How can the nurse facilitate bonding when the infant is transferred to another hospital? This is increasingly the situation as more and more high risk infants are being transferred to regional centers for neonatal care. It is extremely important in this situation for the nursing staff to remain cognizant of the parents' needs. Again, it is important, if at all possible, for the mother to see or touch the infant prior to transport. The transport team should visit with the parents and inform them of their infant's current status and prognosis. The father should be encouraged to visit the regional nursery as soon as possible since he will, in all likelihood, become the intermediary between the mother and the nursery.

This very situation may cause conflict between the mother and father in their personal relationship. The mother may resent the fact that her partner is able to visit the newborn while she is not. She may feel that he is getting to know the baby in ways she is unable to and taking away from her mothering role. She may begin to doubt that her infant's condition really is as her partner relates and may begin accusing him of not being honest. He, in turn, may not confide his fears and anxieties about the infant to her in an effort to support her. What can result is a breakdown in communication between the two partners and destruction of their emotional support systems. And, as stated earlier, problems in the marital relationship or ineffective, weak emotional support systems put the parents at risk for bonding problems. What is left is a situation in which both the infant and the parents are at risk for dysfunctional bonding.

The nurse must be aware of these dynamics and focus on providing support to the parents. Here again, relaying information concerning the infant's condition to both parents simultaneously may prevent some of the discord from developing. Setting up parent support groups is an excellent means of assisting the parents and helping them to recognize that their feelings are normal under the circumstances. In parent support groups, parents with premature or ill newborns meet weekly, or regularly, to discuss their feelings. The nurse can function as a facilitator in allowing the parents to verbalize their concerns and fears and, with the information revealed, is better able to promote bonding and provide support to the family unit.

The mother should be given as much information as possible concerning her infant in a regional center. Photographs are an excellent means of providing the mother with a concrete image of her baby. These snapshots should be made frequently so that the mother is aware of changes in the infant. Placing signs, such as "I love you, Mom," on the Isolette for the taking of the photograph help the mother realize that she is a mother and that there is a bond between her infant and herself, regardless of the distance separating them. Frequent phone calls to the mother from the nursery staff help to keep her informed about her baby.

The mother should be encouraged to visit the regional center as soon as possible. Preparations should be made in advance for this first visit. The infant should be clean and dressed, if feasible, for the visit. A small blue or pink ribbon on the infant's head helps the premature infant to appear more like a "normal" baby. Unnecessary equipment should be removed from around the Isolette. The nurse should be present to explain why lines, intravenous equipment and monitors are attached and to emphasize individual characteristics of the newborn.

——————— CONGENITALLY DEFORMED INFANTS ———————

How can the nurse promote bonding with congenitally deformed infants? This is a sad situation for all concerned. The parents, expecting a normal, healthy infant, begin grieving for the loss of that "perfect" baby. This frequently interferes with the bonding process. Consider this case study:

> Ms. M., a married 30 year old primigravida, delivered an 8 pound male infant with a cleft lip and palate. The delivery room personnel, upon seeing the infant, quickly covered the infant's face and placed the baby in the radiant warmer where the mother could not see it. The father was asked to leave the delivery room without being told why. Ms. M., noticing the apparent anxiety in the staff and the change in their attitude, questioned them about what was wrong with her infant. The reply, *"The pediatrician will talk to you later,"* did nothing to alleviate her anxiety. She imagined she had delivered a "monster" and began crying hysterically.

How could this situation have been avoided? As stated, early events in the bonding process may have long-lasting effects in the parental-infant relationship. Nurses must, from the moment of contact with the parent, be her support person, and assist in facilitating the bonding process with her infant. This must always be cognizant in planning for the patient's care. Frequently, nursing and medical staff are uncomfortable dealing with deformed infants and their parents. Anxieties abound concerning what to say and what not to say. However, these feelings on the part of the staff must be worked through so the staff can be supportive of the parents.

The infant should be shown to the parents as soon as possible after delivery. Emphasis should be given to positive characteristics of the baby— "sweet looking," good cry, lots of hair, long fingers, gender, and the like—so that the parents have something positive and normal to focus on. The infant should be cleaned and wrapped in a blanket before being shown to them to convey the feeling of acceptance by the professional staff. A gentle statement, such as, *"The baby's mouth and lip can be repaired later,"* may have been all that was necessary in the previous situation to alleviate the parents' fears of permanent disfigurement of their infant. Sedatives should be avoided, as they retard the grief process. Nurses should be present during subsequent parental-infant contact since the parents may have more questions and concerns as the initial shock wanes. It must be emphasized that, in general, it is better for the parents to see the anomaly initially than to be allowed to imagine it. Many parents will say, *"I thought it would be worse than that,"* when they are finally shown their infant.

DEATH OR IMMINENT DEATH OF THE NEWBORN

In situations in which the infant dies or death is imminent, the importance of bonding cannot be overemphasized. As stated earlier, it is difficult for parents to attach to their newborn if they are still grieving the loss of another infant. And it is extremely difficult for parents to detach themselves from their newborn who dies if they have not first attached themselves to that infant in some manner. The nurse must do all she can to facilitate bonding and the initiation of the grieving process. With that accomplished, the psychic energy invested in this process can be freed, and the parents can continue with their daily lives in a healthier manner.

What can the nurse do to facilitate bonding when a stillborn is delivered or the infant dies in the delivery room? The atmosphere in the delivery room should be one of unhurried compassion and support. The infant should be cleaned and wrapped in a blanket in such a way that its normal features are emphasized. The parents should be told gently of the death and asked if they desire to see their infant. If they decline initially, they should be informed that they may see the baby later if they change their minds. If the parents had chosen a name for their baby, the child should be referred to by that name. The baby should be described to the parents, whether or not they desire to see him or her. Much tact and compassion must be used in this situation. Frequently a stillborn who had died in utero several days prior appears macerated with distortion of the cranial bones. This should be overlooked and normal physical characteristics emphasized.

> Mrs. P., admitted to labor and delivery pushing and with the cervix fully dilated, delivered a full term, 7 pound, female stillborn. On the basis of physical findings, it appeared that the infant had been dead for several days. The parents had no prior knowledge of the death of their long awaited newborn. The physician gently told the parents of the death. The nurse caring for Mrs. P. cleaned the infant and wrapped her in a pink blanket so that the face was apparent but the cranial distortion was covered.
>
> She asked Mrs. P., *"Had you chosen a name for your daughter?"*
> Mrs. P. replied, *"We were going to name her Sarah."*
> *"Would you like to see Sarah?"*
> *"I don't think so,"* Mrs. P. sobbed.
> *"Sarah is a sweet looking little girl. She looks perfectly normal. Her skin is peeling a little, but that's expected. All of her fingers and toes are perfectly formed. She has light hair and fair skin, just like you and your husband. Her back is nice and straight."*
> *"She looks normal?"*
> *"Yes, she does."*
> *"May I see her?"*
> *"Of course you can."*
> The nurse brought Sarah to her parents and held her for them to view. After a few minutes, Mrs. P. unwrapped the blanket and looked more closely at Sarah. She and her husband both touched their daughter, and Mrs. P. kissed her child good-bye.

At times, because of the uncomfortable situation and anxiety about how best to handle the situation, medical and nursing personnel shy away from initiating this bonding process. However, this is a necessary intervention for the family unit and subsequent childbearing experiences. Frequently, the nurses involved state they have a difficult time controlling their emotions. To reveal sadness or tears in such a situation is not a bad thing for a nurse to do but shows the parents that there is real concern and compassion on the part of the professional staff. The nursing staff should not feel anxiety concerning what to say in consolation; the presence of the nurse, even though silent, is of great comfort to the family.

If death of the newborn is imminent, parents should be prepared as much as possible for the impending death. They should be encouraged to spend as much time as possible with their newborn in an effort to get to know him or her as well as they can. They should be kept informed of the prognosis and called to the nursery when death is pending. They should be allowed as much private time as they desire with their infant. The nursing staff should be supportive to the family in their time of sadness. A follow-up call from the nursery staff to the parents a few weeks after the infant's death helps the parents to feel they were not forgotten and that their experience, although sad, was important to the professional staff.

CONCLUSIONS

Bonding, regardless of the status of the parents or infant is extremely important. Nurses working with obstetrical or neonatal patients have an obligation to foster this family-infant bond that may have such far-reaching effects on the subsequent parent-infant relationship. Interventions should be based on a nursing assessment of both the parents' and the infant's needs. Facilitating this parental-infant bond can be one of the most satisfying aspects of the nursing care given by the nurse caring for obstetrical or neonatal patients.

REFERENCES

1. Bowlby, J.: Attachment and Loss. Vol. 1. New York, Basic Books, 1969.
2. Kennell, J.H., and Klaus, M.H.: Care of mother of high risk infant. Clin. Obstet. Gynecol., *14*:926, 1971.
3. Klaus, M.H., and Kennell, J.H.: Maternal-Infant Bonding. St. Louis, C.V. Mosby Co., 1976.
4. Rising, S.S.: The fourth stage of labor: Family integration. Am. J. Nurs., *74*:870–874, 1974.
5. Rubin, R.: Puerperal change. Nurs. Outlook, *9*:753–755, 1961.
6. Rubin, R.: Maternal touch. Nurs. Outlook, *11*:828–831, 1964.
7. Schaffer, H.R., and Emerson, P.E.: The development of social attachment in infancy. Monogr. Soc. Res. Child. Dev., *29*:196, 1964.
8. Schneirla, T., Rosenblatt, J., and Tobach, E.: *In* Rheingold, H.R. (ed.): Maternal Behavior in Mammals. New York, John Wiley & Sons, 1963.
9. Taylor, P.M., and Campbell, S.G.: Bonding and attachment: Theoretical issues. *In* Taylor, P.M. (ed.): Parent-Infant Relationships. New York, Grune & Stratton, 1980.

CHAPTER 6

NURSING ASSESSMENT AND MANAGEMENT OF THE CHILDBEARING FAMILY IN CRISIS

Joy Hinson Penticuff, R.N., Ph.D.

OBJECTIVES

Upon completion of this chapter, the reader will be able to accomplish the following:

1. List changes in family roles that may occur during perinatal crisis events
2. Describe the impact of family cultural belief systems on reactions to perinatal crisis situations
3. Recognize characteristics of family functioning in crisis situations
4. Describe emotional responses during grief
5. List behaviors to be assessed in determination of the family's level of stress and coping abilities
6. Describe nursing strategies to support family coping in crisis situations
7. Understand the major goal of nursing management for the family experiencing a perinatal crisis

---

The childbearing family in crisis is a family whose members are overwhelmed by loss or threat of loss surrounding childbearing. The concept of crisis implies that the basic behavioral and emotional stability of the family has become significantly disrupted. An example of a crisis would be the birth of an infant with renal agenesis. The mother, upon comprehending that her infant is terminally ill, becomes hysterical and requires sedation. The father goes on a drinking binge. The other two children in the family are cared for by neighbors and are tearful and frightened. Unless prompt, sensitive assistance is given, this family may continue to disintegrate.

Nurses who encounter families experiencing a crisis in childbearing are often in a position to give valuable psychological support as well as assistance in the medical care (Fig. 6–1). Nursing care of the family focuses on the

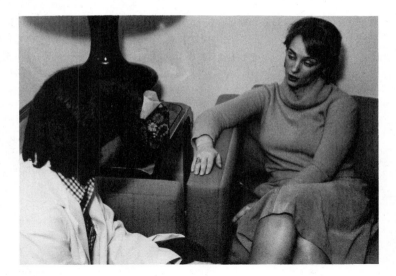

Figure 6-1. Nurses and physicians can support the family by providing information and by allowing them to verbalize their concerns. (Courtesy of Don Shaeffer, Hermann Hospital, Houston, Texas.)

family as a unit rather than on the individual patient whose symptoms have brought the family into the hospital. Nurses may utilize skilled intervention to prevent unresolved crisis, which can, in extreme cases, result in failure of the family to deal realistically with problems and in eventual disintegration of the family unit. Families in crisis have many similarities that will be discussed in detail below. These similarities can be identified and potential problems anticipated so that preventable difficulties need not be added to the family's burden of stress.

Families often do not understand why the crisis event occurred. For example, the woman who presents with hemorrhage due to placenta previa may not understand why she developed this particular medical problem. The causes of premature labor remain obscure, yet families are confused by not being able to obtain answers to the questions, "Why did this happen to me;" "Why did it affect my baby?"

THE NATURE OF CRISIS

Many families find themselves in a crisis situation because a number of things have occurred all at once, with which, taken together, the family is unable to cope. In addition to the medical problem, there may be longstanding family difficulties that make the family as a unit less able to cope with the medical situation. For example, a teenager who is pregnant and whose husband is a young man without a job may be less able to cope with a complication of pregnancy than a woman whose financial situation is more stable. The birth of a physically or mentally handicapped child can contribute to the development of other family problems; for example, the abuse of drugs by one or both of the parents. This can result in deterioration of the family structure and in turn may be a factor leading to child abuse. It can be seen that one crisis situation may trigger a number of crisis situations within the family.

Another characteristic of crisis is the critical nature of the situation. It is critical to the future of the family that the parents are able to cope with the crisis. If they are unable to cope with the crisis, then the family may disintegrate. Divorce and separation are not unusual outcomes when difficulties in childbearing are encountered by families. Divorce and separation rates are approximately four times greater in families of infants who were admitted to neonatal intensive care, regardless of whether or not the infant survived. However, crisis situations are also possibilities for growth and strengthening of the family unit. If the family members are able to communicate with each other and to share their feelings, their thoughts, and their problem solving processes, then there is likely to be growth and increased closeness of the family. Some families are able to communicate and to support each other as they deal with crisis situations. However, other families are simply unable to reach out to each other in crisis and find that they grow further and further apart.

Johnson[4] discusses criteria by which one can evaluate the family's response to a crisis situation. The first is the uniqueness of the situation itself. This has to do with the meaning of the situation to the family. For example, many parents are "shattered" when their child is born with a mental defect. Other families are able to accept intellectual limitations more easily. Some families value physical appearance very much. For them, a child with apparent congenital anomalies would be very difficult to accept. For some families congenital anomalies would be seen as an indication of some type of evil defect in the parents. In their innermost thoughts, some parents may believe that their child is deformed or ill as a result of some sin or unforgivable behavior on their part. Other families do not hold these beliefs about physical deformities or mental impairments. Therefore the family's ideas about the difficulty that the child has or their ideas about reproduction itself will have a significant impact on their ability to cope with the crisis situation. If they are able to see the situation as something that does not label them or their child as irredeemably bad or shameful, then the situation is certainly more hopeful than it would be for parents who view the difficulty as a punishment or sign of evil.

Another aspect of crisis has to do with the parents' relationship before the crisis. Parents who, before the crisis, were able to support each other and communicate their feelings and their thoughts and to solve problems together are certainly more capable of withstanding a crisis situation than are families without open communication patterns.

The last aspect of crisis has to do with the assistance of professionals. Nurses, physicians, social workers, and others can play a valuable part in assisting the family to cope with the crisis situation. As one who encounters the childbearing family in crisis it is important for the nurse to realize that while contact with the family may be of short duration, valuable support can be given if the nurse understands how to recognize families in crisis and how to manage crisis situations.

To function effectively with the family in crisis it is necessary to understand some basic concepts about how families function. In this section are presented basic ideas of family roles, how the family functions as a whole, and cultural influences that may be important when nurses are dealing with families whose cultural heritage is different from their own.

_____ ROLE THEORY _____

One way of understanding families better is to understand role theory. Role theory depicts the behaviors of each individual within the family as these behaviors relate to all the behaviors of the other family members. In other words, the relationship between the father's behaviors and the mother's behaviors is what role theory examines. The roles that are performed by the various members of a family are usually learned from experience and are influenced by cultural heritage. For example, in many white middle class families, it is not unusual for the mother to hold a job of some kind as well as to perform a number of tasks or behaviors that are characteristic of her role. She may, if she has small children, read to her children as she prepares them for bed, she may prepare meals, she may rock her small children before they go to bed, and she may carry out various behaviors that are characteristic of mothering. The father may provide for the family through employment, he may give his wife assistance in the housework, he may read to his children before bedtime, and he may perform a number of the tasks that were traditionally considered to be woman's work. As women have become more and more involved in the work place, the roles of the father in the family have shifted to include behaviors formerly thought to be those for the woman of the house. Thus, the interdependence and reciprocity of roles in the family can be seen.

When a crisis occurs, usually there are major changes in family roles. If the expectant woman is the person who becomes seriously ill, then her medical condition may dictate that she is no longer able to fulfill a variety of tasks that were a part of her role as wife and mother. For example, if she develops severe bleeding during pregnancy and strict bed rest is necessary, she will no longer be able to do household chores. If she was employed, she will have to give up her job, at least temporarily. It will be necessary for other family members to take up the slack. They will have to step in and take over certain tasks that are no longer able to be done by the sick family member. If the sick family member is a newborn, it must be recognized that babies have very significant family roles from their conception through pregnancy and through infancy. Their role is largely a symbolic one in that their parents invest in them certain hopes and aspirations.

If the pregnancy is threatened, then the parents are no longer able to have happy dreams about the unborn baby. Their dreams are more likely to be mixed with feelings of anxiety. If the baby is born with deformities or with serious illness, the parents are not able to have a baby who fulfills the role of the healthy, bouncing baby that friends, relatives, and the parents themselves had expected. Therefore, grieving for the lost perfect baby will occur. Thus it can be seen that even a baby may fail to live up to the expected role within the family.

When a crisis is experienced by the family—either development of high risk complications of pregnancy or birth of a very ill or malformed infant, the effect on family roles is apparent. The usual situation is that when family members are having difficulty in coping with the crisis situation, their roles often lack sensitivity to the needs of other family members. Their roles become less interdependent and more independent so that the family ceases to function as a unit and begins to function more as a group of several unrelated individuals. This results in disorganization of the usual routine of day to day family living, and it intensifies the crisis situation. Adults or older children must learn how to take up the slack in the role if it happens to be a parent who has medical problems and who ceases to function. If one family member is devastated by the crisis and cannot fulfill usual role obligations, then, again, someone else must lend assistance. If the baby requires special time consuming care, the family must recognize that roles may need to be shifted. If the mother will be the one to take special care of the infant, then she may have to quit her job so that she will have the time and energy to meet the needs of the baby.

SYSTEMS THEORY

Systems theory views the family unit as being made up of interdependent parts so that what affects one part will affect all of the parts. This is as true for families in crisis as it is for families in normal situations. If the mother develops a complication of pregnancy that threatens her own health and the health of the fetus, then the entire family's reaction to the complication must be evaluated. The grandparents and any family members or persons who are close to the family will be affected to a certain extent by the situation. Therefore it is not surprising to find that children in the family are often quite upset by the anxiety of the parents when the diagnosis of high risk pregnancy is made or when a child is born with serious illness or defect.

CULTURAL BELIEF SYSTEMS

It is also important to recognize cultural variations in the families with whom the nurse comes into contact. While each family member reacts to the crisis situation in his or her own unqiue manner, cultural beliefs and practices may become extremely important to the family at this time. This is because many of our most powerful traditions and beliefs are those surrounding birth and death. When the nurse is dealing with a family in crisis whose cultural background is different from the nurse's own, it is important to be sensitive and to respect the family's interpretation of the crisis situation in light of their cultural background. Such behaviors as eye contact, touch, eating patterns, and the like are very tied to culture.

Beliefs about the health care system and illness itself are heavily culturally loaded. One must avoid prejudices and cultural biases when working with families of other cultures. It is of benefit for the nurse to acknowledge her own cultural background so that belief systems, values, and life styles that may differ from those of the family can be recognized.

It is necessary to assess the family's view of the crisis situation. This may entail recognizing that the family's interpretation of the crisis event is different from the nurse's. The family may interpret the event as punishment or evil or something to be cured through spiritual rather than physical means. It is also important to recognize that family role changes that may be necessary because of the crisis may not be acceptable to certain families because of their cultural heritage. It is important to attempt to involve all of the family members in decisions about care. However, in some cultures, the father may be the traditional decision maker in the family, and this must be kept in mind. The nurse needs to identify significant others who may influence the family's decision making or who may be supportive to the family. For example, the grandmother may play a very significant role in family life.

It is of critical importance that the family understand instructions and that the family has input into decisions about the nursing plan of care. If an interpreter is needed, it is the responsibility of the health care professionals to see that one is provided so that adequate communication can occur.

CRISIS THEORY

Crisis may be viewed as disorganization of behavior and emotion due to overwhelming stress. One of the most significant characteristics of crisis is that it produces feelings of helplessness and anxiety. The person who is overwhelmed by the crisis situation often has a sense of being totally unable to control what is happening. Another important characteristic of crisis is that during the experience the person may feel that he or she has also lost emotional control. A crisis occurs when the person faces a stressful situation that is so severe that it overwhelms the person's ability to cope.

What defines crisis for one person may not define crisis for another. It is the meaning of the stressful event as well as the strength of the person's coping that determine whether or not that person will experience a crisis. For example, for one parent, admission of the premature newborn to neonatal intensive care may be interpreted as signifying that the infant will not survive. For the other parent it may be interpreted as serious, but not as a crisis situation, because there the baby will receive very careful nursing and medical care. For some parents, use of a mechanical ventilator on the infant is extremely frightening because they feel that the infant must be terribly ill to require ventilatory assistance. However, other families believe that while the infant is receiving mechanical ventilation, continuing vital functioning is assured, and therefore the infant is not in immediate danger of dying. These parents may become more distressed when use of the ventilator is discontinued.

Another factor that influences whether or not an experience will result in a crisis is the coping resources of the parents and the family. If the parents are confronted by overwhelming stress, they may still cope fairly well if they are fortunate enough to have needed resources available and, more importantly, if they can rely on practical assistance and emotional support from family, friends, and health professionals. Practical assistance has to do with the family's ability to "pull together" during difficult times in a constructive, noncritical way. For example, the retired grandfather may volunteer to stay with the other children while the parents visit the seriously ill newborn. Friends may bring food or may do needed housecleaning. Friends and family may provide a nonjudgmental, accepting ear for the parents' expressions of grief and anger. As is often the case, however, friends and even close family members often feel acutely uncomfortable when perinatal loss or the birth of an infant with congenital anomalies occurs. The family may be isolated at just the time when the most support is needed.

It is characteristic of crisis that the families who do become dysfunctional and disorganized to the point of experiencing a crisis are families for whom the stress is so intense that it overwhelms their available support systems and coping resources. It appears that crisis situations are threatening because they involve the feared loss of something important to the family, for example, the loss of the perfect baby that was dreamed of throughout pregnancy or possibly the loss of the mother because of severe pregnancy complications. But it can be seen that crisis situations, with their disorganizing effects on behavior and emotion, are also threatening to the individual's fundamental sense of being able to manage and to cope. The feeling of helplessness is very difficult to deal with and may result in intense anger, depression, and grief.

Crisis situations, therefore, are situations in which the balance between the person's perception of threat and his or her coping resources is lost, and the stressors outweigh the resources. Although the nurse in emergency situations may not deal with the childbearing family in crisis for a prolonged period, the nurse who understands crisis theory and can identify families in crisis is in a position to decrease the unnecessary stress the family has to face. Hospitalization with the diagnosis of threatened loss of the pregnancy or threatened loss of the newborn is a highly emotional situation in which families often lose their ability to comprehend information and to solve problems. Therefore, in crisis situations, the nurse needs to assess the family's reaction to the crisis and determine which person in the family is capable of making those decisions that must be made immediately.

GRIEF RESPONSES

The work of Kübler-Ross[6] in the 1970s demonstrated that most people experience a series of feelings after the loss of a loved one. Grieving may be defined as the emotional response to the loss of anything valued by the individual. Therefore, grieving occurs not only in response to death but also in response to the loss of the hoped for perfect infant or the loss of health and potential. Any medical situation during pregnancy that threatens the development and vitality of the fetus is threatening to the parents who value the prospect of a healthy newborn infant.

STAGES OF GRIEF

Kübler-Ross's work showed that individuals experience grief as a series of feelings, termed "stages," although most grief is some combination of these feelings. The stages are categorized as follows. Denial is the stage in which the individual cannot believe that the painful or threatening reality has occurred. This denial is not a conscious decision on the part of the individual simply to ignore the facts or to ignore the reality of the situation. Denial is an automatic defense mechanism that comes into play to protect the individual from a reality that is too painful to comprehend immediately. Usually, after some time, the reality of the situation is grasped, and slowly families begin to understand what has happened. The next reaction may consist of extreme anger and hostility and a lack of acceptance of the reality. A third phase is bargaining. During this phase the individual "makes deals" for a specific thing by promising to make some sacrifice or to accept the remaining part of the painful situation. For example, if a mother and baby have been separated by the baby's being transported to a neonatal intensive care facility, the mother may bargain, "Please let my baby live long enough for me to hold her in my arms." At some point a sense of acceptance may occur. During this phase depression and withdrawal are not usual. Finally there is a gradual sense of resignation to the inevitable situation and a sense that problems must be dealt with.

One common misunderstanding about the stages of grief is that individuals go through these stages in an orderly sequence. This is not the case. Usually some degree of denial continues in spite of active recognition of the problem and attempts at problem solving by family members. Temporary denial allows a brief respite from high anxiety, although the predominant feeling may continue to be one of intense sadness. Parents may elect to go to a comic movie, for example, to distract themselves from their painful thoughts. The defense of denial enables this restorative process.

Hostility frequently resurfaces after it has been expressed initially. The cycle of acceptance, with the concurrent feelings of sadness, depression, and loss, may spontaneously give way to denial. The bargaining phase may be cycled through again and again with new bargains made as old ones are discarded. Therefore it is important to recognize that acceptance on day six of the crisis may not mean that on day eight the person will not use denial. It appears that there is a psychological protective mechanism in the use of denial that is beneficial in allowing the individual time to collect resources and later face the problem with more strength. However, continued denial distorts the view of the problem and thereby hampers the problem solving activities that the family needs to resolve the crisis situation. It is important for the nurse to realize that there must be readiness on the part of family members to accept bad news. Before the family is able to fully comprehend and solve the problem in a crisis situation, they must have experienced a sense of support either from their own internal strength as a family or from external sources.

GRIEF AS AN EMOTIONAL RESPONSE

Freud[11] also analyzed grieving. The Freudian view of grief is that it is the emotional response to the loss of an attachment object. Therefore, if the individual has invested love or value and there is loss of the loved or valued object, grieving will occur. Threat or loss will produce anxiety.

Very often mixed feelings about the loved object occur. Thus it is possible for parents of a seriously ill infant to be torn between their feelings of love and affection for the struggling infant and their wish not to love the infant so as not to be hurt should the infant die. It is not unusual to find that parents of infants admitted to neonatal intensive care units experience feelings of isolation and lack of affection for the infant so long as the infant is in critical condition. Then with improvement and good prognosis the families are more able to allow themselves the opportunity to realize their love and affection for the infant.

ANTICIPATORY GRIEF

Another aspect of grieving that has received recent attention is the concept of anticipatory grief. In anticipatory grief the family hears bad news that they interpret as meaning that a poor outcome is inevitable. Feelings of imminent loss are experienced. This psychological acceptance of loss, in spite of the continued survival of the infant, may be less difficult for the family to tolerate than the anxiety generated by uncertainty. Anticipatory grief includes a strong sense of impending doom. This feeling of imminent loss is possibly less difficult for the family to tolerate than the total helplessness of uncertainty.

In anticipatory grief the family member becomes convinced that there will be a very bad outcome. The behavior of the family member is consistent with this belief. The family member may not wish to discuss the infant's condition, may withdraw from the infant, or may interact with the infant as though the infant were permanently damaged or not going to live long. Anticipatory grief, in which all reason to hope for a good outcome is taken away, may occur when families are given extremely negative information.

The danger of anticipatory grief is that in cases in which the infant recovers the family may have withdrawn from the infant so thoroughly that their feelings of affection and attachment may be seriously impaired. While it is true that there is a need to present the family with the significant aspects of the infant's condition and prognosis, it has been found that the obliteration of all hope is not appropriate.

FAMILY RESPONSES TO CRISIS

In crisis situations, as was mentioned previously, the emotional responses of the family, especially the individuals within the family, are varied. Some family members will demonstrate external calm and problem solving ability. Others may be less able to control their emotions in the face of severe stress. However, for even the calmest family member, severe and continued crisis will eventually result in disorganization of behavior and emotions. The nurse should be aware that emotion in response to crisis and total apathy in response to crisis are usual in overwhelming stress in humans. Therefore, if the family lashes out at health care personnel, at each other, at the infant, or at whomever happens to be there, their response must be understood in light of the emotional disruption induced by crisis.

COMMUNICATION

Often in crisis situations, communication between family members is strained. Frustration, grief, and possibly physical exhaustion result in increased irritability and preoccupation with one's own feelings. Often men feel that they should not reveal their feelings of helplessness, because of the need to live up to a stereotype of the strong, unemotional male. Wives may resent their husband's apparent lack of feeling in the face of loss. Some of this difficulty in communication has to do with the fact that family members experience grief in highly individualistic fashion. Also, what is perceived as an intolerable threat and therefore highly stress producing for one family member may be perceived as less threatening by another family member.

When one takes into account the variation in perception of the crisis situation, interpretation of the meaning of the threat, and individual differences in both styles of coping with stress and internal and external resources, it can be seen that family members should not be expected to feel and think the same way about crisis situations. For example, one family member may believe that it would be better for a baby to die than to survive but be severely brain damaged. Another family member may strongly disagree. In communicating their feelings and beliefs, it is often difficult for family members experiencing crisis to overcome their own emotion and interpretation of the situation long enough to recognize and support other family members who are also experiencing the crisis.

The emotional derangement that so frequently accompanies crisis can be devastating to family relationships. The husband and wife who were previously able to freely communicate their innermost feelings and thoughts to each other may be so overwhelmed by the crisis that they simply do not have the emotional energy to reach out to each other when overwhelmed by stress. For couples whose communication before the crisis was faulty, crisis situations very often exaggerate the communication difficulties. It is not unusual for marital problems to occur during and after crisis situations.

CHILDREN'S RESPONSE

Children in the family also are caught up in the emotional and behavioral turmoil that accompanies crisis situations. A child may have the mistaken belief that the mother's illness or the new baby's illness was caused by something the sibling did or thought, for instance that the baby should not come home and be a part of the family. A child, especially a preschool child, will easily pick up the emotional disharmony present in the family during a crisis but may not be able to understand that the feelings of anger, sadness, and upset are not due to something that the child did or thought.

It is important that there be adults who can calmly, supportively, and sensitively talk with or otherwise comfort children in the family undergoing crisis. Very often children are displaced from their usual home situation during the crisis situation. They may be cared for by relatives, friends, or neighbors. They need to understand that their parents still love them in spite of the temporary upset and that things will eventually be less difficult.

DISRUPTION OF DAILY FAMILY LIFE

The life of the family in terms of day to day functioning is one of the very first casualties of crisis events. Very often, in talking with family members experiencing crisis, one is struck by the fact that even the most essential elements of daily life have been disrupted. For example, the usual sleep pattern is often significantly changed with prolonged insomnia or prolonged sleeping. Eating habits are disrupted. Family members may have no appetite or may eat voraciously. Very often meals are skipped, or the family no longer sits down to dinner together. Children may be rushed to school or to babysitters without having been fed or properly bathed or clothed. Personal appearance will often suffer.

Perhaps one of the most devastating aspects of crisis, especially when the crisis situation is prolonged over days or weeks, is the exhaustion that sets in partially because of the disruption of sleeping and eating patterns. Of course, the experience of threat and stress is physically as well as emotionally draining.

PROBLEM SOLVING

Problem solving ability of persons in crisis is severely limited, partly because of increased anxiety that decreases the ability to comprehend information. Problem solving is impeded by the fact that at high levels of anxiety concentration is severely disrupted and attention may wander. Persons in an acute crisis situation, with very high levels of anxiety—as evidenced by perspiration, nervous muscular tension, inability to sit still, tachycardia, and increased respiratory rate—are unable to focus on the entire situation at hand. More frequently, such persons will focus on irrelevant minor details of the situation and will not "hear" the gist of what they are being told.

It is essential for the nurse to assist persons in a crisis situation to comprehend essential information so that they can begin to function appropriately. However, often a great deal of support and reassurance will need to be given before the person will be able to focus attention on the problem and comprehend the essential factors involved. Problem solving will be totally ineffective until the situation can be comprehended rationally.

_____ ASSESSMENT IN CRISIS SITUATIONS _____

REALITY TESTING

Reality testing is the term used to describe the ability of the individual to grasp the significant elements of the world around him. In crisis situations, because of the automatic defense mechanism of denial, full perception of threatening aspects of the world around the individual is lost. It can be seen that while this mechanism protects the individual from overwhelming psychological pain and keeps anxiety to a manageable level, continued lack of perception of aspects of the environment causes a distorted view of reality. Therefore in crisis situations it is not unusual for individuals to have poor reality testing. Their comprehension of the significance or the implications of events is lost. This is most often a transitory situation, and comprehension of what is going on will return in time. However, when an individual cannot cope with a very stressful situation, and the anxiety level begins to rise dangerously from a psychological point of view, the mechanism of denial will frequently come into play. When denial is working most effectively, threat is not recognized, and these people have relatively little anxiety. Therefore, if certain family members appear not to comprehend the magnitude of the crisis situation, one may suspect that denial is in effect. However, with continued presentation of the facts in a supportive manner, most individuals will eventually recognize the situation and will respond with emotion and anxiety.

Crisis theory purports that the experience of overwhelming stress has the possibility of either strengthening and making the individual less vulnerable to behavioral and emotional disintegration with succeeding stress or may render the individual more vulnerable to disintegration with succeeding stress. The main factors in determining whether or not disintegration and continued vulnerability will occur are the amount and kind of resources the individual brings to bear in dealing with the crisis.

From the previous discussion it can be seen that assessment by the nurse in crisis situations focuses on whether or not the family is comprehending the full extent of the situation and what their coping resources are.

ANXIETY LEVEL

In evaluating the impact of crisis on family members, it is important for the nurse to assess the level of anxiety being experienced by individuals and their ability to successfully deal with the stress that they are experiencing. Often it is necessary for the nurse to identify those family members who are most capable of problem solving in the situation. In some cases this may be the husband, or it may be one of the grandparents. One of the difficulties of dealing with the situation in this way, however, is that the mother of the sick newborn, or other family members who may not have been consulted in the initial decision making, may feel that their input into the decision was not sought. It is necessary for health team members to explain to the family that in emergency situations some decisions must be made immediately and that as the condition stabilizes, input of all involved persons will be considered.

It is remarkable how frequently health care professionals overlook the very beneficial effects to families of common courtesy and kindness during the crisis. Often families will feel very reassured when they are treated with obvious courtesy and consideration of their feeling, wishes, and needs. Usually families are able to understand the need for staff to be preoccupied with treatment of the medical emergency. The time required for a considerate explanation of what is happening is well spent. Sensitive and considerate communication and support of the family at the onset of the crisis situation can go a long way in assuring the family that their needs will continue to be taken into account by the staff. This fosters a feeling on the part of the family that the staff members are available to them for assistance and that they are giving a high level of professional care. Sometimes families get a wrong impression of nursing and medical care because, in the midst of emergency, no one is available to support them and to explain what is happening. Events surrounding emergencies, especially emergencies of childbearing, produce a great deal of anxiety.

This anxiety further causes the family to be unable to grasp the significant elements of the situation and may easily result in misinterpretation. Once family members have begun to distrust staff and to misunderstand communication with staff, the scene is set for serious difficulties in staff-family relationships.

It may be seen that those families with minimal amounts of emotional support from members within the family and from those outside of the family are the very ones who are the most likely to suffer behavioral and emotional disorganization induced by emotional crisis. Therefore it is important to note the strengths that the family members bring to deal with the crisis. Family members who have experienced serious difficulties in the past but who have been able to support each other, to communicate their thoughts and feelings to each other, to solve problems, and resolve the crisis are often very strong people. While their initial response to the crisis situation may show transient behavioral or emotional disorganization, they are usually able to bring to bear an ability to comprehend the problem, to communicate supportively with each other, and to communicate to staff in such a way as to understand the problem and to begin to solve the problem.

If the problem is one over which the family has no control, then it will be seen that some families will actively seek and readily use outside help, while other families will be wary of intrusion. For example, one mother of a premature infant who had hoped to breast feed but whose infant is very weak and unable to suck adequately will, upon the suggestion that she contact Le Leche for use of an electric breast pump, act on this suggestion. Another mother in the same situation, but who may be younger, inexperienced, and lacking family support for her pregnancy and baby, may have a tendency to give up in the presence of difficulties. Such a mother might make one attempt to contact an outside agency, and if she is unsuccessful on her first try may give up. She may need the nurse's assistance in continuing her efforts to reach the agency, and, indeed, the nurse may actually have to place the call for her. Another mother in the same crisis situation may be so emotionally upset over her infant's serious illness that she is unable to commit herself to the notion of breast-feeding because she cannot believe that the infant will survive. This mother may inform the nurse that she has changed her mind and that she will not continue to pump her breasts in the hope of eventually being able to breast feed her infant. This mother needs a supportive person to whom she can express her fears and frustration. She should receive reassurance that her feelings are understandable. Her sincere wishes about breast-feeding should be clarified and supported.

EVALUATION OF ANXIETY LEVEL

The assessment of the family in crisis includes evaluation of the level of anxiety being experienced by various family members, obviously with a focus on the mother and the father, or the most significant persons in relationship to the mother. The nurse must then recognize that individuals experiencing very high levels of anxiety may be hindered in their ability to understand elements of the medical condition, prognosis, and needed therapy. Attention span will be decreased, and concentration may be lacking. Therefore, communication may include the process of repeating information.

However, the nurse must take care not to give so many details that the family cannot absorb all of the information.

NURSING MANAGEMENT

Nursing management is aimed at reducing the unnecessary stressors with which the family must deal, decreasing unnecessary anxiety, facilitating understanding of the situation, and facilitating coping. It will be realized that coping with stressful events requires the ability to solve problems. A crisis intervention approach focuses on recognition of the possibility for behavioral and emotional disorganization of family members due to overwhelming stress. The nurse attempts to support the family by giving needed information in such a manner that the family can comprehend what is going on. The nurse may need to be somewhat directive in working with the family in the initial phase of a crisis; that is, the nurse may need to tell family members what their options are and, in some cases, to allow the family to draw upon the nurse's knowledge and experience by suggesting which options might be the most beneficial for the family.

INDIVIDUALIZATION

It is also very important that nursing care be individualized for families experiencing extreme stress. Hospital policies and rules should be used merely as guidelines in working with families in the midst of crisis. It is often not appropriate for these families to be treated just like every other family in the hospital. These are people who are under great emotional and physical stress, and their needs may appropriately supersede hospital policy and regulations. The nurse must keep this in mind and use clinical judgment about what can or cannot be allowed in the nursing care of families in crisis.

In the 1960s, for example, it was unusual for fathers to be allowed in delivery suites. Now we recognize how very important the father's presence is in giving support to the laboring woman who desires the father to be with her. This is never more important than in a crisis. In special care nurseries in the recent past, families were banned and could view their infants only through windows. Now health care professionals have become aware of the serious consequences of prolonged separation of parents and newborn. It is certainly true that the family in a crisis situation has even greater needs for support. This is the basis upon which the conclusion is made that hospital rules and regulations may need to be altered for families in crisis situations.

ANTICIPATORY GUIDANCE

Another approach that nurses use in working with families in a crisis situation is anticipatory guidance. This approach provides the family with information about what is likely to happen. For families in a crisis situation the nurse makes decisions about anticipatory guidance so that the family can be prepared for various outcomes but not be so depressed over negative possibilities that they cannot go on. Anticipatory guidance gives information and support so that the family will be optimally prepared to face whatever the future holds.

COORDINATION OF RESOURCES

Another role of the nurse in working with families in crisis has to do with coordination of resources. As mentioned before, the nurse assesses family coping ability, the support that various family members give each other, and the support they receive from health professionals, friends, and community agencies. Many times the nurse is the only person who has a holistic picture of the family. Therefore the nurse is in a position to have input about the number of personnel from other agencies that the family should have to deal with and the need for agencies and services outside of the hospital and can coordinate comprehensive treatment plans involving a number of health disciplines.

COPING WITH CARING

Probably one of the most difficult aspects of nursing the family in a crisis situation is when it involves death of a young mother or permanent injury or death of the newborn infant. Possibly a reason for the emotional upset that often occurs in the nurse in such a situation is that death surrounding birth is so totally unexpected and unacceptable in our modern society. Frequently nurses have difficulty dealing with their feelings during crisis situations such as these.

When families report insensitivity on the part of health care staff they are reporting symptoms that the staff members are not receiving enough support for their work with families confronted with the tragedy of perinatal death. Therefore it is important for nurses to recognize their own emotional responses in such situations so that through this recognition they may be more aware of their ability to be affected emotionally. Sometimes insensitivity toward families may be a reflection of a lack of understanding of exactly what families in crisis are going through. Nurses who work with many families in crisis need to have outlets so that they can have adequate respite from the emotionally draining work that they do. If a situation arises in which the nurse feels emotionally upset, it is important to have a channel to vent the emotion triggered by the crisis situation. If the nurse needs to have some time to reflect and possibly to cry, this is certainly psychologically very healthy. Nurses must come to grips with their feelings and express anger, sadness, and frustration so that they do not become burdened by these feelings. Principles of preventive mental health should be kept in mind by nurses who work with families under stress, because unless the nurse is capable of giving honest emotional support, kindness, consideration, and respect to families in crisis situations, the family will be hindered in coping with it.

_____ CONCLUSIONS _____

It can be seen that nursing assessment and management of the childbearing family in a crisis situation must take into account how families work and the concepts of grief and crisis. The view that family roles are interdependent and reciprocal is an important concept. The influence of cultural background in the way families interpret illness, their valuation of health, and their comfort in interacting with health care personnel should be taken into account.

The nurse should appreciate that during a crisis individuals may have a fear of losing control of their emotions and may feel unable to alter the crisis situation. Family input into decision making is a very effective way to prevent family members from becoming overwhelmed by a feeling of helplessness. Recognition that grief responses occur when something valued or loved is lost or that anxiety occurs with the threat of loss of a valued or loved object is important in working with families in a crisis situation. It is important to recognize that many families initially will respond with denial mixed with a variety of emotions when they begin to comprehend the crisis situation; characteristics such as breakdown in communication, high levels of anxiety, decreased ability to grasp significant aspects of the situation, decreased ability to comprehend the medical condition and prognosis, and feelings of alienation in relationships are usual. Inability to communicate feelings and thoughts may produce much family disharmony. Disruption of activities of daily life such as basic sleeping and eating patterns, resultant exhaustion, and greatly inhibited problem solving are all characteristics of families in a crisis situation.

The nurse assesses the family's grasp of the situation and attempts to enhance understanding through sensitive presentation of facts, assesses the family's coping resources, and suggests appropriate outside help. The nurse must also be aware of her own response to perinatal crisis.

It is hoped that an understanding of crisis theory, family theory, and grief responses will allow the nurse to practice in such a way that working with families in a crisis situation is a professional and personal growth experience. Just as it is possible for families to grow in strength because they have successfully resolved crisis situations, nurses also can grow through their participation in the process of crisis resolution. If families are supported so that they are treated with consideration, respect, and courtesy, they often show surprising strength in coping with very tragic circumstances. Nurses who work closely in such situations with families have the opportunity to experience a real sense of having accomplished something significant.

REFERENCES

1. Bibring, G.L.: Some considerations of the psychological processes in pregnancy. Psychoanal. Stud. Child, *14*:113, 1959.
2. Goosen, G.M., and Bush, H.A.: Adaptation: A feedback process. Adv. Nurs. Sci., *1*:51–65, 1980.
3. Herzog, J.M.: Disturbances in parenting high-risk infants: Clinical impressions and hypotheses. *In* Fields, T.M., Sostek, A.M., Goldberg, S., et al. (eds.): Infants Born at Risk: Behavior and Development. New York, Spectrum Publications, 1979, pp. 357–363.
4. Johnson, S.H.: High-Risk Parenting: Nursing Assessment and Strategies for the Family at Risk. Philadelphia, J.B. Lippincott, 1979.

5. Kübler-Ross, E. On Death and Dying. New York, Macmillan, 1969.
6. Lederman, R.P.: Developmental challenges and conflicts in pregnancy and child-birth. Presented at the American Nurses' Association 52nd Convention, Houston, Texas, June 8-13, 1980.
7. Marshall, R.: Coping with Caring. Philadelphia, W.B. Saunders Co., 1982.
8. Martin, E.P., and Seligman, W.N.: Helplessness: On Depression, Development and Death. San Francisco, W.H. Freeman and Co., 1975.
9. Nuckolls, K.B.: Psychosocial assets, life crisis, and the prognosis of pregnancy. Am. J. Epidemiol., 95:431–441, 1972.
10. Penticuff, J.H.: Psychologic implication of high-risk pregnancy. Nurs. Clin. North Am., 17:69–78, 1982.
11. Schoenberg, B., Carr, A.C., Peretz, D., and Kutscher, A.H. (eds.): Loss and Grief. New York, Columbia University Press, 1970.
12. Snyder, D.J.: The high-risk mother viewed in relation to a holistic model of the childbearing experience. J.O.G.N. Nurs., 8:164–170, 1979.
13. Warrick, L.H.: An aspect of perinatal nursing: Support to the high risk mother. The American Nurses' Association Clinical Sessions. San Francisco. New York, Appleton-Century-Crofts, 1974.

CHAPTER 7

STRESS: THE INFANT, FAMILY, AND NURSE

Shelley Wallisch, R.N., M.S.

OBJECTIVES

Upon completion of this chapter the reader will be able to accomplish the following:

1. Define the concept of stress
2. Identify positive and negative outcomes of stress
3. Compare situational and maturational crises as they relate to high risk perinatal care
4. Identify emotional reactions to high risk situations
5. Describe nursing care for the stressed family during prenatal, intrapartal, and postpartal crises
6. Describe stressors confronting the nursing staff caring for the high risk neonate

Stress is an unavoidable entity in both high risk and critical care settings. Nurses working in such settings are often affected by their own stress, while being called upon to deal objectively with patients' and their families' stresses. Knowledge and insight can help nurses recognize and uncover the sources of stress, enabling them to seek means of avoiding or reducing its effects. In this chapter the identification and management of perinatal stress factors as they affect the infant, family, and nurse will be considered.

STRESS: GENERAL PRINCIPLES AND ITS EFFECTS

Stress is generally thought to be a reaction to a real or perceived threat to physical or emotional well-being. Stress is uncomfortable and so becomes a motivating force in a person's quest to alleviate its source or make adjustments in an attempt to adapt.

Some stress is necessary and beneficial for the maintenance of life and attainment of goals, but a high stress level can be counterproductive. Generally, high stress levels cause a decrease in one's ability to utilize incoming information, to concentrate and problem solve, to master tasks and to make constructive decisions.[20] Events become distorted and exaggerated. Gaps in information may be filled with semifactual data. Stress tends to diminish one's sense of personal effectiveness and self-worth. Thus it can be painful and, like pain, tends to draw the individual inward. Relationships suffer, and family ties are often strained because of the preoccupation with self. A person's sensitivity and response to the personal environment may be diminished until that person appears in a daze, or it may be heightened, leading to distraction, annoyance, or irritation by seemingly insignificant disturbances. Stress is also closely linked with somatic symptoms. Headaches, gastrointestinal disturbances, and fatigue are among the most common stress related physical complaints.

CRISIS: GENERAL PRINCIPLES

When stress is not relieved by the usual coping mechanisms and problem solving techniques, anxiety and disorganization increase. Often the stress begins to interfere with daily functioning, causing a state of crisis.

Every crisis presents both an opportunity for psychological growth and the danger of psychological deterioration. Resolution, either adaptive of maladaptive, generally occurs within 4 to 6 weeks of the precipitating event. The outcome is dependent upon a number of variables: (1) the nature of the crisis event; (2) the state of organization or disorganization of the individual or family at the point of impact; (3) the internal and external resources available; and (4) the individual's or family's previous experience with crisis.[12] An adaptive outcome is one in which the crisis is resolved in a healthy manner. Ultimately there is personal growth and learning from the experience. A maladaptive outcome is resolution to a lower level of functioning at which the individual can no longer cope at the precrisis level.

A person experiencing a crisis 'is more receptive than usual to outside intervention.[2] Family, friends, and professionals can make a great impact at this time.

Crises are often divided into two categories: situational and maturational. A situational crisis is an event not normally occurring in the life cycle (e.g., rape, divorce, bankruptcy), that threatens an individual's or family's biological, psychological, or emotional integrity. A maturational crisis is a normally occurring milestone, or period of change (e.g., infancy, adolescence, pregnancy), in which there is excessive difficulty in attaining the desired or expected goal.[1]

PREGNANCY AND PARENTHOOD: MATURATIONAL CRISES

Pregnancy and parenthood are maturational milestones normally causing stress and occasionally leading to crisis. It is a period of irreversible change, a developmental opportunity for new growth as an individual and as a couple. Some of the usual stresses and concerns for both the husband and wife involve the woman's changing body and her physical symptoms, their changing life style, the reorganization of family roles, and anxiety about the

TABLE 7-1. PREGNANCY AS A MATURATIONAL MILESTONE:
COMMON CONCERNS AND STRESSES

Women	Men
Concerns for baby's health and normalcy	Concerns for baby's health
Fear of harming the baby	Fear of harming the baby
Concerns of body being permanently damaged or changed	Fear of losing wife in childbearing
Fear of unknown (labor, delivery)	
New physical sensations	Acceptance of wife's emotional and physical changes
Body image changes	
Psychological shift inward, emotional lability	Supporting wife emotionally
	Neediness, rivalry toward baby
Changes in expectations and conceptions in role as woman, wife, and mother	Guilt about fantasies involving other women
Changes in sexual desire	Changes in sexual desire
Doubts about abilities as mother	Doubts about abilities as father and provider
Doubts about husband's abilities as father and provider	Doubts about wife's abilities as mother

outcome of the pregnancy. Table 7–1 summarizes some of the usual concerns and stresses of pregnancy.

For women, a common worry is whether the baby will be normal.[17] They wonder whether they can or have hurt their baby by overeating, undereating, smoking, using additives, artificial sweeteners, or even worrying.

Women worry about themselves as well. Particularly during their first pregnancy, women may be concerned about recognizing the first signs of labor, getting to the hospital on time, or losing control during the labor and delivery process. They fear injury, mutilation, or even death during the pregnancy, or especially during childbirth.[17]

Though many women enjoy the early signs of pregnancy and the attention their growing body affords them, many others feel awkward and ugly. As the pregnancy progresses, women may describe themselves as fat, bloated, and distorted. Women who have prided themselves in being attractive and slim may resent the changes in their weight and figure. They commonly express concerns about regaining their former shape after delivery. The support a woman receives from her husband, along with the attitudes she has learned from her mother and other significant people in her life, will influence her adjustment to her changing body.[17]

New physical symptoms and sensations may be disconcerting to the primigravida.[17] Increased breast fullness and sensitivity may cause discomfort. Frequent urination, constipation, fatigue, and nausea may become problems. Favorite foods can now cause heartburn; various smells may be offensive.

The most frequent observation by women about their own mental states during pregnancy is that of over-reaction to events that ordinarily would not affect them. Usually they are unable to pinpoint reasons for their reactions.[17] This emotional liability can strain even the most loving relationships. In addition, the woman experiences a psychological shift inward. As the pregnancy progresses there is increased preoccupation with the self. Husbands often comment on feelings of being pushed aside or left out.

As role expectations and concepts change, anxiety and perhaps resentment grow. Resentment may develop as the mother-to-be ponders the changes her career may take as a result of her increased responsibilities at home. Or the woman may be aware of a growing dependency on her husband and become concerned about his abilities to provide financially and emotionally. An internal conflict between desire for dependence and desire for independence may arise.[17]

Especially in the last months of pregnancy, women report considerable decline in sexual desire. Physical changes, changes in body image and perceived desirability, and concerns about intercourse harming the baby or triggering premature labor have been cited as explanations for this response. However, some women do note an increase in sexual desire and pleasure during pregnancy, and this, too, can become a source of concern.[17]

Following the birth of the baby, readjustment to the nonpregnant state must be attained. Women often long to again be the object of attention, as it is now being lavished upon the infant. Some miss the closeness of the baby in utero. Some cannot reconcile the fact that they are no longer pregnant but they are still "fat." More than expected, they feel confronted with the responsibilities of parenthood and the disruption of their usual life style. Most prospective mothers are unprepared for feelings of annoyance and timidity toward their babies.[18]

Men also undergo stresses and adjustments during their wife's pregnancies and to fatherhood. Initially there is a sense of excitement and pride at the evidence of their virility and potency. But later, concerns surface regarding the current and anticipated changes in their lives and in their relationship with their spouse.

Often feelings of neediness surface along with those of rivalry toward the baby. A sense of isolation may develop as the wife becomes more engrossed in herself and the expected infant. Increased financial and emotional responsibilities may become overwhelming. There may be a sense of panic about being trapped. Because of these conflicts the pregnancy is frequently a time when men engage in fantasies about other women.[17]

Concerns about intercourse during pregnancy are common for men as well as women. They worry that the sperm, the sexual excitement, or the uterine contractions will physically damage the baby, cause bleeding, or initiate labor. Husbands have described feelings that intercourse with a pregnant woman is wrong. Consequently problems may emerge in the couple's sexual relationship. These are usually time limited in nature.[17]

Because our society values the strong, stoical male image, a husband may have difficulty expressing his concerns to his wife, friends, or even to a counselor. The pent-up tension and emotions may inappropriately be released in other situations. Families and professionals who are sensitive to a man's conflicts and concerns during the pregnancy may help rechannel his stress into more appropriate and productive endeavors.

HIGH RISK PREGNANCY: A SITUATIONAL CRISIS

When a situational crisis is superimposed on a maturational crisis, there is even greater potential for disorganization and a maladaptive outcome. Thus the high risk pregnancy creates a double jeopardy for both the individual and her family.

A high risk pregnancy is one in which there is a likelihood that the infant will be stillborn or one in which either the mother or infant is in danger of physical or psychological impairment as a result of the pregnancy. Very few risk conditions affect only the mother or only the fetus. More often, when the mother has a risk characteristic, the physical effect is felt by the fetus, and the emotional impact affects the entire family.[8] A number of high risk characteristics are listed in Table 7-2.

TABLE 7-2. PREGNANCY RISK CHARACTERISTICS

Physical

Age below 16 or above 35	Multiple gestation
Stature and weight	Pre-eclampsia/eclampsia
Height below 60 inches	Rh sensitization
Weight greater than 20%	Hemorrhagic complications
deviation from standard	Polyhydramnios or oligohydramnios
for height and built	Abnormal presentation
Nutritional deficiency	Fever
Multiple pregnancies—more than 5	Premature onset of labor
Previous high risk pregnancy	Premature rupture of membranes
Maternal chronic illness	Fetal distress
Maternal medication and addiction	Prolonged labor, delivery or both
Maternal infection	Precipitous delivery
Exposure to radiation	Complicated delivery
Intrauterine growth retardation	Cord accident
Postmaturity	Placental abruption

Psychosocial

Conflicts or defects in support system
  History of loss of the mother's mother before her own puberty and without adequate substitution of maternal figure
  Chronic conflict with or alienation from one's own mother and other female relatives
  Chronic marital discord, especially if focus of conflict involves childbearing and child rearing
  Poverty or perceived financial distress
Perception that pregnancy will physically cause her harm or permanent damage
Adverse experience during previous or current pregnancy
  Previous birth of damaged child
  Mother reports older child to be emotionally disturbed or behaviorally disordered
  Mother reports experience she fears will damage baby and is resistant to reassurance
Inadequate preparation for childbearing or child rearing
  Mother has no preparation for sexual experience, pregnancy, or motherhood
Concomitant situational or maturational crisis or change
  Adolescence
  Death of a close family member or friend
  Family illness
  Work problems
  Jail sentence

At-risk conditions during the prenatal period produce stress. Stress may leave the mother-to-be feeling unloved or unsupported or may precipitate concern for the health and survival of either her infant or herself. The preoccupation caused by the stress may delay preparation for the infant's arrival and retard bond formation.[11] The stress may have far reaching effects on her family, marriage, or self-esteem. Feelings such as blame, guilt, or failure can disrupt the family's equilibrium and set the stage for maladaptation to parenthood. It has been postulated that stress is not only the result of a high risk pregnancy but it may also play a role in the development of physical complications leading to premature births or low Apgar scores. Studies both supporting and refuting this contention have been presented in the literature.[4,5,9,16,19]

The physical components that created a high risk situation or, more importantly, the woman's perception of having any condition that may be made worse by childbearing or child rearing may interfere with her capacity to accept the pregnancy emotionally and to affiliate with the fetus.[3] Often the existence of physical complications in pregnancy may be met by denial. If the mother does not look or feel sick, the family may not believe there is a risk. Denial is often an effective means of coping with stress at least temporarily, or it may be used as a defense to keep from becoming attached to an infant who may not survive. When a woman fails to seek prenatal care, keep appointments, follow instructions, or acknowledge that a risk situation exists, she may be expressing denial.

Blame and guilt are reactions common to a complicated pregnancy. The mother may feel guilty if her age or health is the cause of the risk situation. The father may experience guilt if he feels responsible for the pregnancy that is now jeopardizing the health of his wife or child. One parent may blame the other. Sometimes the misfortune is viewed as some sort of punishment from God.

In this country the expectation is for pregnancies to end successfully. Therefore the presence of risk conditions or failure to conclude a pregnancy with a normal delivery can lead to feelings of failure. Both parents may feel that their sexual identity is threatened by a poor pregnancy outcome.

Also in the pregnancy at risk, much of the prenatal concern is directed toward providing a safe environment for the fetus, unless the mother's life is imminently endangered. To the already stressed and guilt laden woman, it may seem that only the health of the baby is important. This may confirm her feelings of worthlessness. These feelings may persist after delivery, leading the mother to neglect her own follow-up health care.[8]

Ambivalence and resentment are other common feelings associated with high risk pregnancies. Anger and negative feelings may be directed at the fetus, the marriage partner, other family members, or the health care professional. The mother may resent having to give up her job or reduce her level of activity. The father may resent his wife's increased need for physical and emotional support. The financial strain created by the extra tests and care can also breed resentment.

Because it is often difficult to discuss negative feelings about a pregnancy, hostility may surface in other ways. The mother may smoke more heavily or engage in other health contraindicated activities. The father may work more overtime, stay out late, or drink heavily. Other children may begin to act out as a means of getting their share of attention or to keep their parents from fighting with each other.

Grief can occur at any time during pregnancy if the family feels loss of the child or the mother's health is possible. Grieving that occurs before an actual loss is called anticipatory grief. If the outcome of the pregnancy is normal and healthy, grieving prematurely can lead to a serious aberration in the parent-infant relationship. Sometimes the grief can persist for years and cause an otherwise healthy child to be severely emotionally disturbed.[8]

In addition to real or perceived health concerns there are other life factors that cause a woman and her family a stressful pregnancy. Any event or experience during the current or prior pregnancies that is perceived by the mother as having possible ill effects may increase the stress of this pregnancy.[3] Seemingly insignificant events can take on major proportions in the mind of the stressed woman. A disturbing phone call or an argument with a spouse during the first months of pregnancy may be construed as an omen or thought to have harmed the baby in utero. Past experience with miscarriage or stillbirth will also cause the family to be more anxious and reserved about this pregnancy.

Conflicts or defects in a woman's major support systems, whether past or present, can have serious implications for the pregnant woman and unborn child. Surprisingly, major marital conflicts have less impact than unresolved conflicts involving a woman's mother or other primary female care givers. If the conflict has been lifelong, the woman may feel unsure of herself as a nurturing female.[3] Mothering behaviors are learned from one's mother, and so without intervention, a cycle of maladaptive mothering behaviors can be perpetuated from generation to generation.

Inadequate preparation for childbearing and child rearing, especially for primigravidas, can be quite stressful.[3] Bodily changes, the process of labor and delivery, and infant care can be extremely frightening for the woman with little knowledge and no previous experience.

IDENTIFICATION OF MALADAPTATION TO PREGNANCY

With routine screening by the health professional for "at-risk" responses to pregnancy, further decompensation and maladaptation can perhaps be deterred. Table 7–3 illustrates some lines of questioning that may uncover the mother at risk.[3]

Overt maladaptation to pregnancy is easier to recognize by conventional clinical observation. Most often, decompensation is evidenced by inability to accept the pregnant state and by faulty affiliation with the fetus. Some signs of maladaptation are summarized in Table 7–4.[3]

Rejection and ambivalence toward the pregnancy are normal responses up to a point. In most instances the strongly negative attitudes dissipate around the time of quickening and are almost always resolved by the third trimester. Continued rejection into the third trimester, therefore, is indicative of maladaptation to the pregnancy.

TABLE 7-3. SAMPLE SCREENING QUESTIONS TO ELICIT AT-RISK RESPONSES TO PREGNANCY

Identification of adverse previous experience
  Has anything happened in the past (or during this pregnancy) that might affect the baby?
Major conflict in support system
  Do you plan to raise your children any differently from the way you were raised?
  Is your husband (father of the baby) much help to you?
Lack of prior experience in infant and child care
  How much experience have you had in taking care of children?
Maternal health concerns
  Do you have any condition that you think might be made worse by being pregnant?
Identification of other life changes or life crises
  What are some of the changes you've experienced in your life over the past year?
  Has there been any recent family illness or death?

TABLE 7-4. MALADAPTIVE RESPONSES TO PREGNANCY

Rejection of Pregnancy
  Mother denies, ignores, or constantly overreacts to body and appearance changes.
  Mother is preoccupied with vague unremediable complaints, either physical or emotional.
  At advanced stages of pregnancy, mother dresses and engages in activities that suggest she is not pregnant.

Failure to develop emotional affiliation with the fetus
  There is a minimal or disturbed response to quickening.
  Nesting behavior is absent in the third trimester (particularly in primigravidas).
  Fantasies about the baby are absent or predominately negative.

The onset of quickening usually generates feelings of affiliation with the fetus. This is evidenced by a shift in the mother's attitude toward positive anticipation, a growing acceptance of the pregnancy, and nesting behaviors. The fetus is thought of as a separate person and fantasies of motherhood and the coming infant increase. Failure of these shifts to occur should be interpreted as an early warning signal.

NURSING CARE

No conclusions can be drawn from the appearance of at-risk indicators or from the early signs of maladaptive behaviors. The presence of these signs indicates that further assessment of the situation is in order. Some patients and families might need only more frequent prenatal visits to provide them with the support they need; others may need to utilize community resources, counseling, or psychiatric services.

A consistent, alert, and concerned nurse is probably the most suitable person to evaluate and support the family at risk. During the prenatal visits, encouraging the woman to express her concerns and feelings about pregnancy and her current life situation may be the most expedient and beneficial means of reducing stress. The prospective father and other family members should attend appointments, as well. In this way, the nurse can unveil their concerns and strengthen their support of each other. As an objective listener the nurse can help parents sort out needs and identify and utilize their inner strengths, their friends, and their family supports.

Patient and family teaching is effective in reducing stress. Acquiring awareness of the biological and psychosocial changes that occur in pregnancy can help a family cope with the upsets. Special antenatal tests should be explained thoroughly. A picture from the ultrasound examination or a monitor strip from an oxytocin challenge test showing the baby's normal heartbeat can be very reassuring to nervous parents.

If a mother is hospitalized prior to her labor, every effort should be made for her to see her family. To decrease her feelings of dependence and powerlessness she should be encouraged to participate in the planning of her care. Hospitalization can also provide an excellent opportunity for the nurse to teach and facilitate discussions among the group of high risk mothers.

In addition to direct nursing intervention, the nurse must be prepared to make appropriate referrals. In the event of an unwanted pregnancy, possible genetic complications, or marital conflict, counseling services can be indispensable. For parents unsure about their mothering or fathering skills, child care classes can be sought. Stress on the mother and her family as a result of imposed bed rest or hospitalization can at least be partially relieved by the use of a hired homemaker. The nurse's astute actions and supportive measures during the prenatal period can have far reaching effects in promoting a healthy parent-infant bond.

_____ LABOR AND DELIVERY: WHEN SOMETHING GOES WRONG _____

Labor and delivery make up perhaps the most emotionally charged period during the pregnancy, leaving a lasting impression on the woman. Generally, as labor progresses, anxiety increases. With the increasing discomfort and anxiety, all the woman's attention is focused upon herself. It is difficult for those around her to break through the barrier of this constricted world.

When a life threatening situation arises the barrier may be virtually impenetrable. The woman, if conscious, becomes less able to process information or express her needs. All her energy is directed toward her survival and the impending damage to her body.[15]

Once the mother is transferred from the recovery room to her floor she may feel she is in a surrealistic world. Strange catheters and tubes greet her. Her body does not respond as she expects. Although she knows she has given birth, it may seem unreal. It may be difficult for her to divert her energies to ask of anything more than the sex of the baby. Usually when the mother is ready for active involvement with her infant, she begins to ask about its condition, appearance, and when she might see it.[15]

Non–life threatening complications, such as a fourth degree perineal tear or an elective cesarean section, may have as much or even more impact on the newly delivered mother. Possible explanations may be that the woman whose life was previously endangered is grateful just to be alive or has less available energy to focus on the event.[15]

Mothers sustaining injury during delivery, may have more difficulty interacting positively with their newborns. Some mothers express anger and resentment toward their baby for having been the cause of a complicated delivery or the resulting scar. Pain and potential hemorrhage usually delay the contact between mother and infant past the optimal period for bonding. Also, the measurably lower behavioral and sucking responses that occur when an infant is delivered by cesarean section make it difficult for the mother to feel successful in early mothering tasks.

Premature labor and delivery pose a different set of problems for the mother. The beginning of labor is often an event for which the family is unprepared. The trip to the hospital is disorganized and stressful. At the time of delivery all attention is focused on the infant, who may immediately be hastened to the intensive care unit before the mother can catch a glimpse of it. The mother, in the bustle, is seldom given enough time to ask questions or receive information. If the father is not in the delivery room the mother may be totally without immediate support, and unless there is good communication he will be left to wonder about the outcome of the delivery. Parents frequently respond to a premature delivery with anticipatory grief and gradually withdraw from the relationship already established with the child during the pregnancy.

If the child is born either prematurely or with some type of anomaly, the family will need to grieve for the normal child they were expecting before they can begin to relate to the child they have. The family's grief may be particularly severe if there was little or no advanced warning of this outcome or if they continued to deny there was ever a risk situation. When the child is stillborn or dies shortly after birth, all the hopes, dreams, and fantasies the family had for the child must be buried with it. A long exhausting grief process begins.

Among parents experiencing an abnormal labor, delivery, or neonate, the most common feelings engendered are of shame and failure. There is a deep sense of inadequacy expressed by some women who fail to deliver normally. This lowers self-esteem and may produce a sense of shame. Parents often feel they are not like others, and sometimes this creates a sense of loneliness. If there is permanent disfigurement, such as a scar, or loss, as occurs with hysterectomy, the woman must resolve her feelings toward her changed body image and functioning.

Though maternal death or disability resulting from childbirth is rare, it must be mentioned. Either death or disability of the mother completely disrupts the family structure and often leaves the father in a position of primary care giver for the infant and his other children. This comes at a time when his emotional reserves are the lowest. Both he and his family may deem him responsible for his wife's death or disability. The expenses from the medical treatment, burial, and absenteeism from work will add to the family's stress.

NURSING CARE

Nursing care during the labor, delivery, and early postpartum periods can profoundly influence the family's coping abilities. The most important step the nurse can take in the early postpartal period is to insure an adequate flow of information between medical/nursing staff and the woman's family. If the family is to function supportively during this critical period they must be included as a part of the patient's total care.

The woman who has just endured surgery will need reassurance that she is still intact and will recover. A mother often experiences a loss of self-esteem stemming from her inability to control her body functions. During this period it is particularly important to be sensitive to her bodily needs and concerns. When others respond to her personal needs and hygiene it contributes to her own feelings of self-worth. Setting small attainable goals helps the woman to increase her sense of progress and mastery. A nonthreatening and nonjudgmental atmosphere will help decrease stress.

The new mother needs time to sort through her labor and delivery experiences. She should be questioned as to her perceptions and ideas regarding the circumstances of her abnormal delivery. This provides the nurse with an opportunity to clarify misconceptions and uncover feelings of guilt the woman may be struggling with.

It is important to assure the mother that her infant is receiving good care. Early mother-infant contact is imperative. Even if the mother is not feeling ready to interact, a few brief moments of visual contact are advantageous. This helps to establish the reality of the infant for the mother and may help her readjust some of the fantasies she has had about the outcome of her delivery. When contact cannot be established within the first day or so, a photograph of the infant can prove most beneficial.

After a high risk pregnancy, even of the baby is normal, the family may have countless questions and require extra support to believe the infant will survive. The parents generally need about a week to fully realize they do indeed have a normal, healthy newborn.

Nursing care during the postpartal period should include a continuing assessment of the parents' reaction to the baby. Typically there is a "maternal lag" period, the length varying with the mother's physical condition, but following this, increasing eye and body contact between parent and child is indicative of normal bonding. Some signs that bonding might not be occurring are: (1) The mother cannot describe any distinguishing physical or behavioral characteristics of her offspring; (2) she attributes grossly inappropriate characteristics to it ("the baby's so mean and stubborn, just like my father"); or (3) the mother cannot endow it with an infant status ("the baby looks so intelligent, I just know it's going places").[3] It is dangerous to make an assessment on just one interaction, but one should note the pattern of interactions over time.

If there is a complication with the infant, the sooner the family is presented with the facts, the better able they are to deal with the implications. When there is a deformity the parents should be encouraged to see the baby together as soon as possible, but they need not be forced to interact. Nurses who care for the baby should first become comfortable viewing and handling the deformity themselves before presenting the infant to the family. They should be prepared to point out the normal qualities as well as the abnormalities. When it is possible a rooming-in situation may expedite a mother's acceptance of her child. However, she must not be expected to handle more than she is ready to deal with and should have the option of returning the infant to the nursery should she become overwhelmed. The nurse can be instrumental in helping the mother express her grief over her lost "perfect" child. Gradually, contact with the child should increase.

If the anomaly is reparable, plans for this along with possible outcomes must be presented. All significant family members should be included in this review, both for mutual support and to facilitate their processing of the information. Genetic counseling may be advised, and the parents' blame and guilt must be dealt with.

When the baby is premature and in danger of dying, parents and family must be allowed to retain their hope. They should be encouraged to interact and bond with the infant. This often helps in the grieving process and is undoubtedly beneficial should the baby live. Again, they need an understanding, compassionate nurse to help them deal with their guilt and grief.

When a stillbirth occurs or a nonviable premature infant is born the nurse is often faced with the family's shock and disbelief. There are several steps that can be taken to ease the family's immediate horror and help them mobilize their strengths. One of the most important measures is to physically bring the family together and offer them privacy. They should be given the option of seeing and holding their infant. A photograph can be taken and footprints made as articles of remembrance for the family. If they do not wish to view the baby at the time of death they should be encouraged to reconsider. Often their fantasies can be worse than reality. Parents do change their minds, and until the baby is buried they should have the opportunity to see it. At some hospitals, infants can be retrieved from the morgue, wrapped in a blanket, and shown to the parents in a private room. They are offered the opportunity to hold the baby but cautioned that it will feel cold. It is interesting to note that parents usually remember positive aspects of the baby even if the infant is previable or deformed. Frequently they will point out some familial characteristic or emphasize the baby's normal features.

The nurse can offer emotional support through touching and listening. Like everyone else, nurses often feel awkward when dealing with grief and so simply avoid interacting. Sometimes the nurse's presence is all that is required to reduce the isolation and loneliness the bereaved often feel. Table 7–5 offers some suggestions for those caring for parents who have lost a baby.

The issues arising from a high risk pregnancy or delivery are not resolved when the pregnancy terminates. Therefore the first postnatal visit should include a searching interview to provide an opportunity for parents to settle any "unfinished business." The use of monitors, special medication, or any manipulative procedures often leaves the parents with questions regarding the mother's or the baby's condition. Even if adequate explanations were given in the hospital, stress often distorts their understanding. Interactions with their newborn or their grieving status should also be assessed during this visit. Sufficient time must be allotted to answer questions and listen to concerns.

TABLE 7-5. SUGGESTIONS FOR THOSE CARING FOR PARENTS WHOSE BABY HAS DIED

Encourage them to name the baby.

Give parents the crib card with weight, length, date and time of birth, the I.D. bands, copy of the footprint sheet. Encourage them to send for a copy of the birth certificate.

Honor their request (or offer) to take a picture of the baby.

Encourage both parents to become involved in the burial plans and discussion of the autopsy.

Help parents obtain the information they need, as genetic follow-up. Put them in touch with parent groups formed to share the feelings from a newborn loss.

Provide, if possible, the opportunity for the grieving parents to be together day and night.

Talk about the loss. If parents cry it is not because you made them cry, but because you let them cry.

Include family members, especially grandparents, in the discussion of loss. Let them view and hold the stillborn or infant who dies.

Encourage parents to think about and rehearse how they will share the news with their other children.

Let them know that they might anticipate the resurgence of grief at holiday times and on anniversaries of the baby's birth and death.

Prepare them for things others may unwittingly say, such as:
"Dispose of remains"
"You can have others."
"Was for the best"
"Would have been abnormal anyway"
"Forget about it."

Things to say that may help:
"I'm sorry."
"I know this is a bad time for you."
"Is there anything I can do for you?"
"Is there anyone I can call for you?"

_____ POSTPARTAL CRISIS: THE BABY IN INTENSIVE CARE _____

For some a high risk pregnancy or delivery results in a baby requiring intensive care. Both the environment and what it represents can make the newborn intensive care unit an extremely stressful place. At this point, not only do the parents and family respond to the stress but the infant must be considered as well.

Understandably, little is written about stress from the infant's perspective, but as can be seen by its responses to manipulation and painful procedures, it too is a victim of stress. Birth itself is undoubtedly a stressful event for the neonate, and if labor is long or the passage is difficult the infant can require a prolonged period of recovery. Birth trauma, infection, prematurity, and major congenital anomalies are probably the four broad categories of stressors primarily responsible for an infant's intensive care needs.

In addition to the stress of illness the infant in the neonatal intensive care unit (NICU) is subjected to a number of external stresses, some of them avoidable. Consider the environment: Care is being administered constantly, disturbing the infant's sleep cycle, and needles and wires interfere with comfort and movement. It is bombarded by stimuli. It hears the beeps of the heart monitor and the rush of air and extremely high noise levels under the oxygen hood. The noise levels under an oxygen hood are sufficient to place the baby at risk for later hearing and language impairments.[7] The sudden snapping of the Isolette's portholes as they are closed produces an obvious startle reflex. In addition, overhead fluorescent lights are kept on without variation, interfering with normal circadian rhythms. The oxygen hoods and Isolettes produce visual distortions. Through their plastic angles the adult can have two noses and four eyes. The baby cannot see through misted plastic and cannot bring hands to mouth for exploration and self-comfort. This is the beginning of self-image, and it is distorted.[7]

There are minimal opportunities for human contact in the nursery. When mothering attention is provided it is inconsistent and is often shared by several nurses. Thus, because of the environment in the NICU, the infant is deprived of essential mothering as a result of both physical barriers and inconsistent comforting and care giving measures. Because this is a period in which trust should be established between a mother and infant, there could be far reaching effects on the child's later psychological development.

NURSING CARE

Reducing infant stress in the ICU requires, first, recognition of those events that are stressful and, second, a great deal of ingenuity. Unless the parents are consistently available to the infant a primary nurse is essential for consistent care giving. By having needs met by a caring person, the infant learns to trust. Settings are needed that support intimacy and human tactile, auditory, and visual contact.

Lifting and moving the baby provides visceral and kinesthetic stimulation, and even slight head movement can significantly alter incoming stimuli. Even the most impaired, sick, or unresponsive baby is not unreceptive in terms of sensory-motor experience. Devices have been design to synchronize rocking with the sound of the mother's heartbeat.[7] This has a calming effect on infants. Music seems to sooth infants as well.[13]

The nurse should organize her tasks to minimize interruption of the baby's sleep. All the procedures should be done at one time if possible. If the unit lights must be kept on 24 hours, blankets draped over the tops of Isolettes can produce a darkened effect for the infant without impairing the nurse's vision.

Though nurses are rarely involved in designing the NICU equipment, they are the best observers of the effects it has upon the newborn. NICUs are relatively new, and equipment is still being developed. It is the care providers who specify the technical tools they need. Therefore health professionals must gain environmental awareness to modify and minimize the equipment's adverse effects.

NEWBORN INTENSIVE CARE: THE IMPACT ON THE FAMILY

For parents having endured a high risk pregnancy, the admission of the baby to the NICU has probably confirmed their worst fears and has relentlessly extended their stress. For others, the situation may have come as an unexpected shock, having the power to disrupt their lives. These parents are under extreme degrees of stress, guilt, and frustration. Total care of the high risk neonate must include care of the parents, as they will be the ultimate care givers.

Many of the stresses families face when their infant is premature, ill, or deformed have previously been mentioned. When infant care becomes long term, the problems can mount, and new stresses can surface.

The uncertainty of whether the infant will live or die can be excruciating. Searching for reasons for the illness or prematurity can increase family tension. Guilt, blame, and anger can disrupt the household. The parents may argue or in-laws can criticize. Often the young children at home feel they are the cause of the unhappiness, and little time is afforded them for reassurance.

Separation may become unbearable for the parents. Anxiety increases from secondhand reports and fantasies. They may begin to spend an exhausting amount of time in the unit. Conversely, one frequently encounters the mother or father who, after going to the NICU to see the infant for the first time, makes many excuses not to go again. The sensory overload may be intolerable at certain peaks of stress. Or, if the baby's death seems inevitable, the parents may refuse to risk emotional involvement.

Traveling to and from the nursery becomes both disruptive to the family's routine and exhausting for the parents. Other children may feel they are not getting the attention they deserve and become management problems. Mounting hospital bills add to the strain.

Parents can have very disturbing, ambivalent feelings toward their sick infant. Some parents may express a wish for the baby to die quickly and thus end their anguish. Anger toward the infant is usually directed elsewhere, perhaps to family or staff, because it is felt to be unacceptable. Occasionally, however, these thoughts do surface, and parents need reassurance that they are normal reactions to the stress they are experiencing.

One of the best indicators of the parents' progress is their visiting pattern; their length of stay, their actions and comments during the visit, and their increasing skill in handling the infant. It is of concern when they seem overly optimistic, appear unconcerned about their baby's clinical state, or do not ask questions. The parents who have grappled with the problems seem to adjust better once they take the infant home.[10]

NURSING CARE FOR PARENTS WITH AN INFANT IN NICU

If it is known prior to delivery that a high risk situation exists, it is beneficial in many instances for the parents to meet with the neonatal staff before delivery. If the parents desire they may be invited to the high risk nursery to see the facilities and the care the babies receive. This affords them an opportunity to ask questions and share their fears with professional staff.

In most cases the initial communication with the parents begins shortly after delivery. At this time they need to be given an assessment of the infant's status and a brief description of the therapeutic steps that are being taken. Once the infant's condition is stabilized the father, or perhaps another significant support person for the mother, should be brought into the nursery to see and touch the infant. Both the normal and abnormal signs should be pointed out, and simple description should be given of the tubes and wires surrounding the infant. The neonatologist or primary nurse should then accompany the father (or other support person) to the recovery room where the situation is reviewed for the mother. If a photograph of the infant can be taken it becomes an invaluable tool when describing its size and equipment to the mother. It also serves as a meaningful token or her child's existence while she is confined to her room.

Questions should be answered as honestly and optimistically as is realistic. What parents hear or read into statements during these first critical hours leaves a long lasting impression, and so phrases like "possible brain damage" and "retardation" should not be spoken unless there is absolute certainty.[10]

A nursery information sheet that lists the phone number and visiting hours is helpful. It can also encourage parents to take part in their baby's care. Suggestions for them to bring camera and booties to the nursery may help them begin to assume other parenting behaviors as well.

When the newborn begins to slowly improve, parents should still be spoken to with caution, but with increasing optimism. It helps if one person is consistently assigned to reviewing information with the parents to avoid conflicting reports. The little "graduations" the infant makes (e.g., from warmer to Isolette, or from milk drip to bolus feeds) should be pointed out. Parents should be encouraged to take an increasing role in caring for their infant. It may involve no more than laying a clean diaper under the baby's bottom, but this can be a very significant step for the parents.

When death seems inevitable, parents, grandparents, and other significant family members should be encouraged to spend more time in the nursery. It helps if the family witnesses the care the baby is receiving so they can see that everything possible is being done. If no further measures will be taken the nurse can help the parents make the baby as comfortable as possible. Occasionally parents will ask to hold their dying infant and often, with rearrangement of respirator tubing and intravenous lines, this is possible. Parents need repeated reassurance that they are not at fault. Pointing out how caring and loving they have been to the baby, and how this must have contributed to its comfort, is often helpful in boosting the parents' self-esteem.

After the baby dies, parents need to be told that personnel of the high risk nursery are available for discussion at any time in the future. If the hospital has a grief counselor an appointment can be made for them. Many large cities have parent-run organizations for families experiencing a neonatal death, and parents can be referred to this group. It is important to let them know that they are not alone.

Some babies in the ICU seem neither to improve nor die. The challenge for NICU nurses is to cope with the parents' frustrations as well as their own. Alternating improvement and setbacks can keep the family constantly on edge. They may dread the ring of the telephone. If parents are not able to visit as frequently as they would like because of other children or distance, they should be encouraged to call as often as once a nursing shift if they desire. Often an expected daily phone call from a primary nurse becomes very comforting for a mother. With adequate preparation, some nurseries will allow an occasional visit by siblings, and this is a means of helping the entire family become more involved with the new infant. Parents can endure the hardship and tragedy more easily when they feel others care.

A counseling or a social service referral can help the family deal with secondary problems the crisis has caused. Individual or marital counseling is generally available in the community. Often there are support groups for parents of children born prematurely or with congenital defects. Social workers may be able to help families find resources for their financial needs and involve the parents in future planning for their infant's care.

When an infant in the ICU is finally discharged from the hospital the family may experience yet another crisis or period of disorganization. Taking the infant from a highly skilled staff and a monitored environment to home may be overwhelming, and so a gradual transition is necessary. The infant's discharge should be planned throughout the hospital course. Special procedures can be taught well in advance of discharge and practiced frequently in the unit.

Praise for their increasing skill gives parents the confidence they need to continue to learn about their infant. Some hospitals provide rooming-in for parents for 24 to 48 hours prior to their infant's release. The high risk nursery staff can reassure the parents that they are only a phone call away.

NURSING STRESS

Thus far, only the stresses confronting the parents and infants have been presented. Nurses working in these situations are prone to all the same stress responses as families. It can be assumed that poor management of stress results in poor nursing care, job dissatisfaction, and a lower potential for professional development.

Constant demands are being made upon nurses working in intensive care settings. The constant vigilance, monitors, repetitive exposure to suffering and death, and unique communication problems make the units high risk areas for staff. In addition to the stimulus overload, the nurse must face the typical nursing stresses as well: rotating shifts, understaffing, and standing on the feet most of the day. It is no wonder the nurse turnover in intensive care units is high.

Many staff members have become so accustomed to the environment in which they work that they have reduced ability to recognize the stresses. The stresses in an NICU are similar in many ways to those in other ICUs, but the NICU also has its own unique problems. Physically the unit is often small and crowded with bulky machinery. Monitors alarm, blue bilirubin lights can be annoying to work under, and space per patient is often minimal as a result of the typically high census. The units are designed for optimal communication, leaving no opportunity for a quiet moment. Working in an environment in which one can be constantly observed can produce a subtle but persistent feeling of anxiety.

High census and the frequency and uncertainty of admissions add to anxieties. The sudden death or relapse of a baby who was improving produces a large amount of stress and guilt in the nurse. Sick babies are seldom responsive enough to give nurses the positive rewards they need. When babies do finally become well enough to relate and be cute, they are transferred to an intermediate care nursery. Often their emotionally drained families are not capable of giving the nurses the positive reinforcement they need either.

The infants' families can be another source of stress for the NICU nurses. Often they demand much of the nurses' time by asking the same questions repeatedly. Nurses may be unable to help parents cope with their pain and grief when they perceive them as the source of the baby's illness (e.g., drug addicted infants). Sometimes a subtle rivalry between a nurse and mother is established over the care of the infant.

Nurse-physician relationships are often strained. In many places, pediatric residents rotate through, creating inconsistencies each time a new group begins. In some cases, because they lack experience in such settings, they are insecure and their anxiety permeates the already stressed NICU environment. Because of the number of physicians, ambiguous or conflicting orders and directions can be given. Nurses often complain that physicians ignore their observations or encroach on their jurisdiction. Sometimes the reverse is true, that is, physicians may try to shift their responsibility onto nurses.[6]

Nurses may identify problems with other nurses as well. As with many high pressure jobs, there are peer conflicts and territorial disputes. Many nursing administrators gained their experience before the inception of NICUs and often fail to recognize the unique characteristics and needs of such units.

Bureaucratic-political problems also arise. Nurses may feel defenseless when they have no control over the type or number of patients transported into the unit. Anger may arise when a long term patient is transferred elsewhere because of termination of insurance benefits. Often nurses feel that

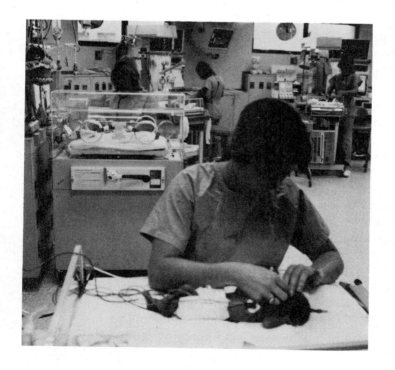

Figure 7-1. The unique characteristics of high risk units must be addressed to alleviate stress producing situations for the nursing staff. (Courtesy of Hermann Hospital, Houston, Texas.)

they do not get the recognition and prestige they deserve within the institution.

Finally, many personal conflicts face the NICU nurse. Because neonatology is a new field the procedures and techniques are constantly changing. Nurses, especially new graduates, sometimes become insecure about their knowledge and competence. Because NICU nurses are difficult to replace on short notice there are feelings of guilt when a personal or family illness forces a nurse to take sick time. The pressure is then on the other nurses to work overtime, causing the individual conflict between helping out on the unit or caring for responsibilities at home.

Ethical-philosophical issues confront the nurse. Who shall be resuscitated and when care shall be terminated are questions each nurse must grapple with. Also, they face the conflict of whether advances in medical science are being made in the interest of or at the expense of human life.

CARE FOR NURSES AT RISK

To retain nurses and a high standard of care in the NICU, administrative and peer support is essential. The majority of stresses cited by nurses in the NICU are psychosocial in nature, indicating where the support is needed most.[6]

Individually, nurses can utilize strategies to reduce their work related tension after hours. A "decompression routine" splits the day into a very distinctive work component and after-work component. Jogging, walking, listening to music, or taking personal time to include an enjoyable routine after work helps the nurse become emotionally distanced from the unit. Days off and vacation time are necessary and should be considered sacred. Nurses must define the boundaries of their own limitations.

Organizational strategies to reduce nurse burnout can be employed. A structured orientation for both nurses and house staff should prepare the staff for the technical and emotional demands if NICU work.[14] Ongoing education to share new information and refresh old skills is important. Either a nurse-educator or a staff nurse given research time off the unit could present relevant topics. Unit policies are necessary to add structure but should be flexible enough to be revised when situations warrant. Staff nurses need to have some involvement in writing the policies. Levels of practice may be a means of giving NICU nurses the recognition they deserve for their added knowledge and expertise.

A support system is perhaps central to the reduction and prevention of burnout among nurses. Interdisciplinary sharing should occur regularly to reduce the "them-against-us" attitude that often arises between nurses and physicians. Nursing support from peers is perhaps the most crucial factor in maintaining staff morale. Group meetings with a well liked and respected outside facilitator have proven effective in some units. Often this helps nurses realize they are not alone in their stress and feelings.

Staffing needs to be adequate enough to allow nurses an occasional mental health day or library day or to make a home visit to a discharged baby. Though rotating to well baby units does not seem to be the solution to giving nurses a break from their routine,[14] perhaps they can develop exchange programs with other hospitals' NICUs or rotate to a position of parent care coordinator, orientation nurse, or in-service instructor to other nurseries, for a month at a time.

Cooperation and creativity are the key elements to an effectively run and supportive NICU atmosphere. If nurses unite and derive support from each other they can then tackle the other problems that plague them daily.

CONCLUSIONS

Any stress occurring during the course of a pregnancy, delivery, or neonatal period has been observed to alter the woman's perception of her infant as a whole and rewarding child to care for.[15] Studies of abused children or those who have suffered failure to thrive syndrome have revealed antecedent factors that may help to identify parents at risk. These factors include profound emotional and physical deprivation of parents, premature birth, birth by cesarean section, and illness during the newborn period.[15] Studies also show that these infants have a grave impact on their family structure. Thirty per cent of the mothers of premature infants were separated from their husbands within 6 months after the mother left the hospital.[15] Neonatal death or deformity can affect the family similarly.

Pregnancy and the early period of parenting are a time for screening and for therapeutic intervention for parents at risk. The nurse's contact with parents during the perinatal period is usually more intimate and more intense than it has been previously or will be again. Nurses are in a position to monitor and intervene in the functioning of the family unit and to help promote and facilitate bonding and early parent-infant interactions. They can challenge and change archaic hospital rules that may interfere with early positive experiences. Early positive experiences lead to attachment, which sets a pattern for lifelong behaviors.

The responses to stress and crisis events are as varied as people. Outcomes depend upon both internal and external resources the individual or family possesses. Following are some possible outcomes of stress and crisis in the perinatal setting.

Family: care givers versus abusers; family harmony and growth versus divorce and resentment

Infant: no learning delay versus handicap; positive interactions, alertness to people and environment versus mental illness

Staff: growth versus burnout

Stress reduction and crisis intervention are important factors in health promotion and prevention, and in individual growth.

REFERENCES

1. Aguilera, D., and Messick, J.: Crisis Intervention, Theory and Methodology. St. Louis, C. V. Mosby Co., 1974.
2. Caplan, G.: Principles in Preventive Psychiatry. New York, Basic Books, 1964, pp. 53-54.

3. Cohen, R.: Maladaptation to pregnancy. *In* Taylor, P. (ed.): Parent-Infant Relationships. New York, Grune & Stratton, 1980, pp. 49–67.

4. Davids, A., and DeVault, S.: Maternal anxiety during pregnancy and childbirth abnormalities. Psychosom. Med., *24*:464–469, 1962.

5. Grimm, E., and Venet, W.: The relationship of emotional adjustment and attitudes to the course and outcome of pregnancy. Psychosom. Med., *28*:34–49, 1966.

6. Jacobson, S.: Stressful situations for neonatal intensive care nurses. Matern. Child Nurs. J., *3*:144–150, 1978.

7. Jones, C.: Criteria for evaluating infant environments in hospitals. J. Assoc. Care Child. Hosp., *7*:3–11, 1979.

8. Jones, M.: The high-risk pregnancy. *In* Johnson, S.H. (ed.): High Risk Parenting. Philadelphia, J.B. Lippincott Co., 1979, pp. 81–93.

9. Kirgis, C., Woolsey, D., and Sullivan, J.: Predicting infant Apgar scores. Nurs. Res., *26*:439–442, 1977.

10. Klaus, M.: Caring for parents. Perinat. Care, *2*:28–30, 1978.

11. Klaus, M., and Kennell, J.: Maternal-Infant Bonding. St. Louis, C.V. Mosby Co., 1976, p. 46.

12. LeMasters, E.E.: Parenthood as crisis. *In* Parad, H. (ed.): Crisis Intervention: Selected Readings. New York, Family Service Association of America, 1965, pp. 111–117.

13. Lindsay, K.: The value of music for hospitalized infants. J. Assoc. Care Child. Health, *9*:104–107, 1981.

14. Marshall, R., and Kasman, C.: Burnout in the neonatal intensive care unit. Pediatrics, *65*:1161–1165, 1980.

15. Mercer, R.: Nursing Care for Parents at Risk. Thorofare, N.J., Charles B. Slack, 1977, pp. 6, 77–99, 108–111.

16. Nuckolls, K., Cassel, J., and Kaplan, B.: Psychosocial assets, life crisis and the prognosis of pregnancy. *In* Schwartz, J. and Schwartz, L. (eds.): Vulnerable Infants, a Psychosocial Dilemma. New York, McGraw-Hill Book Co., 1977, pp. 62–75.

17. Osofsky, H., and Osofsky, J.: Normal Adaptation to pregnancy and new parenthood. *In* Taylor, P. (ed.): Parent-Infant Relationships. New York, Grune & Stratton, 1980, pp. 38–45.

18. Rapoport, R.: Normal crises, family structure and mental health. *In* Parad, H. (ed.): Crisis Intervention: Selected Readings. New York, Family Service Association of America, 1965, pp. 75–87.

19. Schwartz, J.: A study of the relationship between maternal life change events and premature delivery. *In* Schwartz, J. and Schwartz, L. (eds.): Vulnerable Infants, a Psychosocial Dilemma. New York, McGraw-Hill Book Co., 1977, pp. 47–61.

20. Sedgwick, R.: Psychological responses to stress. J. Psychiatr. Nurs., *13*:20–23, 1975.

MATERNAL/FETAL HIGH RISK CARE

CHAPTER 8

ASSESSMENT AND CLASSIFICATION OF THE HIGH RISK MATERNAL-FETAL UNIT

Elissa A. Emerson, M.S., C.F.N.P.

OBJECTIVES

Upon completion of this chapter the reader will be able to accomplish the following:

1. Identify the major causes of maternal risk of morbidity and morality throughout the period of pregnancy and early parenthood
2. Identify major causes of fetal-neonatal risk for morbidity and mortality throughout the perinatal cycle
3. Identify ways to assess risk on initial examination and prenatally, intrapartally, and postpartally
4. Identify the predisposing factors to the major identified risks
5. Identify by signs and symptoms the indicators of the major risk factors in the perinatal cycle
6. Identify tools for assessing risk

A high risk pregnancy is one in which there is increased probability of maternal or perinatal damage or death. Research and experience have permitted identification of characteristics that historically threaten maternal and fetal welfare. Thus half of the pregnancies at risk are identifiable prior to or soon after conception.

Maternal mortality decreased from 660 per 100,000 to 27 per 100,000 births between 1930 and 1971, and fetal mortality decreased comparatively. Thus, use of modern diagnostic measures is increasing the number of preventive and therapeutic successes in reducing morbidity, disability, and death of the mother or fetus before, during, or within 28 days after birth.

The nurse who is aware of deviations from normal and who may be the first or most frequent contact person with the maternal/fetal unit at risk is often the person who identifies and reports potential problems. Nurses and physicians are additionally in a position to educate about life style changes that can minimize risk.

Prenatal care is necessary for assessment and treatment of disorders that jeopardize maternal/fetal well-being. Attention to several major components or intervals in the pregnancy process allows complete identification of the numerous potential risks. This is also true in the intrapartum and postpartum periods. This chapter provides an outline of necessary assessment information in each part of the maternity cycle. It will allow nurses who follow these guidelines an opportunity to identify risk and maximize perinatal outcome.

IDENTIFYING THE WOMAN AT RISK

Twenty to thirty per cent of women account for 50 to 60 per cent of problem pregnancies. Numerous sources identify the following categories, first identified by Wigglesworth[6], as prominently associated with the high risk obstetrical course.

HISTORY

1. Hereditary abnormality (Down's syndrome, osteogenesis imperfecta)
2. Premature or small for dates infant (most recent pregnancy)
3. Congenital anomaly, anemia, blood dyscrasia, preeclampsia-eclampsia
4. Severe social problems (teen pregnancy, drug addiction)
5. Long delayed or no prenatal care

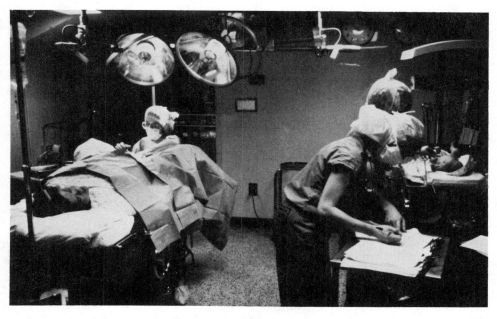

Figure 8-1. Assessment of mother and baby at all times in the perinatal period is essential in identifying risk. (Courtesy of Don Shaeffer, Hermann Hospital, Houston, Texas.)

6. Age under 18 or over 35 years
7. Teratogenic viral illness or use of dangerous drug in the first trimester of pregnancy
8. Fifth or greater pregnancy, especially after age 35 years
9. Prolonged infertility or essential drug or hormone treatment
10. Significant stressful or dangerous event this pregnancy
11. Heavy cigarette smoking
12. Pregnancy within 2 to 3 months of a previous delivery

DIAGNOSIS

1. Height under 60 in. or prepregnant weight 20 per cent over or under standard for age and height
2. Minimal or no weight gain
3. Obstetrical complications (preeclampsia-eclampsia, multiple pregnancy, hydramnios)
4. Abnormal presentation (breech, nonengagement)
5. Fetal failure to grow or disparity between size and length of gestation
6. More than 42 weeks' gestation

IDENTIFYING THE FETUS AT RISK

OBSTETRICAL CONDITIONS

Most perinatal deaths are associated with six obstetrical conditions:

1. Premature separation of placenta
2. Pyelonephritis
3. Preeclampsia-eclampsia
4. Multiple pregnancy
5. Breech presentation
6. Hydramnios

ADDITIONAL HAZARDS

1. Harmful drugs
2. Viral infections
3. Radiation
4. High altitude
5. Personal and social problems (lack of knowledge; poverty)
6. Anesthesia (especially in university medical centers)

FETAL FACTORS

1. Congenital anomalies
2. Short cord (asphyxia)
3. Cord entanglement or compression (asphyxia)
4. Abnormal presentation (trauma, asphyxia)
5. Hydramnios (associated with fetal inability to swallow)
6. Immaturity (in low birth weight infants, mortality is 40 times more

frequent than in term infants; cerebral palsy is 10 times more frequent; malformations, 7 times; and there is 5 times the average occurrence of mental deficiency, visual and hearing problems, and social and emotional disorders)

7. Prematurity (respiratory distress syndrome [RDS], sepsis, intracranial hemorrhage)
8. Fetal infection

NEONATAL FACTORS

These factors, identified during labor and immediately after birth, demonstrate increased risk to the infant and require special treatment.

1. **In the Mother**
   a. Abnormal delivery
   b. Prolonged, difficult labor
   c. Precipitous delivery
   d. Premature labor
   e. Prolonged rupture of membranes (ROM)

2. **Preterm birth (less than 37 weeks)**
   a. Respiratory distress syndrome
   b. Intracranial hemorrhage
   c. Sepsis
   d. Hypoxia-asphyxia (fetal distress)

3. **Birth hypoxia**
   a. Fetal heart rate fluctuations
   b. Meconium staining, aspiration
   c. Fetal acidosis (pH less than 7.2)
   d. Apgar scores less than 7, especially at 5 minutes

4. **Post-term birth (more than 42 weeks), especially with wasting**
   a. At highest risk
      i. Aged primipara
      ii. Preeclamptic-eclamptic patient
      iii. Fetal distress (meconium staining on amniocentesis)
      iv. Urinary tract infection
   b. Dangers
      i. Prolonged labor with cephalopelvic disproportion
      ii. Fetal asphyxia
      iii. Undiagnosed stillbirth

5. **In the fetus or neonate**
   a. Small for dates infant (less than fifth percentile)
   b. Large for dates infants (greater than ninety-fifth percentile)
   c. Any respiratory distress or apnea
   d. Obvious congenital anomalies
   e. Convulsions, limpness, difficulty in sucking or swallowing
   f. Distention or vomiting
   g. Anemia or bleeding tendency
   h. Jaundice with bilirubin greater than 15 mg/100 ml in first 24 hours

Risk may be assigned by biological system and anatomical problem, by signs and symptoms, by history, or by psychosocial danger. The outline of components in the assessment of the maternal-fetal unit delineates "high" and "moderate" risk according to (1) maternal risk and (2) additional relative danger to the fetus.

_____ ASSESSMENT _____

What enters into assessment of the perinatal patient at risk?

1. Initial assessment
    a. Demographical and biological history
    b. Medical history
    c. Reproductive history
    d. Emotional history
    e. Psychosocial examination
    f. Laboratory tests
    g. Initial physical examination

2. Predisposing factors
3. Risk listing by common time interval
4. Antepartal assessment
5. Intrapartal assessment
6. Postpartal assessment
    a. Maternal
    b. Fetal

7. Acute signs and symptoms

_____ ASSESSMENT OUTLINE _____

INITIAL WORK-UP

1. Demographical and biological maternal history
    a. Age
        *i. Less than 15 years (physical and emotional strain)
        *ii. More than 35 years (established biological complications, fatigue)
        iii. Adolescent (15–19 years)
        iv. Maternal age 30–34 years
    b. Weight and size
        i.   Less than 100 pounds
        ii. More than 200 pounds
        iii. Less than 60 in. tall
        iv. More than 20 per cent above or below standard
    c. Race
        i.   Nonwhite
        ii. Social and economic factors that deny optimal reproductive care and performance

    d. Marital status/Living situation
        i. Single
        ii. Without family support
    e. Educational/Occupation
        i. Less than eighth grade
        ii. Unemployed, poverty
    f. Parity
        i. Primigravida (toxemia, dystocia)
        ii. Multiple pregnancy (50 per cent premature deliveries)
        iii. More than 5 pregnancies (rupture of uterus, postpartum atony)
    g. Heavy smoker (anomalies, fetal growth retardation)
   *h. Alcohol or narcotic drug abuse
    i. Venereal disease
    j. Stress

2. Medical History
    a. Inherited disease
    b. Rh negative
    c. Chronic disease, moderate to severe
      *i. Diabetes mellitus, classes B to F
      ii. Diabetes mellitus, class A
    *iii. Renal disease
    *iv. Recurrent urinary tract infections
     *v. Cardiopulmonary disease, cardiovascular accident
    *vi. Hypertension
    vii. Thyroid disease
    viii. Gastrointestinal, liver disease
     ix. Epilepsy, tuberculosis
    d. Rubella
    e. Ulcerative or regional colitis
    f. Poor nutritional status
   *g. Sickle cell disease
    h. Sickle cell trait
   *i. Malignant disease
   *j. Abnormal Papanicolaou smear

3. Obstetrical and Reproductive History
   *a. Two or more previous premature infants
    b. One previous premature infant (7 to 8 per cent of births)
    c. Infant with respiratory distress syndrome
   *d. Diabetes mellitus, classes B to F
    e. Diabetes mellitus, class A
   *f. Two or more fetal losses after 20 weeks
    g. Previous fetal death
    h. Cesarean or difficult delivery
   *i. Previous Rh isoimmunization

---

*High risk (others moderate)

*j. Two or more previous abortions, spontaneous or induced
 k. One previous abortion
*l. Eclampsia
 m. Preeclampsia in two or more pregnancies
 n. Puerperal hemorrhage with transfusion
*o. Infant with anomalies, birth damage, or requiring intensive care
 p. Low birth weight infant (less than 2500 gm) (2 + = *)
 q. Excessive size infant (more than 4000 gm) (2 + = *)
 r. Multiple pregnancy
 s. Abnormal presentation
*t. Previous diagnosis of genital tract anomalies
    i.   Incompetent cervix
    ii. Cervical malformation
    iii. Uterine malformation
*u. Maternal cancer, leiomyomas, ovarian mass
 v. Borderline pelvis
 w. Primigravida
 x. Pregnancy less than 3 months after previous one

4. **Emotional History**
 a. Poor relationship with spouse or significant other
 b. History of inadequate problem solving capacity or coping
 c. Inadequate or no support system
 d. Poor past experience with professional help
 e. Multiple crises (prematurity, cesarean birth, increased risk of child abuse)
 f. Great situational stress
 g. Negative response to diagnosis

5. **Psychosocial Examination**
 a. Personal characteristics
    i.   Ambivalence or lability
    ii. Guilt
    iii. Low self-esteem
    iv. Emotional weariness
    v.   Negative perception of role change
    vi. Fears
        (a) Fetal death or abnormality
        (b) Multiple pregnancy
        (c) Personal danger
        (d) Body image changes
    vii. Inability to express needs
 b. Expected changes in focus
    i.   Self (in early pregnancy)
    ii. Baby (after fetal movement)
    iii. Delivery (final weeks prior to birth)

6. **Laboratory Tests**
 a. Papanicolaou (neoplasm, vaginal infection)
 b. Culture for gonorrhea

---

*High risk (others moderate).

    c. Venereal Disease Research Laboratory (VDRL [syphilis])
    d. Tine PPD (purified protein derivative of tuberculin [tuberculosis])
    e. Rubella titer (exposure in first trimester)
    f. Complete blood count (CBC)
       i. Hemoglobin, hematocrit (anemia)
      ii. White cell count; differential count (infection, virus)
    g. Blood glucose (diabetes mellitus)
    h. Sickledex (sickle cell disease or trait)
    i. Rh and screening for isoimmunization antibodies (erythroblastosis fetalis or neonatorum)
    j. Toxoplasmosis antibody titer
    k. Blood type (for cross matching and isoimmunization)
    l. Urinalysis
       i. Pregnancy confirmation
      ii. Microscopic (infection)
     iii. Glucose (diabetes mellitus, but will normally spill after meals during pregnancy because of tubule overload)
     iv. Acetone (diabetes mellitus, malnutrition)
      v. Protein (preeclampsia, renal dysfunction)
     vi. Culture and sensitivity on urine obtained by clean catch (diabetes, bacteriuria, renal, nutritional; greater than 10^5 reported)
    m. As needed
       i. Blood urea nitrogen (BUN [renal function])
      ii. Creatinine (renal function)
     iii. Sequential multiple analysis (SMA) 12 (liver, renal disease)
     iv. Triiodothyronine T3 (thyroxine T4 [thyroid function])
      v. Hormonal assessment (diabetes, hydatidiform mole)
     vi. Estriols (safety of continuing pregnancy)
     vii. Amniocentesis (direct assessment of fetal growth and well-being, especially with mother over 35 years or diabetic)
    viii. Oxytocin challenge test (OCT [assessment of fetal ability to withstand the stress of labor])
     ix. Placental scanning (for position)
      x. Ultrasonography, radiography (fetal maturity)

7. Initial physical examination
    a. Evidence of hypertension
    b. Circulatory disorder
    c. Cardiopulmonary insufficiency (CHF)
    d. Thyroid disorder
    e. Massive obesity
    f. Urinary tract infection, unresponsive
    g. Confirmation of pregnancy
       i. Nägele's rule (LNMP [last normal menstrual period] −3 months + 7 days)
      ii. Fundal height (FH)
     iii. McDonald's rule (FH x 8/7 = duration of pregnancy in weeks; FH x 2/7 = duration in lunar months)
     iv. Bimanual examination

TABLE 8-1. USING AN ANTEPARTUM RISK SCORING INDEX

Antepartum risk scoring index

Patient's name	Gestational date	Today's date

Value	Condition	Score
Cardiovascular Disorders		
10	Class I heart disease	( )
10	Severe heart disease, classes II–IV	( )
10	Chronic hypertension	( )
	History of preeclampsia	( )
	History of eclampsia	( )
5	Mild preeclampsia	( )
10	Moderate-severe preeclampsia	( )
Renal Disorders		
5	History of GU infection (including acute cystitis)	( )
10	Acute pyelonephritis	( )
10	Moderate-severe renal disease	( )
Metabolic Disorders		
	Family history of diabetes	( )
10	Diabetes: class A or > class A	( )
5	Thyroid disease	( )
	Previous endocrine ablation	( )
History		
10	Therapeutic abortion	( )
5	Habitual abortion	( )
10	Previous stillbirth	( )
10	Previous low birth weight infant	( )
10	Previous neonatal death	( )
10	Previous infant > 10 lb	( )
5	Previous cesarean section	( )
1	Rh negative, nonsensitized	( )
10	Rh negative, sensitized	( )
5	Multiparity > 5	( )
5	Epilepsy	( )
5	Previous fetal anomalies	( )
5	Drug allergy	( )

You often can more precisely measure the degree to which a patient's pregnancy is at risk if you use a risk scoring index rather than rely on clinical impression alone. An antepartum risk scoring index is particularly beneficial in planning appropriate care when tabulated during the first trimester and again early in the third trimester.

To use the index above, adapted from one used at the Cleveland Metropolitan General Hospital, note the value assigned in the extreme left hand column to each condition and enter it in the extreme right hand column as appropriate. The risk factors listed without specific values have not been statistically weighted. Check or leave them blank as appropriate. Consider your findings for these items as additional, though unweighted, risks when tabulating the total score.

TABLE 8-1.   USING AN ANTEPARTUM RISK SCORING INDEX *(Continued)*

Antepartum risk scoring index

Patient's name	Gestational date	Today's date

Value	Condition	Score
Anatomical Abnormalities		
10	Uterine malformation	( )
10	Incompetent cervix	( )
10	Abnormal fetal position	( )
10	Hydramnios	( )
5	Clinically small pelvis	( )
10	Multiple pregnancy	( )
10	Vaginal spotting	( )
Miscellaneous (this pregnancy)		
5	Age < 15	( )
5	Age > 35	( )
5	Weight < 100 lb	( )
5	Weight > 200 lb	( )
1	Mild anemia, 9.0–10.9 hemoglobin	( )
5	Severe anemia, < 9.0 hemoglobin	( )
10	Sickle cell disease or trait	( )
5	Rh sensitized, first time	( )
5	Positive serology	( )
5	Positive PPD	( )
	Viral disease	( )
5	Flu syndrome	( )
5	Vaginitis	( )
	Abnormal cervical cytology	( )
10	Pulmonary dysfunction	( )
10	Post-term (> 42 weeks)	( )
10	Intrauterine growth retardation	( )
	Emotional problems	( )
5	Smoking	( )
5	Alcohol abuse	( )
5	Excessive drug use, nonnarcotic	( )
10	Narcotic use	( )
	No-care patient (no previous medical care late in pregnancy)	( )
Total		

A score of 10 or more on this index indicates a patient is at high risk. However, in assessing your future course of action with each patient, look at absolute scores instead of just the designation of low or high risk. For example, the diabetic with no other problems rates 10 points and therefore is considered at high risk. On the other hand, the obese patient (5) who has a drinking problem (5) and is a heavy smoker (5) scores 15 points; she may be at still greater risk.

    h. Pelvimetry (for evidence of contracted pelvis)
    i. Measurement of uterus
        i. Overextension (hydramnios → postpartum atony → hemorrhage, hydatidiform mole, multiple gestation)
        ii. Insufficient growth (intrauterine growth retardation ([IUGR] → toxemia → poor uteroplacental function → abruptio placentae)
    j. Fetal heart tones (FHTs [greater than 160, less than 120, very irregular, none by 24 weeks, present and now absent, decreased fetal movement])
    k. Presentation, station

FACTORS PREDISPOSING TO RISK

Numerous conditions not diagnosed by history or initial examination may arise later in the pregnancy cycle. Below are listed some of these conditions along with their common precursors. They suggest the necessity of more frequenty visits for appraisal and correction, special treatment, and education and counseling.

1. Antepartum
    a. *Preeclampsia-eclampsia:* primigravida, hypertension, renal disease, multiple pregnancy, hydatidiform mole, age (less than 18, more than 35), race, socioeconomic status
    b. *Diabetes mellitus:* family history, recurrent toxemia, large fetus, polyhydramnios, unexplained fetal death, obesity, persistent glycosuria
    c. *Anemia:* poor nutrition, sickle cell disease or trait, glucose 6-phosphate deficiency (G6PD), urinary tract infections, bleeding tendency, menorrhagia
    d. *Cardiac decompensation:* history of heart disease, stress (anemia, infection, difficult home situation)
    e. *Placenta previa, premature separation (third trimester bleeding):* multiparity, hypertension, multiple gestation, diabetes mellitus, short cord, renal disease, advanced maternal age
    f. *Hyperemesis gravidarum:* gastrointestinal stress reaction, endocrine imbalance, metabolic demands, decreased gastric motility, psychological problems with maternal role
    g. *Extrauterine pregnancy (ectopic):* previous syphilis, gonorrhea, pelvic inflammatory disease (PID), abdominal operations, grand multiparity with pregnancies close together, previous abortions or ectopic pregnancies, IUD in place longer than 3 years
    h. *Fetal death:* diabetes mellitus, renal disease, anomalies, preeclampsia-eclampsia
    i. *Pseudocyesis:* menstrual disturbances, recent body change, fear or wish for pregnancy
    j. *Intrauterine growth retardation:* drug use, hypertension, poor nutrition, preeclampsia-eclampsia, poor uteroplacental functioning

k. *Hydramnios:* diabetes mellitus, fetal inability to swallow in utero
l. *Premature labor:* multiple gestation, polyhydramnios, urinary tract infection, sepsis
m. *Isoimmunization:* Rh negative mother, incompatible parental blood types

2. Intrapartum (see also postpartum factors)

a. *Dystocia (pelvic, uterine, fetal):* primipara, contracted pelvis, inefficient uterine contractions, large infant, exhaustion, advanced maternal age
b. *Cesarean delivery:* contracted pelvis, weak scar, preeclampsia, placenta previa, abruptio placental, dystocia, tumors, maternal herpes or gonorrhea, pelvic fracture, fetal distress, diabetes mellitus, prolapsed cord, hydrocephaly, malpresentation
c. *Prolapse of cord:* prematurity, transverse lie, breech, multiple gestation, polyhydramnios, premature rupture of membranes (PROM), nonengagement
d. *Malpresentation, ruptured uterus:* grand multiparity
e. *Exhaustion, anxiety, infection, dehydration, stress on fetus:* multiple stressors of labor

3. Postpartum

a. *Hemorrhage:* ruptured varices; laceration of birth canal; incomplete placental separation; relaxation of placental site; retained fragments of placenta (subinvolution of uterus); prolonged labor; uterine atony; hematological coagulation problems
b. *Disseminated intravascular coagulation (DIC):* pregnancy; abruption of placenta; eclampsia; retention of fetus longer than 5 weeks after death; amniotic fluid embolism; sepsis; hypertonic labor; difficult delivery; oxytocin induction; meconium staining
c. *Severe preeclampsia-eclampsia:* mild preeclampsia or sudden occurrence with no previous symptoms
d. *Infection, sepsis:* long labor; 24 hours with ruptured membrane; long labor with cesarean delivery, trauma and blood loss requiring aggressive care; exhaustion; problems with placental expulsion; anemia; malnutrition; stasis of ureters; edema of bladder; increased capacity with decreased sensitivity of uterus; anesthesia
e. *Shock:* placenta previa, abruptio placentae, blood loss, loss of circulation to vital organs, infection, operative delivery, aged mother, uterine atony
f. *Mastitis, breast infection:* incomplete emplying of lactating breast; blockage of milk ducts; breast-feeding by infected infant; hospital infection entering via nipples
g. *Trauma:* preexisting medical or surgical conditions
h. *Depression, psychosis:* previous psychiatric diagnosis; difficulty with parental role change; inadequate support system for stresses of pregnancy; anemia; fatigue; complications; low self-esteem; infant at risk

RISK BY MOST COMMON TIME INTERVALS (OVERLAP POSSIBLE)

Risks inherent in the perinatal period can be identified by the time in which they are likely to occur. The following is a list of obstetrical risks as they occur by the time of pregnancy:

1. **Prenatal**
   Early
   Diabetes mellitus
   Hypertension
   Cardiac disease
   Renal disease
   Exposure to teratogens
   Viral illness
   Herpes
   Syphilis, gonorrhea
   Pyelonephritis
   Unresponsive urinary tract infection
   Suspected ectopic pregnancy
   Missed abortion
   Vaginal bleeding
   Hyperemesis
   Isoimmunization
   Need for genetic diagnosis
   Faulty cervix
   Prior transfusions
   Failure of uterus to grow
   Excessive growth
   Trophoblastic disease
   Late
   Diabetes mellitus
   Third trimester bleeding
   Abnormal presentation
   Failure to gain
   Need for growth studies
   Hydramnios
   Unresponsive anemia
   Preeclampsia-eclampsia
   Thromboembolic disease
   Premature labor
   Multiple gestation
   Premature rupture of membranes
   Tumor
   Abnormal oxytocin challenge test
   Induction
   Nonengagement

2. **Intrapartal**
   Previous high risk
   Severe preeclampsia

Eclampsia
Amnionitis
Uterine tetany
Hydramnios
Uterine rupture
Dysfunctional labor
Maternal distress
Abnormal contractions
Arrested dilation
Excessive drugs
Labor more than 20 hours
Second stage more than 1 hour
Precipitous delivery
Meconium staining
Multiple birth
Fetus less than 2500 gm
Fetus more than 4000 gm
No descending part
Fetal distress
Bradycardia
Prolapsed cord
Fetal acidosis
Fetal tachycardia
Shoulder dystocia
Immature L/S (lecithin-sphingomyelin) ratio
General anesthesia

3. **Postpartal**
Cardiovascular compromise
Severe preeclampsia-eclampsia
Infection
Hemorrhage
Urinary tract infection
Trauma
Subinvolution
Breast problems
Abnormal vital signs
Infant respiratory distress–respiratory distress
   syndrome–hyaline membrane disease
Asphyxiation
Preterm (less than 33 weeks)
Post-term (more than 42 weeks)
Weight less than 2500 gm
Weight more than 4000 gm
Cyanotic heart disease
Apnea
Congenital malformation
Convulsions
Shock
Sepsis

Resuscitation
Hypoglycemia-hypocalcemia
Bilirubin more than 10 mg
Apgar less than 5 at 1 minute
Feeding problem
Multiple birth
Failure to gain
Jitteriness
Anemia
CNS depression

ANTEPARTAL ASSESSMENT

1. Frequent regular examinations for progress of pregnancy
2. Repeat of initial bloodwork and urinalysis at intervals (CBC, glucose, rubella titer, Rh titers, gonorrhea culture, urinalysis)
3. History for new symptoms
4. Blood pressure measurement
5. Assessment of fetal growth
   a. Indirect methods
       i. Recalculation of estimated date of confinement (EDC)
      ii. Uterine growth
     iii. Engagement
      iv. Sonography
       v. X-ray for bone maturity
      vi. Fetal activity
     vii. OCT
   b. Direct methods
       i. Amniocentesis
      ii. Amniography
     iii. Cytology

INTRAPARTAL ASSESSMENT

1. Previous risk
2. Cephalopelvic adequacy
3. Choices
   a. Need for fetal monitoring
       i. External
      ii. Internal (scalp)
   b. Analgesia
   c. Duration of labor
   d. Need for induction/augmentation
4. Method of delivery
5. Anesthesia
6. Need for resuscitation

7. Need for newborn transfusion
8. Need for intensive care unit

POSTPARTAL ASSESSMENT

1. Maternal
   a. Observation in delivery room, 1 hour in recovery room
   b. Vital signs, lochia, responses
2. Fetal
   a. Examination in delivery room
   b. Examination and observation in transitional nursery
   c. ICU, 5%
   d. Moderate risk requiring special care, 20%

ACUTE SIGNS AND SYMPTOMS
AND WHAT THEY MAY INDICATE

1. **Bleeding/hemorrhage:** abortion, placenta previa (bright red blood, painless), abruptio placentae (dark red blood, pain), hydatidiform mole (oversized uterus, grapelike vesicles), extrauterine pregnancy, anemia, ruptured uterus, postpartum atony

2. **Blood pressure**
   a. *High:* preeclampsia-eclampsia, kidney disorders or infection, trophoblastic disease (mole)
   b. *Low:* anemia, septic shock, hemorrhagic shock

3. **Blurred vision:** preeclampsia-eclampsia, hypertension

4. **Burning on urination:** urinary tract infection, vaginal infection

5. **Cramping, boardlike abdomen with pain:** abortion, premature separation of placenta

6. **Severe edema:** preeclampsia-eclampsia, renal disease, cardiopulmonary insufficiency, congestive heart failure

7. **Epigastric pain:** severe with severely elevated BP, edema; impending eclampsia; liver rupture

8. **Fever:** infection, sepsis, abortion, eclampsia

9. **Severe headaches:** hypertension, preeclampsia-eclampsia, seizures

10. **Hyperreflexia:** preeclampsia-eclampsia, seizures

11. **Persistent vomiting:** hyperemesis gravidarum, hyperglycemia, hydatidiform mole

12. **Paresis, paralysis, aphasia:** eclamptic cardiovascular accident

13. **Respiratory distress:** congestive heart failure, cardiopulmonary compromise

14.   **Uncontrolled water flow:** rupture of membranes

15.   **Urinary protein, blood:** preeclampsia-eclampsia, urinary tract infection

CONCLUSIONS

By utilizing the information available in this chapter, the nurse is able to assess comprehensively the maternity patient at all periods in the cycle. This will allow the nurse to decide if crisis is imminent and then provide the most appropriate interaction possible. The succeeding chapters will provide the nurse with the information needed to deal effectively with the high risk maternity patient.

REFERENCES

1.   Clark, A.L., and Affonso, D.D.: Childbearing: A Nursing Perspective, 2nd ed. Philadelphia, F.A. Davis Co., 1979.
2.   Gabbe, S., et al.: High-risk pregnancy: Trimester 1. Patient Care, *15*:90–91, 1981.
3.   Jensen, M.D., and Bobak, I.M.: Handbook of Maternity Care: A Guide for Nursing Practice. St. Louis, C.V. Mosby Co., 1980.
4.   Johnson, S.H.: High Risk Parenting. Philadelphia, J.B. Lippincott Co., 1979.
5.   Korones, S.B.: High Risk Newborn Infants: The Basis for Intensive Nursing Care. St. Louis, C.V. Mosby Co., 1972.
6.   Krupp, M., and Chatton, M.: High risk pregnancy. *In* Current Medical Diagnosis and Treatment. Los Altos, Calif., Lange Medical Publications, 1980.

CHAPTER 9

OBSTETRICAL EMERGENCIES

Carole Ann Miller McKenzie, C.N.M., Ph.D.,
and
Sherry A. Gillespie, R.N., M.S.N.

OBJECTIVES

Upon completion of this chapter the reader will be able to accomplish the following:

1. Identify the emergencies that must be handled in the obstetrical area
2. Identify the purposes of the emergency procedures
3. List equipment necessary for the emergency procedures
4. Identify in priority order the actions necessary to accomplish the emergency procedures
5. Explain the rationale for the actions
6. Discuss the importance of the nurse's being able to accomplish these procedures

Because emergencies can occur with such rapidity, threatening mother and fetus, it is essential to isolate that care that deals with the most crucial emergencies. For purposes of this chapter, entities that are synonymous with the most life threatening maternal/fetal emergencies have been detailed. They are not repeated in the procedure appendix (Appendix A). For all of the emergencies detailed here, the precipitating events are discussed and expanded in Chapters 10, 11, and 12.

Because of the nature of these emergencies the nurse is often in a position to assume the responsibilities detailed here. The nurse must be able to initiate these procedures to facilitate maximal maternal/fetal well-being. By following the instructions given here step by step, the nurse is able to render care in an obstetrical emergency in the most effective manner possible.

MATERNAL CARDIAC ARREST

Maternal cardiac arrest may occur in the obstetrical area whenever hemorrhagic or embolic conditions lead to shock. The specific entities that cause the arrest are dealt with in succeeding sections.

Cardiopulmonary resuscitation is begun whenever a patient suffers respiratory and cardiac arrest. Once begun, the procedure is continued until the patient breathes spontaneously or until another qualified person arrives to relieve the nurse.

ETIOLOGY

The etiology of the arrest is dependent upon the entity that has caused the problem in the first place. Shock and arrest occur when the original problem has not been reversed.

ASSESSMENT

1. Clinical presentation
   a. Signs and symptoms
      i. Cessation of life signs
      ii. Fibrillation or flat line on ECG monitor

PROBLEMS AND COMPLICATIONS

1. Fetal death
2. Maternal death

MANAGEMENT

COMMENTS/TIPS/CAUTIONS

1. **Goal**
   a. To restore vital function to mother
      i. Upon discovery of patient, shake her to ascertain whether she is unconscious
      ii. If patient is unconscious, *call for assistance (shout if necessary!)* — Cardiopulmonary resuscitation (CPR) must be started without delay; patient should not be left alone
      iii. Position the patient on a firm, flat surface — To make cardiac compressions more effective
      iv. Check to make sure the patient's airway is patent
         (a) Place hand on patient's forehead and tilt head back slightly — To open airway

(b) Place fingertips of second hand under the lower jaw and gently lift chin

v. Listen for any air movement with your ear placed over her mouth, and watch for chest or abdominal movement up and down

    Opening the airway may have restored spontaneous respirations

vi. If patient has begun to breathe, maintain patient in that position until help arrives

vii. If breathing has not been restored, institute mouth-to-mouth resuscitation

(a) Close the patient's nostrils with the thumb and index finger of the hand placed on her forehead

(b) Take a deep breath and open your mouth wide and place it tightly over the victim's mouth so that no air can escape

viii. Deliver four quick breaths without allowing the victim to exhale

    These four breaths maintain positive pressure in the airway to reinflate the alveoli

ix. Locate the carotid pulse and palpate for 5 to 10 seconds; if pulse is present, do not start cardiac compression; continue to ventilate patient with one breath every 5 seconds

x. If pulse is absent, begin cardiac compression

xi. Locate the lower margin of the rib cage and trace the margin to the notch where the ribs and sternum meet

xii. Place the heel of one hand two fingerbreadths above that notch

    Incorrect placement may fracture a rib or lacerate the patient's liver

COMMENTS/TIPS/CAUTIONS

xiii. Place the other hand over the heel of the first hand; interlock or extend fingers to keep them away from the patient's chest

xiv. Align shoulders over your hands; keep elbows straight and begin compressing downward about 3 to 5 cm at the rate of 60/minute

xv. If only one person is doing resuscitation, perform 15 compressions and then ventilate with two breaths

xvi. Continue for 1 minute and recheck carotid pulse; stop compressions for 5 seconds

xvii. If two persons are performing resuscitation, have one person do five compressions and the other ventilate with one breath after each five compressions

xviii. Continue this procedure until additional assistance arrives or heart beat has been reestablished

xix. If crash cart is available, begin to ventilate patient with Ambu bag

COMMENTS/TIPS/CAUTIONS

Helps to maintain vertical pressure through the heels of the hand

Assures downward, not lateral, compressions; lateral compressions do not deliver sufficient pressure

To see if the victim's heart is beating on its own

HEMORRHAGE AND SHOCK

Hemorrhage in an obstetrical patient is a serious and life threatening event. Nurses must look at each patient as a potential candidate for hemorrhage and be prepared to respond immediately if hemorrhage and shock occur.[4]

ETIOLOGY

Hemorrhage and shock occur in the obstetrical patient when bleeding or coagulation capabilities are compromised to the point of threat to the mother's life.

ASSESSMENT
1. Clinical presentation
  a. Signs and symptoms
- i. Bleeding
- ii. Vital signs increase and then decrease to 0
- iii. Pallor
- iv. Cyanosis
- v. Clamminess
- vi. Decreased urine output
- vii. Decreased level of consciousness

PROBLEMS AND COMPLICATIONS
1. Maternal death
2. Fetal death

PATIENT CARE MANAGEMENT
1. Goals

	COMMENTS/TIPS/ CAUTIONS
a. To identify and assess promptly Assess each patient for any factor that may predispose her to hemorrhage	To keep nurse alert for patients who are more prone to hemorrhage
i. Preeclampsia-eclampsia	
ii. Overdistention of uterus	
(a) Multiple pregnancy	
(b) Polyhydramnios	
iii. Grand multiparity	
iv. Advanced age	
v. Painless vaginal delivery after seventh month	
vi. History of previous hemorrhage, bleeding problem, blood coagulopathy	
vii. Retained placental fragments	
b. To stabilize maternal system if hemorrhage is present	
i. Start IV line with large bore plastic cannula; draw blood for hemoglobin, hematocrit; start IV if needed	To allow rapid replacement of blood
ii. Observe, record, and report blood loss	
(a) Pad count	
(b) Weigh pads and check to more accurately assess loss (1 gm = 1 ml blood)	

iii. Monitor rate and quality of respirations

iv. Measure pulse rates; assess pulse quality by direct palpation

v. Monitor BP every 2 to 5 minutes; compare with normal blood pressure

vi. Monitor urine output
   (a) Insert Foley catheter
   (b) Measure hourly output
   (c) Measure specific gravity

vii. Assess skin for presence of
   (a) Pallor
   (b) Cyanosis
   (c) Coldness
   (d) Clamminess

viii. Frequently assess state of consciousness

c. To restore vital function if shock occurs

   i. Place patient in supine position, not Trendelenburg

   ii. Draw, type and crossmatch, and administer whole blood as soon as possible

   iii. While waiting for whole blood, infuse isotonic fluids, plasma, plasma expanders as ordered by physician

   iv. Administer O_2 by face mask

   v. Assist with insertion and measurement of central venous pressure line

   vi. Continue to monitor output hourly

   vii. Observe for signs and symptoms of disseminated intravascular coagulation (DIC); if present, draw blood immediately for clotting studies

COMMENTS/TIPS/CAUTIONS

When hemorrhage begins respirations increase as a result of sympathoadrenal stimulation

Pulse rate increases as a result of increased epinephrine. Thready pulse indicates vasoconstriction and decreased cardiac output. Changes before drop in BP

Hypotension reflects large loss of circulatory fluid

Decreased output indicates poor perfusion to other vital organs

Indicates the amount of vasoconstriction

Diminished blood flow to brain causes restlessness and anxiety; as shock progresses, state of consciousness decreases

Supine position keeps more blood available to vital centers. Trendelenburg position before delivery shifts uterus against diaphragm and may cause respiratory difficulties

Hypotension results from decreased blood volume

To maintain circulating volume

Increases circulating O_2

Provides estimation of blood volume returning to heart

Provides excellent measure of organ perfusion
1. 50 ml/hour = safe renal perfusion
2. Less than 25 ml/hour = inadequate renal perfusion

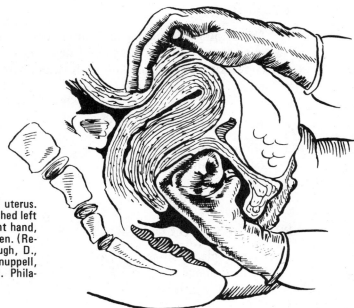

Figure 9-1. Bimanual compression of uterus. Uterus is compressed between the clenched left fist in the anterior fornix and the right hand, which is placed on the patient's abdomen. (Reprinted with permission from Cavanaugh, D., Woods, R.D., O'Connor, T.C., and Knuppell, R.N.: Obstetric Emergencies, 3rd ed. Philadelphia, Harper and Row, 1982.)

	COMMENTS/TIPS/CAUTIONS
viii. If hemorrhage continues, utilize bimanual compression	Bimanual compression of the uterus is a valuable method for controlling uterine atony; it provides twice the amount of uterine stimulation that can be achieved by abdominal massage alone and may allow the nurse to control bleeding until physician arrives
d. To provide emotional support to patient	Fear and anxiety of the patient increase release of catecholamines
e. To control maternal bleeding	
i. Put on sterile gloves	To prevent introduction of bacteria
ii. Insert one fist into the vagina	
iii. Place against cervix and press upward	Places pressure against the anterior walls of uterus
iv. Grasp uterus through abdominal wall with free hand	To allow contact with posterior aspect of uterus
v. Massage uterus between two hands until firm	This provides twice the amount of stimulation and causes venous compression
vi. Infuse oxytocin as ordered by physician[4]	To assist in contraction of uterus

ECLAMPTIC SEIZURE

Preeclampsia may progress to the eclamptic state if left untreated or inadequately assessed. Every preeclamptic patient has the potential for a seizure. As clinical signs indicate a worsening condition, the patient must be protected from injury in the event of a seizure.

ETIOLOGY

The etiology of eclampsia is unknown. Seizures occur when preeclampsia becomes so severe that continued neurological symptoms lead to seizure. It is characterized by vasospasm with vasoconstriction and increased peripheral resistance.

ASSESSMENT

1. **Clinical presentation**
   a. Signs and symptoms
      i. Coma
      ii. Convulsions

PROBLEMS AND COMPLICATIONS

1. Neurological damage
2. Renal damage
3. Maternal death
4. Fetal death

PATIENT CARE MANAGEMENT

Necessary equipment includes oral suction machine, padded tongue blade, oral airway, magnesium sulfate, bath blankets, reflex hammer, and oxygen.

	COMMENTS/TIPS/CAUTIONS
1. **Goals**	
a. To restore maternal equilibrium	
i. Decrease environmental stimuli to the patient	Excessive stimuli may provoke convulsive activities
(a) Dim lights	
(b) Reduce noise	
(c) Reduce number of disturbances to patient	
ii. Place on left side with head slightly elevated	To increase blood flow to uterus and to prevent aspiration
iii. Pad side rails with bath blankets	To prevent injury to patient in event of seizure
iv. Keep oral suction machine, ready for use, at bedside	To prevent aspiration of vomitus
v. Keep padded tongue blade and plastic airway near head of bed	Insertion of tongue blade during seizure may minimize trauma to the mouth
vi. Monitor patient's blood pressure and reflexes closely; observe for twitching of extremities	
vii. Have oxygen available at patient's bedside	Give oxygen to help overcome hypoxemia

———————————— IMPENDING CESAREAN SECTION ————————————

Every obstetrical patient faces the possibility of needing a cesarean section. The decision to do a cesarean section often is made quickly because of danger to mother or baby or both. Nurses must be able to prepare patient quickly and efficiently.

ETIOLOGY

Fetal risk due to anoxia has become so great that delivery must be accomplished immediately. The reasons for this vary according to the clinical entity that is causing the anoxia. The anoxia causes the fetal life support system to be nonfunctional.

ASSESSMENT

1. **Clinical presentation**
   a. Signs and symptoms
      i. Variable decelerations—fetal heart rate
      ii. Various maternal symptoms according to what is occurring
      iii. Absence of or rapid decline of fetal heart rate
      iv. Late accelerations with decreasing variability

PROBLEMS AND COMPLICATIONS

1. Fetal neurological problems
2. Fetal death
3. Maternal problems dependent upon the condition or problem

PATIENT CARE MANAGEMENT

1. **Goals**
   a. To prepare patient for immediate surgery to salvage fetus

	COMMENTS/TIPS/CAUTIONS
i. Draw blood for CBC on patient's admission to labor and delivery; report results to physician	Current status may indicate need to have cross-matched blood available
Upon notification of need for cesarean section	
ii. Draw blood, type and cross-match if ordered	
iii. Prepare abdominal-perineal area as ordered by physician	Decreases chances of infection
iv. Insert Foley catheter to straight drainage bag	To prevent trauma to bladder during surgery and maintain accurate record of output
v. Remove jewelry and nail polish and cover hair with scrub cap	

vi. Give preoperative medication if ordered

vii. Remove scalp electrode and intrauterine pressure catheter before patient is transported to operating room

Prevent introduction of bacteria into the uterus as baby is delivered through the abdomen

If fetal distress or profuse bleeding is the reason for the cesarean section, some pre-operative measures can be deleted (i.e., abdominal-perineal preparation)

If patient must be transported to the operating room, monitor fetal heart tones (FHTs) with Doppler or fetoscope en route

TETANIC CONTRACTIONS

Because tetanic contractions are forceful, they severely decrease the blood and oxygen supply to the fetus and lead to fetal hypoxia. Tetanic contractions may cause uterine rupture or placental abruption.

ETIOLOGY

Forceful contraction of the uterus from vigorous oxytocin stimulation or naturally occurring strong contraction leads to fetal hypoxia.

ASSESSMENT

1. **Clinical presentation**
   a. Signs and symptoms
      i. Forceful contraction of greater than 90 seconds' duration
      ii. Variable deceleration of fetal heart rate
      iii. Rapid decline in fetal heart rate
      iv. Late decelerations with decreasing variability

PROBLEMS AND COMPLICATIONS

1. Fetal death
2. Maternal death
3. Uterine rupture
4. Abruptio placentae

PATIENT CARE MANAGEMENT

1. **Goal**
   a. To stop severe uterine contractions (tetanic [more than 90 seconds])

   i. Turn off oxytocin infusion if on and increase rate of plain IV fluid

Decreases stimulus to the uterus

   ii. Turn patient to left side

Increases blood flow to the uterus

   iii. Give oxygen by face mask to mother at 6 to 8 liters/ minute

Increases available oxygen in the maternal circulating blood, which increases the amount available for exchange at the placental site

iv. Call for physician
v. Administer whiffs of amyl nitrite as ordered by physician until uterus is relaxed

Amyl nitrite relaxes smooth muscles

FETAL HYPOXEMIA AND ACIDOSIS

Fetal scalp sampling is done to aid in identifying fetal hypoxemia and acidosis. Indications for fetal sampling are late decelerations with decreasing variability, smooth baseline with minimal variability, fetal bradycardia or tachycardia, and persistent moderate or severe variable decelerations.

ETIOLOGY

Fetal hypoxemia and acidosis may occur as a result of any condition that compromises the maternal/fetal gas exchange system.

ASSESSMENT
1. **Clinical presentation**
   a. Signs and symptoms
      i. Late decelerations with decreasing variability
      ii. Smooth baseline with minimal variability
      iii. Fetal bradycardia or tachycardia
      iv. Persistent moderate or severe variable decelerations

PROBLEMS AND COMPLICATIONS
1. Fetal neurological problems
2. Fetal death
3. Maternal problems dependent upon the condition or problem
4. Fetal scalp abscess

PATIENT CARE MANAGEMENT

Equipment necessary includes fetal sampling kit, light source, preparation solution, and pH machine.

1. **Goal**
   a. To assess fetal response to labor
      i. The following conditions must be present before procedure can be implemented

      To obtain adequate visualization

      (a) Rupture of membranes
      (b) Adequate cervical dilatation
      (c) Engagement of presenting part

	COMMENTS/TIPS/CAUTIONS
ii. When physician decides to do procedure, obtain all necessary equipment	
iii. Calibrate pH machine if necessary	To assure accurate readings of blood sample
iv. Have patient positioned for vaginal examination (patient may need to move to the end of the bed and prop feet on edge of the bed)	Physician must have room to maneuver endoscope and other equipment
v. Open fetal scalp sampling kit in sterile manner	
vi. Prepare perineal area with Betadine solution	Prevent introduction of bacteria from perineal area into uterine cavity
vii. Physician will insert conical vaginal endoscope in the vagina and through the cervix	Provide adequate visualization of the scalp
viii. Attach light source in the space provided	Provide better visualization
ix. Pour Betadine solution over long cotton tipped applicator to clean the site	Prevent introduction of bacteria present on skin into sampling site
x. Physician will puncture fetal scalp with a 2 × 2 mm microscalpel at the beginning of a contraction.	Fetal blood will flow more freely if the scalp is punctured at beginning of a contraction
xi. Take blood collected in heparinized glass capillary tube directly to the pH machine	Sample must be run quickly before specimen clots
xii. Run specimen according to manufacturer's instructions	
xiii. Normal fetal pH is 7.3 to 7.35. If pH of specimen falls between 7.20 and 7.25, prepare to obtain repeat sample in 15 minutes	This is considered a borderline specimen, and fetus can be watched
xiv. If value falls below 7.20, prepare for immediate low forceps delivery or for emergency cesarean section[4]	Immediate intervention is required to prevent further fetal hypoxia and acidosis and thus to avoid permanent effects

EMERGENCY DELIVERY

Occasionally labor will progress so rapidly that the nurse is faced with delivering the baby before the physician arrives. It is important that the nurse be able to respond in a calm and safe manner.

ETIOLOGY

Emergency delivery may be necessary when the fetus(es) is small and/or when contractions are extremely vigorous. Usual labor patterns are disrupted and labor proceeds very quickly.

ASSESSMENT

1. **Clinical presentation**
   a. Signs and symptoms
      i. Bulging perineum
      ii. Patient says that the baby is coming
      iii. Decreased time in labor pattern
      iv. Vigorous contractions
      v. No physician available

PROBLEMS AND COMPLICATIONS

1. Unsterile delivery: infection of mother and baby
2. Prematurity
3. Multiple gestation
4. Fetal neurological problems
5. Maternal perineal problems
6. Fetal death

PATIENT CARE MANAGEMENT

Equipment necessary includes emergency delivery pack ("precip pack") containing small drape, bulb syringe, two sterile clamps, sterile gloves, sterile scissors, cord clamp, and baby blanket.

	COMMENTS/TIPS/CAUTIONS
1. **Goal**	
a. To maximize positive outcome	
i. Position the woman in a comfortable position	A relaxed patient can assist with delivery more easily
ii. Reassure patient verbally and respond in a calm, relaxed manner; give clear instructions to the woman and praise her for doing a good job	To increase patient's confidence and reduce tension
iii. If time permits, scrub hands and put on sterile gloves. If delivery is imminent, it is more important to control the delivery than to put on gloves.	To decrease chances of infection

iv. If time permits prepare perineum with Betadine solution

Render perineal area as clean as possible

v. Place sterile drape under mother's buttocks

Provide sterile field

vi. As the head begins to appear (crowning):

   (a) Tear the amniotic membrane if it is still intact

Prevent aspiration of amniotic fluid by the baby during the first breath

   (b) Instruct the patient to pant or pant-blow

Decrease the urge to push

vii. Place the flat of the hand on the exposed fetal head and apply *gentle* pressure to prevent the head from popping out too rapidly

Rapid delivery of the head may cause
1. Vaginal or perineal lacerations
2. Rapid change in pressure on the fetal head resulting in subdural or dural tears

viii. Support the perineum and allow the head to be delivered between contractions

Prevent rapid expulsion of the head

ix. Instruct the mother to continue to blow; check for umbilical cord by inserting one or two fingers along the back of the neck

A cord around the baby's neck might tighten or tear during delivery

x. If cord is present around the neck

A loose cord might tighten as the baby's body is born

   (a) Bend fingers like a hook, grasp the cord, and pull it over the baby's head; check to make sure it is not wrapped around with a second loop

   (b) If cord will not slip over head because it is too tight, place two clamps on cord, cut between the clamps, and unwind the cord

xi. Wipe baby's face to remove excess mucus or meconium; use bulb syringe to suction mouth, throat, and nasal passages

Prevent baby from aspirating during breathing

xii. Support the fetal head as restitution (external rotation) occurs

xiii. Place one hand on each side of the head and exert gentle downward pressure until the anterior shoulder emerges under the symphysis pubis

xiv. Apply *gentle* upward pressure to deliver the posterior shoulder

xv. Hold the baby securely while the rest of the body delivers; cradle the baby's head and back in one hand and the buttocks in the other

Baby will be wet and slippery and may be easily dropped

xvi. Hold baby's head down and keep body at the level of the uterus

Facilitate drainage of mucus and facilitate blood flow through the umbilical cord

xvii. Dry the baby rapidly

Prevent heat loss

xviii. When baby's respirations are adequate, place baby on mother's abdomen and cover

Keep baby warm

xix. After pulsation of cord has stopped, place cord clamp near baby and Kelly clamp on umbilical cord and cut cord between the two clamps

xx. Be alert for signs of placental separation
  (a) Slight gush of blood
  (b) Lengthening of cord
  (c) Change in uterine shape from discoid to globular

xxi. Do not pull or tug on umbilical cord

Injudicious traction may tear the cord, separate the placenta, or invert the uterus

xxii. Instruct the mother to push to deliver the placenta; gently ease out the placental membranes

Prevent retention of membrane fragments

xxiii. Check firmness of uterus; gently massage uterus to stimulate contractions and firm uterus

Decrease bleeding

xxiv. Clean the area under the mother's buttocks

Patient's comfort

COMMENTS/TIPS/CAUTIONS

xxv. Monitor mother's condition until further medical
assistance arrives

Detect hemorrhage or other problems before physician arrives

xxvi. Complete necessary records
(a) Identification of infant
(b) Delivery records

xxvii. Allow family opportunity
to bond

CONCLUSIONS

To determine additional nursing care and management of the various entities discussed in this chapter, the nurse should consult the appropriate sections of this book. This chapter contains information only on procedures utilized in extreme emergency. Obviously other procedures and information are necessary to effectively manage the high risk maternity patient. By combining the information available throughout this book the nurse will be able to deal with any obstetrical crisis that arises.

REFERENCES

1. Cavanaugh, D., Woods, R.D., O'Connor, T.C., and Knuppell, R.N.: Obstetric Emergencies, 3rd ed. Philadelphia, Harper & Row, 1982.
2. Jensen, M.D., Benson, R.C., and Bobak, I.M.: Maternity Care: The Nurse and the Family, 2nd ed. St. Louis, C.V. Mosby Co., 1981.
3. Matheny, L.: Emergency! First aid for cardiopulmonary arrest. Nursing '82, 6:34–45, 1982.
4. Olds, S.B., London, M.L., Ladewig, P.A., and Davidson, S.V.: Obstetric Nursing. Menlo Park, Calif., Addison-Wesley-Publishing, 1980.
5. Oxorn, H.: Human Labor and Birth, 4th ed., New York, Appleton-Century-Crofts, 1980.

CHAPTER 10

ANTEPARTAL CRISES

Elaine M. Moore, C.N.M., M.S.N.

OBJECTIVES

Upon completion of this chapter the reader will be able to accomplish the following:

1. Perform a nursing assessment of the antepartal patient admitted to the hospital because of complication of pregnancy

2. Outline the nursing management for the antepartal patient who is bleeding in the first trimester

3. Outline the nursing management for the antepartal patient who presents with bleeding in the second trimester

4. List the predisposing factors for diffuse intravascular coagulation

5. Describe the clinical signs and symptoms displayed with pyelonephritis

6. Describe the problems and complications involved with an active herpes infection in the last trimester of pregnancy

7. List the major risk factors that predispose a pregnant patient to pregnancy induced hypertension

8. Describe the nursing management for mild to moderate pregnancy induced hypertension and the rationale for these actions

9. Outline the emergency treatment for the eclamptic patient

10. Describe the nursing management for the patient with hyperemesis gravidarum

11. Name three tests for fetal well-being that may be used for the class B diabetic patient in the last 2 months of pregnancy

12. List five signs and symptoms displayed by the antepartal patient with cardiac disease

13. State four complications of multiple pregnancy

14. Name the laboratory test that differentiates sickle cell trait, sickle cell disease, and sickle cell–hemaglobin C (SC) disease

The purpose of this chapter is to outline some of the more common high risk conditions that occur as a result of pregnancy or that were present prior to pregnancy but became aggravated because of the pregnant state. One must always keep in mind that for most women pregnancy is a normal physiological process. However, some complications of pregnancy seriously jeop-

153

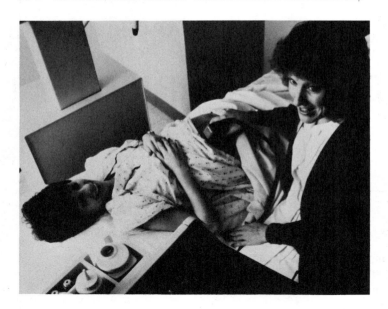

Figure 10-1. Complications of pregnancy may require procedures that necessitate explanations to the patient and her family. (Courtesy of Don Shaeffer, Hermann Hospital, Houston, Texas.)

ardize the health of either the mother or fetus or both. When the expectant mother's health or the fetus' well-being is jeopardized, a crisis results, and hospitalization is necessary. The acute and chronic conditions in this chapter all require hospitalization, and the nursing management will focus on obstetrical nursing care.

Expectant mothers who are hospitalized are extremely concerned about their own health as well as their unborn infant's health. The role of the nurse is to protect and maintain the physiological integrity of both the maternal and fetal systems as well as act as a support person to both the mother and her significant others.

Hospitalization presents a crisis for the whole family, and it is at this time that family members should be encouraged to be together. The nurse caring for the expectant mother must keep in mind that she has two patients, the mother and the fetus, to care for and also has to encourage the family to support the mother during this crisis. This can be accomplished by being astute to the needs of both the mother and the fetus as well as the needs of the significant others. Family members should be kept informed about the status of the mother and unborn infant and encouraged to be with them whenever possible.

Psychological needs as well as physical needs are important at this time. Encouraging the family to express their needs and concerns is important. Explanations to the family as well as to the patient regarding tests, medical procedures, equipment, and nursing procedures may help allay some of the family's anxieties so that they can better support the patient.

ANTEPARTAL ASSESSMENT

When an expectant mother is admitted to the hospital because of a physical crisis, a complete nursing assessment is necessary and includes the following:

IDENTITY

1. Name
2. Age
3. Number of pregnancies
4. Number of living children

CURRENT PREGNANCY

1. Estimated date of confinement (EDC) and last menstrual period (LMP)
2. Number of weeks' gestation
3. Reason for admission to hospital
4. Previous admissions with this pregnancy or previous problems with this pregnancy
5. Treatments for previous problems
6. Presence of
   a. Urinary frequency
   b. Abdominal pain
   c. Headaches
   d. Visual disturbances
   e. Fever or chills
   f. Back pain
   g. Vaginal bleeding or discharge
   h. Fetal movements (if gestation is greater than 20 weeks)

PAST OBSTETRICAL HISTORY

1. Number of years since last delivery
2. Past deliveries normal spontaneous vaginal delivery (NSVD) or cesarean section (CS)
3. Any abnormalities with past pregnancy, delivery, or post partum?
4. Condition, size, and gestational age of baby
5. Abortions: spontaneous or therapeutic, year, problem

MEDICAL AND SURGICAL HISTORY

1. Serious past illness
*2. Known allergies
*3. Drugs taken during this pregnancy
4. Previous operations: type, year, problems
5. Hereditary diseases in family: diabetes, hypertension or sickle cell anemia

ANTEPARTAL RECORD IS AVAILABLE, REVIEW FOR SIGNIFICANT FINDINGS IN:

1. Obstetrical
2. Past medical history
3. Family history

---

*Flag chart with this information

4. Social history
5. Initial physical examination
6. Initial pelvic examination
7. Laboratory data

NURSING PHYSICAL ASSESSMENT

1. **Vital signs**
   a. Temperature
   b. Pulse
   c. Respirations
   d. Blood pressure (BP)
   e. Weight

2. **Chest**
   a. Auscultate heart sounds
   b. Auscultate lung sounds

3. **Abdominal examination**
   a. Lie, presentation, position
   b. Engagement
   c. Fundal height
   d. Estimated fetal weight
   e. Fetal heart tones (FHTs): chart number and location
   f. Abdominal tenderness

4. **Back**
   a. Costovertebral angle tenderness (CVAT)

5. **Extremities**
   a. Upper extremity edema
   b. Ankle or pretibial edema
   c. Quadriceps (knee jerk) deep tendon reflex
   d. Presence of varicosities
   e. Homans' sign
   f. Ankle clonus
   g. Lymphadenopathy

6. **Gynecological examination**
   a. If patient is bleeding, note color, amount, odor, and when last pad changed
   b. Do not do a vaginal examination if patient is bleeding
   c. If patient is not bleeding, do not do a vaginal examination unless you know what you are assessing

PSYCHOSOCIAL ASSESSMENT

1. Assess the mother's feelings regarding this pregnancy.
   a. What pregnancy developmental tasks has she accomplished?
2. Assess the father's feeling regarding this pregnancy.
   a. Is he accepting and supportive of the pregnancy?

3. Socioeconomic status
   a. Culture
   b. Financial problems
4. Educational level of parents
   a. Career plans for mother
5. Problems with this pregnancy that may have affected the relationship between the mother and father
6. Knowledge level of the resources available in community for help if necessary

_____ SPONTANEOUS ABORTION _____

Spontaneous abortion is the termination of pregnancy before the fetus has reached a stage of viability. It carries the risk of life threatening maternal complications.

DIAGNOSIS

In spontaneous abortion there is loss of the products of conception prior to the 20th week of gestation accompanied by vaginal bleeding with or without menstrual-like abdominal cramping or backache.

1. **Incidence**
   a. Occurs in approximately 15 to 20 per cent of all pregnancies
   b. Usually occurs in the second or third month of pregnancy

ETIOLOGY

1. Abnormal embryo or an abnormal trophoblast
2. Acute infection such as pneumonia, pyelonephritis, or influenza
3. Abnormalities of the generative tract such as abnormally short cervix or uterine malformations
4. **Classification of abortion**
   a. *Spontaneous:* the process starts without apparent cause
   b. *Threatened:* occurrence of vaginal bleeding or spotting may or may not be accompanied by abdominal cramping, but the cervix is closed
   c. *Inevitable:* the internal os of the cervix is dilated and accompanied by painful uterine contractions and vaginal bleeding: amniotic fluid may be seen in the vaginal vault, or there may be fluid leaking from the cervix
   d. *Incomplete:* the products of conception have been passed but part, usually the placenta, is retained in the uterus; vaginal bleeding persists until the retained products of conception have been passed
   e. *Complete:* the passage of the products of conception appears to be complete, the uterus is well contracted, and the cervical os may be closed
   f. *Missed:* the products of conception are retained after the fetus is known to have died; the term is usually restricted to cases in which 2 or more months have elapsed between fetal death and expulsion

ASSESSMENT

1. **Clinical presentation**
   a. Signs and symptoms
      i. Vaginal bleeding
      ii. Pelvic cramping and backache may be present
      iii. Membranes may rupture
   b. History
      i. Previous episodes of vaginal bleeding or pelvic cramping with current pregnancy; passage of tissue or clots; EDC; LMP; previous abortions

2. **Biopsychosocial assessment**
   a. Monitor vital signs: TPR and BP
   b. If greatert than 14 weeks gestation monitor FHR with Doppler
   c. Amount and type of vaginal bleeding
   d. Type, onset of, and duration of pain
   e. Mother's emotional state

PROBLEMS AND COMPLICATIONS

1. Hemorrhagic shock
2. Maternal infection
3. Pregnancy loss
4. Psychological trauma due to pregnancy loss

PATIENT CARE MANAGEMENT

	COMMENTS/TIPS/CAUTIONS
1. Goals	
a. To maintain the physiological integrity of the maternal system	
i. Notify physician	
ii. Monitor vital signs every 15 minutes until condition is stable	
iii. If bleeding is heavy	Blood replacement may be necessary if bleeding is excessive
(a) Observe patient for symptoms and signs of shock	
(b) Start IV with large bore catheter	
(c) Place patient in Trendelenburg's position	
(d) Blood: CBC, Rh, type and cross-match immediately	
(e) Palpate for uterus, measure fundus if uterus is palpable; palpate for consistency and tenderness	External blood loss may be deceiving, and uterus may be filling with blood

b. To assess psychological state
   i. Allow father or significant other to remain with mother
   ii. Provide emotional support to mother
   iii. Allow and encourage ventilation of fears and feelings
c. To provide educative information
   i. Prepare patient for possible fetal loss
   ii. Prepare for possible surgery

COMMENTS/TIPS/CAUTIONS

Mother and father should not be separated at this time

Assist the parents to begin grieving if fetal loss is inevitable

DISCHARGE PLANNING/TEACHING

1. Contraception, if loss
2. Emotional support, if loss
3. Plans for future children
4. Care during remaining pregnancy
5. Help with home and family

ECTOPIC PREGNANCY

Ectopic pregnancy, which occurs unexpectedly, is a life threatening event for the mother. Maternal hemorrhage is the most dangerous complication.

DIAGNOSIS

In ectopic pregnancy the fertilized ovum implants in a site other than the endometrial cavity. Implantation may occur in the fallopian tube, abdominal cavity, ovary, or cervix.

1. **Incidence:** 1 in 200 pregnancies in white women and 1 in 120 pregnancies in nonwhite women
2. **Predisposing factors**
   a. Previous pelvic inflammatory disease
   b. Previous pelvic surgery
   c. IUD in place

ETIOLOGY

1. Chronic salpingitis
2. Abnormalities of tubal structure
3. Tubal adhesions
4. Tumors in the pelvic area
5. Previous tubal surgery

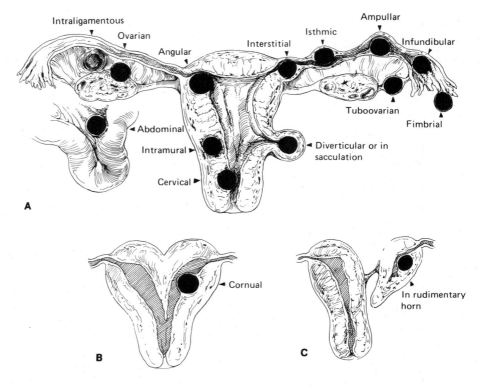

Figure 10-2. Various implantation sites of ectopic pregnancy. (Reprinted with permission from Danforth, D.N.: Obstetrics and Gynecology. Hagerstown, Md., Harper and Row, 1977)

ASSESSMENT

1. **Clinical presentation**
   a. Signs and symptoms
      i. History of missed menstrual period followed by various degrees of vaginal bleeding
      ii. Abdominal or pelvic pain: sharp or dull, constant or intermittent
      iii. Slightly enlarged uterus
      iv. Palpable adnexal mass with pain on movement of the cervix
      v. Shoulder pain in approximately 10 to 15 per cent of patients
      vi. Laboratory data decreased hemoglobin, hematocrit, leukocytosis, positive pregnancy test
      vii. Possibly urinary frequency

2. **Biopsychosocial assessment:** Acute tubal rupture due to ectopic pregnancy: patient in shock with an acute abdominal condition
   a. Vital signs
   b. Blood: CBC, type and cross-match, Rh immediately
   c. Obtain history from patient or significant other
   d. Amount, color, and character of bleeding
   e. Emotional status of mother

PROBLEMS AND COMPLICATIONS

1. Maternal hemorrhage
2. Maternal infection
3. Fetal loss
4. Rarely, maternal death

PATIENT CARE MANAGEMENT

COMMENTS/TIPS/CAUTIONS

1. Goals:
   a. To stabilize physiological integrity of maternal system
      i. Continuously monitor vital signs

      Watch and monitor for signs of shock

      ii. Start IV with large bore catheter
      iii. Prepare for diagnostic tests or surgery
      iv. Gather laboratory data

      All laboratory work ordered stat

         (a) Blood: CBC, Rh, type cross-match
         (b) Urinalysis
      v. Diagnostic procedure if patient is not hemorrhaging

      Only if unsure of diagnosis

         1. Ultrasound
         2. Culdocentesis
      vi. Prepare for surgery if patient is hemorrhaging
         1. Insert indwelling catheter
   b. To provide emotional support to patient and family

   Patient is very uncomfortable and frightened and will require compassionate care

      i. Encourage mother and father to remain together until diagnosis is made and plans for surgery completed
      ii. Explain procedure to parents

      Information about the procedure and what is happening decreases anxiety in both mother and father

      iii. Provide comfort measures to patient

      Stay with patient and position her comfortably; explain why no food or fluid is allowed by mouth

DISCHARGE PLANNING/TEACHING

1. Possibilities of future pregnancies
2. Contraception—*not IUD*
3. Emotional support over loss
4. Help with home and family

Patients who use IUDs have a higher risk of ectopic pregnancy and therefore its use is contraindicated

HYDATIDIFORM MOLE

Hydatidiform mole is threatening to the woman because of possible hemorrhage, anemia, and hypertension and possible malignant sequelae after evacuation of the mole.

DIAGNOSIS

Hydatidiform mole consists of an abnormal placenta without a fetus or fetal tissue. The chorionic villi degenerate and become transparent vesicles containing clear fluid; they have the appearance of clusters of grapes.

1. **Incidence:** 1 in 2000 pregnancies; more frequently in older women

ETIOLOGY

1. Unknown

ASSESSMENT

1. **Clinical presentation**
   a. Signs and symptoms
      i. Vaginal bleeding in almost all patients
      ii. Hyperemesis gravidarum in 30 per cent of patients
      iii. Preeclampsia prior to 24 weeks' gestation
      iv. Hyperthyroidism in approximately 10 per cent of patients
      v. Uterus large for gestational age
      vi. Theca lutein cysts of the ovary possible
      vii. Fluid filled vesicles possibly passed with the bleeding
   b. History
      i. Excessive vomiting, hypertension, and symptoms of pre-eclampsia prior to 24 weeks' gestation; rapidly enlarging uterus

2. **Biopsychosocial assessment**
   a. Vaginal or rectal examinations contraindicated until placenta previa ruled out
   b. No FHTs
   c. Maternal vital signs
   d. Amount, color, and consistency of vaginal bleeding
   e. Palpation of abdomen for uterine tenderness

3. **Diagnostic data**
   a. Increased levels of chorionic gonadotropin after 12 weeks' gestation usually associated with hydatidiform moles
   b. Possibly decreased because of bleeding
      i. Hemoglobin and hematocrit
   c. Ultrasound to confirm diagnosis

PROBLEMS AND COMPLICATIONS

1. Hemorrhage
2. Uterine injury resulting from dilatation and curettage (D&C)
3. Infection

4. Toxemia
5. Development of choriocarcinoma

PATIENT CARE MANAGEMENT

1. Goals

  a. To maintain physiological integrity of maternal system

    i. Assess bleeding

    ii. Monitor vital signs

    iii. Perform nursing actions indicated in care of the preeclamptic patient

    iv. Intake and output

Bleeding may be severe; must watch for signs and symptoms of shock

  b. To prepare patient for surgery

    i. Obtain laboratory studies as ordered

      (a) Blood: CBC, type and cross-match, Rh

      (b) Ultrasound if condition permits

    ii. Explain surgical procedures to patient

Parents need to be together when experiencing a loss

  c. Provide psychological support

    i. Recognize the patient's loss and become involved in grief process

    ii. Allow father to spend time with mother

DISCHARGE PLANNING/TEACHING

1. Provide educational information
2. Stress importance of follow-up care
3. Teach postsurgical care
4. Provide contraceptive information
5. Long term care; subsequent pregnancy

PLACENTA PREVIA

Placenta previa results in painless bleeding in the third trimester. It is considered a grave complication of pregnancy because of the associated risks of hemorrhage and premature birth.

DIAGNOSIS

In placenta previa the placenta is attached in the lower uterine segment and wholly or partly covers the cervical os.

1. Incidence: approximately 1 in 200 deliveries

2. **Predisposing factors**
    a. Increasing age; three times more frequent at age 35 than age 25 years
    b. Increasing parity
    c. Prior uterine scar
    d. Multiple pregnancy

ETIOLOGY

1. **Unknown**

2. **Classification of placenta previa:**
    a. *Total:* the placenta completely covers the internal cervical os
    b. *Partial:* the placenta partially covers the internal cervical os
    c. *Low implantation of placenta:* the placenta encroaches on the region of the internal cervical os and can be palpated on digital exploration about the cervix but does not extend beyond the margin of the internal os

ASSESSMENT

1. **Clinical presentation**
    a. Signs and symptoms
        i. Painless bright red vaginal bleeding usually occurring after 20th week of gestation
        ii. Initial bleeding may be slight or profuse

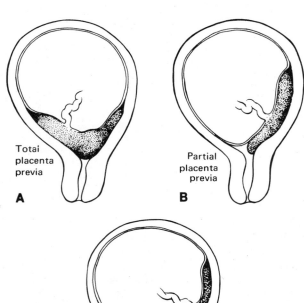

Figure 10-3. Types of placenta previa. Reprinted with permission from Danforth, D.N.: Obstetrics & Gynecology. Hagerstown, Md., Harper and Row, 1977.)

      iii. The first bleeding usually stops spontaneously but reoccurs within hours or days; each subsequent bleeding is more profuse

  b. History

      i. Unengaged presenting part or oblique or transverse lie, EDC, gravidity, parity, previous operations

2. Biopsychosocial assessment admission

  a. FHTs (rate and rhythm)

  b. Fundal height

  c. Presentation, position, and lie of fetus

  d. Number of fetuses

  e. Presence or absence of uterine contractions

  f. Vaginal and rectal examinations are absolutely contraindicated

  g. Monitor vital signs

3. Diagnostic data

  a. Decreasing hemoglobin and hematocrit

  b. Ultrasound

PROBLEMS AND COMPLICATIONS

1. Hemorrhagic shock
2. Prematurity

PATIENT CARE MANAGEMENT (depends on gestational age of fetus and amount of vaginal bleeding)

1. Goals

  a. To maintain physiological integrity of mother and fetus when bleeding is excessive

      i. Start IV with large bore catheter

      ii. Monitor vital signs of mother and fetus

      iii. Assess bleeding and pain (if present)

                                  Check for blood under patient's buttocks as well as what is visible on chux

      iv. Notify physician

        (a) Laboratory studies: Blood: CBC, type and cross-match, Rh

        (b) Prepare for cesarean birth or double setup

                                    If cervix is dilated and uterus is contracting well, occasionally a vaginal delivery will be attempted in the operating room

      i. Abdominal preparation

      ii. Foley catheter

      iii. Notify pediatrician and nursery

COMMENTS/TIPS/CAUTIONS

b. To provide emotional support to parents
   i. Explain procedures to parents
   ii. Encourage father to remain with mother as long as possible
c. To maintain physiological integrity of mother and fetus when bleeding is not excessive or there are significant risks of prematurity
   i. Complete bed rest for mother in hospital
   ii. Pad count
   iii. Physical activity should be restricted — Douching contraindicated
   iv. Vaginal examinations absolutely contraindicated
   v. Vital signs and FHTs
   vi. Palpate abdomen for contractions
   vii. Notify physician if bleeding increases
      (a) Laboratory studies: Blood: CBC, type and cross-match, Rh
      (b) Localization of placenta. Usually by ultrasonography
d. To provide emotional and educational support
   i. Explain procedures to mother and answer questions — This may be the first time patient has been hospitalized
   ii. Encourage parents to spend time together

DISCHARGE PLANNING/TEACHING

1. Diversional activities
2. Help with home and family
3. Economic support

ABRUPTIO PLACENTAE

Painful bleeding in the third trimester is considered a grave complication of pregnancy. Hemorrhagic shock, fetal death, and maternal death can occur.

DIAGNOSIS

In abruptio placentae the normally implanted placenta separates from the uterine wall prior to the third stage of labor.

1. **Incidence:**   approximately 1 in 100 deliveries; higher incidence than normal in women with previous history of placental abruption, abortion, premature labor, antepartal hemorrhage, stillbirth, or neonatal death

2. **Predisposing factors;**
   a. Preeclampsia or hypertensive disorders
   b. High multiparity
   c. Short umbilical cord
   d. Supine hypotensive syndrome
   e. Trauma
   f. Polyhydramnios
   g. Uterine anomaly

ETIOLOGY

1. **Unknown, but relationship with hypertension and increased parity**

2. **Classification of abruptio placentae**
   a. *Mild:* Vaginal bleeding less than 100 ml, uterine activity slightly increased with no FHT abnormalities present, no evidence of shock or coagulopathy
   b. *Moderate:* External bleeding 100–500 ml; increased uterine tone; mild shock; FHTs present or absent; if present may show evidence of fetal distress
   c. *Severe:* External bleeding greater than 500 ml; bleeding may be completely concealed; uterus firm and contracted; moderate to severe shock; fetal death, coagulopathy frequent

ASSESSMENT

1. **Clinical presentation**
   a. Signs and symptoms
      i.   External blood loss (note amount, color, consistency of blood)
      ii. Pain (note onset, duration, and location)
      iii. Abdominal irritability or rigidity and relaxation between contractions
      iv. Maternal vital signs decreased
      v.   FHTs weak or absent
      vi. Increasing fundal height with concealed hemorrhage
   b. History
      i.   Review chart for predisposing factors; review present and prenatal history

2. **Biopsychosocial assessment**
   a. FHTs rate and rhythm
   b. Fundal height

    c. Presentation, position, and lie of fetus

    d. Number of fetuses

    e. Presence or absence of uterine contractions

    f. Vaginal examinations are absolutely contraindicated unless placenta previa has been ruled out

3. Diagnostic data

    a. Ultrasonography to locate placenta

PROBLEMS AND COMPLICATIONS

1. Hemorrhagic shock
2. Fetal death
3. Disseminated intravascular coagulopathy

PATIENT CARE MANAGEMENT

1. Goals

    a. To maintain physiological integrity of mother and fetus when bleeding is severe

      i. Start IV with large bore catheter

      ii. Monitor vital signs of mother and fetus

                           FHTs should be electronically monitored

      iii. Assess bleeding and tolerance to pain

      iv. Prepare for impending surgery

                           May transfer to labor and delivery if condition is stable and until physician arrives

      v. Notify physician

        (a) Laboratory studies: Blood: CBC, type and cross-match, Rh, coagulation studies

      vi. Prepare for cesarean birth

        (a) Abdominal preparation

        (b) Foley catheter

        (c) Notify pediatrician and nursery

    b. To provide emotional support to parents

      i. Explain procedures to parents

                           Do not leave mother alone, she needs nurse's support

      ii. Encourage father to stay with mother as long as possible

COMMENTS/TIPS/CAUTIONS

DISCHARGE PLANNING/TEACHING

1. Long term emotional support, if loss
2. Help with home and family

HEMOLYTIC INCOMPATIBILITY

When a pregnant woman becomes sensitized to produce immunoglobulin G (IgG) antibodies against fetal antigens of the ABO or Rh system, erythrocyte destruction occurs in the fetus and could lead to fetal death.

DIAGNOSIS

In hemolytic incompatibility rising antibody titers may be indicative of Rh sensitization. Maternal titers alone do not accurately reflect the severity of fetal involvement.

1. Rh and ABO blood group antigens account for approximately 98 per cent of all cases of erythroblastosis fetalis
2. The treatment remains the same for severe incompatibility of Rh and ABO
3. Rh incompatibility occurs when the mother is Rh negative and fetus is Rh positive
4. ABO incompatibility occurs when the mother's blood is O positive and that of the fetus is either A or B
5. Hemolytic disease is seen in only about 10 per cent of all cases of ABO incompatibility

ETIOLOGY

1. Antibodies in the mother cross the placenta and enter the fetal vascular system and destroy the fetal antigens of the Rh or ABO system; fetal erythrocyte hemolysis results, causing fetal anemia, congestive heart failure, edema, and ascites

ASSESSMENT

1. **Clinical presentation**
   a. Signs and symptoms
      i. Rising antibody titers in the mother
   b. History
      i. The mother is Rh negative and previously has delivered an Rh positive infant, had an abortion, ectopic pregnancy, or blood transfusion
2. **Biopsychosocial assessment**
   a. Mother at no physiological risk
   b. Assess psychological and emotional status resulting from concerns for fetal welfare
   c. Assess understanding of amniocentesis
   d. Assess FHTs
3. **Diagnostic data**
   a. Amniocentesis
   b. Ultrasonography

PROBLEMS AND COMPLICATIONS

1. Fetal death occurs when erythrocyte destruction becomes extreme

PATIENT CARE MANAGEMENT

1. Goals

a. To provide information about diagnostic tests
   i. Explain ultrasound
   ii. Explain amniocentesis
   iii. Assess fetal status
   iv. Monitor FHTs prior to and immediately after amniocentesis

> COMMENTS/TIPS/CAUTIONS
>
> Knowledge about procedures performed will lower anxiety level of patient

b. To provide emotional support
   i. Encourage parents to be together during hospitalization
   ii. Encourage parents to talk about their fears

> Support family centered maternity care

DISCHARGE PLANNING/TEACHING

1. Help with home and family
2. Subsequent pregnancies
3. Care through remainder of this pregnancy

———— DISSEMINATED INTRAVASCULAR COAGULOPATHY ————

Disseminated intravascular coagulopathy (DIC), a condition that is life threatening to the mother, results from excessive bleeding, usually in the second or third stage of labor.

DIAGNOSIS

DIC may occur after severe hemorrhage due to abruptio placentae, the dead fetus syndrome, amniotic embolism, septic abortion, septic shock, or preeclampsia.

1. Incidence
   a. Unknown
2. Predisposing factors
   a. Abruptio placentae
   b. Intrauterine fetal death with retention of placenta
   c. Preeclampsia
   d. Amniotic fluid embolism

ETIOLOGY

The coagulation process is affected through alterations of the blood clotting mechanisms, and the blood loses its ability to clot.

ASSESSMENT

1. Clinical presentation

    a. Signs and symptoms
      i. Bleeding from site of the IV needle
      ii. Multiple ecchymoses
      iii. Impending shock
    b. History
      i. Any of the above predisposing factors
2. Biopsychosocial assessment
    a. Signs of shock
    b. Bleeding and ecchymosis
    c. Assess emotional status if patient is conscious
3. Diagnostic data
    a. Hypofibrinogenemia
    b. Decreased platelet count
    c. Abnormal thrombin time, prothrombin time (PT), and partial thromboplastin time (PTT)
    d. Increase of fibrin split products and fibrinogen split products

PROBLEMS AND COMPLICATIONS

1. Hemorrhagic shock
2. Transfusion incompatibilities

TABLE 10-1. SYMPTOMS OF SHOCK

	Mild	Moderate	Severe	Irreversible
Respirations	Rapid, deep	Rapid, becoming shallow	Rapid, shallow, may be irregular	Irregular, or barely perceptible
Pulse	Rapid, tone normal	Rapid, tone may be normal but is becoming weaker	Very rapid, easily collapsible, may be irregular	Irregular apical pulse
Blood pressure	Normal or hypertensive	60–90 mm Hg systolic	Below 60 mm Hg systolic	None palpable
Skin	Cool and pale	Cool, pale, moist, knees cyanotic	Cold, clammy, cyanosis of lips and fingernails	Cold, clammy, cyanotic
Urine output	No change	Decreasing to 10–22 cc/hr adult	Oliguric (less than 10 cc) to anuria	Anuric
Level of consciousness	Alert, oriented, diffuse anxiety	Oriented, mental cloudiness or increasing restlessness	Lethargy, reacts to noxious stimuli, comatose	Does not respond to noxious stimuli
CVP	May be normal	3 cm H_2O	0–3 cm H_2O	

Adapted by Clark, A.L., and Affonso, D.D.: Childbearing: A Nursing Perspective, 2nd ed., Philadelphia, F.A. Davis Co., from M.M. Wagner, *in* Royce, J.: Shock: emergency nursing implications. Nurs. Clin. North Am. *8*:380, 1973.

3. Infection
4. Possible maternal death

PATIENT CARE MANAGEMENT

1. **Goals**
   a. To maintain physiological integrity of the mother
      i. Monitor vital signs
      ii. Assist with blood transfusions
      iii. Administer O_2 to mother
      iv. Stabilize mother's condition and prepare for transfer to high risk center
      v. Monitor input and output
      vi. Assist with treatment of underlying disorder, which will arrest the process of DIC
   b. To provide information and support to the family

DISCHARGE PLANNING/TEACHING

1. Help with home and family
2. Long term care

—————————— HYPEREMESIS GRAVIDARUM ——————————

Hyperemesis gravidarum is a risk to both mother and fetus when systemic effects of ketonuria and weight loss lead to dire circumstances such as hypovolemia, dehydration, and death of mother and fetus.

DIAGNOSIS

Hyperemesis gravidarum, or pernicious vomiting of pregnancy, results in dehydration, starvation, and electrolyte imbalance.

ETIOLOGY

1. Unknown; theories proposed
   a. High level of chorionic gonadotropins create an endocrine imbalance
   b. Disturbances of metabolic changes of pregnancy
   c. Decreased gastric motility of pregnancy
   d. Disturbances related to psychological adjustments of pregnancy and the role of mothering

ASSESSMENT

1. **Clinical presentation**
   a. Signs and symptoms
      i. Persistent vomiting after eating
      ii. Weight loss
      iii. Electrolyte imbalance
      iv. Ketonuria
      v. Dehydration with decreased urine output
      vi. Hypovolemia

   b. History
       i. Unplanned or undesired pregnancy; family, financial, or social problems

2. Biopsychosocial assessment
   a. Monitor vital signs
   b. Monitor input and output, including emesis
   c. Evaluate relationships with others

3. Diagnostic data
   a. Ketonuria
   b. Increased specific gravity of urine
   c. Increased hematocrit
   d. Increased BUN
   e. Hyponatremia
   f. Hypokalemia
   g. Hypochloremia
   h. Metabolic alkalosis
   i. Mild increase in bilirubin and liver function

PROBLEMS AND COMPLICATIONS
1. Electrolyte imbalance
2. Ketonuria
3. Dehydration
4. Renal problems
5. Hypovolemia

PATIENT CARE MANAGEMENT

1. Goals

COMMENTS/TIPS/CAUTIONS

   a. To maintain physiological integrity of maternal system with prompt treatment, prognosis is good.
       i. Correct hypovolemia, electrolyte imbalance, and ketosis with IV fluids
       ii. Record input and output
       iii. Daily weight
       iv. Nothing by mouth initially
       v. Provide vitamins and calories to maintain nutrition
       vi. Monitor FHTs with Doppler
       vii. Control environment
       viii. Provide quiet, well ventilated room
       ix. Limit visitors
       x. Offer emotional support
       xi. Recognition of underlying emotional disturbance
       xii. Assess patient's ability to accept pregnancy

To aid in fluid status assessment after vomiting has ceased, begin giving water by mouth and advance diet slowly

After 14 weeks' gestation

Odors from smoking and food may aggravate the vomiting

DISCHARGE PLANNING/TEACHING

1. Diet and vitamins
2. Economic support as needed
3. Help with home and family

——————————— ACUTE PYELONEPHRITIS ———————————

Acute pyelonephritis associated with pregnancy is a serious complication jeopardizing the health of the mother and fetus, requiring hospitalization and intensive treatment.

DIAGNOSIS

Acute pyelonephritis is an infection of the upper urinary tract involving the renal pelvis, renal parenchyma, and the ureter.

1. Incidence
   a. Occurs in 1 to 4 per cent of all pregnant women
   b. May occur in any trimester

ETIOLOGY

1. Usually an ascending infection from symptomatic or asymptomatic bacteriuria
2. The right ureter is compressed during pregnancy as the result of the dextrorotation of the uterus, and compression of the ureter at the pelvic brim causes stasis and slight obstruction of the ureter
3. Causative organisms are usually gram negative organisms normally found in intestine and vagina

ASSESSMENT

1. Clinical presentation
   a. Signs and symptoms
      i. High spiking temperature
      ii. Positive CVAT
      iii. Chills
      iv. Anorexia
      v. Malaise
      vi. Abdominal distention
   b. History
      i. Previous or recurrent symptomatic or asymptomatic bacteriuria, poor feminine hygiene, debility, EDC
2. Biopsychosocial assessment (admission)
   a. Assessment of maternal vital signs
   b. FHTs
   c. Uterine irritability
   d. Input and output
   e. Status of hydration
   f. Degree of pain tolerance

   g. Emotional status
   h. Family situation
3. **Diagnostic data:**
   a. Colony count greater than 100,000
   b. Pus cells in urinary sediment
   c. Increased WBC, and RBC in urine
   d. Proteinuria
   e. CVAT
   f. Increased temperature
   g. Acutely ill appearance

PROBLEMS AND COMPLICATIONS
1. Premature labor
2. High rate of relapse or reinfection
3. Fetal growth retardation or fetal death possible

PATIENT CARE MANAGEMENT
1. **Goals**
   a. To maintain physiological integrity of maternal and fetal systems

      COMMENTS/TIPS/ CAUTIONS

      i. Bed rest with left lateral position

         Minimize obstructive effect of the gravid uterus

      ii. Start IV and add antibiotics per physician's order

         The mother's temperature can reach high limits, and the fetal core temperature is greater than the mother's

      iii. Control temperature with analgesics, antipyretics, and cool sponge baths

      iv. Increase fluids and maintain high urine flow

         To prevent stasis of urine and combat dehydration caused by elevated temperature

      v. Record input and output

         Keep accurate output charts

   b. To provide psychological support
      i. Allow parents to remain together
      ii. Explain procedures and rationale for treatment
      iii. Monitor FHTs

DISCHARGE PLANNING/TEACHING
1. Home care
2. Help with home and family
3. Diversional activities

_____ GENITAL HERPES SIMPLEX VIRAL INFECTION _____

   Genital herpes simplex may necessitate hospitalization during pregnancy if primary or recurrent infection is so severe that excretion of urine is impeded or if pain is so severe that the mother cannot rest. Active infection at the time of delivery can lead to herpes infection in the neonate.

DIAGNOSIS

In herpes genital infection painful lesions on the cervix, labia, or perineum are caused by the herpesvirus and spread by direct person to person contact.

1. **Incidence**
   a. Occurring in epidemic proportions in the general population
   b. The second most common venereal disease, surpassed only by gonorrhea
   c. Occurs in 1 per cent of pregnant females

ETIOLOGY

1. Caused by type I or type II herpesvirus through direct person to person contact
2. Primary lesions appear 2 to 7 days after exposure
3. Fluid filled vesicles can be located on the labia, cervix, vagina, or perineum
4. Illness lasts for 7 to 10 days
5. Pregnant females infected for first time shed virus for 8 to 100 days; patients with recurrences shed virus for 6 to 40 days

ASSESSMENT

1. **Clinical presentation**
   a. Signs and symptoms
      i. Fluid filled vesicles on perineum or labia rupture, forming painful shallow ulcers
      ii. Low grade fever
      iii. Malaise
      iv. Regional adenopathy
      v. Secondary infection of the open lesions may occur, causing erythema and edema around the painful ulcers
   b. History
      i. Usually in young primigravidas; may also have Trichomonas vaginal infection, gonorrhea, or Candida infection

2. **Biopsyhosocial assessment (admission)**
   a. Urinary retention
   b. Extent of edema and inflammation of perineal area
   c. Amount, type, and character of pain
   d. Nutritional status
   e. Vital signs
   f. Emotional state
   g. Educational needs

3. **Diagnostic data**
   a. Tissue culture
   b. Papanicolaou smear

PROBLEMS AND COMPLICATIONS

1. Herpetic infections are associated with increased incidence of abortion and premature delivery
2. If infection is active at term, cesarean section (C/S) delivery is necessary

3. Herpes simplex is transferred to neonate at time of delivery and can be fatal to the newborn
4. Direct fetal scalp monitoring should not be done when mother has had herpes simplex

PATIENT CARE MANAGEMENT

1. Goals

  a. To maintain physiological integrity of maternal system
    i. Monitor urinary output; catheterize if necessary
    ii. Vital signs
    iii. Monitor fluid intake

Temperature elevation usually not very high

  b. To provide comfort measures for pain
    i. Sitz bath qid
    ii. Analgesics for pain
  c. To minimize transmission to health care providers and other patients

Herpetic whitlow is a common complication for health care providers

    i. Use gloves when examining infected area
    ii. Mark all patient utensils, especially sitz bath

DISCHARGE PLANNING/TEACHING

1. Provide educational information to patients
2. Advise against sexual contact when herpes is active
3. Instruct her to inform sexual partners of infection that occurred previously
4. Recurrent infection may be triggered by exposure to sun, local trauma, sexual intercourse, emotional stress, or compromised physical state
5. Acyclovir, a new drug, reduces viral growth and speeds healing of lesions; however, it is not known to be safe during pregnancy

This drug is not a cure for herpes

PREGNANCY INDUCED HYPERTENSION

Pregnancy induced hypertension (PIH) can be life threatening to the fetus and mother; it is often managed by the nurse under the direction of the physician.

DIAGNOSIS

Pregnancy induced hypertension is persistently high BP with elevation to 140/90 or greater or a systolic rise of 30 mm Hg and diastolic rise of 15 mm Hg above the prepregnant BP on two or more occasions 4 hours apart. This BP rise may be accompanied by proteinuria and generalized edema associated with rapid weight gain.

1. **Incidence**
   a. More common in primigravidas
2. Occurs after the week 20 of gestation
3. Occurs in 3 to 4 per cent of all pregnancies
4. Predisposing factors
   a. Family history of hypertension or vascular disease
   b. Obesity or undernutrition
   c. Age extremes in women less than 20 years old and greater than 35 years old
   d. Women with diagnosis of PIH in previous pregnancies
   e. Diabetic mothers
   f. Women with multiple fetuses, hydramnios, hydatidiform mole, large fetus, or fetal hydrops

ETIOLOGY

1. The exact cause is unknown.
2. **Classification of preeclampsia and eclampsia**
   a. *Mild:* mean arterial pressure (MAP) is less than 106 mm Hg (140/90) with an increase in diastolic pressure of more than 20 mm of Hg on two occasions 6 hours apart with the patient at bed rest; proteinuria, edema, or both develop; this definition requires accurate knowledge of the patient's BP readings prior to pregnancy
   b. *Moderate:* MAP is greater than 106 mm Hg (140/90) and less than 126 mm Hg (160/110), or a rise in BP is greater than 30 mm Hg systolic or 20 mm Hg diastolic; this increase in BP is combined with appreciable proteinuria, whereas edema of the lower extremities is usually, but not always, present
   c. *Severe:* MAP exceeds 126 mm Hg (160/110) on at least two occasions 6 hours apart with the patient at bed rest, and urinary protein is greater than 5 gm/24 hours; usually accompanied by headaches and blurred vision; if right upper quadrant or epigastric pain, oliguria, pulmonary edema, or visual or cerebral disturbances occur, severe disease is present; edema of the face, hands, and lower extremities is usually present
   d. *Eclampsia:* this consists of generalized seizures accompanied by hypertension and proteinuria in a pregnant patient; other causes of seizure must be excluded; the seizures may occur postpartally as well as antepartally

ASSESSMENT

1. **Clinical presentation**
   a. Signs and symptoms
      i. Mild-moderate
         (a) Elevation in BP according to above classification
         (b) Proteinuria
         (c) Edema
         (d) Rapid weight gain
      ii. Severe
         (a) Headache
         (b) Visual disturbances
         (c) Epigastric pain
         (d) Hyperreflexia
         (e) Clonus
         (f) Oliguria
         (g) Pulmonary edema
   b. History
      i. Persistent rise in BP above prepregnant levels, prior preeclampsia, funduscopic changes, EDC

2. **Biopsychosocial assessment (admission)**
   a. Blood pressure, TPR
   b. Proteinuria
   c. Edema, degree and location
   d. Weight
   e. Funduscopic changes
   f. Reflex response
   g. Input and output
   h. Mother's emotional status
   i. FHTs
   j. Fundal height: estimated gestational age
   k. Status of membranes

3. **Diagnostic data**
   a. Blood: CBC. Hematocrit may be high because of hypovolemia
   b. Liver enzymes: Should not be increased
   c. 24 hour urine collection for total protein: Total protein should be less than 300 mg/24 hours in normal pregnancy
   d. BUN and serum creatinine
   e. Tests for fetal well-being
      i. Non-stress test: FHR acceleration in response to fetal movements are a reflection of fetal well-being
      ii. Ultrasonography: Determines fetal age, growth, and amount of amniotic fluid and placental location
      iii. Amniocentesis: With worsening PIH to determine the lecithin-sphingomyelin (L/S) ratio for fetal lung maturity

PROBLEMS AND COMPLICATIONS

1. PIH progressing to eclampsia
2. Renal cortical necrosis
3. Hepatic rupture

4. Cerebral hemorrhage
5. Pulmonary edema
6. DIC

PATIENT CARE MANAGEMENT

1. **Goals**
   a. To maintain the physiological integrity of the maternal fetal unit in mild to moderate and severe hypertension

   i. Control the environment for adequate rest

   Limit visitors to family only

   ii. Bed rest in left lateral position

   To decrease pressure on vena cava and increase circulation to uterus

   iii. High protein diet with recommended dietary allowance of (RDA) sodium

   Placenta protein needs replacement because of loss in urine, and restriction of sodium is nontherapeutic

   iv. Maintain fluid intake at 6 to 8 glasses per day

   v. Monitor vital signs q 4 h FHTs if no labor q 8 h

   vi. Daily weight

   vii. Prepare for diagnostic tests and explain procedures

   Medication is usually not prescribed for mild-moderate PIH

   (a) 24 hour urine: Follow procedure as given in hospital laboratory manual

   (b) Schedule ultrasound, non-stress test, and amniocentesis as ordered by physician

   b. To provide emotional support to parents in mild to moderate and severe hypertension

   i. Explain procedures and answer questions

   Decrease fears and anxieties related to tests

   ii. Investigate support system

   If additional problems arise with family the nurse may become involved with family in problem solving

   c. To maintain in addition to the above for severe pregnancy induced hypertension

   i. Seizure precautions, i.e., quiet room, padded tongue blade that is easily accessible

   ii. Adequate hydration; usually patient is receiving an IV

   IV for administration of magnesium sulfate ($MgSO_4$); see procedure for administration of $MgSO_4$; antidote for $MgSO_4$ is calcium gluconate

   iii. Monitor medicinal therapy

  d. To protect patient from injury in eclampsia, a dangerous condition manifested by convulsions and possibly leading to coma

    i. Insert padded tongue blade between patient's teeth to avoid tongue injury

    ii. Maintain side rails in up position and pad with blankets

    iii. Maintain oral airway

    iv. Suction secretion from oral pharynx

    v. Insert oral airway after convulsion terminates

    vi. Support medicinal therapy

    vii. Assist physician to administer drugs

    viii. Physiological management the same as for mild to moderate PIH

COMMENTS/TIPS/CAUTIONS

Tape padded tongue blade to wall at head of bed

Time convulsion; do not leave patient during convulsion

DISCHARGE PLANNING/TEACHING

1. Meet educational needs of mother
   a. Provide nutritional counseling
   b. Instruct regarding signs and symptoms of severe PIH
2. Opportunities for rest
3. Help with home and family
4. Financial support if necessary

DIABETES MELLITUS

Diabetes mellitus associated with pregnancy is a significant factor contributing to perinatal loss or morbidity.

DIAGNOSIS

In diabetes mellitus glucose is unable to enter body cells because of the lack of insulin. This is characterized by hyperglycemia and glycosuria and long term degenerative changes in the vascular system of the body.

1. **Incidence: diabetes (overt or gestational) is reported to complicate 2 to 3 per cent of all pregnancies**

2. **Perinatal mortality is 4 to 5 times higher than in normal pregnancies**

3. **Predisposing factors**
   a. Mother with a family history of diabetes
   b. Obesity
   c. Mother over 40 years of age
   d. Multiparity

ETIOLOGY

1. The exact cause is unknown; it is probably a multifactorial disease
2. Pregnancy is known to unmask diabetes in predisposed individuals; in addition to the predisposing factors listed above, the following may constitute a high risk pregnancy
   a. Glycosuria on two successive occasions
   b. Prior delivery of an infant 9 pounds or greater
   c. Previous stillbirth or infant with congenital anomaly
   d. History of presence of hydramnios
   e. Recurrent Candida infections
3. **White's classification of diabetes[4]**
   a. *Class A:* diabetes appearing during pregnancy but absent in the nonpregnant state (most often restricted to patients with abnormal glucose tolerance tests (GTT) and excluding those with elevated fasting blood sugar (FBS) levels.
   b. *Class B:* Overt diabetes, onset after age 20 years, duration less than 10 years; no vascular disease
   c. *Class C:* Onset between age of 10 and 20 years or duration 10–19 years; no vascular disease
   d. *Class D:* Onset before age of 10 years or duration more than 10 years; benign retinopathy
   e. *Class E:* Calicification present in pelvic vessels (this category no longer used by most authorities)
   f. *Class F:* Diabetic nephropathy (proteinuria, decreased creatinine clearance)
   g. *Class R:* Proliferative retinopathy
   h. *Class RF:* Nephropathy plus retinopathy
   i. *Class H:* Arteriosclerotic heart disease

ASSESSMENT

1. **Clinical presentation**
   a. Signs and symptoms
      i. Polydipsia, polyphagia, polyuria
      ii. Weight loss
      iii. Blurred vision
      iv. Orthostatic dizziness
      v. FBS greater than 120 mg/100 ml.
   b. History. See Diagnosis: Predisposing Factors, and Etiology
2. **Biopsychosocial assessment (admission)**
   a. Assess classification of diabetes
   b. Review antepartal history for predisposing factors
   c. Review antepartal record for

   i. Gestational age
   ii. Presence of glycosuria, ketonuria, or proteinuria
   iii. Baseline vital signs
   iv. Results of FBS or GTT
   v. Funduscopic changes
  d. Assess dietary intake
  e. Assess insulin requirements
  f. Assess patient's knowledge of condition and reason for hospitalization
  g. Assess mother's emotional status
  h. Assess FHTs if gestation greater than 14 weeks

3. Diagnostic data
  a. FBS and 2 hour postprandial blood sugar tests
  b. Check urine for glucose and ketones
  c. Oral or IV GTT

PROBLEMS AND COMPLICATIONS

1. Increased incidence of abortion in early pregnancy
2. Increased incidence of preeclampsia
3. Increased incidence of perinatal mortality and morbidity such as stillbirth, respiratory distress syndrome, congenital anomalies, and birth trauma due to macrosomia

PATIENT CARE MANAGEMENT

1. Goals

  a. To determine the dietary needs of the mother in early pregnancy
   i. Provide dietary counseling
   ii. Monitor blood sugar and urine sugar
   iii. Calculate daily insulin requirements if needed

  b. To provide education in early pregnancy to patient and family concerning diabetes and pregnancy
   i. Explain signs of hypoglycemia and hyperglycemia
   ii. If insulin is necessary, teach patient how to administer.
   iii. Prepare patient for management of pregnancy in last trimester

COMMENTS/TIPS/CAUTIONS

Weekly visits to obstetrician for non-stress tests, ultrasound, and amniocentesis

   iv. Be an active listener and investigate fears and anxieties expressed by patients

c. To schedule diagnostic tests and report results to physician in early pregnancy

    i. Prepare for tests and explain procedures

d. To manage most class A and well controlled class B and C diabetics in third trimester of pregnancy on an outpatient basis unless complications develop

    i. Uncomplicated class A diabetics at 40 weeks' gestation

        (a) Weekly OCT

        (b) Serum or 24 hour urine estriol determination two or three times a week

        (c) Fetal movement records

These are all tests for fetal well-being

    ii. Uncomplicated class B and C diabetics; intensive fetal surveillance should begin at 32 weeks' gestation

        (a) Weekly OCT

        (b) Fetal movement counts

        (c) Serum and urinary estriol determination three times a week

        (d) Admit to hospital near term

These can be done on an outpatient basis

e. To determine fetal maturity prior to delivery (through L/S ratio obtained by amniocentesis)

L/S ratio of 2 or greater indicates fetal lung maturity and delivery is usually scheduled

DISCHARGE PLANNING/TEACHING

1. Dietary counseling
2. Emotional support
3. Financial support if needed
4. Help with home and family

HEART DISEASE

Heart disease is considered a major risk factor during pregnancy because it is the fourth leading cause of maternal morbidity.

DIAGNOSIS

Congestive heart failure demonstrates that the maternal heart can no longer meet the demands of pregnancy.

1. Incidence
   a. Has decreased in the past several decades as a result of antibiotic therapy and modern cardiovascular surgery to repair congenital defects
   b. Occurs in patients with previously diagnosed rheumatic fever

ETIOLOGY

1. Classification for the severity of heart disease by the New York Heart Association (Table 10–2)

ASSESSMENT

1. Clinical presentation
   a. Signs and symptoms
      i. Rales heard at the base of the lung with a stethoscope
      ii. Progressive generalized edema
      iii. Dyspnea upon exertion
      iv. Frequent cough (with or without hemoptysis)

TABLE 10–2.   CLASSIFICATION FOR THE SEVERITY OF CARDIAC DISEASE*

Classification	Criteria—Patient Behaviors
Class I	No limitation on physical activities. Normal physical activity causes no discomforts. No symptoms of cardiac insufficiency or anginal pain
Class II	Slight limitation on physical activities. Normal physical activity causes fatigue, dyspnea, or anginal pain.
Class III	Moderate to marked limitation of physical activity. Less than ordinary activity creates excessive fatigue, palpitation, dyspnea, or angina pain.
Class IV	Unable to carry out physical activity without experiencing discomforts, symptoms of cardiac insufficiency, or angina pain even at rest

Women in classes I and II usually emerge with a normal childbearing experience while those in classes III and IV are more vulnerable to complications.

*Excerpted from Diseases of the Heart and Blood Vessels—Nomenclature and Criteria for Diagnosis, 5th ed. Boston, Little, Brown and Company, copyright 1955 by the New York Heart Association, Inc. These classifications are not included in the 7th ed., revised 1973, or the 8th ed., revised 1979.

        v. Episodes of palpitations
       vi. Difficulty in breathing or sense of smothering
  b. History
        i. Rheumatic fever or rheumatic heart disease, congenital heart defects, or cardiac surgery

2. **Biopsychosocial assessment**
  a. Antepartal history, EDC, gestational age
  b. Complications of pregnancy
  c. Current medications
  d. Admission vital signs
  e. FHTs
  f. Emotional status and anxiety
  g. Physical examinations
        i. Heart and lung sounds
       ii. Dyspnea
      iii. Presence of cough
      iv. Presence of edema

3. **Diagnostic data**
  a. ECG
  b. Chest roentgenogram

PROBLEMS AND COMPLICATIONS

1. Progressive congestive heart failure
2. Premature delivery
3. Infection
4. Fetal anoxia resulting from maternal anoxia
5. Increased incidence of intrauterine growth retardation

PATIENT CARE MANAGEMENT

1. **Goals**
  a. To maintain the physiological requirements of the mother
        i. Administer O_2
       ii. Promote rest
      iii. Provide adequate nutrition and fluids
      iv. Protect from infection
  b. To monitor fetal well-being
        i. FHTs
       ii. Non-stress test

COMMENTS/TIPS/CAUTIONS

Quiet environment; limit visitors to family members
Increase protein and iron when not in acute distress; additional energy required to combat infection

DISCHARGE PLANNING/TEACHING

1. Meet educational needs
2. Explain need for frequent rest
3. Teach mother to avoid anything that requires sudden increase in cardiac output

4. Help with home and family
5. Information regarding subsequent pregnancies
6. Diet
7. Financial support, if needed

MULTIPLE PREGNANCY

Multiple pregnancy carries an increased risk of prenatal mortality and morbidity for the mother and the fetus.

DIAGNOSIS

In multiple pregnancy two or more embryos develop in the uterus at the same time.

1. Incidence
   a. White race, 1 in 95 pregnancies
   b. Black race, 1 in 78 pregnancies
2. Predisposing factors:
   a. Woman a twin
   b. Increased age
   c. Increased parity
   d. Endogenous gonadotropin
   e. Infertility drugs

ETIOLOGY

1. Monozygotic twins develop from one ovum and one sperm and divide into two identical parts
2. Dizygotic twins develop from two ova and two sperm

ASSESSMENT

1. Clinical presentation
   a. Signs and symptoms
      i. Uterus large for gestational age
      ii. Two fetuses are palpable
      iii. Two fetal heart tones heard
      iv. Hydramnios
   b. History
      i. Family history of twins, excessive weight gain, hydramnios
      ii. Increased evidence of preeclampsia, lower extremity edema, anemia, hemorrhoids, varicosities
2. Biopsychosocial assessment
   a. Review antepartal record on admission
   b. Maternal vital signs
   c. Emotional status
   d. Nutritional status

    e. FHTs

    f. Status of membranes

3. Diagnostic data (if twin pregnancy not confirmed)
   a. Ultrasound

PROBLEMS OR COMPLICATIONS

1. Anemia
2. Pregnancy induced hypertension
3. Hydramnios
4. Premature delivery
5. Difficult delivery
6. Possible cesarean section

PATIENT CARE MANAGEMENT

1. Goals

    a. To maintain physiological integrity of maternal system

        i. Provide rest — *Control environment so patient can get rest*

        ii. Monitor vital signs

        iii. Meet nutritional needs — *Six small meals tolerated better than three large meals*

    b. To maintain physiological integrity of fetal system

        i. Monitor FHTs every 4 hours unless mother is sleeping

        ii. Meet the educational needs of mother — *Prepare mother for care of two infants*

        iii. Meet the emotional needs of the mother — *Prepare for labor; encourage father to be supportive during labor and delivery*

COMMENTS/TIPS/CAUTIONS

DISCHARGE PLANNING/TEACHING

1. Help with home and family
2. Financial support if needed
3. Long range planning for babies

ANEMIAS

    Hereditary anemias such as sickle cell anemia and sickle cell–hemoglobin C disease (SC anemia) are complicated by pregnancy and place the patient at risk.

DIAGNOSIS

Sickle Cell Disease

    In sickle cell anemia the inheritance pattern (SS) is homozygous; erythrocytes become sickle shaped and have decreased O_2 carrying capacity. It occurs in 0.7 per cent of the American black population.

Sickle Cell Trait

In sickle cell trait the inheritance pattern is heterozygous; AS hemoglobin is present. It is present in 8.4 per cent of the American black population.

Sickle Cell–Hemoglobin C

In sickle cell–hemoglobin C disease (SC) the inheritance pattern is heterozygous. It occurs in 0.15 per cent of the American black population.

The disease is quiescent in the nonpregnant state but gives rise suddenly in pregnancy to a variety of complications, namely, hemolytic crisis, particularly in the third trimester, marked by bone pain and sudden death.

ETIOLOGY

All three anemias are caused by inheritance patterns.
1. Patients with SC disease may be symptom free until pregnancy occurs.
2. Mothers with AS hemoglobin usually do not have a crisis but are more prone to urinary tract infection and pyelonephritis.

ASSESSMENT

1. **Clinical presentation (hemolytic crisis)**
   a. Signs and symptoms
      i. Marked bone pain and abdominal pain
      ii. Hemoptysis
      iii. Hematuria
      iv. Fever and chills
   b. History
      i. SS Hemoglobin, SC hemoglobin

2. **Biopsychosocial assessment**
   a. Review prenatal record for EDC; hemoglobin electrophoresis; gestational age; fundal height; vital signs; previous complications of pregnancy
   b. Review prenatal laboratory data
   c. Assess pain and vital signs, especially temperature
   d. Assess emotional status of mother
   e. Assess for skin hemorrhages and jaundice
   f. Assess fetal status—FHTs

3. **Diagnostic data**
   a. Hemoglobin electrophoresis
   b. Blood: CBC, type and cross-match, Rh

PROBLEMS AND COMPLICATIONS

1. Abortion
2. Premature birth
3. Fetal death

PATIENT CARE MANAGEMENT

1. Goals

a. To maintain the physiological integrity of the maternal system

  i. Assist with transfusion of packed cells

  ii. Provide adequate rest

  iii. Administer O_2

  iv. Encourage proper nutritional intake

  v. Protect against infection

b. To meet educational and emotional needs of family

  i. Information about disorder

  ii. Emotional support

COMMENTS/TIPS/CAUTIONS

Signs and symptoms of transfusion reaction
1. Urticaria
2. Dyspnea
3. Cyanosis
4. Chills
5. Nausea and vomiting
STOP transfusion at once if these occur.

DISCHARGE PLANNING/TEACHING

1. Diet, vitamins
2. Help with home and family
3. Financial assistance, if needed
4. Subsequent pregnancies

CONCLUSIONS

The primary responsibility of the nurse during an antepartal crisis is to stabilize the physiological systems of the mother and fetus. Basic nursing knowledge is necessary and must be practiced safely before the nurse attempts to provide more advanced nursing management. Once the physiological needs have been met, the nurse must focus her attention on the psychological, emotional, and educative needs of the patient. In many circumstances these needs are not adequately addressed, and no interpretations are provided the patient or family regarding the reason for procedures that are performed or diagnostic studies ordered. Both the mother and her significant others have a right to an explanation regarding their care in the hospital. The ultimate goal in managing an antepartal crisis is to provide safe nursing care to both mother and fetus with inclusion of the father of the baby in the care as much as possible.

REFERENCES

1. Bettoli, E.: Herpes: Facts and fallacies. Am. J. Nurs., 82:924-929, 1982.
2. Clark, A.L., and Affonso, D.D.: Childbearing: A Nursing Perspective, 2nd ed. Philadelphia, F.A. Davis Co., 1979.
3. Danforth, D.N.: Obstetrics and Gynecology. Hagerstown, MD., Harper & Row, 1977.
4. Niswander, K.R.: Manual of Obstetrics. Boston, Little, Brown & Co., 1980.
5. Perez, R.H.: Protocols for Perinatal Nursing Practice. St. Louis, C.V. Mosby Co., 1981.
6. Reeder, S.J., Mastroianni, L., and Martin, L.L.: Maternity Nursing. Philadelphia, F.A. Davis Co., 1979.
7. Sharp, E.S., and Willis, S.E.: Hypertension in pregnancy: Prenatal detection and management. Am. J. Nurs., 82:798-808, 1982.
8. Willis, S.E.: Hypertension in pregnancy: Pathophysiology. Am. J. Nurs., 82:792-797, 1982.

CHAPTER 11

INTRAPARTUM CRISES

Sherry A. Gillespie, R.N., M.S.N.

OBJECTIVES

Upon completion of this chapter the reader will be able to accomplish the following:

1. List the parameters to be assessed for every woman admitted to labor and delivery

2. Discuss the hypertensive disorders of pregnancy and their management during the intrapartum period

3. Discuss the five major complications of labor and their management during the intrapartum period

4. Identify the major complications of the intrapartum period related to the fetus

5. Identify the major causes of fetal distress and the appropriate treatment measures

6. Identify the major bleeding disorders of the intrapartum period prior to delivery

7. Identify the major causes and predisposing factors to postpartum hemorrhage

8. Identify the obstetrical conditions associated with disseminated intravascular coagulation

9. Identify the two life threatening emergencies related to uterine complications

10. Identify the most common emergencies in obstetrical analgesia and anesthesia

---

The crises that arise during the intrapartum period include hypertensive complications, complications relating to labor or the fetus, hemorrhagic problems, and uterine complications. The most common obstetrical analgesic and anesthetic emergencies will also be mentioned.

The intrapartum period usually progresses normally with no problems for the mother or the baby. When complications do occur, however, they arise quickly and may have devastating effects on the mother or baby or both. Therefore nurses who work with obstetrical patients must be aware of the major complications and how to recognize warning signs and institute treatment measures effectively.

Often during these crisis situations all of the attention is focused on the mother and baby. It is important to remember that this is a family experience. The nurse needs to handle the emergency in a calm, efficient manner and still offer support and comfort to the husband and any other support person. If they receive the support they need then they can continue to function as a source of support and comfort to the laboring woman. The experience can still be a family centered one to the limits of the complication. The nurse is in an excellent position to facilitate a positive experience.

The most important activity of the nurse during the intrapartum period is assessment. The condition of every woman admitted to labor and delivery should be thoroughly assessed. Many of the complications discussed in this chapter can be detected by the nurse through careful assessment of the patient's past history, current physical status, and labor progress. The assessment will then allow the nurse to deal more knowledgeably with any complications as they occur.

_____ PATIENT IN LABOR _____

ADMISSION ASSESSMENT

1. **Review prenatal record**
   a. Obstetrical history
      i. Age
      ii. EDC
      iii. Gravidity, parity, and previous obstetrical problems (type of labor, abortions, stillbirths)
      iv. Baseline maternal vital signs
      v. Results of laboratory tests
         (a) Blood: Rh and type
         (b) VDRL (Venereal Disease Research Laboratory)
         (c) Rubella
         (d) Gonococcal culture
         (e) Hematocrit
         (f) Urinalysis (glucose, acetone, protein)
      vi. Type of analgesia/anesthesia requested
      vii. Any problems during pregnancy
   b. Significant personal data
      i. Type of childbirth preparation
      ii. Family support
      iii. Feeding preference
      iv. Special birth requests

2. **Initial examination of patient**
   a. Determine onset of labor
   b. Assess duration, intensity, frequency, and regularity of contractions
   c. Determine the status of the membranes
   d. Assess vaginal discharge: amount, odor, character
   e. Determine time and consistency of last meal or oral intake

3. **Physical assessment**
   a. Check vital signs, BP, and fetal heart rate (FHR)

    b. Check for edema of the legs, face, hands
    c. Fundal height measurement (see Appendix A)
    d. Leopold's maneuvers to determine fetal presentation, lie, position, and engagement (see Appendix A)
    e. Vaginal examination during labor (see Appendix A) to assess
       i. Effacement and dilatation
      ii. Presentation and position of fetus
     iii. Station
     iv. Degree of molding
    f. Deep tendon reflexes and presence of clonus (see Appendix A)

4. Laboratory assessment
    a. Dipstick urinalysis for protein, glucose, ketones
    b. Complete blood count (CBC)

5. Psychosocial assessment
    a. Evaluate woman's general appearance and demeanor
    b. Verbal interaction
    c. Anxiety level
    d. Energy level
    e. Discomfort or pain with contractions

ASSESSMENT OF PROGRESS IN LABOR

1. Progress in labor is assessed by evaluation of the physical and emotional factors that are summarized in Table 11-1.

_____ PREGNANCY INDUCED HYPERTENSION COMPLICATIONS _____

Pregnancy induced hypertension is the third leading cause of maternal death in the United States. It is a major cause of perinatal mortality and is often associated with fetal growth retardation.

DIAGNOSIS

Pregnancy induced hypertension (PIH) occurs in 5 to 7 per cent of all pregnancies.

1. Preeclampsia: Hypertension with proteinuria and/or edema developing after 20 weeks' gestation
2. Eclampsia: Preeclampsia with grand mal seizures occurs in 1 in 2000 pregnancies
3. Chronic hypertension
    a. Persistent high blood pressure from any cause
    b. Present at any stage of gestation
    c. More common in pregnant black women
4. Chronic hypertension with superimposed preeclampsia
    a. Occurs after week 20

TABLE 11-1. ASSESSMENT IN LABOR

| Phase of Labor | Physical Assessment | | | | | Behavioral Assessment | | Nursing Implications |
	Dilatation (cm)	Contractions Frequency in min.	Duration in sec.	Intensity	Station	Show	Patient Behaviors	Anxiety Level	
Early	0–3	5–30	10–30	Mild	Primigravida 0 multipara 0 to –2	Scant, brownish mucus plug; pink mucus	High energy level Contentment, excitement Smiling, laughing, talking	Mild (enhances perception)	Excellent time for teaching (i.e., breathing techniques) Time to assess expectations of labor and delivery Excessive anxiety in early phase is usually related to environment, procedures, or behaviors of staff members
Active	4–7	3–5	30–60	Moderate	Primigravida +1 to +2 multigravida +1 to +2	Scant to moderate; pink to bloody mucus	Decreased attention to environment; less talking, more preoccupied with self Physical changes: flush, GI distress—nausea and vomiting—pallor, dry mouth Verbalizations about feelings of	Moderate to severe	Provide quiet, relaxing environment Meet dependency needs by anticipation: check bladder, mouth care, perineal care, back rubs Remain with patient as much as possible, since she has more difficulty in following directions

Transition	8-10	1-3	60-90	Strong, expulsive	+2 to +3	Copious, bloody show	Fatigue and exhaustion	Severe—panic
							Withdrawal from environment: less responsive to questions, less aware of stimuli, amnesic between contractions, frequent dozing Aggressive behaviors Physical changes: shaking, chills, nausea and vomiting, beads of perspiration on forehead and upper lip, feeling of need to defecate	helplessness Increased dependency needs manifested by frequent demands, complaints

Respond in calm, quiet voice
Let patient rest between contractions
Praise efforts to cope
Orient patients to reality
Accept aggressive behaviors without retaliation

Adapted from Affonso, D.: The crisis of labor and birth. *In* Maturational Crises of Childbearing. Honolulu, University of Hawaii Press, 1972; Jensen, M.D., Benson, R.C., and Bobak, J.M.: Maternity Care: The Nurse and the Family, 2nd ed. St. Louis, C.V. Mosby Co., 1981; Clark, A., and Affonso, D.D.: The Childbearing Family: A Nursing Perspective, 2nd ed. Philadelphia, F.A. Davis Co., 1979.

    b. Elevation of BP (rise of 30 mm Hg systolic or 15 mm Hg diastolic) on top of already elevated BP

        i. Incidence higher in certain groups: primigravidas and low socio-economic groups (10 to 30 per cent), and those with poor nutritional status

        ii. Recurs in subsequent pregnancies in up to 33 per cent of patients

        iii. Affects women at extremes of the reproductive years (less than 20 and more than 35 years of age)

        iv. May be present in multigravidas who have

            (a) Uterine overdistention (twins, hydramnios)

            (b) Vascular disease, including essential chronic hypertension and diabetes

            (c) Chronic renal disease

        v. Occurrence before week 20 usually associated with hydatidiform mole

        vi. Commonly associated with intrauterine growth retardation

        vii. Severe cases may be associated with disseminated intravascular coagulation (DIC)[12]

ETIOLOGY

1. Not fully known
2. Characterized by vasospasm with vasoconstriction and increased peripheral resistance (causes decreased delivery of oxygen and glucose to'body tissues)
3. Hypovolemia: Plasma volume lost to the interstitial space, causing edema
4. Proteinuria: Loss of efficiency in filtration system of the kidneys

ASSESSMENT

1. Clinical presentation

    a. Signs and symptoms

        i. Preeclampsia

            (a) BP: 140/90 or increase of 30 mm Hg systolic or 15 mm Hg diastolic over baseline readings

            (b) Edema: usually limited to face and hands, present in the morning (associated with rapid weight gain)

            (c) Proteinuria: 500 mg or more protein in 24 hour urine specimen; 2+ protein in a random sample (late symptom)

        ii. Severe preeclampsia

            One or more of the following

            (a) Systolic pressure higher than 160 mm Hg systolic or 110 mm Hg diastolic on two occasions 6 hours apart

            (b) Proteinuria: 5 gm/24 hour specimen; +3 to 4+ on random sample

            (c) Cerebral or visual disturbances

                (1) Altered consciousness

                (2) Headache

        (3) Scotomata
        (4) Blurred vision
    (d) Intrauterine growth retardation
    (e) Danger signs
        (1) Epigastric or upper quadrant pain
        (2) Thrombocytopenia or impaired liver function
        (3) Cyanosis and pulmonary edema
  iii. Eclampsia
    (a) Grand mal seizures
    (b) May occur up to 72 hours after delivery
  iv. BP very labile; peak pressure occurs during night
   v. Rise in hematocrit[9]
b. History
   i. Age, parity
  ii. Multiple pregnancy
 iii. Chronic hypertension, chronic renal failure, diabetes
 iv. Race, socioeconomic status
  v. Nutritional history

PROBLEMS AND COMPLICATIONS

1. Coma
2. Fetal death or disability; prematurity
3. Abruptio placentae
4. Renal failure
5. Stroke
6. Detached retina, temporary blindness
7. Maternal death

PATIENT CARE MANAGEMENT

1. Goals in severe preeclampsia

a. To prevent preeclampsia from becoming more severe (early detection)

   i. Review past medical and obstetrical history for predisposing factors

COMMENTS/TIPS/ CAUTIONS

Preeclampsia may recur

  ii. Review current prenatal history for
    (a) Baseline BP and presence of proteinuria throughout pregnancy
    (b) Amount and rate of weight gain

Weight gain of 5 pounds or more per week may be early sign of preeclampsia

    (c) History of headache, blurred vision, or edema (particularly of hands and face)

iii. Take BP on admission; *if BP elevated,* place patient on her left side and repeat measurement in 15 minutes

Diastolic pressure is better indicator or severity of condition

iv. Evaluate for presence of edema
v. Check for hyperactive reflexes and the presence of clonus (see Appendix A)
vi. Check first voided specimen of urine with dipstick for presence of protein

Helps evaluate severity and progression of preeclampsia

b. To prevent seizures
   i. Provide proper environment
      (a) Admit patient to a quiet labor room
      (b) Dim lights
      (c) Keep noise level down
      (d) Restrict number of disturbances to patient
      (e) Place in left lateral position
   ii. Monitor BP at least every hour, more frequently if unstable
   iii. Check reflexes every hour

Helps determine the level of muscle and nerve irritability

   iv. Record intake and output every hour

If patient cannot void easily or frequently, insert Foley catheter to straight drainage

   v. Assess patient for
      (a) Severe headaches
      (b) Visual problems
      (c) Epigastric pain
      (d) Irritability or restlessness
   vi. Institute seizure precautions (see Chapter 9); *do not leave patient alone*
   vii. Give patient nothing orally
c. To prevent progression to eclamptic state
   i. Administer IV magnesium sulfate as ordered by physician (see Chapter 9)
2. Goals in eclampsia
   a. To protect patient from injury during eclamptic seizure
      i. Place tongue blade or airway in patient's mouth

To maintain airway and to prevent patient from biting tongue; *do not attempt to insert with force*

ii. Turn woman on left side; suction nasopharynx as necessary

Remove mucus and prevent aspiration

iii. Administer IV magnesium sulfate as ordered

iv. Administer oxygen to mother

v. Monitor fetal status

Oxygen supply to fetus is decreased during seizure

vi. Note type and length of seizure

b. To detect abruptio placentae early
  i. Evaluate for
    (a) Vaginal bleeding
    (b) Uterine tenderness
    (c) Change in fetal activity and FHR
    (d) Sustained abdominal pain

c. To provide emotional support to patient and family
  i. Explain procedures fully
  ii. Keep family informed of progress
  iii. Reassure patient; be honest
  iv. Encourage expression of emotion

PREMATURE LABOR

Prematurity, the greatest single problem in obstetrics today, is responsible for a large number of neonatal deaths from respiratory distress syndrome and intraventricular hemorrhage. Approximately 80 per cent of perinatal mortality is attributable to low birth weight infants (less than 2500 gm).[1] Prematurity is responsible for almost two thirds of neonatal deaths.

DIAGNOSIS

Premature labor is the onset of regular uterine contractions accompanied by cervical effacement or dilatation before 37 weeks' gestation.[8]

1. **Incidence**
   a. In United States, 6 to 7 per cent
   b. In black population, 10 to 11 per cent

2. **Predisposing factors**
   a. Spontaneous rupture of membranes
   b. Incompetent cervix

    c. Uterine anomalies, preventing expansion

    d. Overdistention of uterus (multiple pregnancy, polyhydramnios, large fetus)

    e. Anomalies of the products of conception

    f. Faulty placentation

    g. Retained intrauterine device

    h. Previous preterm delivery or late abortion

    i. Serious maternal disease (preeclampsia, anemia, chronic renal diseases, acute febrile illnesses)

    j. Elective induction of labor[9]

ETIOLOGY

The precise cause is unknown in 50 per cent of cases.

1. Factors associated with premature labor

    a. Low socioeconomic status

    b. Certain ethnic backgrounds (black population)

    c. Small size

    d. Smoking

    e. Bacteriuria

    f. Poor prenatal care[8]

ASSESSMENT

1. Clinical presentation

    a. Signs and symptoms

        i. Uterine contractions at least once every 10 minutes lasting for 30 seconds or more

        ii. Effacement or dilatation

        iii. Fundal height

    b. History

        i. Gestational age

        ii. Previous premature delivery

        iii. Febrile illness

        iv. Abdominal surgery

        v. Maternal injury

        vi. Abruptio placentae

2. Biopsychosocial assessment

    a. Palpation of uterus during contractions

    b. External fetal monitoring to record frequency and duration of contractions

    c. Vaginal examination to determine status of effacement and dilatation

    d. Estimation of fetal weight

3. Diagnostic data

    a. Urinalysis (clean catch; to rule out urinary tract infection)

    b. Real-time study (to confirm gestational age)

    c. Vaginal aspiration of amniotic fluid for determination of L/S ratio

PROBLEMS AND COMPLICATIONS

  a. Premature delivery

  b. Attendant complications of premature birth

PATIENT CARE MANAGEMENT

1. Goals

  a. To establish definitive diagnosis of labor

      i. Connect patient to external monitor, if available, to determine frequency and duration of contractions

> Have patient tell nurse (you) when she is having a contraction (mark on strip), since in extreme prematurity toco-dynamometer may not accurately record contractions

      ii. Palpate fundus to determine strength of contractions

> Remember external tracings do not reflect strength of contractions

     iii. Perform sterile vaginal examination to determine cervical effacement and dilatation

> Usually no attempt to stop premature labor if dilatation is 4 cm or more

     iv. Check obstetrical history to determine accurate gestational age:

        (a) EDC

        (b) Rate of fundal growth

      v. Assist with obtaining additional data to establish accurate gestational age

        (a) Real-time study

        (b) Vaginal aspiration of amniotic fluid (if amniotic membranes rupture) for L/S ratio

  b. To determine any preexisting factors that may predispose to premature labor

      i. Obtain urine by clean catch for routine studies and culture

> Urinary tract infection often associated with premature labor

      ii. Obtain careful history

     iii. Hydrate patient as ordered by physician

> Maternal dehydration associated with premature labor

  c. To attempt to inhibit premature labor as specified by physician

      i. Administer ritodrine, magnesium sulfate (see Chapter 9), or ethanol as ordered by the physician (see Appendix A)

> Ethanol IV is no longer considered the drug of choice for premature labor (see Appendix A)

d. To provide emotional support to parents
  i. Assess parents' behavior and knowledge of condition
  ii. Provide information to assist with reduction of guilt feelings
  iii. Keep woman and husband informed of fetal status
  iv. Inform patient of preparations for baby if labor cannot be stopped
e. To prepare for premature delivery if labor cannot be halted
  i. Do not leave patient alone
  ii. Coach woman through each contraction; keep analgesia to a minimum
  iii. Notify pediatrician of imminent delivery
  iv. Transfer patient to delivery room
  v. Have forceps available for physician's use
  vi. Coach patient to facilitate efforts in *controlling* pushing
f. To establish maternal-infant bond
  i. Provide opportunity for mother to see and touch infant before it is taken to the nursery (if baby's condition will permit)
  ii. Relay information to parents about infant's condition
  iii. If baby is in critical condition, make arrangements for parents to see baby; provide emotional support
g. If baby dies, to provide parents with emotional support; make arrangements for parents to see and hold baby, if they desire

Premature labor may progress rapidly, thus allowing precipitate delivery. Delivery of head must be controlled to prevent trauma to fetus

If physician does not arrive, be prepared to do emergency delivery (see Chapter 9)

If baby is in another hospital, encourage frequent communication, pictures of baby, visits by father

PREMATURE RUPTURE OF MEMBRANES

Premature rupture of the membranes (PROM) is associated with an increased rate of maternal and fetal infection. While maternal infection from premature rupture is not serious, sepsis in the fetus is a leading cause of death in newborns.

DIAGNOSIS

Rupture of the membranes is considered premature if it occurs 1 hour or more before the onset of labor irrespective of duration of gestation.

1. **Incidence**
   a. Occurs in 10 to 12 per cent of pregnancies
2. 20 per cent of babies born after premature rupture weigh less than 2500 gm
3. Increased incidence of prolapsed cord, especially in premature infants
4. Frequently associated with malpresentation of fetus (i.e., breech)

ETIOLOGY[8]

1. Unknown
2. 50 to 70 per cent of patients with PROM go into spontaneous labor within 48 hours
3. Length of latent period (between rupture of membranes and onset of labor) influenced by
   a. Gestational age
   b. Latent period shorter when fetus is large
   c. Latent period longer in primigravidas
   d. Intrauterine infection shortens latent period

ASSESSMENT

1. **Clinical presentation**
   a. Signs and symptoms
      i. Large amounts of fluid flowing from vagina
      ii. Absence of contractions
   b. History
      i. Gestational age
      ii. Time of rupture of membranes and quality of fluid
      iii. Fetal movement after rupture
2. **Biopsychosocial assessment**
   a. Sterile speculum examination
   b. Temperature, pulse, respiration
   c. Presentation
   d. FHR
   e. Fundal height and estimated fetal weight
   f. *Do not do digital examination.* This increases risk of infection
3. **Diagnostic data**
   a. Nitrazine test
   b. Fern test
   c. Group B beta streptococcus cultures (positive culture a contraindication to continuing pregnancy)
   d. Vaginal aspiration of fluid for L/S ratio
   e. Blood: CBC

PROBLEMS AND COMPLICATIONS

1. Prematurity
2. Infection: maternal and fetal
3. Prolapse of cord
4. Malpresentation
5. Fetal prognosis depends on
   a. Fetal maturity
   b. Presentation (breech presentation has the worse prognosis, especially if premature)
   c. Fetal mortality increased in intrauterine infection (the longer the rupture, the higher the incidence of infection)

PATIENT CARE MANAGEMENT

1. **Goals**
   a. To confirm diagnosis of ruptured membranes
      i. Perform sterile speculum examination
      ii. Obtain specimen for nitrazine and fern testing (see Appendix A)
      iii. Obtain specimens for group B beta hemolytic streptococcus cultures from vagina and rectum
      iv. *Do not perform vaginal examination* — Examinations should be kept to a minimum to decrease the risk of infection
      v. Notify the physician
   b. To accurately assess gestational age
      i. Take accurate history
      ii. Calculate EDC
      iii. Measure fundal height and estimate fetal weight
      iv. Assist physician with real-time study if available
   c. To recognize signs and symptoms of amnionitis promptly
      i. Take patient's temperature and pulse on admission and every hour thereafter — Elevated temperature may be indication of infection
      ii. Monitor fetal heart tones — Fetal tachycardia may be an early sign of infection
      iii. Note color and odor of fluid
      iv. Evaluate patient for uterine tenderness

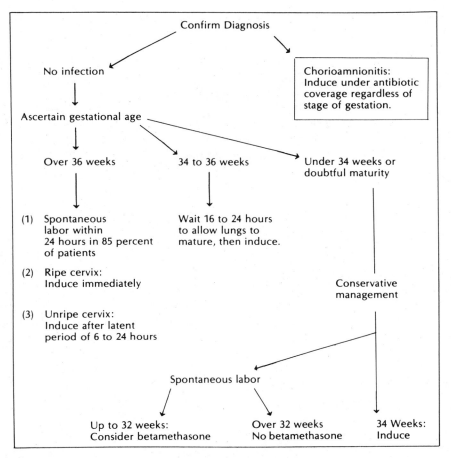

Figure 11-1. Premature rupture of membranes. (Reprinted with permission from Oxorn, H.: Human Labor and Birth, 4th ed. New York, Appleton-Century-Crofts, 1980.)

    d. To facilitate successful outcome
        i. See Figure 11-1
       ii. Provide emotional support
      iii. Referral to social service for
           any assistance needed

PROLAPSE OF CORD*

Prolapse of the cord is life threatening to the fetus. It occurs unexpectedly and is most often recognized and managed by the nurse until the physician arrives.

DIAGNOSIS

Prolapse of the cord is premature expulsion of the umbilical cord during parturition. Prolapse of the cord is usually diagnosed after rupture of mem-

---

*This section on prolapse of the cord is by Carole Ann Miller McKenzie, C.N.M., Ph.D.

branes (ROM) but prior to the delivery of the fetus. The cord is compressed with every contraction.

1. **Incidence**
   a. 1 in 400 pregnancies
2. **Predisposing factors**
   a. Breech presentation
   b. Multiple pregnancy
   c. Prematurity or baby small for gestational age (SGA)
   d. Lack of engagement of presenting part

ETIOLOGY

1. Mechanical causes: poor fit of passenger into pelvis
2. Abnormal presentation
3. Inadequate pelvis
4. Premature rupture of membranes
5. High station
6. Traumatic ROM after examination or enema
7. Life threatening condition for fetus due to compression of cord. Impairment of oxygen transfer from mother to fetus, leading to fetal anoxia

ASSESSMENT

1. **Clinical presentation**
   a. Signs and symptoms
      i. Station 0 → -4
      ii. ROM
      iii. Cord at introitus, or palpable during examination
      iv. FHR accelerates slightly (180 to 200)
      v. Rapid, sharp drop in FHR (200 to 0 if no treatment)
   b. History
      i. Persistent breech or other abnormal presentation
      ii. SGA or breech

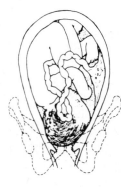 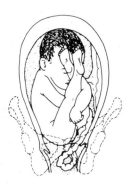 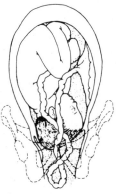 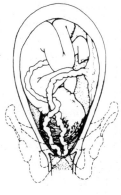

| A | B | C | D |

Figure 11-2. Prolapse of cord. Note pressure of head on cord, which endangers fetal circulation. *A,* Occult prolapse of umbilical cord. *B,* Breech with prolapsed cord. *C,* Complete prolapse of umbilical cord. *D,* Forelying umbilical cord. (Reprinted with permission from: Jensen, M.D., et al.: Maternity Care: The Nurse and the Family, 2nd ed. St. Louis, The C.V. Mosby Company, 1981.)

      iii. Multiple gestation
      iv. Inadequate pelvis
       v. ROM
      vi. Enema
     vii. LMP, EDC
    viii. Any measures to determine gestational age
      ix. Parity

2. **Biopsychosocial assessment**
   (On admission)
   a. Station
   b. Dilatation
   c. Fundal height and estimated fetal weight
   d. FHR
   e. TPR

   (At time of prolapse)
   f. Assess condition of cord (whether intact)
   g. Feel for pulsation of cord for FHR (pulsation is the major indicator of fetal welfare)
   h. Mother's emotional status

3. **Diagnostic data**
   a. FHR monitor strip, if available
   b. Fetal blood gas determination, if means available (may not be practical from time or logistical standpoint to obtain these)

PROBLEMS AND COMPLICATIONS

The quicker the nurse acts, the less likely problems and complications will occur.

1. Fetal death
2. Traumatic delivery
3. Fetal anoxic episode leading to long range complications
4. Infection (maternal or neonatal or both)

PATIENT CARE MANAGEMENT

1. **Goals**

   COMMENTS/TIPS/
   CAUTIONS

   a. To maintain physiological integrity of fetal system
      i. Keep hand in vagina and push presenting part away from cord

      Once hand is in vagina, it *cannot* be removed for any reason. Position of hand with presenting part pushed away from cord must be maintained through contractions and until delivery

      ii. Continuously assess fetal welfare from pulsation of cord and call out FHR to other personnel, as available
      iii. Call for assistance

      Calls for assistance may be at "top of your lungs" if necessary

      iv. Assist patient to knee-chest

or Trendelenburg's position, maintaining hand position at all times

v. Administer O_2 to mother

vi. Deliver fetus as quickly as possible

b. To prepare patient for immediate delivery

i. Have physician notified

ii. Have staff prepare for immediate cesarean section (C/S)

(a) Blood: CBC, type and cross-match

(b) Foley catheter (if time)

iii. Call out station, dilatation, position, presentation, FHR, cord condition to physician or other staff

c. To provide psychological support to parents

i. Reassure parents of welfare of fetus via cord pulsation

ii. Explain to parents what will happen

iii. Allow father or other support person opportunity to stay to provide support to mother

iv. Continuously provide family with supportive comments

Preparation for C/S should proceed at great speed; Foley catheter can be inserted later

C/S is usually treatment of choice; occasionally fast forceps or vacuum extraction will be attempted if patient is multiparous and completely dilated; if any other complications ensue, e.g., shoulder dystocia, vaginal delivery was inappropriate choice

If cord is compressed for 5 minutes or longer, central nervous system damage or death of the fetus will result

Father is usually asked to leave during complications; it appears much more appropriate to allow him to stay to provide support during the crisis

DYSFUNCTIONAL LABOR

Prolonged labor is associated with increased perinatal and maternal morbidity. There is a marked increase in maternal infection and hemorrhage. Fetal injury and death are the most serious outcomes of this disorder.

DIAGNOSIS

Dysfunctional labor is labor that lasts longer than 24 hours without the cervix becoming fully dilatated.[8]

1. **Incidence**
   a. 1 to 7 per cent
2. **Predisposing factors**
   a. Primigravidity
   b. PROM when cervix is closed and uneffaced
   c. Excessive analgesia or anesthesia in latent phase

TABLE 11-2. COMPARISON OF DYSFUNCTIONAL LABOR PATTERNS

	Hypotonic	Hypertonic
Characteristics		
Onset	During active labor	Onset of labor (latent phase)
Contractions	Brief, mild irregular	Colicky, sharp pains frequent, poor resting tone
Treatment		
Oxytocin	Indicated	Contraindicated
Sedation	May be indicated	Indicated

Adapted from Reeder, S., Mastroianni, L., and Martin, L.: Maternity Nursing, 14th ed. Philadelphia, J.B. Lippincott, 1980.

d. Overdistention of uterus (multiple pregnancy or hydramnios)
e. Grand multiparity
f. Missed or delayed labor
g. False labor or prodromal stage of labor
h. Uterine abnormalities[8,10]

3. **Classification**[11] (Table 11-2)
a. *Hypertonic:* inefficient uterine contractions that may be perceived by the patient as stronger than the amount of work that the contraction accomplishes; there may be increased uterine resting tone, and the strength of the contraction is not centered in the fundus
b. *Hypotonic:* contractions of very poor tone or intensity; 15 mm Hg too little pressure to dilate cervix

ETIOLOGY

1. Fetopelvic disproportion
2. Malpresentations and malpositions
3. Inefficient uterine action, including rigid cervix
4. Occurrence less frequent because of advances in treatment[10]
a. Recognition that prolonged labor is associated with increased perinatal mortality
b. Ability to administer minute amounts of oxytocin to treat uterine dysfunction
c. More frequent use of C/S than midforceps deliveries

ASSESSMENT

1. **Clinical presentation**
a. Signs and symptoms
(Hypertonic dysfunction)
i. Occurs at onset of labor
ii. Force of contraction is centered in location other than fundus; constant tension in muscle (high resting tone 15 mm Hg) but quality of contractions poor

TABLE 11-3. LENGTHS OF PHASES OF LABOR

	Primigravidas		Multiparas	
	Average	*Upper normal*	*Average*	*Upper normal*
Latent phase	8.6 hours	20 hours	5.3 hours	14 hours
Active phase	5.8 hours	12 hours	2.5 hours	6 hours
First stage of labor	13.3 hours	28.5 hours	7.5 hours	20 hours
Second stage of labor	57 minutes	2.5 hours	18 minutes	50 minutes
Rate of cervical dilatation during active phase	Under 1.2 cm/hour is abnormal		Under 1.5 cm/hour is abnormal	

Reprinted with permission from Oxorn, H.: Human Labor and Birth, 4th ed. New York, Appleton-Century-Crofts, 1980.

    iii. Latent phase greater than 20 hours in primigravida or 14 hours in multigravida

    iv. Extremely painful contractions

    v. Appearance of fetal distress early in labor

    vi. Does not respond favorably to oxytocin

    vii. Sedation often helpful

(Hypotonic dysfunction)

    i. Contractions decrease in strength (less than 50–60 mm Hg)

    ii. Contractions less frequent

    iii. Resting tone less than normal (8–12 mm Hg)

    iv. Uterus can be indented at peak of contraction

    v. Occurs during active phase (cervix dilated at least 3 cm)

b. History

    i. Onset of contractions, contraction pattern

    ii. Uterine abnormalities or operations

    iii. Medications, sensitivity to analgesia or anesthesia

    iv. History of pregnancies

    v. ROM (time, quality)

    vi. Multiple pregnancy

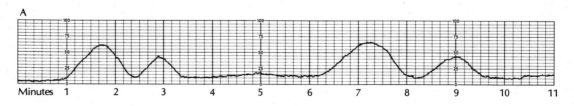

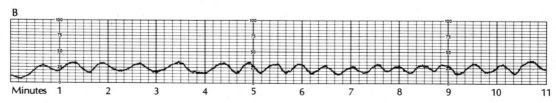

Figure 11-3. Incoordinated uterine motility: *A,* first degree; *B,* second degree. (Reprinted with permission from Olds, S.B., et al.: Obstetric Nursing. Menlo Park, California, Addison-Wesley Publishing Co., 1980.)

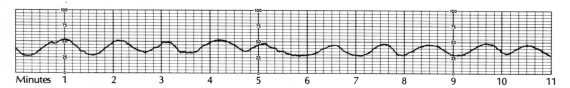

Figure 11-4. Hypertonic uterine motility. (Reprinted with permission from Olds, S.B., et al.: Obstetric Nursing. Menlo Park, California, Addison-Wesley Publishing Co., 1980.)

2. **Biopsychosocial assessment**
   a. Quality and strength of contraction
   b. Uterine basal tone on monitor
   c. Patient's response to contractions
   d. Indentation of uterus during contraction
   e. Maternal temperature and pulse (increases indicate maternal dehydration)
   f. Graphic analysis of labor (Friedman curve)
   g. State of cervix
   h. Station
   i. Position, fundal height, number of fetuses, hydramnios
   j. Failure to progress[8]

PROBLEMS AND COMPLICATIONS

The quicker the diagnosis is made, the less likely problems and complications will occur.

1. Fetal injury and death
2. Intrauterine infection
3. Maternal exhaustion
4. Increased need for operative intervention
5. Maternal dehydration
6. Psychological sequelae for mother (difficult labor has definite deleterious effect upon future childbearing)
7. Decreased placental perfusion and fetal hypoxia[9]

PATIENT CARE MANAGEMENT

1. **Goals**
   a. To avoid and/or intervene with occurence of abnormal progress in labor
      i. Systematically appraise and record
         (a) Frequency, strength, duration of contractions
         (b) Cervical effacement and dilatation (chart on Friedman graph)
         (c) Station (failure to descend)

COMMENTS/TIPS/
CAUTIONS

Have internal pressure catheter inserted to accurately appraise contractions

(d) Position

(e) FHR

b. To ensure favorable perinatal outcome

    i. Monitor vital signs every hour

    ii. Observe patient's level of fatigue and ability to cope with contractions

    iii. Watch patient for signs of dehydration (dry cracked lips)

    iv. Check for bladder distention; catheterize if necessary

    May look like small balloon over symphysis

c. To attempt to correct dysfunctional labor, as ordered by physician

(Hypertonic dysfunction)

    i. Administer sedative as ordered (i.e., morphine 10 to 15 mg IM)

    ii. Maintain adequate IV infusion to prevent dehydration

    iii. Do not give oxytocin to anyone with hypertonic contractions

    May cause tetanic contractions that may lead to abruptio placentae or uterine rupture

    iv. Discontinue oxytocin if being administered (see procedure for Tetanic Contractions, Chapter 9)

    v. Be alert for precipitous delivery (see Chapter 9)

    Do not leave patient; have "precip pack" in room

(Hypotonic dysfunction)

    i. Administer sedative as ordered if hypotonic dysfunction occurs during prolonged latent phase

    ii. Begin oxytocin augmentation of labor as ordered by physician (see Appendix A)

d. To provide psychological support to patient and family

    i. Provide information about progress of labor to patient and family

    ii. Provide comfort measures

COMMENTS/TIPS/CAUTIONS

(e.g., back rub, cool cloth) to assist with relaxation
iii. Respond in a calm, accepting manner; coach patient with breathing techniques
iv. Accept patient's frustration and anger

AMNIOTIC FLUID EMBOLISM

Amniotic fluid embolism is an extremely rare but almost invariably fatal complication. Approximately 50 per cent of patients die at the time of embolization, and more than 50 per cent of the survivors die subsequently.[1]

DIAGNOSIS

An amniotic fluid embolus occurs when a large amount of amniotic fluid is infused into the maternal circulation. Multiple tiny emboli are formed and occlude the pulmonary capillaries. Rapid respiratory distress and shock occur.

1. **Incidence**
   a. 1 in 37,000 deliveries
2. **Predisposing factors**
   a. Multiparity
   b. Hypertonic uterine contractions
   c. Oxytocin induction or stimulation of labor
   d. Traumatic delivery
   e. Meconium in amniotic fluid
   f. Large baby
   g. Age over 30 years
   h. Intrauterine fetal death
   i. Operative delivery

ETIOLOGY

All of the following must be present for development of amniotic fluid embolism:
1. Rent through the amnion and chorion
2. Opened maternal veins (marginal separation of placenta, laceration of uterus or cervix)
3. Pressure gradient (vigorous labor, including that induced with oxytocin)
4. Toxic elements in amniotic fluid (meconium, cytolytic products from dead fetus)

ASSESSMENT

1. **Clinical presentation**
   a. Signs and symptoms
   (Premonitory)
      i. Shaking chill

   ii. Sweating
  iii. Anxiety
   iv. Coughing
    v. Vomiting
   vi. Convulsions
(Cardinal)
  vii. Respiratory distress
 viii. Cyanosis
   ix. Cardiovascular collapse
    x. Hemorrhage
   xi. Coma
(If patient survives initial episode)
  xii. Bleeding (secondary to DIC)
 xiii. Uterine atony
 b. History
    i. Meconium stained fluid
   ii. Multiparity
  iii. Large fetus
   iv. Intrauterine fetal death
    v. Induction or augmentation of labor

2. **Biopsychosocial assessment**
 a. Hypertension
 b. Tachycardia
 c. Pink, frothy sputum
 d. Dyspnea
 e. Cyanosis
 f. Massive hemorrhage

PROBLEMS AND COMPLICATIONS

There may be nothing the nurse can do.

1. Maternal death
2. Fetal death

PATIENT CARE MANAGEMENT

1. **Goals**
 a. To anticipate patients at risk
    i. Screen all patients for pre-disposing factors (see Diagnosis)
 b. To prevent and recognize impending amniotic fluid embolism
    i. Notify physician if patient experiencing chest pain, cyanosis, frothy sputum, tachycardia, hypotension, massive hemorrhage

COMMENTS/TIPS/CAUTIONS

In patients in whom delivery is being induced, watch very closely for occurrence of intra-uterine fetal death; two risk factors are combined

Always report at first sign; amniotic fluid embolism is often fatal

	COMMENTS/TIPS/CAUTIONS
c. To maximize successful outcome	
i. Call for assistance	Someone must remain with patient
ii. Administer oxygen under pressure	
iii. Assess fetal status	One nurse should monitor fetal status, and one should assist physician to stabilize condition of mother
iv. Monitor patient for cardiac or respiratory arrest	
v. Institute cardiopulmonary resuscitation immediately in event of arrest (see Chapter 9)	There may be nothing the nurse can do
vi. Prepare for immediate delivery	
vii. Continue to monitor maternal status	
viii. Prepare for immediate transfusion	
d. To provide emotional support to family and patient	
i. Explain what is happening	
ii. Reassure and be honest	
iii. Provide family with supportive comments	

MALPOSITION OF FETUS

Malpositions are responsible for prolonged labor, particularly of the second stage. Prolonged labor is associated with an increased incidence of maternal and fetal infection.

DIAGNOSIS

Malpositions are normal vertex presentations in which the occiput has failed to rotate into the anterior position.[1] Malpositions are either occiput transverse or occiput posterior.

1. **Incidence**
   a. Occurs in 10 per cent of all vertex presentations; 25 per cent of these require medical intervention
   b. More common in primigravidas

ETIOLOGY
1. Fetal head engaged in occiput posterior position
2. Cephalopelvic disproportion
3. Abnormal pelvic shape

ASSESSMENT
1. **Clinical presentation**
   a. Signs and symptoms

        i. Back labor
       ii. Prolonged labor
      iii. Maternal exhaustion
       iv. Leopold's maneuvers suggest malposition
        v. Always suspect posterior presentation when patient complains
           of back labor
   b. History
        i. Previous malposition
       ii. Estimated size of fetus
      iii. EDC
       iv. Previous CS

2. Biopsychosocial assessment
(Right occiput posterior [ROP])
   a. Abdominal examination reveals
        i. Vertical lie
       ii. Head at or in pelvis
      iii. Fetal back on right side
       iv. Small parts easily palpable on left side
        v. Breech in fundus
       vi. Cephalic prominence on left but not easily palpated
   b. FHT heard on right side but indistinctly
   c. Vaginal examination (see Fig. 11–5)[8]

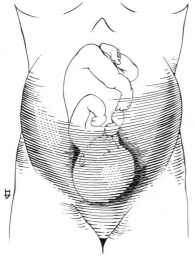

A. Abdominal view.

Figure 11-5. Right occiput posterior: *A,* abdominal view; *B,* vaginal view. (Reprinted with permission from Oxorn, H.: Human Labor and Birth, 4th ed. New York, Appleton-Century-Crofts, 1980.)

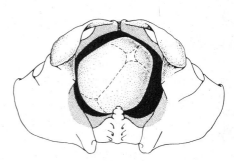

B. Vaginal view.

(Left occiput transverse [LOT])
  a. Abdominal examination reveals
      i. Longitudinal lie
     ii. Head at or in pelvis
    iii. Back on left side
     iv. Small parts on right, and usually can be felt easily
      v. Breech in fundus
     vi. Cephalic prominence on right
  b. FHT heard loudest in left lower quadrant
  c. Vaginal examination (see Fig. 11–6)[8]

PROBLEMS AND COMPLICATIONS

1. Prolonged second stage of labor
2. Increased maternal discomfort
3. Fetal distress
4. Cessation of descent
5. Molding

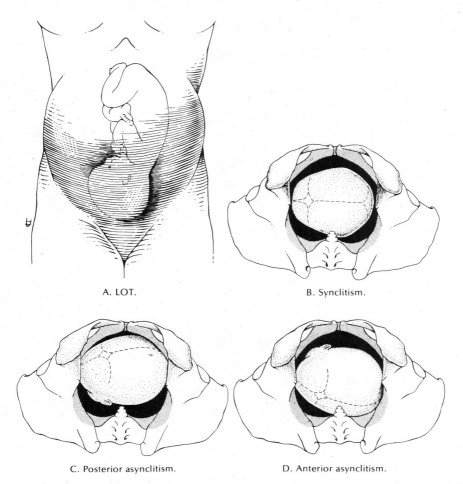

A. LOT.   B. Synclitism.

C. Posterior asynclitism.   D. Anterior asynclitism.

Figure 11-6. Left occiput transverse: *A*, LOT; *B*, synclitism; *C*, posterior asynclitism; *D*, anterior asynclitism. (Reprinted with permission from Oxorn, H.: Human Labor and Birth, 4th ed. New York, Appleton-Century-Crofts, 1980.)

PATIENT CARE MANAGEMENT

1. Goals
   a. To avoid maternal exhaustion
      i. Supportive measures to reduce discomforts of pregnancy

      Don't forget to offer support to the coach; make sure coach eats and takes breaks also

         (a) Back rubs, counterpressure
         (b) Frequent changes of position
         (c) Cool compresses
      ii. Observe patient for signs of dehydration
         (a) Cracked lips
         (b) Dry skin
         (c) Elevation of temperature
      iii. Encourage pushing efforts

      Once fetal head can be seen, positioning a mirror so patient can observe perineum may encourage her pushing efforts

   b. To proceed with delivery as quickly as possible
      i. Prepare patient for possibility of forceps delivery
      ii. Encourage patient to empty bladder

      If patient cannot empty bladder, make sure straight catheter is added to delivery table so physician can empty bladder before forceps application

      iii. Assist patient with relaxation techniques during forceps application
      iv. If forceps marks are present after delivery, explain their presence to parents and that they will go away

---

MALPRESENTATION

Malpresentation is a serious complication of obstetrics. Fetal injury during the delivery process may have long term effects. Labor may be prolonged, resulting in maternal and fetal complications.

DIAGNOSIS

Malpresentation is any presentation of the fetus other than vertex, i.e., breech, face, shoulder, and brow.

PROBLEMS AND COMPLICATIONS

1. **Effects on Labor**
   a. Associated with reduced efficiency of labor
   b. Incidence of fetopelvic disproportion is higher
   c. Prolonged labor common
   d. Presenting part remains high
   e. Frequent premature rupture of membranes

2. **Effects on Mother**
   a. Maternal exhaustion common because of prolonged labor
   b. More lacerations
   c. Bleeding more profuse
   d. Greater incidence of infection caused by
      i. Premature rupture of membranes
      ii. Excessive blood loss
      iii. Tissue damage
      iv. Frequent vaginal examination
   e. Patient's discomfort seems out of proportion to strength of contractions

3. **Effects on Fetus**
   a. Excessive molding
   b. Increased incidence of anoxia, brain damage, asphyxia, and intra-uterine death
   c. Prolapse of cord more common[8]

PATIENT CARE MANAGEMENT

1. **Goals**
   a. To detect abnormal presentation
      i. Perform Leopold's maneuvers (see Appendix A) on admission to labor and delivery room
      ii. Evaluate presentation and position during each vaginal examination

      COMMENTS/TIPS/CAUTIONS

      Nurse often first person to detect abnormal presentation

   b. To facilitate medical management of patient
      i. Prepare patient for whatever delivery deemed appropriate (vaginal, forceps, cesarean)
   c. To provide emotional support to parents
      i. Explain what is happening
      ii. Allow verbalization of feelings regarding possible loss of vaginal delivery

      It is normal to grieve for loss of expected normal vaginal delivery

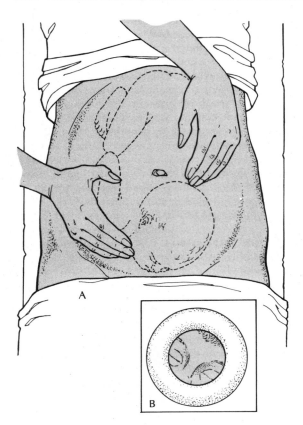

Figure 11-7. Face presentation: *A,* palpation of the maternal abdomen with the fetus in RMP; *B,* vaginal examination may permit palpation of facial features of the fetus. (Reprinted with permission from Olds, S.B., et al.: Obstetric Nursing. Menlo Park, California, Addison-Wesley Publishing Co., 1980.)

MALPRESENTATION: FACE PRESENTATION

DIAGNOSIS
1. **Incidence**
   a. 1 in 600 pregnancies
   b. More frequent in multigravidas
2. Face the presenting part
3. Longitudinal lie with complete extension of the head
4. Not usually recognized until onset of labor
5. Anterior presentations frequently deliver vaginally
6. Persistent posterior presentations cannot delivery vaginally[8,9]

ETIOLOGY
1. Any factor favoring extension or previous flexion of the head
    a. Contracted pelvis
    b. Large fetus
    c. Pendulous abdomen, present in some multiparas
    d. Multiple coils of cord around the neck
2. Anencephaly

ASSESSMENT
1. **Clinical presentation**
(Anterior face presentation)

a. Signs and symptoms
    i. Prolonged labor (face a poor dilator)
    ii. Early rupture of membranes
b. History: none significant

2. Biopsychosocial assessment
a. Abdominal examination
    i. Difficult to outline back of fetus
    ii. Deep furrow can be palpated between occiput and back
b. FHTs heard on side of small parts
c. Vaginal examination
    i. Absence of round, even vertex
    ii. Softer and irregular presenting part palpated
    iii. Identification of facial features, particularly nose and gums[8]

PROBLEMS AND COMPLICATIONS

1. Baby's face very edematous and possibly bruised
2. Mother more prone to lacerations during delivery
3. Cesarean section

MALPRESENTATION: BROW PRESENTATION

DIAGNOSIS
1. Incidence
a. 1 in 1000 to 1 in 3000 pregnancies
2. Occurs when head is partially extended instead of flexed
3. Forehead the presenting part
4. Usually will not deliver vaginally (brow is broadest diameter of fetal head)

ETIOLOGY
1. Cephalopelvic disproportion
2. Fetal conditions that prevent flexion (i.e., tumors of neck, nuchal cord, fetal anomalies)
3. Increased fetal mobility (polyhydramnios, small, or premature rupture of membranes)
4. Premature rupture of membranes before engagement
5. Abnormal placental implantation
6. Lax abdominal and pelvic musculature[7,8]

ASSESSMENT
1. Clinical presentation
a. Signs and symptoms
    i. Leopold's maneuvers suggest malpresentation
    ii. Prolonged labor
b. History
    i. Previous brow presentation
    ii. Estimated fetal weight

        iii. Fundal height, EDC

        iv. Previous cesarean section

2. Biopsychosocial Assessment

    a. Abdominal examination

        i. Occiput and chin easily palpated

        ii. Cephalic prominence on the same side as fetal back

    b. Vaginal examination

        i. Diamond shaped fontanelle on one side

        ii. Orbital ridges and root of nose on other side[8]

PROBLEMS AND COMPLICATIONS

1. Cesarean delivery required in most cases
2. Prolonged labor
3. Perineal lacerations that may extend into vaginal fornices
4. Fetal mortality increased because of injuries received during delivery and infection due to prolonged labor

———— MALPRESENTATION: BREECH PRESENTATION ————

DIAGNOSIS

1. Incidence

    a. Occurs in 3 to 4 per cent of pregnancies

    b. Decreases near term

    c. Increases before term

2. Fetus in longitudinal lie
3. Buttocks and/or feet or knees lie closest to cervix
4. Incidence of prolapsed cord increased
5. Largest part of fetus delivers last
6. Classification of breech

    a. Frank: buttocks alone are presenting part

    b. Complete: buttocks and feet together are presenting part

    c. Incomplete: feet (single or double) or knees are presenting part[8]

ETIOLOGY

1. Prematurity
2. Hydramnios
3. Multiple pregnancy
4. Placenta previa
5. Contracted pelvis
6. Hydrocephalus
7. Large baby[8]

ASSESSMENT

1. Clinical presentation

    a. Signs and symptoms

        i. Patient feels movements in lower abdomen

      ii. Engagement prior to labor uncommon
     iii. Prolapsed cord
     iv. Prolonged labor, since breech a poor dilator
  b. History
      i. Past obstetrical history
     ii. LMP, estimated fetal size
     iii. Previous pelvic findings

2. Biopsychosocial assessment
  a. Abdominal examination
      i. Longitudinal lie
     ii. Soft, irregular mass lying over pelvis
     iii. Head in fundus, often ballotable
     iv. No cephalic prominence
  b. FHTs often heard loudest at or above umbilicus
  c. Vaginal examination must be done at time of rupture of membranes to make certain cord has not prolapsed
      i. High presenting part
     ii. Absence of head with its suture lines and fontanelles
     iii. Presenting part soft and irregular
     iv. Foot may be palpated[8]

3. Diagnostic data
  a. X-ray pelvimetry and flat plate x-ray of the abdomen for any patient who has not delivered a mature infant without difficulty
  b. Real-time study to confirm diagnosis and measure biparietal diameter

PROBLEMS AND COMPLICATIONS

1. Fetal mortality increased as result of
  a. Intracranial hemorrhage (major cause of fetal mortality)
  b. Prematurity
  c. Congenital anomalies
  d. Prolapse of cord
  e. Fetal asphyxia from other causes
  f. Fetal injury
2. Increased incidence of
  a. Cerebral palsy
  b. Epilepsy
  c. Mental retardation
  d. Hemiplegia[8]

MALPRESENTATION: SHOULDER PRESENTATION (TRANSVERSE LIE)

DIAGNOSIS

Shoulder presentation is the situation of fetus during labor when its long axis and that of the mother are at right angles to one another.

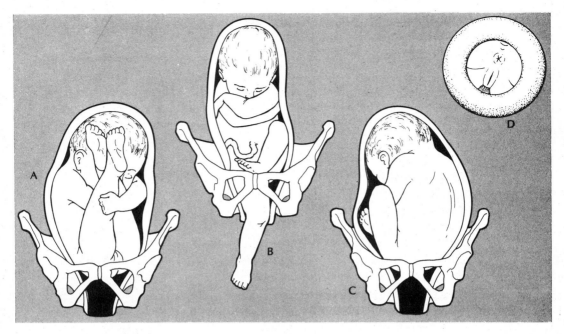

Figure 11-8. Breech presentation: *A,* frank breech, *B,* incomplete (footing) breech; *C,* complete breech in LSA position; *D,* on vaginal examination the nurse may feel the anal sphincter, which grips the finger; the tissue of the fetal buttocks feels soft. (Reprinted with permission from Olds, S.B., et al.: Obstetric Nursing. Menlo Park, California, Addison-Wesley Publishing Co., 1980.)

1. **Incidence**
   a. 1 in 500 deliveries
   b. Increases with parity

ETIOLOGY[9]

1. Unusual laxity of abdominal musculature resulting from grand multi-parity
2. Prematurity
3. Placenta previa
4. Contracted pelvis
5. Multiple pregnancies
6. Polyhydramnios[9]

ASSESSMENT

1. **Clinical presentations**
   a. Signs and symptoms
      i. Abdomen appears widest from side to side
      ii. Fundus of uterus barely extends above umbilicus
   b. History
      i. Previous cesarean section
      ii. Malpresentation

2. **Biopsychosocial assessment**
   a. Abdominal examination
      i. No presenting part in fundus or over symphysis
      ii. Head may be palpated on one side and breech on the other

        iii. Position of back is readily identified
    b. FHTs are usually heard just below midline of umbilicus (no diagnostic significance in position)
    c. Vaginal examination
        i. Neither head nor breech can be felt
        ii. If presenting part can be felt, it is usually ribs, shoulder, hand, or back

3. Diagnostic data
    a. X-ray pelvimetry

PROBLEMS AND COMPLICATIONS

1. Prolapse of cord
2. Uterine rupture
3. Prolonged labor
4. Infection

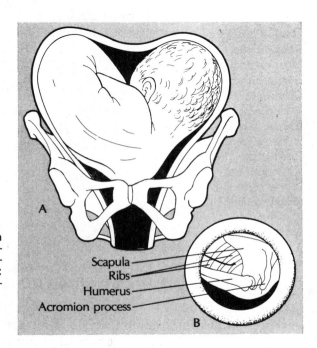

Figure 11-9. *A,* Shoulder presentation. *B,* On vaginal examination the nurse may feel the acromion process as the fetal presenting part. (Reprinted with permission from Olds, S.B., et al.: Obstetric Nursing. Menlo Park, California, Addison-Wesley Publishing Co., 1980.)

_____ SHOULDER DYSTOCIA _____

    Shoulder dystocia is a serious complication of labor. The fetal head is delivered, but the shoulders cannot be delivered by usual methods. By this time the umbilical cord has been drawn into the pelvis and is being compressed, leading to hypoxia and asphyxiation of the baby.

DIAGNOSIS

    Shoulder dystocia consists of inability to deliver the shoulders by normal means following delivery of the head.

1. Incidence
    a. Less than1 per cent (0.15 per cent)
2. Prolonged second stage and midforceps delivery may be warning sign (incidence increases to 4.57 per cent)

ETIOLOGY

1. Dystocia associated with
   a. Maternal obesity
   b. Excessive weight gain
   c. Oversized infants (more than 4 kg)
   d. History of large siblings
   e. Diabetes
2. Causes of dystocia after birth of head
   a. Short umbilical cord
   b. Abdominal or thoracic enlargement of infant
   c. Locked or conjoined twins
   d. Uterine constriction ring
   e. True shoulder dystocia[8]

ASSESSMENT

1. Clinical presentation
   a. Signs and symptoms
      i. Prolonged second stage (more than 2 hours)
      ii. Recoil of head against perineum
      iii. Restitution of head not spontaneous
      iv. Traction from below and pressure from above fail to deliver child
   b. History
      i. Birth weight of previously delivered infants
      ii. Estimation of fetal weight

PROBLEMS AND COMPLICATIONS

1. Fetal
   a. Death, intrapartum or neonatal
   b. Birth injury; brachial plexus palsy, fractured clavicle
   c. Late neuropsychiatric abnormalities in child
   d. Fetal anoxia
   e. Hemorrhagic effusions in fetus
   f. Irreparable fetal brain damage
2. Maternal
   a. Lacerations of birth canal

PATIENT CARE MANAGEMENT

1. Goals
   a. To recognize warning signs of shoulder dystocia
      i. Notify physician of warning signs (prolonged second stage and recoil of head against perineum during delivery)
   b. To maximize successful neonatal outcome by assisting physician with delivery of shoulders
      i. Provide suprapubic pressure when requested to collapse diameter of shoulders

      (a) Place flat of one hand over flat of the other
      (b) Keep arms straight
      (c) Apply downward pressure
  c. To detect trauma in neonate early
      i. Assess for neonatal abnormalities

MULTIPLE PREGNANCY

Maternal morbidity and perinatal morbidity and mortality are greatly increased with multiple pregnancy because of increased medical and obstetrical complications.

DIAGNOSIS

In multiple pregnancy there is more than one fetus in the uterus at one time.

1. Incidence
  a. Twins: 1 in 100 pregnancies
  b. Triplets: 1 in 10,000 pregnancies
  c. Quadruplets: 1 in 750,000 pregnancies
  d. More common in multigravidas and in black population

2. Other possible complications
  a. Anemia (greater demand for iron by fetuses)
  b. Polyhydramnios
  c. Premature labor
  d. Placenta previa
  e. Preeclampsia-eclampsia[8,9]

ETIOLOGY

1. Not proven
2. Monozygous twins (25 per cent): genetic factors
3. Dizygous twins (75 per cent): multiple ovulation due to excessive gonadotropic stimulation

ASSESSMENT

1. Clinical presentation
  a. Signs and symptoms
      i. Uterus and abdomen seem larger than expected
      ii. Uterine growth more rapid than normal
      iii. Unexplainable weight gain
  b. History
      i. Family history
      ii. EDC
      iii. Fundal height
      iv. Estimated fetal weight

2. **Biopsychosocial assessment**
    a. Palpation of two heads or two breeches
    b. Two fetal hearts auscultated at the same time by two observers and differing in rate by 10 beats/minute
3. **Diagnostic data**
    a. Roentgenogram of abdomen: reveals two skeletons
    b. Ultrasound: reveals two skulls

PROBLEMS AND COMPLICATIONS

1. Polyhydramnios
2. Increased incidence of preeclampsia
3. Anemia prevalent in mother
4. Excessive weight gain
5. Maternal complaints of fetal overactivity
6. Increased incidence of malpresentation
7. Fetal mortality increased (4 times greater than that of singletons); prematurity major cause of death)
8. Risk to second twin greater than to first
    a. Greater incidence of operative deliveries
    b. Too long interval between deliveries
    c. Second twin usually occupies less favorable position (incidence of malpresentation increased)
9. Overstretching of uterus leads to premature labor, early rupture of membranes, slow progress in labor, increased risk of postpartum hemorrhage[8]

PATIENT CARE MANAGEMENT

1. **Goals**
    a. To detect presence of twins, triplets, promptly
        i.   Perform Leopold's maneuvers (see Appendix A) on admission
        ii. Try to auscultate two heart tones when fundal height is extremely large
        iii. Assist physician with real time study, or transport patient to x-ray room to confirm diagnosis
    b. To deliver multiple pregnancy safely
        i.   Notify pediatricians of imminent delivery
        ii. Transport patient to delivery room before complete dilatation

COMMENTS/TIPS/
CAUTIONS

Second stage of labor usually rapid for first twin; all preparations for delivery need to be conducted in a calm, organized manner

iii. Prepare additional infant warmer for use in delivery room

iv. Obtain additional emergency equipment (i.e., Ambu bag, laryngoscope) for use with second twin

v. Place additional cord clamp and bulb syringe on instrument table

vi. Prepare bottle of IV fluid with oxytocin 20 units, connect to infusion pump, and place in delivery room

vii. Have additional nursing personnel available to assist with delivery and to assist pediatrician

viii. Be prepared to assist with resuscitation of babies

ix. Monitor patient closely for postpartum hemorrhage

c. To provide emotional and physical support to parents

i. Provide encouragement and praise during pushing efforts

ii. Facilitate bonding experience; make sure mother gets to hold (or at least to see) both babies before they are transported to nursery

iii. Facilitate rest and relaxation following delivery

COMMENTS/TIPS/CAUTIONS

Obtain when patient admitted to unit so warmer will be available in event of precipitous labor

Labor may have to be augmented for delivery of second twin

Second twin frequently has suffered more hypoxia, is often delivered in a malpresentation, and therefore is more depressed at birth

Woman is often exhausted after delivery of first baby

FETAL DISTRESS

Fetal distress during the intrapartum period is a serious emergency. The fetus can tolerate only a certain amount of hypoxia before it succumbs. Neurological deficits may occur as a result of continued or repeated hypoxic episodes.

In fetal distress evidence such as a change in the fetal heart rate pattern or activity indicates that the fetus is in jeopardy. It may be due to meconium staining of the amniotic fluid (except when fetus is a breech presentation) or abnormalities of the FHR (decelerations or changes in beat to beat variability).

FETAL DISTRESS DUE TO
———— MECONIUM STAINING OF THE AMNIOTIC FLUID ————

ETIOLOGY

1. Passage of meconium is caused by hyperperistalsis of the colon and relaxation of the anal sphincter resulting from hypoxia
2. Fetal hypoxia may occur without presence of meconium
   a. In infants of less than 34 weeks' gestation
   b. In Rh sensitized infants with severe anemia[1]

ASSESSMENT

1. Clinical presentation
   a. Signs and symptoms
      i. Green or yellow stained amniotic fluid
         (a) Fresh meconium: bright green
         (b) Old meconium: less bright, orange brown

2. Biopsychosocial assessment
   a. Observation of meconium stained fluid coming from vagina

PROBLEMS AND COMPLICATIONS

1. Aspiration of meconium by fetus

PATIENT CARE MANAGEMENT

1. Goals
   a. To prevent aspiration of meconium by infant at birth
      i. Provide DeLee suction apparatus for physician to use at delivery

      COMMENTS/TIPS/CAUTIONS

      Keep DeLee suction apparatus in delivery room and with each "precip pack"

      ii. Coach mother to pant after delivery of head while mouth and nose are being suctioned

      Allows physician adequate time to suction before delivery of body and baby's first breath

      iii. Using laryngscope, visualize baby's vocal cords as quickly as possible after delivery (preferably before the baby's first breath). Suction any meconium from cords

      With baby's first deep breath, the meconium will be aspirated into lungs

      iv. Assist with intubation if meconium is present below the cords to allow deep suctioning

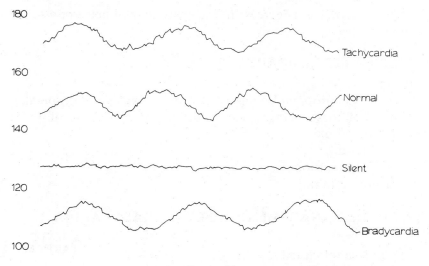

Baseline fetal heart rate.

Figure 11-10. Fetal heart patterns: baseline heart rate. (Reprinted with permission from Oxorn, H.: Human Labor and Birth, 4th ed. New York, Appleton-Century-Crofts, 1980.)

FETAL DISTRESS DUE TO ABNORMALITIES OF THE FETAL HEART RATE*

Fetal tachycardia is a rise in the baseline fetal heart rate to greater than 160 beats/minute.

ETIOLOGY OF FETAL TACHYCARDIA
1. Fetal hypoxia and tachycardia (an early sign)
2. Drugs induced: atropine and scopolamine block parasympathetic nervous system, resulting in increase in heart rate; ritodrine and isoxsuprine (Vasodilan) stimulate fetal heart, increasing the rate
3. Prematurity
4. Maternal anxiety
5. Maternal fever
6. Fetal infection
7. Fetal movement and stimulation
8. Fetal cardiac arrhythmia

PATIENT CARE MANAGEMENT IN FETAL TACHYCARDIA
1. Goals

COMMENTS/TIPS/
CAUTIONS

   a. To reduce fetal heart rate
      i. Begin to administer oxygen by face mask at 8 liters/minute
     ii. Take mother's temperature
    iii. Notify physician

IV rate may need to be increased if mother has fever

*From Litchfield, M.L.: Intrapartum fetal monitoring. Intrapartum Assessment and Management Module, Charleston, Medical University of South Carolina, Perinatal Education Program, 1982.

Fetal bradycardia is a decrease in the baseline fetal heart rate to less than 110 beats/minute.

ETIOLOGY OF FETAL BRADYCARDIA

1. Fetal hypoxia
2. Drug induced: propranolol; agents for producing epidural, spinal, pudendal anesthesia; oxytocin, which causes hyperstimulation of the uterus, resulting in hypoxia
3. Prolapsed cord
4. Maternal hypotension
5. Maternal hypothermia

PATIENT CARE MANAGEMENT IN FETAL BRADYCARDIA

	COMMENTS/TIPS/ CAUTIONS
1. Goals	
a. To relieve fetal bradycardia	
i. Begin to administer oxygen by face mask at 8 liters/ minute	Continued fetal bradycardia may necessitate an immediate C/S
ii. Change maternal position	Change in maternal position facilitates increased blood flow
iii. Discontinue oxytocin if infusion is being given	
iv. Notify physician immediately	

Early deceleration is a transitory decrease in fetal heart rate caused by compressions of fetal head. Compression of fetal head stimulates vagus nerve to decrease heart rate. Early deceleration is not considered a sign of fetal distress.

DIAGNOSIS OF EARLY DECELERATION

1. Uniform shape of deceleration on fetal monitor strip
2. Begins at beginning of contraction and ends with end of contraction

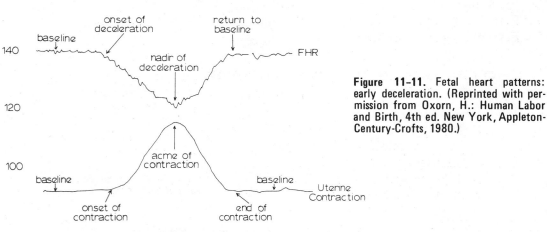

Figure 11-11. Fetal heart patterns: early deceleration. (Reprinted with permission from Oxorn, H.: Human Labor and Birth, 4th ed. New York, Appleton-Century-Crofts, 1980.)

Early deceleration.

3. Depth of decelerations is related to intensity of contraction
4. Deceleration rarely goes below 110 beats/minute

ETIOLOGY OF EARLY DECELERATION

1. Sterile vaginal examination
2. During second stage of labor with pushing efforts
3. During application of scalp electrode
4. In cephalopelvic disproportion
5. In vertex presentations

PATIENT CARE MANAGEMENT IN EARLY DECELERATION

COMMENTS/TIPS/
CAUTIONS

1. No treatment necessary   Early decelerations may be first sign that cervix is
completely dilated

Variable decelerations consist of transitory decreases in fetal heart rate caused by compression of umbilical cord. Variable decelerations are not associated with poor fetal outcome if baseline heart rate remains stable and variability is not decreased.

DIAGNOSIS OF VARIABLE DECELERATION

1. Variable shape (often V or U shaped) of deceleration on fetal monitor strip
2. Variable onset: may begin at any time in relation to contraction
3. Heart rate may fall below 90 beats/minute; variable decelerations below 60 beats/minute are severe
4. Variable duration (greater than 40 to 60 seconds = prolonged deceleration)
5. Occur more frequently in active labor

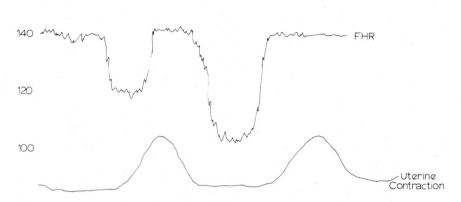

Variable deceleration.

Figure 11-12. Fetal heart patterns: variable deceleration. (Reprinted with permission from Oxorn, H.: Human Labor and Birth, 4th ed. New York, Appleton-Century-Crofts, 1980.)

ETIOLOGY OF VARIABLE DECELERATION

1. Prolapse of cord
2. Nuchal cord (cord around the neck)
3. Cord occlusion (true knot)

PATIENT CARE MANAGEMENT IN VARIABLE DECELERATION

1. Goals

a. To relieve compression of umbilical cord

    i. Change mother's position

        (a) Back to side

        (b) Side to side

        (c) Knee-chest

    ii. Perform sterile vaginal examination

    iii. Begin to administer oxygen by face mask at 8 liters/minute

    iv. Notify physician

    v. Discontinue oxytocin if decelerations severe and prolonged

    vi. Document treatment on strip graph and labor record

    vii. Assist physician in obtaining fetal scalp sample for pH determination (see Chapter 9)

COMMENTS/TIPS/CAUTIONS

Use knee-chest position only for prolapsed cord or a severe prolonged deceleration not relieved by other position changes

It is important to rule out prolapse of cord

Late deceleration is a transitory decrease in fetal heart rate caused by uteroplacental insufficiency; uteroplacental insufficiency means that there is decreased blood flow to the fetus. *All late decelerations are ominous.* Hypoxia is present.

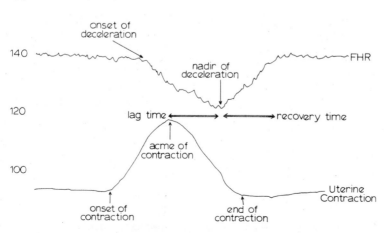

Late deceleration.

Figure 11–13. Fetal heart patterns: late deceleration. (Reprinted with permission from Oxorn, H.: Human Labor and Birth, 4th ed. New York, Appleton-Century-Crofts, 1980.)

DIAGNOSIS OF LATE DECELERATION

1. Uniform shape of deceleration on fetal monitor strip
2. Begins after onset of contraction and ends after contraction completed
3. Often begins with peak of contraction
4. Depth of deceleration related to intensity of contraction

ETIOLOGY OF LATE DECELERATION

1. Hematological disorders: anemia, sickle cell disease, Rh isoimmunization
2. Bleeding disorders: abruptio placentae, placenta previa
3. Hypertensive disorders
4. Placental dysfunction: infarcts, postmature
5. Diabetes
6. Maternal hypotension
7. Uterine hyperstimulation and tetanic contractions

PATIENT CARE MANAGEMENT IN LATE DECELERATION

1. Goals

    a. To minimize the effects of late deceleration

	COMMENTS/TIPS/CAUTIONS
i. Turn patient to her left side	Will increase blood flow to the uterus
ii. Discontinue oxytocin administration	Will decrease uterine activity and maximize blood flow to uterus
iii. Begin to administer oxygen by face mask at 8 liters/minute	Increase amount of oxygen available for fetus
iv. Increase IV fluids	
v. Notify physician	
vi. Document treatments on strip graph and labor record	Remember that strip graph is part of medical record

In *decreased variability* the change in fetal heart rate is less than 5 beats/minute with little or no fluctuation around the baseline. Decreased variability is very ominous if associated with late deceleration or severe or prolonged variable deceleration.

ETIOLOGY OF DECREASED VARIABILITY

1. Hypoxia and acidosis
2. Fetal sleep (should last only 20 to 30 minutes)
3. Drug induced: narcotics, i.e., meperidine (Demerol); anesthetic agents; barbiturates; magnesium sulfate; alcohol; ritodrine
4. Prematurity
5. Fetal cardiac arrhythmias

PATIENT CARE MANAGEMENT IN DECREASED VARIABILITY

1. Goals

    a. To minimize the effects of decreased variability

      i. Rule out benign cause, i.e., drugs, fetal sleep
     ii. Begin to administer oxygen by face mask at 8 liters/ minute
    iii. Institute treatment for any deceleration
    iv. Notify physician immediately

INTRAUTERINE FETAL DEATH

A mother in whom intrauterine fetal death is diagnosed faces a tremendous emotional crisis. When labor does not start spontaneously she then must undergo induction of labor with its associated risks and complications. She also is at risk for complications when intrauterine death is prolonged.

DIAGNOSIS

Intrauterine fetal death is the death of the fetus in utero after 20 weeks' gestation.

1. Predisposing factors
   a. Maternal diabetes after 38 weeks' gestation
   b. Rh sensitized mothers

ETIOLOGY

1. Unknown
2. Trauma
3. Abruption of placenta

ASSESSMENT

1. **Clinical presentation**
   a. Signs and symptoms
      i. Cessation of fetal movement
      ii. Absence of fetal heart tones
   b. History
      i. Diabetes
      ii. Rh sensitization of mothers
      iii. Trauma
      iv. Cessation of fetal movement

2. **Biopsychosocial assessment**
   a. Palpation of overlying sutures during vaginal examination

3. **Diagnostic data**
   a. Flat plate x-ray of the abdomen reveals overlying suture
   b. In real-time study no cardiac movement detected

PROBLEMS AND COMPLICATIONS

1. Amniotic fluid embolus
2. Disseminated intravascular coagulation (DIC) more likely if dead fetus has been retained in utero longer than 5 weeks (incidence 1 in 4)[1]

PATIENT CARE MANAGEMENT

1. **Goals**

   a. To prevent development of coagulation defect

      i. Obtain baseline clotting studies on admission and obtain serial determinations as ordered by physician

         As labor progresses the DIC process may begin to manifest itself

      ii. Evaluate condition of patient for signs of abnormal bleeding process, i.e., bleeding from gums, nose, or puncture sites

   b. To expedite delivery with minimal discomfort

      i. Begin induction of labor as ordered by physician

         (a) *Oxytocin:* watch patient and do not allow contraction pattern to become hyperstimulated

            Risk of amniotic fluid embolism already increased

         (b) *Prostaglandin suppositories:* premedicate patient to counteract major side effects of the drug: nausea and vomiting, diarrhea, and elevation of temperature

            Warn patient of common side effects so that she will be prepared

      ii. Administer medication for pain as needed by patient

         Larger than usual doses of pain medication may be given, since fetus is dead

   c. To help mother and family begin grieving process

      Most important role of nurse is to facilitate grieving process

      i. Assess mother's and family's response to fetal death and stage of grieving process

         Remember that patient's culture influences how she will handle and respond to this loss

      ii. Assess mother's support system

         Should begin in labor and delivery room and be communicated to postpartum staff

      iii. Encourage parents to see and hold baby

         Parents often imagine that baby looks far worse than it does; prepare them for the abnormalities; if parents refuse to see baby, take a picture of baby and give to another close family member in case parents later express regrets about not seeing baby

      iv. Prepare them for how the baby looks

	COMMENTS/TIPS/CAUTIONS
v. Clean baby and make as attractive as possible; wrap in baby blanket and take to parents	Emphasize the normal features of infant
vi. Remain with parents as needed to facilitate grief, or allow them time alone if they desire	It is all right to let them see you cry or show emotion; it lets them know you care
vii. Do not try to minimize experience for them by stating that they can always have other children	Parents must be able to accept this loss before they can consider future
viii. Provide information to parents about normal phases in grieving process	Parents frequently feel anxious and confused about how they are feeling; they may even feel that they are going crazy

ABRUPTIO PLACENTAE

Abruptio placentae is a serious complication of pregnancy. In severe cases associated with fetal death, the maternal mortality is 10 per cent. Abruptions account for about 15 per cent of all perinatal deaths. Perinatal mortality occurs in over 50 per cent of cases of abruptio placentae.[1,3]

DIAGNOSIS

Abruptio placentae is premature separation of the normally situated placenta from its uterine site of implantation after 20 weeks' gestation and before delivery of the fetus. Bleeding, apparent or concealed, always accompanies abruption.

1. **Incidence**
   a. 1 in 250 pregnancies[1]
   b. Tends to recur in subsequent pregnancies

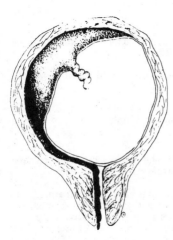

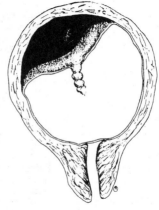

Figure 11-14. Abruptio placentae: *A,* external or apparent; *B,* internal or concealed. (Reprinted with permission from Oxorn, H.: Human Labor and Birth, 4th ed. New York, Appleton-Century-Crofts, 1980.)

A. External or apparent.   **B.** Internal or concealed.

Abruptio placentae. Revealed and concealed hemorrhage.

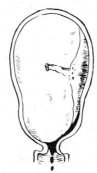

Revealed hemorrhage

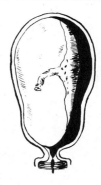

Concealed & revealed hemorrhage

Figure 11-15. Abruptio placentae: *A,* revealed hemorrhage; *B,* concealed and revealed hemorrhage; *C* and *D,* concealed hemorrhage. (Reprinted with permission from Cavanaugh, D., et al.: Obstetric Emergencies, 3rd ed. Philadelphia, Harper and Row, 1982.)

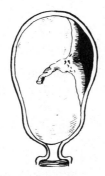

Concealed hemorrhage

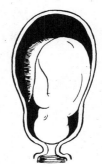

Premature separation of placenta with concealed hemorrhage

   c. Approximately 50 per cent of abruptions occur before week 36 of pregnancy

2. Predisposing factors
   a. Hypertension of any origin
   b. Increased parity
   c. External trauma
   d. Overdistention of uterus, including multiple pregnancy
   e. Short umbilical cord
   f. History of reproductive loss (abortion, premature labor, stillbirth, neonatal death)

ETIOLOGY

1. Exact cause is unknown
2. Often associated with DIC[1,8,9]

3. Classification
   Abruptions are classified in two ways:
   a. By grade
      i. *Grade O:* diagnosed only after delivery when a small dark clot is found adhering to a segment of placenta; patient is usually asymptomatic

  ii. *Grade 1:* External bleeding is often present, but uterine tetany and tenderness may not be noted; no shock or fetal distress occurs

  iii. *Grade 2:* External bleeding may be observed together with uterine tetany and tenderness; fetal distress is present, and fetal death may occur

  iv. *Grade 3:* External bleeding may or may not be evident; uterine tetany, maternal shock, fetal death, and DIC are typical[3]

 b. By degree

  i. Total: complete separation of the placenta

  ii. Partial: separation of a portion of the placenta so that maternal bleeding occurs between the uterine wall and the placental surface

ASSESSMENT

1. Clinical presentation

 a. Signs and symptoms

  i. Apparent (revealed) hemorrhage

   (a) Vaginal bleeding (bright red or dark clotted)

   (b) Slight uterine irritability

   (c) Uterus relaxes poorly between contractions

  ii. Concealed hemorrhage

   (a) No vaginal bleeding

   (b) Extreme pain produced by accumulation of blood behind placenta; may be of sudden onset

   (c) Increase in uterine size

   (d) Rigidity of uterus; uterus fails to relax between contractions

   (e) Fetal distress; absence of fetal heart tones[8,9]

 b. History

  i. Trauma

  ii. Polyhydramnios

  iii. Uterine anomalies

  iv. Multiparity

  v. Hypertension

  vi. Rh factor

  vii. Fundal height

2. Biopsychosocial assessment

 a. Amount of vaginal bleeding

 b. Signs of shock (rapid pulse, dyspnea, yawning, restlessness)

 c. Uterine tone between contractions

 d. Uterine size

3. Diagnostic data

 a. Blood: CBC, clotting studies

 b. Real-time study

PROBLEMS AND COMPLICATIONS

1. Maternal death

2. Fetal death
3. DIC
4. Renal failure
5. Neurological damage to infant
6. Postpartum hemorrhage[8]

PATIENT CARE MANAGEMENT

1. Goals

COMMENTS/TIPS/
CAUTIONS

   a. To promptly recognize patients with factors predisposing to abruption

      i. Assess patient for

         (a) Hypertension

         (b) Multiple gestation

         (c) Diabetes

         (d) Multiparity

         (e) Advanced maternal age

   b. To promptly detect signs of premature separation of placenta

      i. Notify physician of any sudden changes in behavior, i.e., aching pain in abdomen, regional tenderness)

      ii. Report any vaginal bleeding to physician

Remember that bleeding may be concealed

      iii. Evaluate uterine relaxation between contractions

Concealed hemorrhage may cause the uterus to become boardlike

      iv. Measure fundal height and mark on abdomen with a pen if suspicious of abruption: reevaluate every hour

Increase in fundal height is indicative of concealed hemorrhage

      v. Institute measures for treatment of hemorrhagic shock if signs of shock occur (see Chapter 9) and prepare for immediate delivery (see Chapter 9), vaginal or cesarean

      vi. Notify physician of abnormalities in FHR

   c. To deliver fetus safely and stabilize maternal condition

      i. Assist physician with rupture of membranes with a membrane trocar or spinal needle

Gradual drainage of amniotic fluid decreases intrauterine tension, reduces extravasation of blood into the myometrium, and decreases chance of amniotic fluid embolus

      ii. Prepare to induce labor if bleeding is not severe and

FHTs are stable (see Oxytocin [Pitocin] Induction, Appendix A)

(a) Be prepared to help perform cesarean section if necessary: have blood typed and cross-matched and ready for immediate transfusion

ii. Observe patient for signs of DIC: bleeding from mouth, nose, or puncture sites

iii. Notify pediatrician to be present for delivery

d. To provide emotional support to parents

i. Explain what is happening

ii. Reinforce positive aspects of mother's condition, i.e., stable FHTs, decreased bleeding

iii. After delivery provide information about baby's condition

COMMENTS/TIPS/CAUTIONS

Infant may need attention because of hypoxia, prematurity, or birth trauma

PLACENTA PREVIA

Placenta previa is the most common cause of bleeding during the latter months of pregnancy and presents a severe threat to the mother and baby if profuse hemorrhage occurs.

DIAGNOSIS

In placenta previa the placenta is implanted in the lower uterine segment so that it adjoins or covers the internal os of the cervix.

1. **Incidence**
   a. 1 in 200 pregnancies
   b. Increases with parity
   c. More common in women over 35 years of age
   d. Incidence of malpresentation increases

2. **Predisposing factors**
   a. Multiparity
   b. Advancing maternal age
   c. Faulty implantation
   d. Previous uterine scarring (especially of the lower segment)
   e. Endometritis after a previous pregnancy
   f. Large placenta

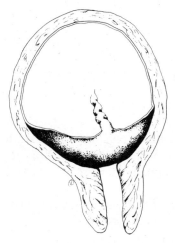

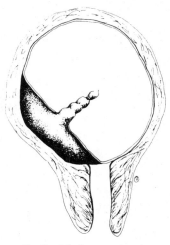

A. Total placenta previa.

B. Partial placenta previa.

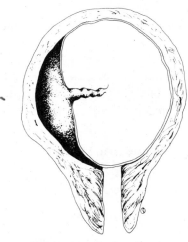

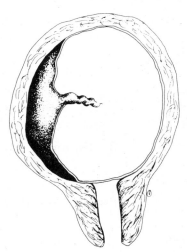

C. Marginal placenta previa.

D. Low lying placenta.

Figure 11-16. Placenta previa: *A,* total placenta previa; *B,* partial placenta previa; *C,* marginal placenta previa; *D,* low lying placenta. (Reprinted with permission from Oxorn, H.: Human Labor and Birth, 4th ed. New York, Appleton - Century - Crofts, 1980.)

3. **Classification**

Classification is based upon anticipated placement of placenta at full dilatation of cervix

a. *Total:* internal os covered completely by placenta
b. *Partial:* internal os partially covered by placenta
c. *Marginal:* edge of placenta at margin of internal os
d. *Low lying placenta:* region of internal os encroached upon by placenta so that placental edge may be palpated by examining finger when introduced through cervix[9]

ETIOLOGY

1. Precise cause unknown
2. As cervix effaces and dilates, there is a degree of separation of placenta from the wall of the uterus; this is associated with rupture of the underlying blood vessels[8]

ASSESSMENT

1. Clinical Presentation
   a. Signs and symptoms
      i. Painless hemorrhage, which usually does not appear until early third trimester
     ii. Bright red bleeding
    iii. Uterus remains soft.
    iv. First episode of bleeding often while patient is asleep
     v. Presenting part often found floating above symphysis pubis
    vi. First hemorrhage almost never catastrophic
   b. History
      i. Painless vaginal bleeding during last trimester
     ii. Maternal age, parity
    iii. Malpresentation
    iv. EDC, estimated fetal weight, fundal height

2. Biopsychosocial Assessment
   a. Manual examination is not done except under double setup conditions
   b. BP, vital signs
   c. Amount and character of bleeding (pad count)
   d. Visualization of placenta on speculum examination
   e. Presence of malpresentation

3. Diagnostic data
   a. Ultrasound or real-time scan

PROBLEMS AND COMPLICATIONS

1. Shock following massive hemorrhage
2. Failure of engagement
3. Abnormal presentation (breech or transverse lie)
4. Congenital anomalies
5. Placenta accreta
6. Postpartum hemorrhage
7. Prematurity[8]

PATIENT CARE MANAGEMENT

1. Goals
   a. To promptly recognize and evaluate signs and symptoms of placenta previa and rule out abruptio placentae
      i. Observe and assess any external bleeding: count pads, weigh pads and linen savers, assess color
     ii. Assess patient for presence of pain

COMMENTS/TIPS/CAUTIONS

Placenta previa frequently will have been diagnosed prior to admission to labor and delivery

Bright red bleeding usually associated with placenta previa rather than abruptio placentae

TABLE 11-4. DIFFERENTIATION OF PLACENTA PREVIA
AND ABRUPTIO PLACENTAE

	Placenta Previa	Abruptio Placentae
Onset	Quiet and sneaky	Sudden and stormy
Bleeding	External	External and concealed
Color of blood	Bright red	Dark venous
Anemia	= Blood loss	> Apparent blood loss
Shock	= Blood loss	> Apparent blood loss
Toxemia	Absent	May be present
Pain	Only labor	Severe and steady
Uterine tenderness	Absent	Present
Uterine tone	Soft and relaxed	Firm to stony hard
Uterine contour	Normal	May enlarge and change shape
Fetal heart tones	Usually present	Present or absent
Engagement	Absent	May be present
Presentation	May be abnormal	No relationship

Reprinted with permission from Oxorn, H.: Human Labor and Birth, 4th ed. New York, Appleton-Century-Crofts, 1980.

	COMMENTS/TIPS/CAUTIONS
iii. Assess uterine contractility and relaxation	
b. To control bleeding and stabilize maternal condition	
i. Do not give anything orally	Surgery a distinct possibility
ii. Do not perform rectal or vaginal examination	May stimulate profuse hemorrhage
iii. Do not give enema	
iv. Place patient in semi-Fowler's position	Fetal body may act as a tamponade against the placenta
v. Monitor maternal and fetal status	
c. To deliver a viable neonate	
i. Prepare for double setup (see Appendix A)	
d. To provide emotional support to parents	
i. Explain what is happening	Give rationale
ii. Encourage verbalization of concerns and questions	
iii. Prepare couple for possibility of surgical delivery	Allow support person to remain with mother if possible

PLACENTAL DISORDERS

Retention in the uterus of part (fragments) or all of the placenta interferes with contraction and retraction, keeps the blood sinuses open, and leads to postpartum hemorrhage. Retained placenta is caused by partial separation of a normal placenta; entrapment of partially or completely separated placenta by a constriction ring of the uterus; or abnormal adherence of entire placenta or portion of placenta to uterine wall.[3]

PLACENTAL DISORDERS: ──────── ABNORMAL ADHERENCE OF THE PLACENTA ──────────

DIAGNOSIS

1. **Incidence**
   a. 1 in 540 to 1 in 93,000 deliveries
2. **Predisposing factors**
   a. Increased maternal age
   b. Multiparity
   c. Uterine scar
   d. Previous curettage
   e. Previous manual removal of placenta
   f. Previous endometritis
   g. Placenta previa
   h. Implantation of placenta in cornual area[8]
3. **Classification**
   Abnormal adherence of the placenta is classified in two ways:
   a. By extent
      i. *Complete:* entire placenta is adherent to the myometrium
      ii. *Partial:* one or more cotyledons are adherent
   b. By depth
      i. *Placenta accreta:* placenta is adherent to the myometrium
      ii. *Placenta increta:* chorionic villi have penetrated the uterine muscle
      iii. *Placenta percreta:* the villi penetrate wall of the uterus[8]

ETIOLOGY

1. **Maternal factors**
   a. Increased maternal age
   b. Multiparity
2. **Uterine factors**
   a. Uterine scar
   b. Previous curettage
   c. Previous manual removal of placenta
   d. Previous endometritis
3. **Placental factors**
   a. Placenta previa
   b. Implantation of placenta in the cornual area

ASSESSMENT

1. **Clinical presentation**
   a. Signs and symptoms
      i. Retention of placenta

      ii. Postpartum hemorrhage, particularly when physician attempts manual removal of placenta
- b. History
  - i. Antepartum bleeding
  - ii. Previous uterine surgery

2. Biopsychosocial assessment
- a. Heavy bleeding
- b. Passing of clots
- c. Failure of placenta to separate

PROBLEMS AND COMPLICATIONS

1. Uterine inversion
2. Uterine rupture
3. Postpartum hemorrhage
4. Maternal infection

PATIENT CARE MANAGEMENT

1. Goals
- a. To minimize the effects of placental disorders
  - i. Institute measures to combat hemorrhagic shock
  - ii. Contact anesthesiologist and have operating room ready for possible operation
  - iii. Help patient relax during uterine exploration
  - iv. If complete placenta accreta is found, prepare patient for hysterectomy

_____ DISSEMINATED INTRAVASCULAR COAGULATION _____

The presence of DIC in any patient is an extreme emergency. If DIC is not treated immediately and effectively, the end result is often maternal death.

DIAGNOSIS

DIC is a pathological form of clotting that is diffuse rather than localized; it consumes clotting factors, such as fibrinogen, so that massive external and internal hemorrhage occurs.[3]

1. Incidence
- a. Not known

2. Predisposing factors[3]
- a. Abruptio placentae
- b. Intrauterine dead fetus syndrome
- c. Amniotic fluid embolism
- d. Preeclampsia-eclampsia
- e. Hemorrhagic shock

    f.   Rupture of uterus
    g.   Tumultuous labor

ETIOLOGY

Stimuli likely to initiate DIC (occurs with abruption, intrauterine fetal death, amniotic fluid emboli)

1. Infusion of tissue extract
2. Endothelial damage
3. Bacterial debris or endotoxins (septic shock)
4. Chemical and physical agents
5. Hemolytic processes
6. Immune reactions
7. Thrombocytopenia[1,3]

ASSESSMENT

1. Clinical presentation
    a.   Signs and symptoms
        i.   Abnormal bleeding, usually heavy vaginal bleeding
        ii.   Hematuria
        iii.   Bleeding from gums and nose
        iv.   Prolonged oozing from injection sites
    b.   History
        i.   Abruption
        ii.   Intrauterine fetal death (particularly of more than 5 weeks' duration)
        iii.   Preeclampsia-eclampsia
        iv.   Postpartum hemorrhagic sepsis
        v.   Tumultuous or hypertonic labor
        vi.   Difficult delivery

2. Diagnostic data
    a.   Reduced platelets
    b.   Reduced fibrinogen
    c.   Prolonged prothrombin time
    d.   Prolonged partial thromboplastin time
    e.   Increased fibrin split products

PROBLEMS AND COMPLICATIONS

1. Maternal death
2. Fetal death

PATIENT CARE MANAGEMENT

1. Goals
    a.   To recognize symptoms of DIC promptly
        i.   Evaluate for the presence of any predisposing factor

ii. Observe for any signs of abnormal bleeding

iii. Note any signs of tachycardia, diaphoresis, restlessness with anxiety

b. To remove causative factor

i. Assist physician as directed to institute treatment

c. To control shock

i. Institute procedure for hemorrhagic shock

ii. Administer whole blood as needed to maintain hematocrit at 30 per cent and urinary output at 30 cc/hour

iii. Administer blood components as needed: platelets, cryoprecipitate

iv. Report laboratory values to physician

COMMENTS/TIPS/CAUTIONS

Prolonged oozing from puncture sites may be one of the first signs of beginning DIC

One unit of platelets raises the adult level by 5000; this replaces elements depleted because of coagulation defects

_____ **RUPTURE OF THE UTERUS** _____

Rupture of the uterus continues to be one of the most dangerous complications of pregnancy. It is responsible for 5 per cent of all maternal deaths, and infant death occurs in 50 to 75 per cent of cases.[1,10]

DIAGNOSIS

Rupture of the uterus is the tearing of previously intact uterine musculature or of an old uterine scar. It may occur during pregnancy but is more frequent during labor.

1. **Incidence**
   a. 1 in 2000 pregnancies

2. **Predisposing factors**
   a. Previous cesarean section
      i. If classic incision was used, rupture more likely to occur during last trimester of pregnancy
      ii. If lower segment incision was used, rupture more likely to occur during labor
   b. Grand multiparity (a thin uterine wall)
   c. Malpresentation
   d. Minimum cephalopelvic disproportion
   e. Pendulous abdomen
   f. Trauma to the abdomen[1]

ETIOLOGY

1. **Classification**
   a. *Complete:* Rupture extends through entire uterine wall, and uterine contents spill into abdominal cavity
   b. *Incomplete:* Rupture extends through endometrium and myometrium, but peritoneum surrounding uterus remains intact
2. Rupture of weakened cesarean section scar, usually from a classic incision (most common cause)
3. Mismanagement of oxytocin induction or stimulation of labor
4. Prolonged or obstructed labor
5. Malpresentation or fetal abnormality (i.e., hydrocephalus)
6. Excessive fetal size
7. Traumatic vaginal delivery—such as internal version, midforceps delivery, shoulder dystocia, or breech extraction—when the cervix is not completely dilated or effaced[10]

ASSESSMENT

1. **Clinical presentation**
   a. Signs and symptoms
      i. *Overt rupture*
         (a) Intense, sharp, shooting pains in lower abdomen
         (b) Sensation of internal tearing
         (c) Immediate cessation of contractions and dissipation of pain (torn muscle can no longer contract)
         (d) Vaginal bleeding, usually slight
         (e) Abdominal palpation reveals fetus beside uterus
         (f) Fetal bradycardia occurs, or fetal heart tones may be lost
         (g) Signs of maternal hypovolemic shock[3,7]
      ii. *Impending rupture*
         The following may indicate that the lower uterine segment is becoming acutely thin:
         (a) Restlessness and anxiety because of severe pain
         (b) No progress in cervical dilatation
         (c) A ridge or "ballooning out" of uterus above the symphysis pubis
         (d) A contraction (retraction) ring may be evident between the upper and lower uterine segments (manifested by an indentation across the lower abdominal wall with acute tenderness above the symphysis)
         (e) Tetanic contractions (over 90 seconds' duration)
         (f) Nausea and vomiting
         (g) Fetal distress[3,7]
   b. History
      i. Previous cesarean section
      ii. Malpresentation
      iii. Some degree of cephalopelvic disproportion
      iv. Oxytocin administration

v. Parity

vi. Sudden abdominal pain with nausea and vomiting

2. Biopsychosocial Assessment

a. Hypotension

b. Rapid pulse rate

c. Skin cold, clammy, and pale

d. Abdominal examination indicates generalized tenderness with "rebound"; distention

e. Absence of fetal heart tones

f. Ascent of presenting part on vaginal examination when compared with previous examination

g. Palpation of fetus beside uterus

PROBLEMS AND COMPLICATIONS

Treatment must begin immediately to avert the following:

1. Irreversible shock and maternal death
2. Fetal death
3. Fetal anoxia leading to long range complications
4. Peritonitis

PATIENT CARE MANAGEMENT

1. Goals

a. To prevent tetanic contractions (lasting more than 90 seconds) or hyperstimulation during labor

i. Monitor frequency and length of uterine contractions

ii. Monitor baseline uterine tone during oxytocin administration

iii. If tetanic contractions or hyperstimulation occurs, institute immediate treatment (see Chapter 9)

b. To promptly recognize signs of impending rupture

i. Assess patient for signs of restlessness and anxiety

ii. Assess patient's description of pain

iii. Palpate uterus for presence of contraction ring

c. To promote a more successful outcome by prompt treatment

COMMENTS/TIPS/CAUTIONS

Patients may have hyperstimulatory contractions naturally without labor being augmented or induced with oxytocin; baseline uterine tone should not exceed 25 mm Hg

Patient will begin to describe the pains as different

<table>
<tr><td>

i. Call for assistance and have physician notified

ii. Institute measures outlined for treatment of hemorrhagic shock (see Chapter 9)

iii. Prepare patient for immediate laparotomy

iv. Continue to monitor maternal vital signs and fetal heart tones

</td><td>

COMMENTS/TIPS/ CAUTIONS

Prompt surgical intervention is the only hope for the fetus

</td></tr>
</table>

d. To provide emotional support to family

    i. Respond in a calm, organized fashion — *Anxiety is contagious*

    ii. Explain to parents what will happen

    iii. Remain with patient until anesthesia has been given — *To provide some measure of reassurance to patient*

    iv. Provide support to father and other family members while surgery is in progress

---

INVERSION OF THE UTERUS

Inversion of the uterus after delivery is a critical intrapartum complication. Profound shock occurs, and if treatment is not instituted immediately, maternal mortality may reach 30 per cent; even among recognized and treated cases, mortality is about 10 per cent.[1,3]

DIAGNOSIS

Inversion of the uterus is a turning inside out of the uterus so that the fundus intrudes into the cervix or vagina (caused by too vigorous removal of the placenta before it is detached by the normal process of labor).

1. **Incidence**
   a. 1 in 5000 deliveries
   b. Occurs more often in primigravidas

2. **Predisposing factors**
   These can be subdivided into abnormalities of the uterus and its contents and functional condition of the uterus.
   a. Adherent placenta
   b. Short umbilical cord
   c. Congenital anomalies
   d. Weakness of uterine wall at placental site
   e. Fundal implantation of placenta
   f. Neoplasm of uterus

    g. Relaxation of myometrium

    h. Disturbance of contractile mechanism[1,8]

3. Mismanagement of the third stage of labor

ETIOLOGY

1. Attempts to hasten third stage of labor by combined traction on cord and improper fundal pressure on relaxed uterus
2. Manual removal of placenta
3. Increase in abdominal pressure (coughing, sneezing)[1,8]
4. Pathological stages of inversion
    a. Acute inversion (occurs immediately after birth of baby or placenta before cervix has begun to contract)
    b. Cervix and lower uterine segment contract around encircled portion of uterus
    c. Edema
    d. Reduction of blood supply
    e. Gangrene and necrosis
    f. Sloughing[8]

ASSESSMENT

1. Clinical presentation
    a. Signs and symptoms
        i. Signs of shock out of proportion to amount of bleeding observed
        ii. Traction being exerted on the cord
    b. History
        i. Previous uterine inversion
        ii. Previous retained placenta

2. Biopsychosocial Assessment
    a. Large, red, rounded mass protrudes 20 to 30 cm outside introitus (complete inversion)
    b. Smooth mass can be palpated through dilated cervix (incomplete inversion)
    c. Inability to locate uterine fundus on abdominal palpation[3]

PROBLEMS AND COMPLICATIONS

1. Irreversible shock and maternal death
2. Hysterectomy
3. Infection

PATIENT CARE MANAGEMENT

1. Goals
    a. To promote more successful outcome by prompt institution of treatment
        i. Institute measures outlined in Chapter 9 for hemorrhagic shock

COMMENTS/TIPS/
CAUTIONS

Shock presents greatest immediate danger

ii. Notify anesthesiologist and assist with intubation as directed
iii. Administer oxytocin as directed by physician
iv. Assist physician as directed during attempt to replace uterus manually
v. Prepare for surgery if manual replacement unsuccessful

COMMENTS/TIPS/ CAUTIONS

Do not use methylergonovine (Methergine) or ergonovine (Ergotrate), since they cause cervical as well as uterine contraction

OBSTETRICAL ANALGESIA AND ANESTHESIA

Of every 100 maternal deaths in the United States, 6 to 10 are directly related to anesthesia. Ninety per cent of these deaths are preventable and result from unwise choice of anesthetic, improper technique, or excessive dosage. Unfortunately the baby is also affected.[1] The morbidity from prolonged fetal and maternal hypoxia is considerable.

OBSTETRICAL ANALGESIA

Analgesia is the reduction or relief of pain without loss of consciousness.

AGENT

1. Barbiturates (Seconal, Nembutal, Amytal): most effective in latent phase of labor
2. Narcotics (Demerol): most effective in active phase of labor
3. Ataractics (Phenergan, Largon, Vistaril): most effective in latent phase of labor

PATIENT CARE MANAGEMENT

1. Ascertain patient allergies
2. Explain action of drug to patient and family
3. If intravenous medication is prescribed, administer it during a uterine contraction to decrease transfer of drug to fetus
4. Raise side rails
5. Document amount, route of administration, and time on labor record and baby check list

PROBLEMS AND COMPLICATIONS

1. Drug reaction
2. Depression of neonate

_____ OBSTETRICAL ANESTHESIA _____

Anesthesia is partial or complete absence of sensation with or without loss of consciousness.

AGENTS FOR GENERAL ANESTHESIA

1. Nitrous oxide: produces local or general loss of sensitivity to touch, pain, or other stimulation
2. Thiopental (Pentothal) sodium: produces rapid induction of anesthesia; depresses neonate
3. Halothane: relaxes uterus quickly; used to facilitate intrauterine manipulation, version, or extraction[3]
   a. Anesthetic agents reach fetus in about 2 minutes
   b. Amount of fetal depression is related to depth of maternal anesthesia
   c. Greatest danger is aspiration of vomitus with respiratory obstruction, aspiration pneumonitis, and cardiac arrest (most common cause of maternal death).

PATIENT CARE MANAGEMENT IN GENERAL ANESTHESIA

1. Note time and quality of last meal on admission of patient
2. Do not give patient anything by mouth during labor
3. Assist with intubation as directed by anesthesiologist
4. During immediate postpartum period monitor patients closely who have received halothane (more prone to uterine atony)

PROBLEMS AND COMPLICATIONS OF GENERAL ANESTHESIA

1. Laryngospasm
2. Aspiration of vomitus
3. Respiratory depression
4. Cardiac arrest

AGENTS FOR REGIONAL ANESTHESIA

1. Procaine (Novocain)
2. Lidocaine (Xylocaine)
3. Bupivacaine (Marcaine)
4. Tetracaine (Pontocaine)
5. Mepivacaine (Carbocaine)

TYPES OF ADMINISTRATION OF REGIONAL ANESTHESIA

1. Pudendal block: injection of a local anesthetic at the pudendal nerve root to produce numbness of the genital and perianal region
2. Epidural: injection of an anesthetic on top of (or over) the dura through third, fourth, or fifth lumbar interspace; may be given as a single injection or continuously
3. Saddle (low spinal): injection of anesthetic agent into the subarachnoid space where the medication mixes with cerebrospinal fluid

PROBLEMS AND COMPLICATIONS OF REGIONAL ANESTHESIA

1. Hypotension (hypotension from spinal anesthesia the second most common cause of maternal anesthetic death)
2. Respiratory depression
3. Convulsions[1]

PATIENT CARE MANAGEMENT IN REGIONAL ANESTHESIA

1. Note any history of allergy to local anesthetic agents
2. Hydrate patient with 500 ml lactated Ringer's solution before giving spinal or epidural anesthesia
3. Check BP every minute for 5 minutes after administration of spinal or epidural anesthesia; continue BP checks
4. If hypertension occurs
   a. Increase rate of IV infusion
   b. Elevate the patient's legs 90 degrees
   c. Turn patient to left lateral position (to remove pressure of the uterus from the inferior vena cava)
   d. If hypertension continues, give ephedrine 12.5 mg IV
   e. Give oxygen by face mask[1]
5. *Someone must monitor mother with spinal anesthesia at all times.* Respiratory arrest can occur if spinal anesthesia goes too high.

CONCLUSIONS

As has been noted, many of these complications are extremely rare and will never be encountered by the majority of nurses. With the information provided in this chapter, however, the nurse has a solid knowledge base on which to interact with intrapartum patients. Recognition of predisposing

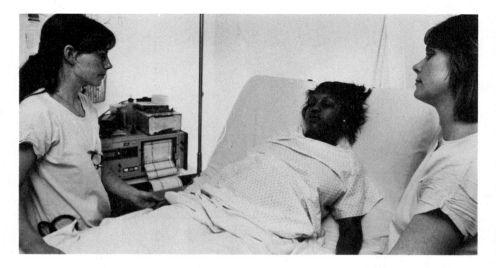

Figure 11-17. Nurses who care for the intrapartum patient in the high risk center appreciate follow-up by staff in the outreach center. (Courtesy of John Clark, Medical University of South Carolina College of Medicine, Charleston, South Carolina.)

factors can guide the nurse in giving care and being more vigilant in observing the patient and significant changes in her. Prompt recognition is the key to preventing harmful sequelae in both mother and infant.

Many of these complications require treatment and follow-up in a tertiary perinatal center. The nurse in the outreach center has the crucial task of stabilizing the condition of the patient and preparing her for transport to the high risk center. The goal of care should be to provide the tertiary center with the most thorough assessment of the patient's history and present condition as is possible. A copy of her prenatal chart and current hospital record should accompany the patient. A family member should be encouraged to accompany her.

Follow-up of the patient's condition and outcome is appreciated by the family and by the nursing and medical staffs at the tertiary center and provides positive feedback to the nurses in the regional center. Communication between the nursing and medical staffs in each center assists the family in effectively reconciling the experience.

REFERENCES

1. Cavanagh, D., Woods, R.E., O'Connor, T.C., and Knuppel, R.A.: Obstetric Emergencies, 3rd ed. Philadelphia, Harper & Row, 1982.
2. Clark, A.L., and Affonso, D.D.: Childbearing: A Nursing Perspective, 2nd ed. Philadelphia, F.A. Davis Co., 1979.
3. Jensen, M.D., Benson, R.C., and Bobak, J.M.: Maternity Care: The Nurse and the Family, 2nd ed. St. Louis, C.V. Mosby Co., 1981.
4. Kelly, M., and Mongiello, R.: Hypertension in pregnancy: Labor, delivery, and postpartum. Am. J. Nurs., 82:813, 1982.
5. Litchfield, M.L.: Intrapartum fetal monitoring. Intrapartum Assessment & Management Module. Charleston, Medical University of South Carolina, Perinatal Education Program, 1982.
6. Matheny, L.: Emergency: First aid for cardiopulmonary arrest. Nursing '82, 12:34, 1982.
7. Olds, S.B., London, M.L., Ladewig, P.A., and Davidson, S.U.: Obstetric Nursing. Menlo Park, Calif., Addison-Wesley Publishing, 1980.
8. Oxorn, H.: Human Labor and Birth, 4th ed. New York, Appleton-Century-Crofts, 1980.
9. Pritchard, J.A., and MacDonald, P.C.: Williams' Obstetrics, 16th ed. New York, Appleton-Century-Crofts, 1980.
10. Reeder, S.J., Mastroianni, L., and Martin, L.L.: Maternity Nursing, 14th ed. Philadelphia, J.B. Lippincott Co., 1980.
11. Varney, H.B.: Nurse-Midwifery. Boston, Blackwell Scientific Publications, 1980.
12. Willis, S.E.: Hypertension in pregnancy: Pathophysiology. Am. J. Nurs., 82:792, 1982.

CHAPTER 12

POSTPARTAL CRISES

Carole Ann Miller McKenzie, C.N.M., Ph.D.

OBJECTIVES

Upon completion of this chapter the reader will be able to accomplish the following:

1. List the components of postpartum assessment
2. Identify the educational needs of the postpartum patient
3. Discuss the data necessary to obtain a thorough postpartum assessment
4. Identify the defense, definition, predisposing factors, etiology, clinical presentation, biopsychosocial assessment, problems and complications, and patient care management of the following postpartal crises: postpartum hemorrhage, thrombophlebitis, puerperal infection, and psychological risk
5. Differentiate between the types of hemorrhage that can occur post partum
6. Differentiate the types of puerperal infection by sites and signs and symptoms

---

A crisis in the postpartal period may be a continuation of a crisis beginning antepartally or intrapartally, or it may be a crisis that begins and ends during the 6 week postpartum period. Regardless of the genesis of the crisis and even though the fetus is not physically affected, the ramifications of a postpartal crisis are most serious. Family integrity may be disrupted, and the integration of the new family member may be hindered. If the crisis is continued from the antepartal or intrapartal periods, the neonate may be experiencing physiological aftereffects. The mother herself may be in grave danger, and her psychological well-being may be compromised. In all, while a postpartal crisis may physiologically affect only the parturient, the long range effects may be staggering not only on her but on the entire family.

It is essential for the nurse to maintain as much positive family centered care as possible while dealing with the crisis to minimize the long range ramifications. By so doing, the nurse is encouraging the family to deal with the crisis in the most efficient manner possible. Although something has occurred to render the experience abnormal, the family needs to maximize the normal aspects of the experience in a positive way.

This chapter will deal only with those entities in the postpartal period that are life threatening or extremely serious. Because of the rapid equaliza-

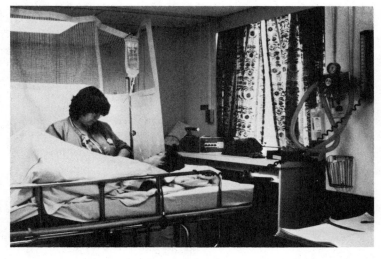

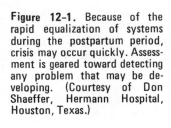

Figure 12–1. Because of the rapid equalization of systems during the postpartum period, crisis may occur quickly. Assessment is geared toward detecting any problem that may be developing. (Courtesy of Don Shaeffer, Hermann Hospital, Houston, Texas.)

tion of systems during this period, crisis is possible at every point. Even when the experience is normal, the possibility of a rapidly evolving threat to well-being is present. The assessment process in the postpartal period is geared to detect rapidly any entity that may be developing. The first portion of the chapter will deal with that assessment process. After assessment, the chapter will include cardiovascular risk, infections in various body systems, and psychological risk.

POSTPARTUM ASSESSMENT

Postpartum assessment is done to determine any abnormality of body systems during the postpartum adaptation process. It is particularly useful in assessing infections occurring at the numerous portals of entry after delivery. Starting at the head and working to the toe of the patient will assist in ensuring a complete assessment.

At each point of the assessment process, teaching can be utilized. Even in an emergency the nurse can make note of educational needs and plan to educate the patient and family as part of anticipatory guidance. The third column of Table 12–1 lists educational needs of patients during the normal postpartum process. In a crisis, additional, specific needs for education are superimposed on the usual educational needs.[5]

POSTPARTUM HEMORRHAGE

Hemorrhage is the leading cause of maternal deaths. Hemorrhage poses two dangers: (1) The anemia resulting from hemorrhage lowers the woman's resistance and predisposes her to puerperal infection. (2) If the hemorrhage is not arrested, death will be the final result.[6]

DIAGNOSIS

Postpartum hemorrhage is blood loss greater than 500 ml following delivery.

1. **Incidence**
   a. Occurs in 5 per cent of all deliveries

TABLE 12-1. POSTPARTUM EDUCATIONAL NEEDS

Body Part	Characteristics	Educational Needs
Vital signs	TPR, BP	How to take a temperature and its importance
Breasts	Contour, temperature, texture, masses, character of veins, pain; nipples: everted, cracks or fissures Types of neonatal feeding problems	Self examination of breasts, breast support, neonatal feeding, breast care
Abdomen	Diastasis recti, CVA tenderness, distention	Postpartum exercises, support
Fundus	Texture, position, pain, midline	Fundal massage, control of bleeding
Elimination	Bladder: distention, pain, amount of voiding, frequency Bowel: bowel movement, pain, bleeding	Fluids, diet, exercise, rest, overdoing
Lochia	Character, amount, odor, clots	Counting pads, too much bleeding, reporting abnormal odor and amount
Perineum	Healing of episiotomy, hematoma, inflammation, temperature, pain, hemorrhoids	How to sit, Kegel exercise, heat to perineum and sitz baths, appropriate way to wipe and apply perineal pads, perineal care, treatment and prevention of hemorrhoids
Legs	Homans' sign, edema, character of veins	Abnormalities to report
Emotional status	Nonverbal and verbal: Dependency, happiness, family support, feelings about neonate and labor experience	What to expect, skills for caring for neonate, changes in familial relationships, where to get help

   2. Can often be predicted in advance of delivery
   3. Blood loss often underestimated
   4. **Classification**
      a. *Early*. Hemorrhage occurring within 24 hours of delivery
      b. *Late*. Hemorrhage after 24 hours

ETIOLOGY

   1. Mismanagement of third stage of labor (incomplete placental separation)
   2. Uterine atony
   3. Lacerations of birth canal
   4. Hematological disorders (DIC)
   5. Complications of pregnancy (inversion of uterus, placenta accreta)
   6. Tumors of cervix or uterus

PROBLEMS AND COMPLICATIONS

   1. Hypovolemic shock
   2. Death
   3. Anemia
   4. Puerperal infection
   5. Thromboembolism

TABLE 12-2. CONDITIONS THAT PREDISPOSE TO POSTPARTUM HEMORRHAGE

Antedating Pregnancy	Arising During Pregnancy and Labor
Previous postpartum hemorrhage	Placenta previa
Grand multiparity	Abruptio placentae
Fibroids	Multiple pregnancy
Idiopathic thrombocytopenia purpura	Polyhydramnios
Von Willebrand's disease	Precipitate labor
Leukemia	Prolonged labor
	Chorioamnionitis
	Forceps delivery
	Cesarean section
	General anesthesia
	Mismanagement of third stage of labor
	Acute coagulation defect

Reprinted with permission from Cavanaugh, D., et al.: Obstetric Emergencies, 3rd ed., Philadelphia, Harper & Row, 1982.

POSTPARTUM HEMORRHAGE DUE TO UTERINE ATONY

Uterine atony is failure of the uterus to contract well or maintain its contraction following delivery. It is the primary cause of early postpartum hemorrhage.

1. **Predisposing factors**
   a. Grand multiparity
   b. Hydramnios
   c. Large fetus
   d. Delivery of twins or triplets
   e. Red haired patients
   f. Deep inhalation anesthesia
   g. Exhaustion from prolonged labor[6]

ETIOLOGY

The uterus is "overstretched" and poorly contractile, thus allowing brisk venous bleeding. The control of postpartum bleeding is by contraction and retraction of the myometrial fibers.

ASSESSMENT

1. **Clinical presentation**
   a. Signs and symptoms
      i. Dark blood
      ii. Boggy, soft uterus
      iii. Expulsion of clots

POSTPARTUM HEMORRHAGE DUE TO LACERATIONS

Lacerations of the perineum, vagina, and cervix are sometimes responsible for rapid, profuse blood loss.

1. **Predisposing factors**
   a. Operative delivery
   b. Aseptic or unattended spontaneous delivery

    c. Precipitous delivery

    d. Size, presentation, and position of the uterus[6]

ASSESSMENT

1. Clinical presentation

    a. Signs and symptoms

        i. Bright red arterial bleeding

        ii. Hard, firmly contracted uterus

————— POSTPARTUM HEMORRHAGE DUE TO HEMATOMA —————

A hematoma is a collection of blood in pelvic tissue due to damage to a vessel wall without laceration of the tissues. Blood loss may be severe enough to result in hemorrhagic shock.

Vessel trauma results from:

1. Pressure of the presenting part on the pelvic structures
2. Forceps manipulation
3. Excessive external fundal pressure on the uterus
4. Paracervical or pudendal anesthesia

ASSESSMENT

1. Clinical presentation

    a. Signs and symptoms

        i. Increasing pelvic and perineal pain

        ii. Inability to void

        iii. Tense, ecchymotic areas

        iv. Signs of shock in the absence of significant external bleeding

PATIENT CARE MANAGEMENT

1. Goals

    a. To control bleeding and stabilize maternal condition in hemorrhage due to atony

	COMMENTS/TIPS/CAUTIONS
i. Massage uterine fundus	To promote contraction of the uterus
ii. Prepare intravenous infusion of oxytocin	
iii. If physician is not available, perform bimanual compression of the uterus (see Chapter 9)	
iv. Administer methylergonovine (Methergine) or ergonovine (Ergotrate) IM or IV (see Appendix A) as ordered by physician	Should not be given to patients with elevated BP unless absolutely necessary
v. Monitor vital signs	
vi. Institute measures for treatment of hemorrhagic shock (see Chapter 9)	

b. To provide emotional support to parents in hemorrhage due to atony
   i. Explain procedures to parents
   ii. Respond in a calm, organized manner

Anxiety is contagious

c. To discover promptly all lacerations causing hemorrhage
   i. Assist patient with relaxation techniques to promote better visualization of perineal area
   ii. Provide proper sutures for correct repair of lacerations
   iii. Monitor vital signs every 15 minutes or every 5 minutes if bleeding is profuse
   iv. If symptoms of shock occur, implement procedure for hemorrhagic shock
d. To recognize hematomas quickly and institute treatment
   i. Investigate patient's complaints regarding increasing perineal discomfort
   ii. Note any areas of swelling when patient is removed from delivery table and evaluate for increase in size
   iii. Monitor patient's ability to void after delivery; insert Foley catheter if needed
   iv. Assist physician with evacuation of hematoma

Patients who have been able to void and then cannot void should be suspected of having a hematoma

THROMBOPHLEBITIS

Thrombophlebitis may lead directly to pulmonary embolism. An embolus may occlude the pulmonary artery, leading to death of the mother, because the circulatory processes of the lung are obstructed.[1]

DIAGNOSIS

Thrombophlebitis is an inflammatory process of the lining of a vein associated with formation of a thrombus. It may involve the veins in the leg or the pelvis. Sometimes it is called milk leg.

When inflammation is not present the process is called phlebothrombosis.

1. **Incidence**
   a. 16 cases reported in 29,770 pregnancies[7]
   b. 0.5 per cent in vaginal delivery
   c. 1–2 per cent in cesarean section
   d. 50 per cent of emboli originate in pelvic vessels[4]

2. **Predisposing factors**
   a. Stasis the greatest single factor
   b. Use of oral contraceptives before pregnancy
   c. Working at a job during pregnancy that requires sitting for long periods[7]
   d. Obesity
   e. Hemorrhage
   f. Cesarean section or operative delivery
   g. Varices
   h. Anemia
   i. Heart disease
   j. Prolonged labor; intrapartum (third stage) complications
   k. Toxemia of pregnancy
   l. Postdelivery pelvic infection

ETIOLOGY

1. Blood stasis due to formation of thrombi at the placental site or over-stretching of the vessels
2. Increased coagulability of blood post partum
3. Vascular abnormality
4. Infection

ASSESSMENT

1. Clinical presentation
    a. Signs and symptoms
        i. Homans' sign positive unilateral or bilateral
        ii. Temperature elevated to 105°F
        iii. Chills
        iv. Pain in leg
        v. Leg hot to the touch
        vi. Swelling and tenderness
        vii. Redness along affected vein
        viii. Leg white (arterial circulation constricted)
        ix. Severe pain in groin
        x. Inability to sleep
        xi. Unexplained elevation of pulse rate
        xii. Extreme swings in temperature (105°F to normal)
        xiii. Hypotension (from bacterial shock)
        xiv. Slight leg pain from walking, before severe leg pain
    b. History
        i. Noted between 10th and 20th postpartum day
        ii. Type of labor and delivery
        iii. Age

      iv. Parity

      v. Weight

      vi. Predisposing factors

2. Biopsychosocial assessment

   a. TPR

   b. BP

   c. Homans' sign

   d. Weight

   e. Hemoglobin and hematocrit

   f. Sleeping patterns

   g. Pain perception

3. Diagnostic data

   a. Hemoglobin and hematocrit

   b. Phlebography, if available

PROBLEMS AND COMPLICATIONS

1. Pulmonary embolism: Cardiac pain; dyspnea; pulse irregular or difficult to obtain; pallor and cyanosis; increased apprehension; hemoptysis; tachycardia; rales; tachypnea; air hunger; sobbing
2. Additional instances of thromboembolism
3. Death

PATIENT CARE MANAGEMENT

1. Goals

	COMMENTS/TIPS/CAUTIONS
a. To prevent occurrence of embolism	
i. Anticoagulants: low dose heparin, warfarin (Coumadin)	Avoid aspirin and products containing aspirin
ii. Bed rest/immobilization, elevation of affected limb	Prevent pressure on bed clothes
iii. Antibiotics if infectious process present	
iv. Massage of extremities prohibited	Maintain minimal postpartum bleeding, fundus well contracted
v. Observe for signs and symptoms of embolism	
vi. Oxygen as necessary	
vii. Sedatives as necessary	
viii. Treatment for shock if necessary (see Chapter 9)	
ix. Fluids	
x. Elastic stockings	
xi. Oral contraceptives prohibited	(Contraception necessary to avoid pregnancy)
b. To maintain comfort	
i. Moist heat to extremities	

ii. Explanation of importance
of treatment
iii. Sedatives as necessary
c. To provide emotional support
i. Diversionary activities
ii. Explanations of and opportunity to talk about what
is happening
iii. Let patient know how children are doing in her ab-
sence
iv. Explain to family what is
happening

Will depend on patient's interests

DISCHARGE PLANNING/TEACHING

1. Caution about aspirin use with
anticoagulant therapy
2. Rest
3. Contraceptive use
4. Arrange for household help, if necessary
5. Arrange for financial help, if necessary

Oral contraceptives contraindicated

INFECTIONS IN VARIOUS BODY SYSTEMS

Puerperal infections by themselves are not life threatening. However,
they may lead to thrombophlebitis, pulmonary embolism, and hemorrhage
as a result of subinvolution and eventually in maternal death.

DIAGNOSIS

Puerperal infection is defined as an infection accompanied by a temperature of 100.4°F on any 2 days post partum, exclusive of the first 24 hours,
when taken orally at least four times a day.[8] It is also known as childbed or
childbirth fever, postpartum fever, and puerperal sepsis.

1. **Incidence**
   a. Occurs in 6 per cent of deliveries in the United States

2. **Predisposing factors**
   a. Hemorrhage
   b. Trauma during labor and delivery
   c. Labor longer than 24 hours
   d. Premature rupture of membranes
   e. Retention of placental fragments
   f. Manual removal of placenta
   g. Severe anemia
   h. Malnutrition
   i. General debilitation

    j. Many vaginal examinations during labor
    k. Droplet infection in hospital personnel
    l. Sexual intercourse after rupture of membranes
    m. Hematomas
    n. Diabetes
    o. Breaks in aseptic technique and hand washing
    p. Improper perineal care
    q. Intrauterine manipulation or operative delivery

ETIOLOGY

1. Portals of entry following delivery
   a. Site of placental attachment
   b. Perineal body, episiotomy, or lacerations
   c. Urinary tract
   d. Vagina
   e. Breasts
   f. Lymphatic system along uterine veins (open to bacteria when cervix dilated; placental site; and fallopian tubes)
2. Portals of entry are moist and dark and susceptible to bacterial invasion
3. Multiple species of bacteria are found, both anaerobic and aerobic *(Bacteroides, Peptostreptococcus, Clostridium, Peptococcus, Escherichia coli)*

ASSESSMENT

1. **Clinical Presentation**
   a. Signs and symptoms
      i. Involving perineum, vulva, vagina, or cervix
         (a) Pain
         (b) Burning on urination
         (c) Sensation of heat
         (d) Discoloration of tissues
         (e) Edema
         (f) Purulent discharge
         (g) Elevated temperature (100.4 to 101°F)
         (h) Urinary retention
         (i) Chills
         (j) Repaired edges red and inflamed
         (k) Wound separation or dehiscence (bursting open)
         (l) May progress to ulceration if untreated
      ii. Uterine symptoms (infection at site of placental attachment: endometritis; muscle of uterus: metritis; pelvic connective tissue: parametritis)
         Mild symptoms
         (a) Temperature elevated: 101 to 103°F (48+ hours post partum)
         (b) Pulse rate increased (100 to 140)
         (c) Chills
         (d) General malaise

       (e)   Anorexia

       (f)   Headache

       (g)   Uterine tenderness extending laterally

Severe symptoms

       (h)   Prolonged or recurrent afterbirth pains

       (i)   Subinvolution

       (j)   Slight abdominal distention

       (k)   Scanty, odorless lochia or moderately heavy, foul, bloody, seropurulent lochia

       (l)   White blood cell count elevated

       (m) Occurs 3–5 days post partum unless organism is beta hemolytic streptococcus in which case onset is more precipitous

       (n)   Temperature elevated 104 to 105°F

       (o)   Uterus tender and enlarged

       (p)   Repeated chills and sweats

       (q)   Unilateral or bilateral abdominal pain extending laterally

Severe symptoms preceded by mild uterine symptoms (a to g)

       (r)   Deep flank pain

       (s)   Fixation of uterus

       (t)   Skin in inguinal region reddened, edematous, and tender with fluctuation

       (u)   May include signs of peritonitis[8]

  iii. Peritonitis

       (a)   Temperature elevated: 103 to 105°F

       (b)   Chills

       (c)   Pulse rate increased (140+); weak

       (d)   Severe pain

       (e)   Paralytic ileus

       (f)   Diarrhea

       (g)   Rapid, shallow, chest breathing

       (h)   Frequent projectile vomiting, possibly with feces

       (i)   Abdominal distention with extreme tenderness and rigidity

       (j)   Face flushed, then pale, gray, cold, and sweaty with sunken eyes

       (k)   Anxious expression and restlessness

       (l)   Excessive thirst

       (m) Foul breath

       (n)   Dry, brown tongue

       (o)   Severe decrease in urinary output

       (p)   Delirium

       (q)   Unconsciousness

       (r)   If untreated, last two symptoms will lead to death[8]

  iv. Bacteremia

       (a)   Temperature elevated: 103 to 104°F

       (b)   Pulse rate increased (120+)

       (c)   Chills

       (d)   Rapid, shallow respirations

       (e)   Profuse, foul lochia

(f)   Skin pale with cyanosis in fingers and lips
(g)   Signs and symptoms of peritonitis[8]
v. Cystitis
(a)   Temperature elevated: 100 to 101°F
(b)   Pain or burning or both upon urination
(c)   Tenderness over bladder
(d)   Urinary frequency
(e)   Urinary urgency
(f)   Hematuria
vi. Acute pyelonephritis
(a)   Signs and symptoms of cystitis
(b)   Temperature elevated: 100°F+
(c)   Costovertebral angle (CVA) tenderness
(d)   Lumbar pain
(e)   Shaking chills
(f)   Loss of appetite
(g)   Nausea and vomiting
vii. Engorgement
Engorgement is not an infectious process per se but is frequently a precursor of mastitis.
(a)   Bilateral breast enlargement and distention
(b)   Breast hard and sensitive to touch
(c)   Throbbing pain
(d)   Temperature elevated: 99 to 100°F
viii. Mastitis
Precursor symptoms
(a)   Marked engorgement of breast
(b)   No signs and symptoms first postpartum week, then slight fever
(c)   Mild pain in one segment of breast, especially when baby nurses
(d)   Breast fluctuation[8]
Acute symptoms
(e)   Temperature elevated: 103 to 104°F
(f)   Chills
(g)   General malaise
(h)   Pulse rate increased
(i)   Hard, red, tender, irregular mass in one or both breasts
(j)   Severe and acute tenderness and pain in one or both breasts
(k)   Headache
Abscesses
(l)   Remittent fever with chills
(m) Swollen and extremely painful breasts
(n)   Large, hard mass with area of fluctuation
(o)   Bluish tinge to skin (location of abscess)
(p)   Discharge of pus[8]
b. History
i. Nutritional status, weight

      ii. Previous infections and type

     iii. Type of labor and delivery

     iv. Anemia

      v. Time of ROM

     vi. Number of examinations during labor, trauma during labor and delivery

    vii. Diabetes

   viii. Date of delivery

    ix. Type of infant feeding

     x. Temperature during labor and delivery

    xi. Sexual history

   xii. Chronic disease

2. Biopsychosocial assessment

  a. Usual postpartum assessment to determine any areas of abnormality

  b. TPR, BP

  c. Weight

  d. Intake and output

  e. CVA tenderness

  f. Homans' sign

  g. Observation of infant feeding, if breast

  h. Bowel movements

  i. Discharge

  j. Lochia; observe pads and technique of perineal care

  k. Assess pain and tenderness and areas of warmth

3. Diagnostic data

  a. Urinalysis

  b. Culture and sensitivity tests as necessary of urine, wound, lochia, breast milk, cervix, vagina, vulva, blood

  c. Complete blood count with special attention to white blood cells and hemoglobin and hematocrit

  d. Blood sugar determination

PROBLEMS AND COMPLICATIONS

1. Maternal death
2. Thrombophlebitis
3. Pulmonary embolism
4. Neonatal infection
5. Hemorrhage
6. Subinvolution
7. Sterility
8. Chronic kidney disease
9. Septic shock
10. Disseminated intravascular coagulation

PATIENT CARE MANAGEMENT

1. Goals

  a. To prevent infection from resulting in more serious complications

Prompt recognition and treatment

    i. Culture and sensitivity tests

    ii. Antibiotics as appropriate

    iii. Isolation and aseptic technique as appropriate

    iv. Correction of any underlying condition

Continuing assessment

    v. Vital signs at least four times a day or more often if necessary

    vi. Condition of patient

    vii. Measure intake and output   *Catheterize only as last resort*

    viii. Check for progress of involution

    ix. Semi-Fowler's position to facilitate drainage

    x. Preparation for surgery or emergency procedures as necessary   *Incision and drainage may be carried out*

b. Provide patient with comfort measures

    i. Adequate nutrition   *Patient may require innovative, high calorie snacks if appetite poor*

    ii. Adequate fluids, IV or oral   *2000 to 3000 cc/24 hours*

    iii. Good hygiene

    iv. Oral care

    v. Frequent linen changes

    vi. Leg exercises if appropriate   *To increase circulation*

    vii. Promote rest and sleep   *Quiet environment, visitor restriction*

    viii. Breast hygiene, perineal care   *Use good technique and teach patient*

    ix. Breast support-binder, bra   *Be sure bra is supportive*

    x. Heat applications   *In patient with mastitis only if she is breast feeding*

    xi. Cold applications to breasts   *In patient with engorgement if she is not breast feeding*

    xii. Analgesics as necessary

    xiii. Keep breasts empty, only if patient is breast feeding   *Patients do not need to stop breast feeding, but it will be painful and may increase afterbirth pains; administer medication 20 minutes before*

    xiv. Cocoa butter to breasts: fissures and nipples

    xv. Facilitation of complete bladder emptying

c. To provide patient with support and education

    i. Assist in maintaining family contact

    ii. Keep patient and family informed

iii. Educate patient about transmission of infection and ways to minimize
iv. Preparation for procedures

COMMENTS/TIPS/CAUTIONS
Staff should also be very aware of asepsis and throat cultures and should not work with droplet infection

PSYCHOLOGICAL RISK

Psychological risk may take the form of depression, psychosis, or schizophrenia, all of which are serious psychological problems. The ramifications of these entities can be life threatening to mother and child. If the disease interferes with the maternal-infant attachment process, child abuse may result. If the depression is severe enough, suicide may result.

DIAGNOSIS

Postpartum depression and psychosis are maladaptations to the conflicts of the postpartal period. Usual defense mechanisms are not as efficient as normal. Decreased self-esteem may also contribute to an emotional letdown. Psychosis is a severe disturbance in thinking, feeling, and behavior manifested by distortion or detachment from reality.

1. **Incidence**
   a. Major psychiatric complications occur in 3 in 1000 pregnancies
   b. "Nervous breakdowns" account for 15 per cent; 60 per cent of these patients develop manic-depressive or schizophrenic reactions

2. **Predisposing factors**
   a. Previous psychological problems
   b. Neurosis, psychosis, schizophrenia
   c. Low self-esteem
   d. Poor pregnancy or labor and delivery experience
   e. Drug addiction
   f. Excessive analgesia
   g. Serious metabolic disorders
   h. Alcoholism
   i. Syphilis
   j. Poor tolerance to stress or excessive amounts of stress
   k. Psychiatric problems during pregnancy
   l. Family history of manic-depressive psychosis
   m. Non–family centered childbirth experience

ETIOLOGY

1. Generally unknown
2. May be related to hormonal changes after delivery
3. Diminished methods of coping
4. Decreased efficiency of defense mechanisms

5.   Existing personality traits
6.   Unconscious conflicts
7.   Unresolved and unmet maturational needs
8.   Baby not the cause, but the catalyst
9.   Psychological and physiological stressors of pregnancy
10. New obligations of parenthood

ASSESSMENT
1. Clinical presentation
   a. Signs and symptoms
       i. Increased irritability
      ii. Inability to sleep
     iii. Anorexia
     iv. Extreme depression
      v. Suspiciousness
     vi. Agitation and tenseness
    vii. Total rejection of and hostile feelings toward baby and significant others
   viii. Delusions; may deny existence of baby
     ix. Avoidance of contact or any interpersonal exchange with the infant
      x. Crying spells and "blues"
     xi. Obsession that baby will replace her in spouse's affections
    xii. Guilt regarding aversion to pregnancy, attempted abortion, or other personal conflicts
   xiii. Excitement, with rhyming or punning
   xiv. Disinterest in personal care
    xv. Appearance of helplessness
   xvi. Self-accusatory
   xvii. Expression of strange or inappropriate thoughts or feelings
  xviii. Suicidal, may wish infant dead
   xix. Hallucinations
    xx. Hostility to medical staff
   xxi. Abandonment of reality
   b. History
       i. How pregnancy went and date of delivery
      ii. Childbirth experience
     iii. Life stressors
     iv. Physical problems
      v. Psychosocial, economic, and family pressures
     vi. Difficult labor and delivery
    vii. Drug and alcohol usage
   viii. Venereal disease
     ix. Analgesia in labor and post partum
      x. Chronic metabolic disorders
     xi. Psychiatric history
    xii. Family history of manic-depressive psychosis

2. Biopsychosocial assessment
   a. Eating patterns

    b. Interaction with baby and family and staff
    c. Sleep patterns
    d. Amount of relaxation
    e. Psychological profile
    f. Assessment for dehydration
    g. Plans for baby and family
    h. Coping mechanisms, stress tolerance, and self-esteem

3. Diagnostic data
    a. VDRL (Veneral Disease Research Laboratory) test
    b. Metabolic screening tests
    c. Blood levels of drug and alcohol

PROBLEMS AND COMPLICATIONS:

1. Severe psychiatric illness
2. Suicide
3. Child abuse and infanticide
4. Destruction of family relationships

PATIENT CARE MANAGEMENT

1. Goals
    a. To identify the crisis state promptly
        i. Assess mother with infant, by herself, and with family and staff
        ii. Assess mother's plans for infant and for herself
        iii. Assess sleep and eating patterns
        iv. Assess dehydration
        v. Assess psychological state and behavior
    b. To provide support to mother
        i. Assist mother with parenting skills
        ii. Give criticism in positive way and praise positive actions
        iii. Accept mother's feelings
        iv. Reinforce reality in a nonjudgmental way
        v. Support strengths of family unit
        vi. Listen to family's expression of feelings
        vii. Assist family to adjust to crisis

   viii. Convince family not to re-
         ject patient as bad wife
         and mother
     ix. Provide information
  c. To maintain safe environment
      i. Remove harmful objects
     ii. Stay with patient when
         baby is there
    iii. Do not allow drugs to be
         in room; be sure patient
         completely takes all drugs
  d. To provide physiological sup-
     port for problem
      i. Psychiatric consultation
     ii. Tranquilizers
    iii. Electroconvulsive therapy
     iv. Transfer to psychiatric in-
         patient service
      v. Psychotherapy

Especially important to have a
primary care giver who will
not reject the baby

DISCHARGE PLANNING/TEACHING

1. Provide optimal discharge environment
2. Contraception
3. Emotional support
4. Facilitation of parental and parent-infant relationships
5. Help with family and home
6. Financial assistance if necessary

CONCLUSIONS

   This chapter on postpartal crises has encompassed only those entities
that are life threatening or extremely serious, but there are many other
things that may occur to the parturient and her family. Although the postpartum period is primarily a normal, non–life threatening time, integrating
a new baby into the family and adapting to the body's return to its prepregnant state can be considered a crisis of mammoth proportions. It is important for the nurse to realize that even though there is a life threatening
crisis, these "normal" crises are also taking place and cannot be ignored. It is
also crucial to realize that the postpartum patient, although usually normal,
has many needs that the nurse is in a unique position to assess and meet.
Whatever the situation, it is hoped that the nurse will respond to the fact
that the postpartum family is not just a family that is all right but that it
provides the nurse an opportunity to practice nursing at its fullest. The
varied adaptations that must take place to allow the family to be at its fullest
potential provide the nurse with great challenges. It is hoped that the challenges will be met.

_____ REFERENCES _____

1. Anderson, B.A., Camacho, M.E., and Stark, J.: Interruptions in Family Health During Pregnancy, 2nd ed. New York, McGraw-Hill Book Co., 1979.
2. Butnarescu, G.F., Tillotson, D.M., and Villarreal, P.P.: Perinatal Nursing. Volume 2: Reproductive Risk. New York, John Wiley & Sons, 1980.
3. Cavanaugh, D., Woods, R.E., O'Connor, T.C., and Knuppel, R.A.: Obstetric Emergencies, 3rd ed. Philadelphia, Harper & Row, 1982.
4. Jensen, M.D., Benson, R.C., and Bobak, I.M.: Maternity Care: The Nurse and the Family, 2nd ed. St. Louis, C.V. Mosby Co., 1979.
5. McKenzie, C.A., Canaday, M.E., and Carroll, E.: Comprehensive care during the postpartum period. Nurs. Clin. North Am. $17:23-48$, 1982.
6. Oxorn, H.: Human Labor and Birth, 4th ed. New York, Appleton-Century-Crofts, 1980.
7. Pritchard, J.A., and MacDonald, P.C.: Williams' Obstetrics, 16th ed. New York, Appleton-Century-Crofts, 1980.
8. Varney, H.: Nurse-Midwifery. Boston, Blackwell Scientific Publications, 1980.

HIGH RISK
NEONATAL CARE

CHAPTER 13

ASSESSMENT AND CLASSIFICATION OF THE HIGH RISK NEONATE

Cornelia B. Dewees, C.N.M., M.N.

OBJECTIVES

Upon completion of this chapter the reader will be able to accomplish the following:

1. List the criteria to be assessed in the Apgar scoring system
2. State the points assigned for each item on the Apgar score
3. Identify the risk level of the neonate as determined by the 1 minute Apgar score
4. Identify factors in the maternal/fetal history that predispose the neonate to health problems
5. Identify physical characteristics that may indicate that a neonatal problem exists
6. Identify neurobehavioral characteristics that may indicate that a neonatal problem exists
7. Describe neonatal classification in terms of size and gestational age
8. Describe steps for estimating the neonate's gestational age with the Dubowitz scoring system

The nursing members of the perinatal health team are vital in the assessment and management of the neonate at risk. Beginning with immediate contact in the delivery setting and continuing throughout the neonatal period, the nurse must perform skillful assessments upon which to base nursing interventions. Data obtained as a part of the newborn's complete data base are also vital as a basis for the plan of medical management.

The first systematic assessment of every newborn is the Apgar score. It provides a rapid evaluation of the neonate's status and is the objective determination upon which decisions about immediate supportive and resuscitative measures will be based. Repeated scoring is an evaluation of the neonate's response to these measures and of success in adapting to extrauterine life.

When immediate life threatening conditions have been managed and the infant's condition has begun to stabilize, it is necessary to make a more thorough assessment, including physical, neurobehavioral, and maturity-gestational age classifications. These, along with the Apgar scores and immediate stabilization measures employed, will provide a basis for decisions about the level of care needed by the neonate and whether transport to another setting is indicated. The nurse must have repeated experiences in handling, observing, and assessing neonates to differentiate normal characteristics and common benign deviations from serious or life threatening conditions. The written word is only one modality for learning, and simply reading this chapter cannot impart the discriminatory skills necessary for accurate assessment. Each nurse who is employed in a situation that could entail caring for a neonate at risk should seek out opportunities to perform neonatal assessments with the guidance of a skillful practitioner.

_ ASSESSMENT AND CLASSIFICATION OF THE HIGH RISK NEONATE _

Assessment is the first step in the nursing process providing the data upon which all neonatal care and management decisions are based.

DIAGNOSIS

A high risk neonate is an infant between birth and the end of the 28th day of life who is affected by a condition that may pose a considerable hazard to life and health.

1. Predisposing factors

Conditions that threaten the neonate's health may arise from one or several of the following. Examples of common predisposing conditions are included.

   a. Factors in family history
       i.   *Inherited disorders:* cystic fibrosis, sickle cell trait, phenylketonuria
       ii. *Communicable disease:* tuberculosis
   b. Factors in mother's past medical-surgical history
       i.   Anomalies of the reproductive system, diabetes mellitus, herpes simplex type II
       ii. Surgery of the reproductive-endocrine system, Rh sensitization in a previous pregnancy or by blood transfusion
   c. Mother's past obstetrical history
       i.   Prematurity, stillbirths, congenital anomalies, previous neonatal complications
   d. Maternal-fetal conditions in this pregnancy
       i.   *Maternal:* preeclampsia, premature rupture of membranes, rejection of pregnancy, malnutrition
       ii. *Fetal/placental:* Rh incompatibility with sensitization, abruptio placentae, placenta previa
   e. Intrapartal factors
       i.   *Fetal:* Fetal distress, large or very small fetus

ii. *Maternal:* Precipitate or prolonged labor, prolonged rupture of membranes, dehydration, cephalopelvic disproportion

iii. *Obstetrical:* Analgesia, anesthesia, oxytocics, forceps delivery, cesarean section

ASSESSMENT

1. **Immediate**
   a. Apgar scoring (Table 13–1)
      i. Score at 1 minute is basis for immediate resuscitation or stabilization efforts
         (a) High risk (0–3): severely depressed; full resuscitative efforts indicated
         (b) Moderate risk (4–6): moderately depressed; some resuscitative efforts indicated
         (c) Low risk (7–10): adapting fairly well; supportive care indicated
      ii. Score at 5 minutes evaluates progressive adaptation to extrauterine life and efforts at stabilization
      iii. Scoring may be repeated every 5 minutes until stabilized to evaluate resuscitative efforts
      iv. Refer to appendix for directions for scoring each item in the Apgar score

2. **Physical**
   a. A systematic approach is mandatory to assure that nothing is overlooked
   b. General appearance is evaluated first, then specific systems
   c. Care must be taken to avoid stresses that could worsen neonate's condition
      i. Examine in a warm environment, under a radiant warmer, or in an enclosed incubator

TABLE 13-1. APGAR SCORE CHART

Characteristic	Score		
	0	1	2
Heart rate	Absent	Less than 100	100 or greater
Respiratory effort	Absent	Slow, irregular, weak	Lusty cry
Muscle tone	Flaccid	Some flexion of extremities	Well flexed, active
Reflex irritability	No response	Grimace, some motion	Vigorous cry, active withdrawal
Color	Cyanotic, pale	Body pink, extremities cyanotic	Entirely pink

ii. Group procedures and assessment to conserve infant's strength and to minimize oxygen consumption
iii. The more obviously ill or premature the infant, the briefer and more cursory the assessment must be at any one time
iv. Physical assessment and gestational age assessment and classification (see next section) may be performed simultaneously but are presented separately for clarity
v. Throughout assessment be alert for changes in infant's condition and adjust assessment as necessary
vi. Proceed with assessment in systematic manner as outlined in Table 13–2.
vii. See Table 13–5 for a list of equipment needed

3. **Gestational age**
   a. Gestational age may be determined from length of mother's pregnancy or by examination and scoring with the Dubowitz system
      i. Length of pregnancy
         (a) A term infant is one born between 38 and 42 weeks' gestation
         (b) A preterm infant is one born before 38 weeks' gestation
         (c) A post-term infant is one born at 42 weeks' gestation or later
      ii. The Dubowitz tool may be used to classify an infant of uncertain gestational age; it uses a combination of neurobehavioral and physical characteristics; some items are of limited use in very ill or preterm infants, but a close estimation may usually be obtained; if scoring is done carefully, a gestational age within 2 weeks' accuracy may be obtained; proceed with scoring according to the signs in Figure 13–1 and Table 13–3.

After scoring all items carefully, add the score and determine the estimated gestational age by referring to the graph in Figure 13–2.

   b. The infant is next classified by the two parameters of gestational age and birth weight; by this maneuver the infant is placed in a category of size-gestational age that carries with it known risks for the infant (see Fig. 13–3)
      i. *Appropriate for gestational age (AGA):* the infant ranks between the 10th and 90th percentile of weight for the particular gestational age
      ii. *Small for gestational age (SGA):* the infant ranks below the 10th percentile for the particular gestational age
      iii. *Large for gestational age (LGA):* the infant ranks above the 90th percentile for the particular gestational age
   c. SGA infants and LGA infants each are susceptible to a series of common problems for the particular classification; when assessing the infant the nurse should observe carefully for signs of these problems (Table 13–4)

**TABLE 13-2. NEONATAL CHARACTERISTICS
AND INDICATORS OF PROBLEMS**

Characteristic	Indicative of problem
General appearance: assess by observation alone	
Posture	Lack of flexion of extremities
Symmetry	Asymmetry of posture or any body part; some asymmetrical head molding can be normal
Size	Large or very small
Spontaneous movements	Absence of movement, asymmetry, paralysis, jittery or jerky movements, repetitive or rhythmic convulsive movements of one or more extremities
Respirations	Intercostal, substernal, sternal, supraclavicular retractions; grunting, stridor, asymmetry
Color	Pale, cyanotic, bright red, mottled
Cry	Shrill, weak, none, catlike
Urine	If none after 24 hours, may indicate blockage, anomaly, or dehydration
Odor	Musty odor associated with metabolic diseases
Heart: assess by observation, palpation, auscultation while infant quiet	
Localized pulsation may be visible at 4th intercostal space	Excessive chest heave with each beat
Apical impulse palpable at 4th intercostal space midclavicular line	Thrill
Rate 100–180; varies with activity; some irregularities may be normal	Gross irregularity of rhythm; murmurs: usually heard at left sternal border, 3rd interspace; rarely at apex; rate less than 100; over 180
Blood pressure (55 systolic in term baby)	Hypertension, hypotension
Lungs: assess by observation, percussion, auscultation	
Abdominal breathing with some movement	"Seesaw" chest to abdomen pattern
Rates 30–60 breath per minute, normally somewhat irregular	Rate less than 20–30, over 60, or grossly irregular with periods of apnea
Equal filling, symmetry, clear breath sounds to diaphragm	Unequal filling, silent areas, dullness, shallow respirations
A few coarse rales normal in the first minutes of life until alveolar fluid resorbs	Rales, ronchi, wheezing, grunting; excessive tympany, overinflation, barrel chest
Percussion, clear	Flaring of alae nasae, retractions, "worried facies" with labored respirations

TABLE 13-2. NEONATAL CHARACTERISTICS
AND INDICATORS OF PROBLEMS *(Continued)*

Characteristic	Indicative of Problem
Body proportions: assess by observation and measurement	
Head circumference largest diameter (33–35 cm)	Large or small
Chest circumference at nipple line (30–33 cm)	Larger than head
Flexed back, extremities	Flaccid; rigid in extension, asymmetry
Length. Term: 19–21 inches	
Weight. Term, average: 2600–3800 gm	
Skin: assess by observation and palpation	
Skin temperature (axillary) 97.7–98.6°F	Hypothermia, hyperthermia
Vernix caseosa in skin folds, on back	Excess vernix: preterm (34–36 weeks' gestation) Little or no vernix: preterm (early third trimester) or post-term
Color pink with some acrocyanosis	Pale, cyanotic, jaundiced, plethoric (red), mottled
Capillary fillings. Blanch with pressure, should refill rapidly	Slow capillary filling associated with compromised cardiac status or vasoconstriction
Lanugo on shoulders, back, forehead	Covers body on prematures
Milia on nose, chin	Birth trauma may be evidenced by wide variety of findings, including ecchymoses, localized cyanosis petechiae Edema, soft or firm swellings of specific parts
Hemangiomas, nevi, mongolian spots	Usually not serious but should be noted for later evaluation
Vesicles: erythema toxicum (red rash with vesicles): no apparent untoward significance	Rash, pustules with clear or purulent drainage
Subcutaneous fat layer	Lack of fat in prematures Excess in large infant (e.g., of diabetic mother)
Hydration	Skin peaks or wrinkles in dehydration Edema or shiny skin in fluid overload or cardiac failure
Head and neck: assess by palpation and observation	
Symmetry of head. Some molding and overriding of sutures normal	Excessive molding, large overlap
Mild caput succedaneum	Extreme caput succedaneum Cephalhematoma, bruising
Fontanels: fluctuant Anterior: diamond shaped (5 cm x 5 cm—or less)	Large or tense associated with increased intracranial pressure

TABLE 13-2. NEONATAL CHARACTERISTICS
AND INDICATORS OF PROBLEMS *(Continued)*

Characteristic	Indicative of Problem
Posterior: triangular (1.5 cm or less), may be fingertip only because of molding	Soft bones, fractures
Hair: normal pattern of hairline and brows	Low hairline, bushy brows, excess sworls, bald patches
Ears: normal position (top of ear above level of corner of eye), firm cartilage, patent canal; preauricular pits or tags should be noted	Low-set, rotated backward Absence of part or all of pinna or canal Soft cartilage associated with prematurity
May blink or cry to loud noise	If absent, recheck later Hearing evaluation in ill young infant is imprecise
Face: symmetrical Mandible: symmetrical Nasal bridge: somewhat flat	Asymmetry, paralysis Protruding or receding Collapsed
Eyes: symmetry Some lid edema due to silver nitrate is normal	Wide set (4.5 cm between pupils), narrow set, asymmetry Excess edema, epicanthal folds; ecchymosis
Pupils equal, react equally to light	Pupils unequal, nonreactive; abnormalities of iris
Red reflex present	Cataracts, cloudy cornea
Subconjunctival hemorrhage: usually benign, resolves	
Pseudostrabismus	Setting sun sign (each pupil or iris drops below lower lid) (if brief, may be normal)
Blink reflex to bright light	Absence may indicate visual impairment
Nose: nares patent (check by occluding first one, then other) Septum midline, straight Sneeze reflex normal	Nonpatency Deviated, fracture
Mouth: Symmetry and movement Lips and hard and soft palate intact Smooth gums, no teeth; minor deviations can be normal Tongue: normal size, shape, placement	Asymmetry Cleft lip, palate Natal teeth pose danger of aspiration Large or very small tongue; normal tongue with short mandible may appear large.
Neck: normal range of motion	Frenulum very short Limitation of motion Masses: Nodes, enlarged sternocleidomastoid muscle (torticollis), hemotoma; extra skin folds, webbing, edema; branchial clefts, sinuses, cysts, venous distention
Chest: assess by observation, palpation, measurement	
See Lungs. Symmetry, bellshaped	Asymmetry of structures or movement Barrel shaped

TABLE 13-2. NEONATAL CHARACTERISTICS
AND INDICATORS OF PROBLEMS *(Continued)*

Characteristic	Indicative of Problem
Clavicles	Crepitus or cry on palpation is associated with fracture
Ribs: flexible, symmetrical	Crepitus, asymmetry, splinting
Nipples: symmetry, breast tissue present in term baby; spacing	No breast nodule: associated with preterm; wide spaced ($>$ 28% of chest circumference): supernumerary nipples (not pathological but may be associated with other conditions)
Abdomen: assess by inspection, auscultation, palpation, percussion	
Cylindrical, may protrude, soft on palpation	Tense, distended, bulging flanks, engorged blood vessels
Auscultate bowel sounds (normally present after 10–15 minutes of life)	Masses, enlarged organs; percuss for hollow or fluid filled masses; absence of bowel sounds
Palpate liver at right costal margin	Liver $>$ 3 cm below costal margin
Palpate kidneys (before feeding)	Enlarged, absent
Palpate spleen (barely palpable or impalpable)	Enlarged
3 vessels in umbilical cord, bluish white Wharton's jelly	2 vessels in cord, foul odor of cord, meconium stained or jaundiced cord; erythema at base of cord; umbilical hernia; bladder distention
Femoral pulse: present, equal bilaterally, approximately equal in intensity to brachial pulses	Asymmetry, weaker than brachial pulses, absence of pulses
Male genitalia: assess by observation and palpation	
Penis: meatus at end of glans	Epispadias, hypospadias
Testes in scrotum, normal rugae	Undescended (cryptorchidism); hydrocele, edema; absence of rugae (premature); dimpling of scrotum associated with testicular torsion
Smooth perineum	Dimple, sinus
Patent anus	Imperforate anus
Female genitalia: assess by observation	
Labia majora: well developed in term	Labia minora protrude more in preterm; labial fusion
Clitoris normal	Enlarged
Urethral meatus behind clitoris	Displaced
Hymenal tags, white discharge normal; vagina patent Pink tinged discharge	Hymen sealed over vagina
Anus patent	Imperforate anus

TABLE 13-2.   NEONATAL CHARACTERISTICS
AND INDICATORS OF PROBLEMS *(Continued)*

Characteristic	Indicative of Problem
Back: assess by palpation and observation	
Straight, symmetrical	Winging of scapula
Palpate for intact vertebrae	Curved spine, missing (or partial) vertebrae Masses, protrusion from spine (myelomeningocele)
Pilonidal dimple (can visualize bottom of opening)	Pilonidal sinus or cyst
Normal hair pattern on sacrum, lanugo	Excess or absence of hair
Extremities: assess by palpation, observation	
Count all digits, palpate all long bones for completeness and intactness	Phocomelia, amelia, deletions or fusion of digits; extra digits, fractures of long bones
Nails well formed	Missing or malformed nails; edema
Normal palmar creases	Simian crease (Down's syndrome)
Plantar creases cover about half of foot at term	Sole creases covering a third or less associated with preterm Great toe widely spaced from others (Down's syndrome)
Resistance to extension, firm plantar and palmar grasp	Poor muscle tone, no resistance; weakness or absence of grasp reflexes
Brachial, popliteal, pedal pulses present, approximately equal	Weak, absent, asymmetrical
Some tibial curvature normal	Excess tibial torsion
Feet and ankles move easily, may be flexed and incurved because of in utero position	Abnormal position of foot, inability to easily correct to normal position
Patellar tendon reflex, brachial tendon reflex present	Absence of reflexes
Ankle clonus: a few beats are normal	Sustained clonus
Hips move through full range of motion	Click present on abduction; limitation of abduction
Skin folds symmetrical on buttocks and thighs	Asymmetry of skin folds associated with congenital hip dislocation
Neurobehavioral responses: assess by observation, percussion, palpation, manipulation, moving from least aversive to more aversive	
For obviously ill or premature infant, testing a few reflexes will suffice: rooting, sucking, swallowing, palmar grasp, plantar grasp, Babinski (positive in normal neonate)	Weakness or absence of any of these may be related to infant's state (sleep, waking, crying) or degree of satiety; a poor response should be retested later

TABLE 13-2. NEONATAL CHARACTERISTICS AND INDICATORS OF PROBLEMS *(Continued)*

Characteristic	Indicative of Problem
Observe infant's general responses to stimuli in the environment such as handling, light, noise	General poor response may be associated with central nervous system trauma, central depression, or immaturity Asymmetry of response often associated with local trauma Hyperactive and hypoactive responses may indicate problems

TABLE 13-3. SCORING SYSTEM FOR EXTERNAL PHYSICAL CRITERIA

External sign	Score*				
	0	1	2	3	4
Edema	Obvious edema of hands and feet; pitting over tibia	No obvious edema of hands and feet; pitting over tibia	No edema		
Skin texture	Very thin, gelatinous	Thin and smooth	Smooth, medium thickness; rash or superficial peeling	Slight thickening; superficial cracking and peeling, especially of hands and feet	Thick and parchment-like; superficial or deep cracking
Skin color	Dark red	Uniformly pink	Pale pink; variable over body	Pale; only pink over ears, lips, palms, or soles	
Skin opacity (trunk)	Numerous veins and venules clearly seen, especially over abdomen	Veins and tributaries seen	A few large vessels clearly seen over abdomen	A few large vessels seen indistinctly over abdomen	No blood vessels seen
Lanugo (over back)	No lanugo	Abundant; long and thick over whole back	Hair thinning, especially over lower back	Small amount of lanugo and bald areas	At least half of back devoid of lanugo
Plantar creases	No skin creases	Faint red marks over anterior half of sole	Definite red marks over > anterior half; indentations over < anterior third	Indentations over > anterior third	Definite deep indentations over > anterior third
Nipple formation	Nipple barely visible; no areola	Nipple well defined; areola smooth and flat, diameter < 0.75 cm	Areola stippled, edge not raised diameter > 0.75 cm	Areola stippled, edge raised, diameter < 0.75 cm	
Breast size	No breast tissue palpable	Breast tissue on one or both sides, < 0.5 cm diameter	Breast tissue on both sides, one or both 0.5-1.0 cm	Breast tissue on both sides, one or both > 1 cm	
Ear form	Pinna flat and shapeless, little or no incurving of edge	Incurving of part of edge of pinna	Partial incurving whole of upper pinna	Well-defined incurving whole of upper pinna	
Ear firmness	Pinna soft, easily folded, no recoil	Pinna soft, easily folded, slow recoil	Cartilage to edge of pinna, but soft in places, ready recoil	Pinna firm, cartilage to edge; instant recoil	
Genitals Male	Neither testis in scrotum	At least one testis high in scrotum	At least one testis right down		
Female (with hips half abducted)	Labia majora widely separated labia minora protruding	Labia majora almost cover labia minora	Labia majora completely cover labia minora		

*If score differs on two sides, take the mean.

Reprinted with permission from Dubowitz, L.M.S., Dubowitz, V., and Goldberg, C.: Clinical assessment of gestational age in the newborn infant. J. Pediatr., 77:1-10, 1980.

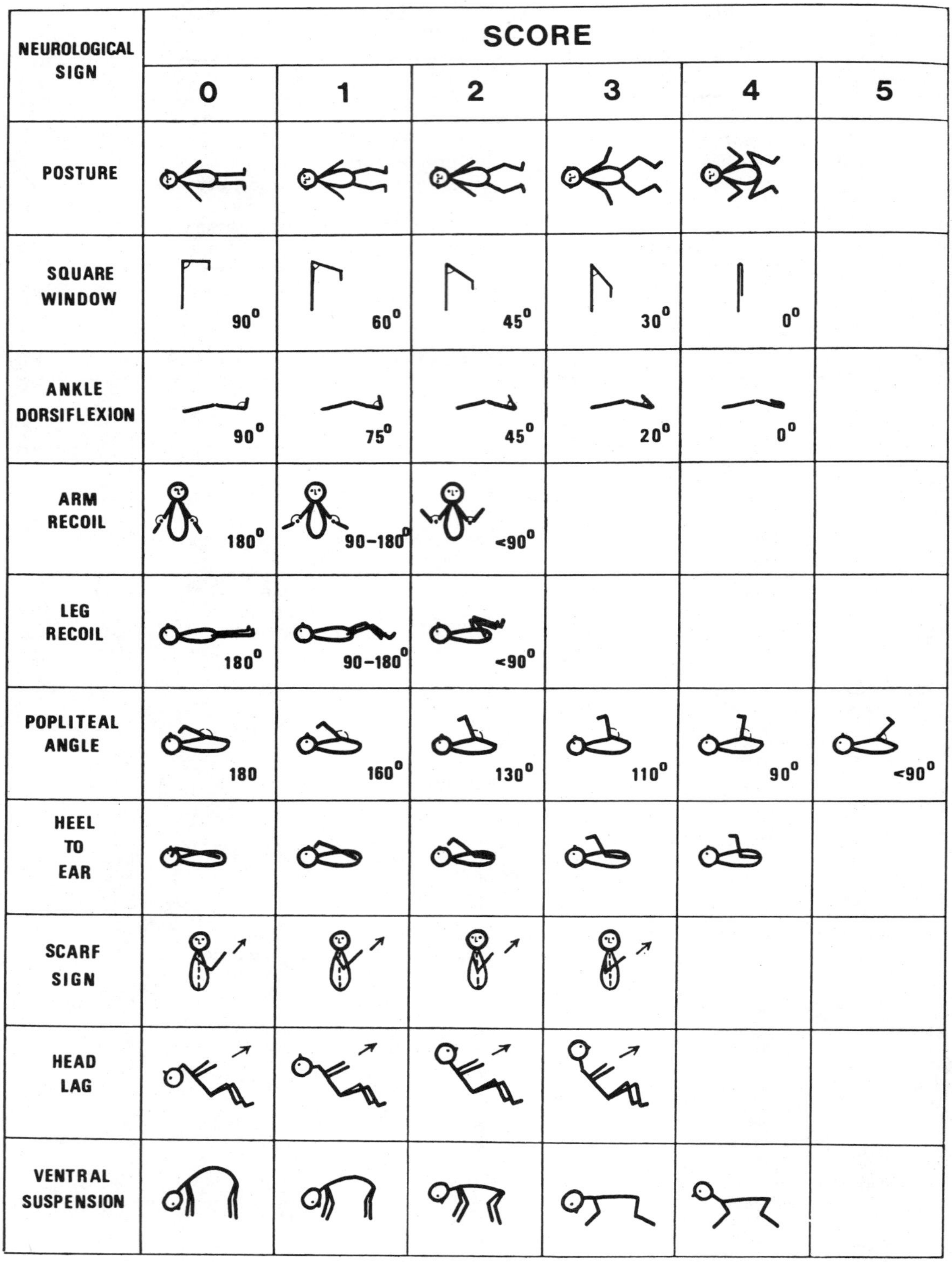

NEUROLOGICAL SIGN	SCORE 0	1	2	3	4	5
POSTURE						
SQUARE WINDOW	90°	60°	45°	30°	0°	
ANKLE DORSIFLEXION	90°	75°	45°	20°	0°	
ARM RECOIL	180°	90–180°	<90°			
LEG RECOIL	180°	90–180°	<90°			
POPLITEAL ANGLE	180	160°	130°	110°	90°	<90°
HEEL TO EAR						
SCARF SIGN						
HEAD LAG						
VENTRAL SUSPENSION						

Figure 13-1. Techniques of assessment of neurological criteria. (Reprinted with permission from Dubowitz, L.M.S., Dubowitz, V., and Goldberg, C.: Clinical assessment of gestational age in the newborn infant. J. Pediatr., *77*: 1-10, 1970.)

SOME NOTES ON TECHNIQUES OR ASSESSMENT OF
NEUROLOGICAL CRITERIA

POSTURE: Observed with infant quiet and in supine position. Score 0: Arms and legs extended; 1: Beginning of flexion of hips and knees, arms extended; 2: Stronger flexion of legs, arms extended; 3: Arms slightly flexed, legs flexed and abducted; 4: Full flexion of arms and legs.

SQUARE WINDOW: The hand is flexed on the forearm between the thumb and index finger of the examiner (Fig. 3). Enough pressure is applied to get as full a flexion as possible, and the angle between the hypothenar eminence and the ventral aspect of the forearm is measured and graded according to diagram. (Care is taken not to rotate the infant's wrist while doing this maneuver.)

ANKLE DORSIFLEXION: The foot is dorsiflexed onto the anterior aspect of the leg, with the examiner's thumb on the sole of the foot and other fingers behind the leg (Fig. 4). Enough pressure is applied to get as full flexion as possible, and the angle between the dorsum of the foot and the anterior aspect of the leg is measured.

ARM RECOIL: With the infant in the supine position the forearms are first flexed for 5 seconds, then fully extended by pulling on the hands, and then released. The sign is fully positive if the arms return briskly to full flexion (Score 2). If the arms return to incomplete flexion or the response is sluggish it is graded as Score 1. If they remain extended or are only followed by random movements the score is 0.

LEG RECOIL: With the infant supine, the hips and knees are fully flexed for 5 seconds, then extended by traction on the feet, and released. A maximal response is one of full flexion of the hips and knees (Score 2). A partial flexion scores 1, and minimal or no movement scores 0.

POPLITEAL ANGLE: With the infant supine and his pelvis flat on the examining couch, the thigh is held in the knee-chest position by the examiner's left index finger and thumb supporting the knee. The leg is then extended by gentle pressure from the examiner's right index finger behind the ankle and the popliteal angle is measured (Fig. 5).

HEEL TO EAR MANEUVER: With the baby supine, draw the baby's foot as near to the head as it will go without forcing it. Observe the distance between the foot and the head as well as the degree of extension at the knee. Grade according to diagram. Note that the knee is left free and may draw down alongside the abdomen (Fig. 6).

SCARF SIGN: With the baby supine, take the infant's hand and try to put it around the neck and as far posteriorly as possible around the opposite shoulder. Assist this maneuver by lifting the elbow across the body. See how far the elbow will go across and grade according to illustrations. Score 0: Elbow reaches opposite axillary line; 1: Elbow between midline and opposite axillary line; 2: Elbow reaches midline; 3: Elbow will not reach midline.

HEAD LAG: With the baby lying supine, grasp the hands (or the arms if a very small infant) and pull him slowly towards the sitting position. Observe the position of the head in relation to the trunk and grade accordingly. In a small infant the head may initially be supported by one hand. Score 0: Complete lag; 1: Partial head control; 2: Able to maintain head in line with body; 3: Brings head anterior to body.

VENTRAL SUSPENSION: The infant is suspended in the prone position, with examiner's hand under the infant's chest (one hand in a small infant, two in a large infant). Observe the degree of extension of the back and the amount of flexion of the arms and legs. Also note the relation of the head to the trunk. Grade according to diagrams.

If score differs on the two sides, take the mean.

Figure 13-1 *(Continued)*

TABLE 13-4. COMMON PROBLEMS OF INFANTS
SMALL OR LARGE FOR GESTATIONAL AGE

Classification	Common Problems
Small for gestational age	Congenital anomalies Hypoglycemia (blood glucose < 30 mg/dl, term; < 20 mg/dl preterm Hypocalcemia (serum calcium > 7.5 mg/dl) Polycythemia ($> 65\%$ hematocrit in a central venous sample) Birth asphyxia (pH 7.2 or less) Respiratory distress syndrome Meconium aspiration (particularly in post-term SGA) Intrauterine infection Hyperbilirubinemia
Large for gestational age	Birth trauma Hypoglycemia Hypocalcemia Hyperbilirubinemia Respiratory distress syndrome Meconium aspiration Polycythemia

TABLE 13-5. EQUIPMENT FOR ASSESSMENT OF THE NEONATE

Equipment	Purpose
Infant scale in grams	Weighing infant
Regular thermometer or electronic thermometer	Measuring temperature
Measuring tape in centimeters (paper, disposable, or plastic)	Measuring length, circumference
Stethoscope	Heart, lung, abdominal examination
Ophthalmoscope	Eye examination
Flashlight	Testing blink reflex, oral examination
Tongue blade	Oral examination
Alcohol wipes	To clean equipment commonly used by many babies (stethoscope, ophthalmoscope, flashlight)
Neonatal size blood pressure cuff and Doppler apparatus	Measuring blood pressure

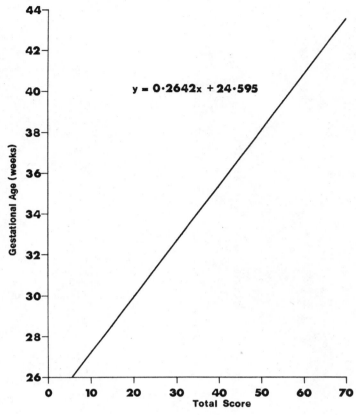

$$y = 0.2642x + 24.595$$

Figure 13-2. Graph for reading gestational age from total score. (Reprinted with permission from Dubowitz, L.M.S., Dubowitz, V., and Goldberg, C.: Clinical assessment of gestational age in the newborn infant. J. Pediatr., *77*:1-10, 1970.)

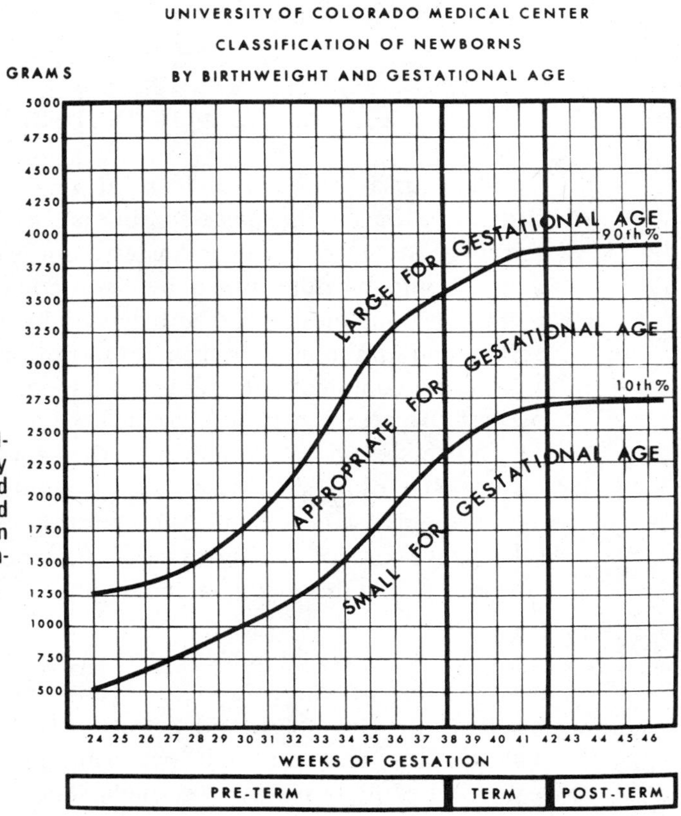

UNIVERSITY OF COLORADO MEDICAL CENTER

CLASSIFICATION OF NEWBORNS

BY BIRTHWEIGHT AND GESTATIONAL AGE

Figure 13-3. University of Colorado Medical Center classification of newborns by birthweight and gestational age. (Reprinted with permission from Battaglia, F.C., and Lubchenco, L.O.: A practical classification of newborn infants by weight and gestational age. J. Pediatr., *71*:159-163, 1967.)

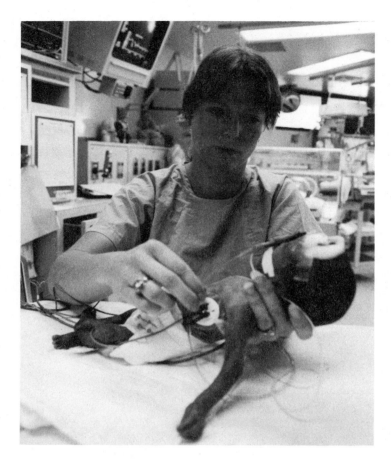

Figure 13-4. Frequent assessment of the neonate at risk is a primary responsibility of the nurse. (Courtesy of Hermann Hospital, Houston, Texas.)

CONCLUSIONS

The nurse should make careful, repeated assessments of the neonate at risk, beginning with Apgar scoring and continuing until the infant is transferred or discharged. General assessment is ongoing, and the extent of assessment should be determined by the neonate's condition and ongoing treatment. Thoroughness must be balanced by attention to conserving the baby's energy and minimizing oxygen consumption.

Once a complete data base is obtained it must be shared with other members of the neonatal health care team by systematic reporting and recording. The nurse should be familiar with the charting format of the particular institution. Recording should be descriptive, detailed, and complete if it is to be of maximum use to all concerned with the infant's care. It is particularly useful to have a record in narrative of the sequence of events, assessment, resuscitation, and stabilization immediately after birth in case the infant must be transported.

It is extremely important that the nurse who must evaluate and care for newborn infants develop skills in assessment. Further study of characteristics of normal neonates and deviations will assist the nurse to identify problems quickly. Experience in performing assessments with a skilled clinician as teacher is the best way to refine assessment skills.

—————————————— REFERENCES ——————————————

1. Barness, L.A.: Manual of Pediatric Physical Diagnosis. Chicago, Year Book Medical Publishers, 1974, pp. 197–214.
2. Clark, A.L., and Affonso, D.D.: Childbearing: A Nursing Perspective, 2nd ed. Philadelphia, F.A. Davis Co., 1979, pp. 563–598.
3. Klaus, M.H., and Fanaroff, A.: Care of the High-Risk Neonate, 2nd ed. Philadelphia, W.B. Saunders Co., 1979, pp. 66–93.
4. Korones, S.B.: High-Risk Newborn Infants: The Basis for Intensive Nursing Care. St. Louis, C.V. Mosby Co., 1981, pp. 103–106.

CHAPTER 14

NEONATAL EMERGENCIES*

Alice F. Illian, R.N., B.S.N.

OBJECTIVES

Upon completion of this chapter the reader will be able to accomplish the following:

1. Identify the life threatening potential of the following neonatal emergencies: asphyxia, shock, air block, and tracheoesophageal fistula
2. Describe the principles of neonatal resuscitation
3. Identify common drugs used in resuscitation
4. Identify equipment necessary for resuscitation and stabilization
5. Explain the emergencies identified and the rationale involved in their management

This chapter will be devoted to specific life threatening emergencies common to newborns. There are many circumstances that constitute emergencies with eventual life threatening sequelae but that cannot be classified as immediately life threatening. For example, an imperforate anus is a serious defect, and requires surgery as soon as possible, but is not immediately life threatening. The purpose of this chapter is to provide the perinatal health care provider with practical guidelines that will enhance early recognition and treatment of a life threatening emergency. Even though the cause or type of the emergency varies, the basic steps (or "ABCs") in resuscitation are always the same. The infant must have a patent airway, adequate oxygen exchange, and cardiovascular and metabolic support. Treatment methods change according to the nature of the emergency, but the basics must be accomplished to optimize the outcome.

The subjects to be discussed will include resuscitation in asphyxia, shock, air block, and surgical emergencies that cannot be postponed, such as severe diaphragmatic hernia and tracheoesophageal fistula.

A basic consideration for all emergency care is equipment and its readi-

---

*The author wishes to thank Margo Cox, M.D., for her assistance in reviewing this manuscript.

ness. Any hospital or birthing center should have the basic tools to enable the nurse provider to handle emergencies effectively. These items must be checked regularly for proper functioning. Being prepared for emergencies is often the difference between a good outcome and a disaster. Refer to Table 14–1 for a complete list.

ASPHYXIA

Asphyxiated newborns are in a life threatening position in which seconds count. Their condition is evident at birth or shortly thereafter, and their obvious compromised state is easily recognized by the delivering physician and the nurse.

DIAGNOSIS

Asphyxia is a condition in which there has been a lack of oxygen to the infant in utero, resulting in a transient to prolonged hypoxial insult with accompanying acidosis. It can begin in labor, in the transitional phase, or just after birth. Asphyxia results in primary to secondary apnea or ultimate failure to breathe, or in death if not promptly treated.

1. **Incidence**
   a. Occurs to some degree in roughly 20 per cent of all births

TABLE 14–1.   EQUIPMENT LIST FOR NEONATAL RESUSCITATION

1. Radiant heat source (warmer) with Servo control
2. Oxygen supply with blender and flowmeter connected
3. Vacuum supply with regulator connected
4. Cardiac monitor, neonatal model
5. Clock (preferably with timer device)
6. Bulb syringe
7. DeLee trap suction devices, size 8 or 10 French
8. Suction catheters, sizes 6, 6.5, and 8 French
9. Laryngoscope with size 0 and 1 straight blades, extra batteries, and extra bulbs
10. Endotracheal tubes sizes 2.5 (up to 1000 gm), 3.0 (1000 – 2500 gm), 3.5 (2500 gm – 4000 gm), and 4.0 (over 4000 gm)
11. Stylet
12. Magill or bayonet-style forceps
13. Stethoscope
14. 500 cc bag and mask, connected to O_2 source
15. Umbilical catheter tray

Iris scissors	Stopcock
Straight scissors	Scalpel handle and blade
4 mosquito clamps	Medicine cup
Curved iris forceps without teeth	Sterile 4 × 4 bandages
Small Addison tissue forceps	2 or 3 sterile towels
Small needle holder	3-0 or 4-0 silk sutures

b. Most frequent in infants of mothers who have been classified as high risk

ETIOLOGY

1. **Depression of the fetal central nervous system (CNS) due to**
   a. Analgesia or anesthesia during labor and delivery
   b. Birth trauma

2. **Classification of major factors contributing to asphyxia**
   a. Maternal
      i. Compression of the inferior vena cava and aorta during active labor, occluding the arterioles and therefore affecting the oxygen–carbon dioxide exchange to the fetus
      ii. Hypotension acquired after administration of regional anesthesia (epidural or caudal), directly affecting the infant's respiratory center; general anesthesia severely depresses the CNS
      iii. Sudden abruptio placentae
      iv. Placenta previa
      v. Prolapsed cord
      vi. Uterine rupture
      vii. Eclampsia uncontrolled by medication
      viii. Sudden maternal temperature spikes complicated by suspected sepsis
   b. Fetal
      i. Lung disease as seen in premature infants less than 36 to 37 weeks of gestational age
      ii. Lung disease as a result of pneumonia acquired in utero
      iii. Airway obstruction from mucus, vernix, or meconium
      iv. Congenital disorders such as choanal atresia, laryngeal web, or hypoplastic lung with or without surgical defects of the trunk wall
      v. Birth trauma
         (a) Mid or high forceps delivery with or without rotation procedures
         (b) Use of suction extractors, causing direct pressure to infant's head
         (c) Cervical spine injuries, such as transection of the cord or severe vertebral compression
         (d) Laceration of the cord during cesarean section, resulting in severe blood loss
         (e) Cord around the neck
         (f) Severe blood loss due to placenta previa, abruptio placentae, or fractured cord

ASSESSMENT

1. **Clinical Presentation**
   a. Signs and symptoms
   The signs and symptoms of asphyxia may start early in labor and continue throughout parturition.

TABLE 14-2. RELATIONSHIP BETWEEN 5 MINUTE APGAR SCORE
AND EXPECTED DEGREE OF ASPHYXIA

Apgar Score at 5 Minutes	Degree of Asphyxia
7–9	None
3–6	Moderately depressed
0–2	Severely depressed

(During labor)
  i. Meconium stained amniotic fluid
  ii. Late or variable fetal heart decelerations as seen on the fetal monitor strip
  iii. Complete loss of fetal heart tones or heart rate
  iv. Sudden obstetrical emergencies as mentioned earlier
(Upon delivery)
  v. A low Apgar score at 1 and 5 minutes (Table 14–2)
     (a) Cyanosis or a pale gray color
     (b) Gasping respirations or apnea
     (c) Heart rate below 60 beats/minute
     (d) Little or no reflex activity
     (e) Decreased tone
  vi. Cool to touch (especially extremities) with poor peripheral perfusion as seen by sluggish or no capillary refilling

PROBLEMS AND COMPLICATIONS

1. Infant with these clinical signs should be immediately resuscitated (Fig. 14–1) (the sooner effective resuscitation is initiated the more favorable the outcome, both short and long term)

2. Some early problems related to resuscitation
   a. Inability to provide adequate ventilation
   b. Inability to provide adequate cardiovascular function
   c. Inability to correct respiratory or metabolic acidosis
   d. Additional physical trauma to the infant

3. Long term problems relate to varying degrees of cerebral ischemia sustained
   a. In severe asphyxia, infant will probably develop seizure disorders

PATIENT CARE MANAGEMENT

1. **Goals**
   a. To provide smooth transition from intrauterine life to extrauterine life
      i. Place newborn infant onto a radiantly warmed work surface and begin to rub dry.

COMMENTS/TIPS/CAUTIONS

Cold stress is as dangerous to newborns as any other illness; as temperature decreases, oxygen consumption increases, as does metabolic acidosis; hypoglycemia and neurological insult may also occur[20]

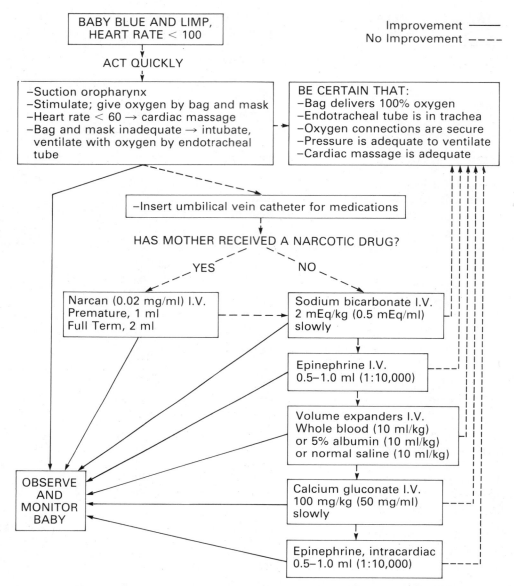

Figure 14-1. Resuscitating the newborn infant. (From Perinatal Continuing Education Program, Division of Neonatal Medicine, Department of Pediatrics, University of Virginia Medical Center, Charlottesville, Virginia, 1982.)

Rubbing provides two functions
(a) Prevents excess heat and calorie loss due to evaporation
(b) Provides cutaneous stimulation, which in itself may stimulate respiration
b. To provide patent airway

COMMENTS/TIPS/CAUTIONS

Be sure the work surface is adequate; this provides quick and easy access to the child

Do not hold a compromised infant to show it until infant has been dried and its status adequately assessed; recognizing the much documented need for parental-infant bonding is important, but an extra few seconds of simple and conscientious care may well be the difference between no illness and severe impairment

i. Hyperextend neck of new-born

ii. Clear nasopharynx with a DeLee trap or wall suction until airway is clear of mucus, vernix, or meconium

iii. An assistant should hold oxygen source to the infant's nose and mouth area

c. To assess and provide ventilation

i. Initiate ventilation if there is no evidence of spontaneous respiration or if the infant is only gasping

ii. Use a bag and mask apparatus that is attached to an oxygen source

iii. If the infant does not start to breathe or gasp after use of bag and mask for 1 to 2 minutes, then the infant must be orally intubated and the bag squeezed at a rate of 60 to 80 times a minute (refer to Appendix B for intubation)

d. To assess the cardiac status and augment circulation

i. Feel the umbilical cord for pulsation, which is the heart rate; if heart rate is greater than 100, infant will usually continue in transition without problems

ii. Call out the heart rate or tap the rate as you feel it so that other team members know status of the infant

iii. If heart rate is less than 60 beats/minute institute cardiac massage immediately at rate of 180/minute; proper ratio is 3 compressions to 1 ventilation. Place two fingers over the midsternal area or encircle the infant's chest with both hands (lace

COMMENTS/TIPS/ CAUTIONS

Nasopharyngeal suction can stimulate the vagus nerve, which can cause significant bradycardia; suctioning should be fast and thorough with enough time between passes to allow accommodation in the infant

If the infant is stained with meconium do not initiate respiration until the meconium has been cleared from the trachea (unless the heart rate is less than 60)

During resuscitation, speed is absolutely essential; orotracheal intubation is quick and does not require the skill of nasotracheal intubation; after the condition of the infant has been stabilized, a nasotracheal tube may be placed if continued mechanical ventilation is required

Lack of a stethoscope should never hinder accurate assessment of the heart rate; the heart rate can be assessed quickly and must be done in tandem with all the steps of resuscitation discussed

fingers in back, compress sternum with thumbs)—either is appropriate

e. To correct and maintain optimal metabolic homeostasis

   i. If infant continues to be unresponsive, it is appropriate to provide metabolic and cardiovascular support. Be prepared to administer the following four basic drugs (see also Table 14–3 and Fig. 14–2)

      (a) $NaHCO_3$ (sodium bicarbonate), 0.5 to 1.0 mEq/kg every 1 to 2 minutes as long as heart rate less than 70

      (b) Epinephrine, 1:10,000, 0.1 to 0.5 cc/kg/dose

      (c) Calcium chloride, 10 per cent, 0.15 cc/kg/dose

      (d) Glucose, 25 per cent, 2 cc/kg

f. To provide an entry port for passage of drugs, fluids, and volume expanders

   i. When it has become apparent that medications are required during resuscitation, the fastest way to give them is by inserting an umbilical venous or umbilical arterial catheter (see Appendix B for technique)

g. To determine the status of the metabolic component and to assess adequacy of ventilation

   i. Be prepared to obtain the following laboratory tests

      (a) Arterial blood gas (see Appendix B)

COMMENTS/TIPS/CAUTIONS

During asphyxia, infant's pH drastically decreases, glucose consumption increases, and cells use much more oxygen; if pH and glucose status are corrected, oxygen carrying capacity of the blood improves and the pulmonary pressure decreases, allowing more optimal oxygenation of lung and brain tissue

Bicarbonate, an alkali, will increase pH of blood; when given in tandem with glucose, gasping is prolonged, indicating that respiratory efforts are enhanced and cardiovascular collapse is delayed

The glucose acts as a source for replacing energy used by the cells in increased oxygen consumption[18]

Provides easy and rapid access for administering medications and a port for fast and reliable blood sampling; may be attached to a physiological pressure transducer for direct central pressure monitoring

A central line is preferable during resuscitation, since time could be wasted trying to insert a peripheral line when the peripheral perfusion is shut down, as it is in asphyxia

Umbilical vessels are easy to cannulate because asphyxia causes vasodilatation; once oxygenation takes place these vessels constrict and cannulation becomes more difficult

Blood gases will tell exact status of patient; critical things to look for during resuscitation in the immediate newborn period are:
  pH: If it is less than 7.05 to 7.20, administration of sodium bicarbonate must then be considered; however, overuse of alkali should be avoided for several reasons
1. Marked metabolic acidosis is the true indication for alkali administration; alkali can contribute to carbon dioxide retention as sodium bicarbonate breaks down into water and carbon dioxide; patients must be ventilated effectively when alkali is given during resuscitation[2,6,12]
2. As a hyperosmolar solution, alkali may produce pressure and volume changes in cerebrospinal fluid; intraventricular hemorrhage and cerebral edema may be associated with administration of alkali solution because of the metabolic alteration in the cells;[2,12] kidney damage may also occur

If the P_{O_2} is less than 50 torr, administration of oxygen by hood must be considered once the infant arrives in the nursery, especially if central cyanosis and tachypnea are present

If P_{CO_2} is greater than 60, along with decreased pH and decreased P_{O_2}, continuous mechanical ventilation is indicated

TABLE 14–3. MEDICATIONS USED IN RESUSCITATION

Name, Source, Synonyms, Preparations	Dosage and Administration	Uses	Action and Fate	Side Effects	Nursing Implications/ Remarks
Sodium bicarbonate 4.2% 0.5 mEq/cc (also available in 8.4% but must be diluted 1:1 with sterile water)	1–2 mEq/kg/ dose, or 0.5–1 mEq/kg/ min of arrest IV push	For severe acidosis (pH < 7.05 and base deficit of 15 mEq/ liter	Reverses myocardial failure and low cardiac output that occur with severe asphyxia and pulmonary vasoconstriction that occurs with acidosis	May be associated with intracranial hemorrhage; may cause CO_2 retention	Draw up in 6 cc syringe IV extravasation causes skin slough; give through a patent IV
Aqueous epinephrine 1:10,000 0.1mg/cc	0.05 mg/dose, (0.5 cc) IV push or intracardiac	Asystole or profound bradycardia	Excreted by kidneys Adrenergic action	Tachycardia, arrhythmia	Draw up in TB syringe
Calcium gluconate 100 mg/cc	100 mg/kg/ dose 1cc/kg IV push	↓ Calcium		Bradycardia; sloughs if IV infiltrates	Draw up in 3 cc syringe give slowly
Calcium chloride 10% 100 mg/cc	0.15 cc/kg IV push	Cardiac arrest	Potentiates digitalis	Gastric irritation; potentiates digitalis	Draw up in TB syringe, give slowly
Atropine	0.01 cc/kg 0.01–0.03 mg/kg IV push or endotracheal	Severe bradycardia; second- or third-degree heart block	Vagal suppression	Hyperthermia, urinary retention, tachycardia	Draw up in TB syringe, give slowly
Glucose $D_{10}W$ undiluted $D_{25}W$ 1:1 with sterile water	2–4 cc/kg		Easily metabolized Source of calories	Rebound hypoglycemia	D_{25} causes skin slough if IV is not patent
Naloxone (Narcan) 0.4 mg/cc—dilute 0.1 cc with 0.9 cc sterile water for 0.04 mg/cc	0.01–0.15 mg/ kg/dose IV or IM only	Narcotic induced depression			Draw up in TB syringe; rapid acting
Isoproterenol (Isuprel) —dilute to 0.2 mg/cc	0.05–0.1 mg/ kg/min for continuous low blood pressure IV flow 0.5–1 cc IV push, very slow, of dilute solution	Severe bradycardia Cardiac arrest	Beta-adrenergic action	Hypotension; arrhythmia with overdose	Usually given in drip solution Observe heart rate closely

PEDIATRIC RESUSCITATION MEDICINES

Weight: _____   Height: _____   BSA: _____

ET tube size: _____   Length: _____

DRUG & STRENGTH	DOSE	AMOUNT TO BE GIVEN
Tidal volume	10-15 ml/kg	_____
NaHCO$_3$ - approx. 1mg/ml	1 meq/kg. dilute 1:1 w/ sterile H$_2$O in newborns	_____
D$_{50}$W-Glucose 50% 50 gm/100ml	0.5 gm/kg	_____
Adrenalin 1:10,000 (Epinephrine)	0.1 ml/kg. IV or Intracardiac*	_____
Atropine .1 mg/ml BRISTAJET .4 mg/.5 ml AMPULE	0.01 mg/kg*	_____
Ca Chloride 10% 100 mg/ml	0.2 ml/kg. give slowly and monitor heart rate	_____
Dopamine	Drip: 2-5 mcg/kg/min. initially Titrate to clinical condition	See Infusion Chart
Isoproterenol	Drip: 0.1 mg/kg/min Titrate to clinical condition	See Infusion Chart
Lidocaine 1% 20 mg/ml BRISTAJET	Bolus: 0.5-1 mg/kg/dose* Drip: 0.020-0.05 mg/kg/min	_____
Narcan Neonatal 0.02 mg/ml Adult 0.4 mg/ml	0.01 mg/kg Titrate to clinical contition	_____
DC counter shock	2 watt-seconds/kg maximum 4 watt-seconds/kg	_____

*May be diluted with sterile water and given per ET tube if unable to establish if line.

Admitting Date: _____   Time: _____

_____
INTERN   Date: Time:

_____
PRIMARY NURSE

Figure 14-2. Worksheet for resuscitation medications. Appropriate dosages for resuscitation can be calculated on admission and kept with the baby for ready access. (Courtesy of Hermann Hospital, Houston, Texas.)

(b) Hematocrit determination from blood obtained from a central line or a heel stick.

(c) A Dextrostix determination from heel stick blood

ii. Continue with the code procedure until the infant has been transported to the ICU or triage nursery. The procedure must be accurately documented throughout (see Figure 14–3)

iii. Once the infant is in the nursery, use a cardiorespiratory monitor and ventilator or hood as needed; then prepare for transport to a tertiary center if your facility cannot provide level III care

COMMENTS/TIPS/ CAUTIONS

A hematocrit of less than 40 ml/dl in combination with low blood pressure is a fair indicator of shock; blood or other volume expanders may be administered with caution at a rate of 5 to 10 cc/kg per injection as their overuse may also compromise the cerebral outcome; injections should be given rapidly enough to correct perfusion but slowly enough to prevent abrupt pressure changes; vascular beds, particularly in the brain, dilate in response to hypotension; if the pressure rises too fast, there is no time for this vasculature to partially reconstrict—therefore the capillaries are stressed by the high pressure and may rupture, resulting in edema or hemorrhage or both[1,3,5,10]

A Dextrostix reading of 40 ml/dl or less will probably be the case (most probably 0 to 25 will be the finding); prepare to administer glucose (see Table 14–3) and to start IV administration of $D_{10}W$ for maintenance fluids

When to stop attempts to resuscitate an infant is often a difficult decision; many "rounds" of resuscitation drugs may be used without response

It is not appropriate for the decision to stop to be made in the delivery room; remember that any infant born with an Apgar score of 1 or above is considered a live birth; since resuscitation in itself is the treatment of a live patient, the infant must be admitted to the nursery

Complications of treatment may include:
1. Trauma from handling (bruised chest, extremities)
2. Pneumothorax (inappropriate pressures with bag or ventilator)
3. Medication overdose
4. Death

SHOCK

Shock is any condition in which perfusion is inadequate to meet the tissue's needs. Shock in itself is a dangerous situation for which monitoring should be continuous. The key to understanding shock is to comprehend the mechanisms behind it.

There are several forms or classifications of shock. The type of shock the patient is experiencing is usually related directly to the diagnosis. For example, the patient with congenital heart disease needs to be monitored for cardiogenic shock; likewise the patient with sepsis may well develop septic shock.

Four categories of shock will be discussed: hypovolemic, hypoglycemic, septic, and cardiogenic. Note that many of the clinical manifestations of the four categories overlap and appear to follow the same course. The key to managing shock is to understand the patient's history, that is, to understand why the patient developed the shock condition.

Shock in itself may be an end stage condition. How quickly and effectively shock is treated will have a direct effect on the patient's survival, both physically and neurologically. The longer shock persists, the more likely are the chances the patient will sustain kidney and brain damage in the form of necrosis. The renal necrosis in newborns is often reversible; the brain necrosis

CARDIOPULMONARY RESUSITATION WORKSHEET
HERMANN HOSPITAL / *The University Hospital*

DATE OF ARREST | CODE CALLED ☐ YES ☐ NO | RESUS. START ___ AM PM | PRE ARREST DIAGNOSIS

TYPE OF EMERGENCY

☐ SEIZURE
☐ APNEA
☐ SHOCK
☐ CARDIAC ARREST RHYTHM UNKNOWN
☐ AIRWAY OBSTRUCTION
☐ OTHER

INITIAL EKG

☐ BRADYCARDIA
☐ ASYSTOLE
☐ VENTRICULAR FIBRILLATION
☐ VENTRICULAR TACHYCARDIA
☐ ELECTRO MECHANICAL DISOCIATION

METHOD OF VENTILATION

☐ MOUTH TO MOUTH
☐ VENTILATOR
☐ BAG/MASK

METHOD OF CIRCULATORY ASSISTANCE

☐ EXTERNAL CLOSED
☐ INTERNAL OPENED

PROCEDURES DONE

☐ O₂ STARTED
☐ I.V. INSERTED
☐ CVP INSERTED
☐ SUCTIONED
☐ PACEMAKER INSERTED
☐ ABG'S ___ TIME
☐ INTUBATION ___ TIME

	TIME	BP	PULSE/RESP	TIME	BP	PULSE/RESP	TIME	BP	PULSE/RESP	TIME	BP	PULSE/RESP	TIME	BP	PULSE/RESP AM PM	TIME	BP	PULSE/RESP AM PM	TIME	BP	PULSE/RESP AM PM
V S I T G A N L S															SIZE			DONE BY			TIME
R P H E Y R H C M G	TIME		PATTERN	TIME		PATTERN	TIME		PATTERN	TIME		PATTERN	TIME		PATTERN	TIME		PATTERN	TIME		PATTERN
D E F I B	TIME		WATT/SEC	TIME		WATT/SEC	TIME		WATT/SEC	TIME		WATT/SEC	TIME		WATT/SEC	TIME		WATT/SEC	TIME		WATT/SEC

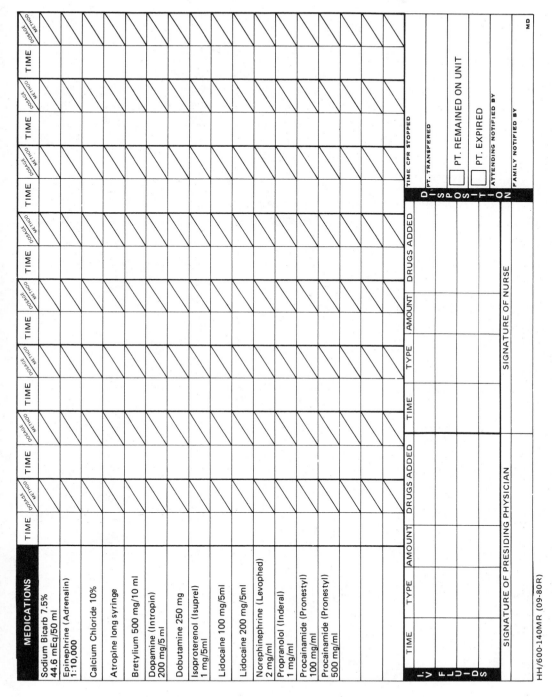

Figure 14-3. A CPR record is essential for determination and evaluation. (Courtesy of Hermann Hospital, Houston, Texas.)

305

is irreparable. The long term neurological outcome should therefore be considered foremost by the health care professional.

HYPOVOLEMIC SHOCK

Hypovolemia, due to a maternal or fetal disorder or trauma, is frequently seen at birth. It is also seen anytime after admission when there has been blood loss or a hypoxic insult (e.g., brain hemorrhage) resulting in a decrease in the hematocrit value to less than 40 ml/dl. This is one of the most common types of shock in the newborn.

DIAGNOSIS

Hypovolemic shock is a condition in which there has been an acute loss of volume (blood) to the extravascular space ultimately resulting in inadequate tissue perfusion.

1. **Incidence**
   a. 1 in 1000 live births[6]
2. Hematocrit less than 40 ml/dl
3. Blood pressure less than 40 mm Hg
4. Central venous pressure less than 4 cm H_2O

ETIOLOGY

1. **Maternal factors**
   All of these factors will contribute to intrapartum asphyxia:
   a. Abruptio placentae
   b. Placenta previa
   c. Placental laceration at cesarean section
   d. Uterine rupture
   e. Maternal-fetal transfusion

2. **Fetal factors**
   a. Twin to twin transfusion
   b. Severe erythroblastosis
   c. Avulsion of umbilical cord
   d. Fracture of umbilical cord
   e. Laceration of umbilical cord

ASSESSMENT

1. **Clinical presentation**
   a. Signs and symptoms
      i. Hematocrit less than 40 ml/dl
         (a) Signifies remarkable blood loss or dilution due to decreased peripheral perfusion; peripheral perfusion is shut down as the body automatically shunts blood to the more important areas such as the brain, heart, liver, kidney, and lungs

      ii. Cyanosis
- (a) Due to decreased oxygen carrying capacity of the blood resulting from lack of cells (hemoglobin) and also due to peripheral vasoconstriction

    iii. Tachycardia (heart rate above 180 beats per minute)
- (a) Due to infant body's attempt to compensate for decreased perfusion by increasing the heart's pump action to circulate what oxygen carrying cells are available

    iv. Tachypnea (respiratory rate above 60)
- (a) The infant body's need for more oxygen results in rapid breathing in attempting to gain it; rapid breathing also assists in expiration of carbon dioxide

     v. Hypotension (systolic blood pressure less than 40 mm Hg)
- (a) Due to decreased circulating volume

    vi. Temperature instability
- (a) Due to stress to the hypothalamus and to autoregulation; CNS depression also results in temperature instability

   vii. Acidosis
- (a) Due to lactic acid build-up resulting from anaerobic metabolism in poorly perfused, poorly oxygenated tissues

  viii. Decrease muscle tone
- (a) Due to cellular loss of glycogen '
- (b) Due to CNS depression from a decrease in circulation of glucose in the blood

b. History
- i. Infant pale, cool, or mottled, seemingly unresponsive
- ii. Irregular respiratory pattern or apnea
- iii. Sudden low or progressively decreasing blood pressure, weak pulse, and poor peripheral perfusion

PATIENT CARE MANAGEMENT
1. Goals

	COMMENTS/TIPS/CAUTIONS
a. To provide an accessible and stable environment	
i. Place infant on radiant warmer to Servo control of 36.5°C	A warmer provides good work surface as well as stable temperature, therefore reducing cold stress; cold stress uses up depleted glycogen stores and increases oxygen consumption
b. To assess infant's condition and to determine the cause of the hypovolemia	
i. Check vital signs and observe for different patterns from previous checks	
ii. Pay particular attention to blood pressure	Continue until blood pressure returns to a more normal level; be sure infant is attached to cardiorespiratory monitor
(a) If the BP less than 40 mg Hg prepare for volume resuscitation using a bolus of 10 to 20 cc/	

kg/dose of one of the following:

    (1) Fresh frozen plasma

    (2) Normal saline

    (3) 25 per cent albumin diluted 1:4 with sterile saline; or 5 per cent albumin followed by either:

    (4) Whole blood or parked red blood cells (O negative)

iii. Record vital signs and blood pressure immediately and every 15–30 minutes as needed

iv. Assess infant for lacerations or trauma after delivery

Review of the maternal history may reveal intrapartum accident such as cord fracture that would cause the infant to be hypovolemic at birth

v. Check all IV lines, especially central lines, to be sure they have not become disconnected: tape all connections

It is not unusual for infant's central lines to become disconnected, causing quick blood loss

vi. Continuously monitor the infant's respiratory status; clear airway of any mucus or other obstructing debris

Suction as discussed previously—quickly without too much vagus nerve stimulation

vii. Draw blood for type and crossmatch

Not only is blood useful for volume expansion, it is also an alternate source for blood carrying hemoglobin molecules

viii. Arterial blood gas (ABG) determination

ABG determinations are essential for monitoring the pH and Pco_2; acidosis is probable and should be corrected; increased CO_2 may indicate the need for assisted ventilation

ix. Determine blood glucose level with Dextrostix immediately, record, and repeat every hour until the infant's condition is stable

Hypoglycemia will probably occur; hypoglycemia potentiates hypovolemia and acidosis

c. To prevent neurological stress

i. Handle infant minimally and with caution

Handling, changing position, and suctioning can raise the intracranial pressure, thereby placing stress on the brain capillaries, and may contribute to intraventricular hemorrhage

ii. Do not push fluids rapidly or give too many fluids

In addition to the following complications of treatment, death of the infant may occur
1. Over expansion of the vascular volume
2. Pulmonary edema from a high level of fluids on board
3. Death

HYPOGLYCEMIC SHOCK

Hypoglycemic shock occurs when the circulating blood glucose level has become so low that the CNS becomes depressed, therefore depressing respiration, decreasing cardiac output, and shutting down peripheral circulation. The infant with hypoglycemic shock will very often have seizures and hypoxia. Long term follow-up in transient symptomatic neonatal hypoglycemia has shown a 30 to 50 per cent incidence of neurological impairment.[11]

DIAGNOSIS

Hypoglycemic shock is the condition resulting when the blood glucose level is less than 40 mg/100 ml in the term infant and less than 30 mg/100 ml in the preterm infant.

1. **Incidence**
   a. Unexplained hypoglycemia occurs transiently in about 4 per cent of normal term infants in the first 3 days of life.
2. **Predisposing factors for hypoglycemia**
   a. Asphyxia at birth
   b. Prematurity
   c. Postmaturity
   d. Infant of diabetic mother (IDM)
   e. Infant large or small for gestational age (LGA, SGA)
   f. Infant with sepsis
   g. Respiratory distress syndrome
   h. Infants who have had cold stress
   i. Metabolic disorders

ETIOLOGY

Common causes of hypoglycemia include the following:
1. Hyperinsulinism (e.g., IDM)
2. Decreased liver glycogen stores (e.g., prematurity, SGA)
3. Poor mobilization of liver glycogen stores

ASSESSMENT

1. **Clinical presentation**
   a. Signs and symptoms
      i. Tachypnea (respiratory rate greater than 60/minute)
         (a) Due to hypoxia, carbon dioxide retention, and acidosis
      ii. Tachycardia (heart rate greater than 180/minute)
         (a) Due to low blood pressure
      iii. Low temperature (less than 36.5°C)
         (a) Due to CNS depression
      iv. Low blood pressure (less than 40 mm Hg)
      v. Acidosis
         (a) The product of anaerobic metabolism in hypoxic tissues is lactic acid; it circulates, therefore causing acidosis
      vi. Decreased muscle tone, weak cry, stupor, jitteriness
         (a) All due to CNS depression

      vii. Diaphoresis
        (a) Due to excessive secretion of epinephrine in response to hypoglycemia
     viii. Seizures
        (a) CNS irritability; diffuse necrosis of cortical neurons and damage to the cerebellum[18]
  b. History
    i. Lethargy or irritability
    ii. Cool or sweaty
    iii. With or without a high risk history

PATIENT CARE MANAGEMENT

COMMENTS/TIPS/CAUTIONS

1. Goals

  a. To provide the "ABCs"
    i. Clear airway
    ii. Assess respiratory (breathing) mechanism
    iii. Support cardiovascular and metabolic component

Hypoglycemia mimicks respiratory distress; therefore, rapid assessment is required; in profound hypoglycemia, both cardiorespiratory arrest and seizure may occur and be followed by long term neurological damage

  b. To determine glucose level
    i. Obtain a Dextrostix reading via blood from heel stick, toe prick, or finger prick

Be careful not to make direct contact between the strip and the surface pricked; and extremely fine membrane may be crushed, invalidating the reading

    ii. If Dextrostix reading is less than 45 mg/100 ml obtain a serum glucose determination immediately

The Dextrostix method is reliable as a rule, but the serum value can confirm hypoglycemia

    iii. If Dextrostix reading is in range of 0 to 25 mg/100 ml, therapy should begin immediately

Blood samples should be carried to the laboratory within 30 minutes or false readings may be obtained, because macrophages in the blood consume the available glucose; false low results may be obtained and inappropriate treatment given

  c. To provide an entry port for glucose administration
    i. A large bore (22, 23, or 24 gauge) intravenous catheter should be inserted peripherally or in the scalp area; insertion of an umbilical venous catheter may be necessary

In an infant left too long with hypoglycemia, peripheral perfusion will probably have shut down and an umbilical line will therefore be required; the advantage of a central line is that high concentrations of glucose can be safely given

  d. To reestablish normal serum glucose levels
    i. Prepare to administer
      (a) $D_{10}W$ 2 to 4 cc/kg per slow IV injection
      (b) D_{25} 1:1 with sterile water 2 to 4 cc/kg per IV injection

These protocols may work well for infant with transient neonatal hypoglycemia

e. To evaluate and maintain therapy

    i. Continued IV administration of $D_{10}W$ at 75 to 100 cc/kg/24 hr or more if clinically indicated

    ii. Obtain a Dextrostix reading every 30 minutes initially and then every hour until readings of 45 to 90 mg/100 ml are consistently obtained (at least three times), then check every 4 hours until stable

    iii. Be prepared to administer hydrocortisone (Solu-Cortef) 5 mg/kg/day in two divided doses IV or orally[2,4] or prednisone 2 mg/kg over 24 hours

f. Determine why hypoglycemia persists and determine what diagnostic work-up is indicated

COMMENTS/TIPS/CAUTIONS

These protocols may work well for infant with transient neonatal hypoglycemia

The Dextrostix reading must also be watched closely when the infant is being weaned from high concentration dextrose

Infants requiring these drugs usually have a genetic or metabolic disorder rather than transient neonatal hypoglycemia; they require close diagnostic work-ups with metabolic or genetic specialists

Complications of treatment
1. Skin irritation or sloughing due to the high osmolarity of glucose
2. Rebound hypoglycemia

SEPTIC SHOCK

The presentation of septic shock is similar to that of hypovolemic shock and hypoglycemia shock, but blood, plasma, and glucose alone will not correct the problem. In infants with shock immediately at birth sepsis must be considered in addition to asphyxia.

DIAGNOSIS

Septic shock occurs in an infant when infection is present.

1. Incidence

a. The incidence of sepsis neonatorum is 4 per 1000[4]

2. Predisposing factors

Infants can become infected in utero or after several days of life for a wide variety of reasons. Close attention to the maternal history will give some indication of sepsis risk factors.

a. Prolonged or premature rupture of the membranes (more than 24 hours prior to birth)

b. Maternal sepsis, urinary tract infection

c. Amnionitis

d. Fever during labor

       e. Repeated vaginal examination
       f. Difficult delivery requiring instrumentation
       g. Mother who had no prenatal care
       h. Prematurity
       i. Infants of diabetic mothers
3. Onset is usually from birth to 24 hours of age
4. Initially infant is thought to have acute respiratory distress
5. Chest radiograph may reveal pneumonitis
6. Ventilation will be very difficult to manage
7. Later onset of sepsis with shock may be seen in infants who acquire meningitis or develop surgical problems such as bowel perforation often seen in necrotizing enterocolitis

ETIOLOGY

1. Group B beta hemolytic streptococcus is one of the main gram positive organisms causing the fulminating sepsis that presents precipitously with shock; *E. coli* is the most common gram negative organism that presents with gram negative shock and sepsis

ASSESSMENT

1. **Clinical presentation**
    a. Signs and symptoms
      i. Temperature instability (less than 97.6°F or greater than 99.0°F)
       (a) Due to CNS irritability and poor metabolic reserves
      ii. Lethargy, irritability, and seizures
       (a) Due to CNS irritability and hyponatremia[4]
      iii. Hypoglycemia (glucose levels less than 40 mg/100 ml)
       (a) Due to poor metabolic reserves and increased peripheral utilization of glucose
      iv. Tachycardia (heart rate above 180) or bradycardia (heart rate less than 120), tachypnea, or apnea
       (a) Due to CNS depression, hypoglycemia, increased carbon dioxide, and acidosis
      v. Hypotension (BP<40 mm Hg)
       (a) Due to CNS depression, fluid leaking out of the intracellular space, and other effects of endotoxins
      vi. Disseminated intravascular coagulation (DIC)
       (a) Incidence 66 per cent[4]
      vii. Jaundice
       (a) Due to hemolytic anemia from red cells breaking as they pass through areas of vessels that have been affected by thrombin build-up as seen in DIC
      viii. Hypoxia
       (a) Due to build-up of lactic acid, leading to decrease of oxygen uptake by cells; further worsened by hypoglycemia and electrolyte imbalance

(b) Vascular injury induced by hypoxia may also contribute to DIC[6]

ix. Petechiae

(a) Due to low platelet count (less than 50,000 cu mm), seen with severe infections from endotoxin producing organisms

b. History

i. Infant cold, mottled, lethargic, and possibly jaundiced

ii. Gradual to worsening signs of respiratory distress, apnea, or both

iii. Infant may or may not display seizure activity

PATIENT CARE MANAGEMENT

1. Goals

a. To provide rapid assessment and treatment, institute ABCs

This step a prerequisite for further treatment

i. Place infant on a radiantly heated warmer on Servo control and connect a cardiorespiratory monitor; the ECG rhythm strip will be a valuable indicator of electrolyte problems

(a) Peaked T waves may occur with elevated potassium levels

ii. Clear airway

iii. Provide for respiration and oxygen exchange

iv. Give cardiac support

v. Give drugs if needed

vi. Obtain and record the vital signs, blood pressure, and central venous pressure (if available)

Recording establishes baseline data

vii. Manage hypotension as described in the section on hypovolemic shock.

Be aware that hypovolemia (particularly when the infant has necrotizing enterocolitis) occurs because of massive fluid shifting in the abdomen secondary to the inflammatory response to bowel necrosis; BP will be low; blood, plasma, or crystalloids should be administered to maintain the BP and urinary output; whole blood stays in the vascular space, but other expanders can leak through damaged capillaries, increasing interstitial edema; corticosteroid (Solu-Cortef 50 mg/kg stat; then 50 mg/kg/day divided every 6 hours) stabilizes endotoxic damaged membranes and increases cardiac output and peripheral perfusion[9]

b. To decrease abdominal distention

i. Insert nasogastric or Replogle tube and connect to source of low continuous or intermittent suction

c. To assess and support the hematological and metabolic status

Gastric dilatation further compromises respiratory effort; decompression of bowel prevents aspiration if the infant vomits

i. Be prepared to obtain the following laboratory tests

	COMMENTS/TIPS/CAUTIONS
(a) CBC with differential and platelet counts	Platelets may be less than 20,000/cu mm, necessitating transfusions of platelets
(b) Prothrombin time and partial thromboplastin time	Both may be prolonged; this finding along with a low platelet count, indicates DIC,[6] prepare to give transfusions of fresh whole blood immediately and fresh frozen plasma 10 cc/kg every 4 to 6 hours
(c) Blood: Type and cross-match	Occasionally in infants with profound sepsis bleeding will continue even though there have been many trials of therapy; exchange transfusions with fresh whole citrated or heparinized blood are sometimes given along with continued transfusions of platelets and fresh frozen plasma; whole blood provides specific factors enhancing the phagocytic properties of the infant's leukocytes and may also provide small amounts of specific antibodies.[9] Fresh frozen plasma can add clotting factors as well as increase the vascular volume, thereby increasing BP
(d) Glucose	Hypoglycemia will be present (glucose less than 40 mg/100 ml), and IV fluids will be required; remember to monitor blood glucose frequently with the Dextrostix until the level is stable
(e) Electrolytes	Sodium level will be low (less than 130 mEq/liter); potassium may be elevated (more than 6.4 mEq/liter); calcium may be low (less than 7–8 mg/100 ml); electrolyte disorders contribute to potential shock and left untreated may contribute to profound seizures
(f) Arterial blood gases	There may be some respiratory acidosis that will be corrected with ventilation and sodium bicarbonate, but the overall acidosis is metabolic and requires close monitoring
(g) Blood culture	Obtain with a venipuncture after double povidone-iodine (Betadine) preparation; it is very important to obtain cultures before antibiotics are administered to prevent masking of organisms; this is a common error and is easily preventable
(h) Cerebrospinal fluid for cell count and culture	The physician may choose to delay this procedure (lumbar puncture) during acute shock; be prepared to resuscitate the infant—infants with sepsis do not tolerate this procedure well when in shock
d. To provide an entry port for fluids and medications i. Prepare to assist with insertion of an umbilical artery catheter or a central line if one is not already in place	Arterial and central venous pressure (CVP) lines provide access and allow direct pressure monitoring. CVP readings reflect the hydration status of the heart; these lines also allow administration of hyperosmolar medications such as sodium bicarbonate and high concentration glucose; drugs such as these are more effective when given through a central line because they are taken up more quickly; extravasation of these caustic drugs into peripheral tissues is then prevented
ii. Insert the largest bore peripheral line possible for additional access	Peripheral lines may be used for antibiotics; refer to Appendix B for medications used for sepsis Complications of treatment may include: 1. Fluid overloading 2. Tissue sloughing from caustic medications 3. Death

CARDIOGENIC SHOCK

Acute cardiogenic shock is not seen in neonates as often as other types of shock such as hypoglycemic shock or hypovolemic shock; however, it is important to acknowledge it.

DIAGNOSIS

Cardiogenic shock may be considered primary pump failure.

1. Chest radiograph will show cardiomegaly
2. The ECG may show ST and T wave anomalies and low voltage QRS complexes, indicating rapid heart dilatation

ETIOLOGY

There are several causes for cardiogenic shock, including the following:

1. Heart disease
2. Myocarditis due to sepsis, viral disease, or asphyxia
3. Overloading of fluids

ASSESSMENT

1. **Clinical presentation**
   a. Signs and symptoms
      i. At presentation infant is cold, mottled, apparently dying
      ii. Tachypnea with a shallow breathing pattern, usually first sign noticed
      iii. Tachycardia: Heart rate more than 160 beats/minute
         (a) Due to heart's attempt to maintain cardiac output and to compensate for low blood pressure
      iv. Hypothermia
         (a) Due to low cardiac output and CNS depression
      v. Acidosis
         (a) Secondary to hypoxia and consequent lactic acidosis
      vi. Hypotension: BP less than 40 mm Hg, central venous pressure greater than 12 cm H_2O^4
         (a) May not be present if shock is of rapid onset
      vii. Hepatosplenomegaly
         (a) Due to venous congestion and edema in the liver and spleen
      viii. A murmur with or without arrhythmia
      ix. Wheezing or rales on auscultation
   b. History
      i. Previous respiratory distress, hypoglycemia, or asphyxia
      ii. Shock symptoms, possible manifestation of asymptomatic and undiagnosed heart disease

PATIENT CARE MANAGEMENT

1. **Goals**
   a. To provide rapid assessment and treatment
      i. Institute ABCs
      ii. Obtain and record the vital signs

COMMENTS/TIPS/CAUTIONS

Attach infant to a cardiorespiratory monitor

(a) Maintain temperature

(b) Assess the heart rate and QRS complex

iii. Take, record blood pressure

iv. Take and record the central venous pressure (if the line is available)

b. To assess and support the metabolic component

   i. Obtain the following laboratory values to establish the baseline

     (a) Glucose

     (b) Electrolytes

     (c) Arterial blood gases

c. To decrease the stress to the heart

   i. Prepare to restrict fluid intake

   ii. Prepare to administer the following drugs

     (a) Digoxin (Lanoxin), total digitalizing dose (TDD): preterm 0.03 to 0.06 mg/kg/24 hr[2,6]; term, 0.04 to 0.08 mg/kg/24 hr[2,6]; give ½ TDD and then repeat ¼ dose every 8 to 12 hours twice; then give 1/8 dose every 12 hours as maintenance

     (b) Furosemide (Lasix), 1 to 3 mg/kg IV every 8 hours, given as a single dose over 3 minutes

     (c) Isoproterenol (Isuprel), 1 mg/100 cc in D_5W drip, dose to be titrated (1 mg/100 cc = 10 μg/cc); pump at about 1 μg/kg/minute until the desired effect is obtained

     (d) Dopamine (Intropin) may be considered for low blood pressure; dose of 1 to 10 mcg/kg/min until the desired effect is obtained; dilute this medication in D_5W

COMMENTS/TIPS/CAUTIONS

Place on a radiant warmer on Servo control; cold stress aggravates the shock entity

If the infant is already being monitored, trends or changes in the voltage of the QRS can be detected quickly by placing a small piece of tape on the oscilloscope; mark the peak and the lowest deflection of the QRS complex on the tape—sudden or subtle changes can be quickly assessed

Central blood pressures are always preferable, particularly when peripheral perfusion has shut down; if only peripheral monitoring devices are available, however, the pressure may be taken in two ways; by palpation, or by Doppler

Cuff sizes are important. The cuff should be half to two thirds of the length of the infant's upper arm; cuffs that are too small or too large will decrease the accuracy of the reading and therefore possibly cause a change in the therapy

A CVP of greater than 12 indicates cardiogenic shock; a CVP of less than 4 indicates that the shock may be related to hypovolemia or septic shock[4]

The heart fails because it can no longer handle the volume load

Errors in administration of digitalis are the most common and the most devastating errors made in treating neonates because of the fractional amounts used; *always double check* the order and your calculations *before* giving the dose; with evidence of myocarditis some cardiologists use even smaller TDD

Diuresis should occur within an hour

Assess specific gravity of the urine after every voiding; this indicates the kidney's ability to concentrate

Carefully monitor the serum sodium and potassium levels, as these electrolytes become depleted after repeated diuretic therapy

Check heart rate frequently

Watch for arrhythmias, which are common with toxic isoproterenol levels

Monitor the QRS and BP constantly, as dose should be enough to keep up the heart rate and cardiac output without causing fluid overload[6]

Should be given in a separate peripheral line from Isuprel

Increases cardiac output, increases BP, and increases renal output[4]

_____ AIR BLOCK _____

Air block, especially under tension, is a life threatening condition requiring immediate treatment. Tension pneumothorax is sudden accumulation of air in the pleural space; 0.5 per cent of all newborns may experience pneumothorax. Pneumothorax may involve the mediastinal area and may even dissect into the pericardial sac. Air block is often associated with pulmonary interstitial emphysema which is a progressive entity.

DIAGNOSIS

In air block, air in the distal alveoli extravasates (or ruptures) into the perialveolar space and eventually into the pleural space.

1. Anterior-posterior, lateral, decubitus, and cross-table lateral chest radiographs will show a darkened area (almost black) in the location of the lesion; the lung may be outlined along the edge of the lesion, and there may be mediastinal shift
2. Pneumomediastinum will be particularly evident in the lateral view; the darkened area will be directly between the sternum and the heart, and the anterior-posterior film may show an indistinct halo around the heart
3. In pneumopericardium there will be a distinct black halo around the heart
4. Pneumoperitoneum appears as a defined black space between the abdominal wall and the peritoneal area

ETIOLOGY

Other major factors in air block:

1. Underlying lung disease such as hyaline membrane disease, which is characterized by stiff and brittle lungs that require peak high inspiratory pressures
2. Meconium aspiration, in which a ball-valve effect of the meconium in the distal airways traps air into the alveoli by inhibiting air flow in exhalation, thereby causing the alveoli to rupture
3. Iatrogenic causes, such as those due to overly vigorous squeezing of ventilation bag during mechanical ventilation with pressures over 40 to 60 mm Hg, or ventilator accidents (knobs accidentally turned the wrong way)

Acute clinical results of air block:

1. Sudden decrease in pH and PO_2
2. Devastating compression of the thoracic organs
3. Severely compromised ventilation
4. Decreased venous return
5. Diminished cardiac output
6. Shock

ASSESSMENT

1. Clinical presentation
   a. Signs and symptoms

     i. On auscultation breath sounds may be unequal, diminished on one side, or completely absent on both sides

    ii. The chest wall may become asymmetrical with a mediastinal shift

   iii. The cardiac apex will shift toward the unaffected side

   iv. Large areas of light will be visible around the tip of the transilluminator applied to the suspected side

    v. There may be sudden worsening of the clinical condition with cyanosis and acidosis

b. History

     i. The infant has a sudden unexplained change in color and respiratory effort

    ii. There may be a precipitous decrease in heart rate and blood pressure

   iii. Breath sounds may be distant or not heard at all

PATIENT CARE MANAGEMENT

	COMMENTS/TIPS/CAUTIONS
1. Goal	
a. To provide immediate assessment and resuscitation	Manage the emergency in the usual way and try to determine the cause
i. Institute ABC procedure	Breath sounds should be checked immediately when the clinical condition suddenly crashes
ii. Perform a rapid physical assessment	
iii. Obtain and record vital signs and blood pressure	Provides baseline data
b. To confirm suspicion of air block	
i. Obtain chest radiograph immediately; a decubitus or cross-table lateral film may also be ordered	Positioning for radiographs is important as rotation of the infant's body may hide the exact location of the air leak. See also Diagnosis
ii. Transilluminate the chest	A large diffuse air pocket will surround the light source
c. To evacuate air from the pleural space to reexpand the lung and reestablish effective ventilation	
i. Prepare the skin over the suspected (or confirmed) area with povidone-iodine (Betadine)	
ii. Be prepared to insert a 21 gauge butterfly needle or intravenous catheter into the affected area	The needle may be placed directly into the site at a 40 degree angle over the top of the ribs
iii. Attach a stopcock and a 35 to 60 cc syringe and aspi-	This may be all that is required, especially with pneumopericardium; if the clinical

rate gently until air is removed

iv. Prepare the infant by properly restraining for immediate chest tube placement

v. Open the thoracotomy set and arrange a chest drainage evacuation (Pleurevac) or bottle setup (see procedure for thoracotomy in Appendix B for details)

vi. Stabilize the chest tube and attach to a draingE set and suction.

   (a) Direct wall suction may be used with Pleurevac devices; however, thoracic suction units must be used with traditional bottle type setups

d. To assess the effectiveness of the chest tube

i. Repeat radiographs

ii. Auscultate chest frequently for evidence and quality of breath sounds

iii. Observe for bubbling or fluctuation in the chest drainage system

iv. Continue to monitor vital signs and blood gases

COMMENTS/TIPS/CAUTIONS

status does not improve or air leak is continuous, a chest tube must be inserted

A purse string suture and tincture of collodion for sealing are excellent for stabilizing; a small piece of 1 inch adhesive tape to anchor the tube to the infant's skin may be placed 2 to 3 cm above the distal end of the tube, all connections should be taped shut to prevent accidental disconnection

Although placement of tube may be correct, air may still be present and necessitate an additional tube

Breath sounds may still be diminished but should be audible

Indicates patency; large amounts of bubbling may be indicative of a leak in the connecting tubing

Acidosis should improve and blood pressure should stabilize; in the case of pneumopericardium the bradycardia will be corrected

Complications of treatment may include:
1. Hemorrhage from accidentally knicking the arteries under the ribs during needle aspiration or chest tube placement
2. Reaccumulation of air
3. Cardiac perforation (with pneumopericardium) or tamponade or both
4. Death

TRACHEOESOPHAGEAL FISTULA
(WITH ESOPHAGEAL ATRESIA)

There are several types of tracheoesophageal defects (Fig. 14–4). Tracheoesophageal fistula is an anatomical anomaly that occurs in the third to sixth week of embryonic life.

DIAGNOSIS

The diagnosis can be made promptly from the following:

1. A history of polyhydramnios and the symptoms displayed by the infant (excessive salivation)
2. Inability to pass a nasogastric tube to the stomach

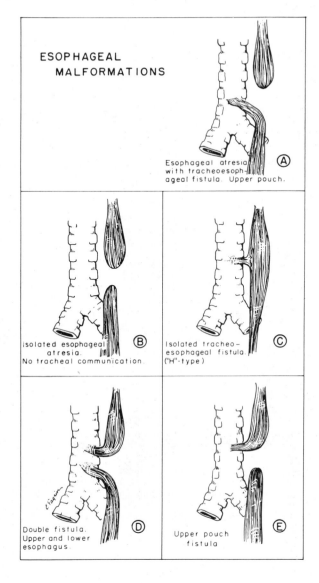

ESOPHAGEAL
MALFORMATIONS

Esophageal atresia
with tracheoesoph-
ageal fistula. Upper pouch. Ⓐ

Isolated esophageal Ⓑ
atresia.
No tracheal communication.

Isolated tracheo- Ⓒ
esophageal fistula.
("H"-type)

Double fistula. Ⓓ
Upper and lower
esophagus.

Upper pouch Ⓔ
fistula

Figure 14-4. Esophageal malformations. Representation of the various forms of esophageal malformations shown in the order of frequency in which they occur. (Reprinted with permission from Nardi, G.L., and Zuidema, L.D.: Surgery, 4th ed. Boston, Little, Brown and Co., Copyright ©1982.)

3. A chest radiograph that reveals a curled nasogastric tube in a pouch near the tracheal area

4. Contrast dye studies will clearly outline the defect, but they are highly controversial because of the great risk of pneumonia due to aspiration of the contrast material

1. **Incidence**
    a. 1 in 3000 to 4500 live births[4]
    b. Of these infants 21 per cent are premature and 19 per cent are small for gestational age[4]

ETIOLOGY

The etiology of tracheoesophageal fistula (TEF) is unknown. As a result of the defect, there may have been polyhydramnios; 33 per cent of mothers with polyhydramnios have children with TEF, and 82 per cent of these children have esophageal atresia not involving the trachea.[8]

ASSESSMENT

1. Clinical presentation
   a. Signs and symptoms
      i. Excessive mucus in the upper airway
      ii. Choking and coughing
      iii. Cyanosis with feeding
      iv. Abdominal distention due to air passing from the trachea to the stomach through the distal fistula
      v. Rales and rhonchi
      vi. Pneumonia-like chest radiographic findings due to gastric secretions that flow back into the lungs and cause chemical irritation

PATIENT CARE MANAGEMENT

1. Goals

COMMENTS/TIPS/CAUTIONS

   a. To maintain the vital signs and to institute the ABCs of treatment as appropriate
      i. Place the infant on a radiant warmer
      ii. Attach to cardiorespiratory monitor

   Elevating the head of the bed or having the infant in an infant seat will assist in keeping the proximal pouch decompressed and in decreasing backflow of gastric juices into the lungs

   b. To provide relief from respiratory distress
      i. Elevate the head of the bed
      ii. Place Replogle tube in proximal pouch
      iii. Provide adequate oxygen
      iv. Monitor for and be prepared to treat respiratory failure

   Since 21 per cent of these infants are premature, they may also have lung disease; these infants almost always require some form of assisted ventilation after surgery if not before

   c. To maintain the hydration status
      i. A parenteral $D_{10}W$ solution may be started at a rate of 65 to 80 cc/kg/day, since the infant cannot be given anything by mouth

   If an arterial or venous line is not already in place, a large bore catheter such as a 22 or 24 gauge intravenous catheter is suggested prior to surgery, having the access line inserted in the unit will decrease the anesthesia preparation time in the operation room

   d. To prepare the infant for surgery as soon as possible, preferably within 12 hours
      i. Obtain blood for type and cross-match; CBC, differential and platelet counts; prothrombin and partial thromboplastin times; glucose and electrolyte determinations

ii. Obtain a consent form from the parents for operation

e. To prevent sepsis

    i. Antibiotic therapy should be initiated after blood cultures have been obtained

f. To maintain ventilation

    i. Close attention to arterial blood gases

    ii. Close observation of the respiratory status

g. To prepare for postoperative care

    i. Prepare to care for a gastrostomy

    ii. Be prepared to care for a chest tube

Support for the family is very important; an explanation of the defect and simple drawings demonstrating how the surgical procedure will correct the defect are concrete concepts that parents deal well with; not only will they benefit from the explanation, but they will have something tangible to refer back to

Several weeks are needed for proper healing of the repair; a gastrostomy tube is inserted for feeding

Repairs of tracheoesophageal fistula are commonly done through a lateral thoracic incision; a chest tube is inserted prior to closing to evacuate blood and serous fluid once the procedure is over

Complications of treatment include
1. Sepsis
2. Leaking of the anastomosis
3. Dysmotility of the lower esophageal segment
4. Unilateral diaphragmatic paralyisis
5. Stricture of the anastomosis
6. Respiratory distress
7. Pneumonia

h. To prevent extubation and trauma to the repair sites

    i. Do not suction the trachea below the repair site

    ii. Restrain the infant

Maintaining a patent endotracheal tube is paramount—however, damage may occur with inappropriate suctioning; suctioning should be limited to just long enough to clear the tube; excessive chest physiotherapy is not indicated immediately postoperatively

Many infants are active after their operation and can easily extubate themselves or pull out their gastrotomy tube

CONCLUSIONS

Life threatening emergencies can be caused by a variety of conditions, but their critical management remains constant. The "ABCs" should be second nature to all nurses. Advanced life support measures are also important, and practitioners in critical care areas should be well versed in their use. Patient outcome is largely dependent on the correct institution of the ABCs. The nurse's role in emergency care of the neonate begins at birth and continues until the baby's health problems have been resolved. Knowledge of emergency care is fundamental to positive outcome for the high risk neonate.

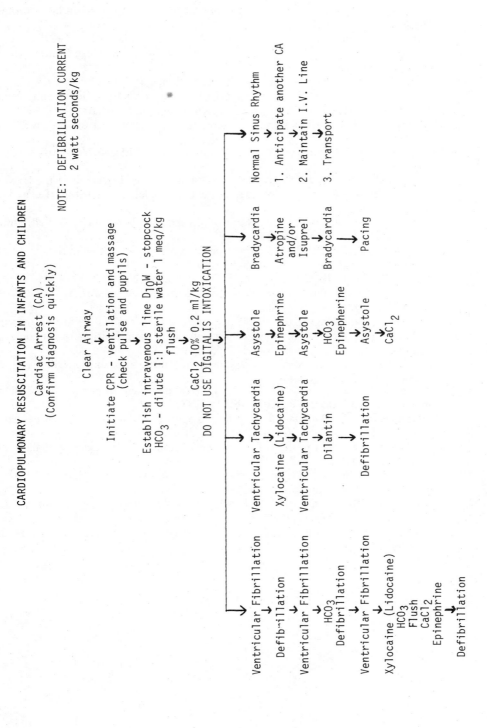

Figure 14-5. Quick reference guide to CPR. When printed on a small card, this chart is readily available to all personnel. (Courtesy of Hermann Hospital, Houston, Texas.)

REFERENCES

1. Apgar, V.: A proposal for a new method of evaluation of the newborn infant. Anesthesiol. Analg., *32*:260, 1953.
2. Avery, G.B.: Neonatology, 2nd ed. Philadelphia, J.B. Lippincott Co., 1981.
3. Bada, H.S., et al.: Changes in intracranial pressure during exchange transfusion. J. Pediatr., *94*:1, 1979.
4. Behrman, R.E.: Neonatal-Perinatal Medicine. St. Louis, C.V. Mosby Co., 1977.
5. Cerebral blood flow in the newborn infant: Relation to hypoxic-ischemic brain injury and periventricular hemorrhage, editor's column. J. Pediatr., *94*:1, 1979.
6. Cloherty, J.P., Stark, A.R.: Manual of Neonatal Care. Boston, Little, Brown & Co., 1980.
7. Harper, R.G., and Yoon, J.J.: Manual of Neonatology. Chicago, Yearbook Medical Publishers, 1974.
8. Hoelzer, D.J.: Tracheo-esophageal fistula—Grand Rounds. Presented at the University of Texas Medical School, Department of Pediatrics, Houston, Texas, December 1981.
9. Klaus, M.H., and Fanaroff, A.A.: Care of the High-Risk Neonate, 2nd ed. Philadelphia, W.B. Saunders Co., 1979.
10. Lou, H.C., et al.: Impaired auto regulation of cerebral blood flow in the distressed newborn infant. J. Pediatr., *94*:118-121, 1979.
11. Nugent, S.K., et al.: Raised I.C.P. Am. J. Dis. Child., *33*:260-262, 1974.
12. Perog, S.H., and Ferrara, A.: Medical Care of the Sick Newborn. St. Louis, C.V. Mosby Co., 1976.
13. Raju, T.N.K., Vidyasagan, D., and Papazafiratou, C.: Cerebral perfusion pressure and abnormal intracranial pressure wave forma: Their relation to outcome in birth asphyxia. Crit. Care Med., *9*:449-453, 1981.
14. Raju, T.N.K., et al.: Intracranial pressure during intubation and anesthesia in infants. J. Pediatr., *96:*860-861, 1980.
15. Reppert, S.M., Ment, L.R., and Todres, I.D.: The treatment of pneumopericardium in the newborn infant. J. Pediatr., *90*:115, 1977.
16. Sheldon, R.E., and Dominak, D.S.: The expanding role of the nurse in neonatal intensive care. New York, Grune & Stratton, 1980.
17. Shenkin, H.A., and Bouzarth, W.F.: Clinical methods of reducing intracranial pressure. N. Engl. J. Med., *282*:26, 1970.
18. Vaughan, V.C., McKay, R.J., and Behrman, R.E.: Textbook of Pediatrics, 11th ed. Philadelphia, W.B. Saunders Co., 1979.
19. Vestal, K.W.: Pediatric Critical Care Nursing. New York, John Wiley & Sons, 1981.
20. Volpe, J.J., and Pasternak, J.F.: Parasagittal cerebral injury in neonatal hypoxic-ischemic encephalopathy: Clinical and neurological features. J. Pediatr., *91*:472-476, 1977.

CHAPTER 15

RESPIRATORY CRISES

Adita Lynn Root, R.N., Ph.D.

OBJECTIVES

Upon completion of this chapter the reader will be able to accomplish the following:

1. Describe the two leading hypotheses central to the development of respiratory distress syndrome
2. Identify the signs and symptoms of the clinical presentation of respiratory distress syndrome
3. Identify the predisposing factors to meconium aspiration
4. Describe the signs and symptoms of the clinical presentation of meconium aspiration
5. Differentiate respiratory distress syndrome from transient tachypnea through physical assessment of the neonate
6. Define an apneic episode
7. Identify six common causes of apnea
8. Identify three main methods of assessment to properly identify pneumothorax
9. Describe the treatment and complications of pneumothorax
10. Discuss the etiology of diaphragmatic hernia
11. Describe proper management of an infant for whom a ventilator is being used
12. Describe proper feeding management of the infant with choanal atresia

The most profound physiological change required in the neonate is transition from fetal or placental circulation to independent respiration. The loss of the placental connection means the loss of complete metabolic support, the most important and essential function being the supply of oxygen and the removal of carbon dioxide. The neonate's adjustment to extrauterine life is a complex physiological process. The first 24 hours are the most critical, since during this time respiratory distress and circulatory failure can occur rapidly and with little warning.

The most critical and immediate physiological change in the neonate is the onset of breathing. The promptness of this transition is initiated by sudden exposure to stimuli in the exterior environment. Sudden chilling of the infant probably excites peripheral sensory impulses in the skin, which are transmitted to the respiratory center. Undoubtedly the rapid decrease of temperature from the uterus to the delivery room is a powerful stimulus. Chemical factors also trigger the respiratory center, and tactile stimulation has been considered as contributing significantly to the initiation of respiration.

Initial entry of air into the lungs is opposed by the surface tension of the viscid fluid that fills the alveoli. Because respiratory movements occurred before birth, fluid filled the lungs, which were largely nonfunctional since exchange of oxygen and carbon dioxide occurred through the process of diffusion via placental circulation. For respiration to occur, this surface tension must be opposed by a negative pressure greater than 25 mm Hg to open the alveoli for the first time. The first cry of the newborn exerts a negative pressure of up to 50 mm Hg. Once the alveoli are opened, further respiration of less force maintains alveolar stability.

The most common and immediately most important emergencies related to the newborn infant in the delivery room are failure to initiate respiration and failure to maintain satisfactory respiration.

Disorders of respiration in the newborn infant can be categorized in two general groups: respiratory failure or depression of the respiratory center (central nervous system failure) and interference with the alveolar exchange of oxygen and carbon dioxide (peripheral respiratory difficulty).

Disturbances of respiration manifested in the immediate postnatal period may have had their origin in utero, in the delivery room, or in the nursery. A wide variety of pathological lesions may be responsible. They are manifested by one or more of the signs of respiratory distress (Table 15–1).

If respiratory embarrassment is severe, pallor or cyanosis may also be present, and it is occasionally difficult to distinguish cardiovascular from respiratory disturbances on the basis of clinical findings alone.

When problems with respiration are anticipated, preparations can be made for intensive care during the periods of greatest threat, and, through this care, the incidence of neonatal mortality can be significantly reduced. Assessment and prompt intervention in life threatening emergencies often make the difference between a favorable outcome and a lifetime of disability. The nurse in the newborn nursery is familiar with the characteristics of the neonate and recognizes the significance of benign and serious deviations from expected observations.

RESPIRATORY DISTRESS SYNDROME
(HYALINE MEMBRANE DISEASE)

Respiratory distress syndrome is the major cause of death in the newborn period and also carries the highest risk in terms of long term neurological complications. This disorder is associated with 30 per cent of all neonatal deaths and 50 to 75 per cent of the deaths of premature infants in the United States.

TABLE 15-1. DISORDERS OF RESPIRATION IN THE NEONATE

Type	Manifestations	Clinical Entity
Central nervous system failure	Apnea Slow, irregular, gasping respiratory efforts	Narcosis Prenatal or perinatal anoxia Intracranial hemorrhage or trauma CNS anomalies
Peripheral respiratory difficulty	Rapid respiratory rate Increasing respiratory rate Chest lag Intercostal retraction Subcostal retraction Xiphoid retraction Chin tug Expiratory grunt Frothing at lips	Primary atelectasis Congestive pulmonary failure Idiopathic respiratory distress (hyaline membrane) syndrome Aspiration of amniotic fluid containing formed elements Pneumonia Diaphragmatic hernia Lung cysts Lobar emphysema Pneumothorax Aspiration of food or mucus

From Vaughan, V.C., and McKay, R.J.: Nelson's Textbook of Pediatrics, 10th ed. Philadelphia, W.B. Saunders Co., 1975.

DIAGNOSIS

Respiratory distress syndrome is seen almost exclusively in preterm infants, infants of diabetic mothers, and infants born by cesarean section and is due to a deficiency of surfactin, a surface tension lowering lipid formed in the walls of alveoli. The tendency of the lungs of affected infants to collapse is correlated with high surface tension and the absence of surfactin.

1. **Incidence**
   a. 10 per cent of all prematures may have the disease, with 70 to 80 per cent of the infants weighing less than 2500 gm
   b. 20 to 30 per cent mortality, with most deaths occurring within 72 hours of birth
2. Major factors producing respiratory distress are listed in Table 15-2.

ETIOLOGY

There are two leading hypotheses central to the development of respiratory distress syndrome.

1. **Pulmonary surfactant deficiency**
   a. Little synthesis of lecithin, a major constituent of surfactin, in fetuses prior to 20 weeks of gestation
   b. Alteration of lecithin could result in atelectasis, decreased lung compliance, increased work of breathing, and eventually insufficient ventilation with asphyxia, hypoxia, and acidosis

TABLE 15-2. RESPIRATORY DISTRESS

Cause	Effect
Increased surface tension of alveoli (surfactant deficiency)	Alveolar collapse; atelectasis; increased work of breathing
Impaired gas exchange	Hypoxemia and hypercapnia with respiratory acidosis
Increased pulmonary vascular resistance	Hypoperfusion of pulmonary circulation
Hypoperfusion (with hypoxemia)	Tissue hypoxia and metabolic acidosis
Increased transudation of fluid into lungs	Hyaline membrane function
	Impaired gas exchange

Reprinted with permission from Whaley, L.M., and Wong, D.: Nursing Care of Infants and Children. St. Louis, C.V. Mosby Co., 1979.

   c. Pulmonary arterial vasoconstriction with increased vascular resistance and shunting through the foramen ovale and ductus arteriosus is thus produced
       i. Pulmonary blood flow would be reduced with injury to cells producing lecithin
      ii. Injury to vascular bed would result in an effusion of proteinaceous material into the alveolar spaces

2. Pulmonary hypoperfusion

Intrauterine or neonatal asphyxia with hypoxia and mixed respiratory and metabolic acidosis leads to increased pulmonary vascular resistance and systemic hypotension
   a. Venous blood bypasses the lungs through the foramen ovale and ductus arteriosus
   b. Ischemia of the alveolar lining cells that produce surfactin or lecithin or both
       i. Compromise of surfactant production
      ii. Atelectasis and hypercalia from a deficiency of surface tension lowering lipids
     iii. Effusion of plasma and red cells from injured cepillaries leading to formation of fibrin in the air spaces

ASSESSMENT

1. Clinical presentation

Begins with rapid, shallow respirations, which usually increase to 60/minute or more within 2 hours of birth

Signs and symptoms
       i. Substernal retractions
      ii. Tachypnea (respiratory rate increasing to 80 to 120 breaths/minute)

   iii.   Flaring of the external nares
   iv.   Audible expiratory grunt
    v.   Cyanosis appears but can usually be abolished by a 40 to 50
         per cent concentration of ambient oxygen
   vi.   Infant flaccid, inert, and unresponsive
  vii.   Frequent apneic episodes

2. **Biopsychosocial assessment**
    a. Clinical estimate of gestational age
    b. Age
    c. Vital signs: TPR; blood pressure
    d. Prenatal and delivery history
    e. Respiratory pattern
    f. Color
    g. Peripheral perfusion
    h. Muscle tone and reflexes (sucking, Moro)
    i. Activity level
    j. Auscultation
    k. Parents' understanding and reactions to infant's illness
    l. Support mechanisms: intrinsic and extrinsic
    m. Transport of infant to perinatal center will add stress to separation to
        family unit
    n. Observe separation of mother and father from infant and its impact
        on process of bonding

3. **Diagnostic data**
    a. Chest roentgenogram
         i.   Cardiac anatomy
         ii. Lungs
    b. Arterial blood gas
         i.   Hypoxemia: PO_2 less than 60 in 100 per cent forced inspira-
              tory oxygen (FiO_2)
         ii. Acidemia: pH less than 7.30
    c. Serum glucose
    d. Hematocrit: Hyperviscosity can cause or contribute to pulmonary
        blood flow
    e. White cell count

PROBLEMS AND COMPLICATIONS

1. Neonatal death within 72 hours of birth
2. Pneumothorax
3. Bronchopulmonary dysplasia (chronic lung disease)
4. Recurrent pulmonary infections
5. Intracranial hemorrhage
6. Neurological impairment
7. Retrolental fibroplasia (complication of oxygen therapy)

PATIENT CARE MANAGEMENT

1. **Goals**
   a. To maintain adequate oxygenation and ventilation
      i. Place infant in neutral thermal environment to minimize oxygen requirement
      ii. Correct acidosis by IV administration of sodium bicarbonate or tromethamine to dilate pulmonary vessels and reduce constriction response
      iii. Provide additional fractional inspired oxygen content by increasing ambient oxygen concentration
      iv. Assist or control ventilation
      v. Monitor arterial blood gases at frequent intervals (every hour or more often)
      vi. Clear mucus obstructed passages
   b. To support vital functions
      i. Monitor vital signs: TPR; blood pressure
      ii. Monitor aortic blood pressure through umbilical artery
   c. To maintain hematocrit, hemoglobin and blood volume for tissue perfusion and oxygenation
      i. Record amounts of blood withdrawn from infant
      ii. Recheck hematocrit when volume of blood lost is 10 per cent of infant's estimated blood volume or less than 45 per cent
   d. To maintain physiological equilibrium
      i. Provide neutral thermal environment to maintain temperature within normal range with minimal heat

Oxygen should be ordered by concentration and not flow

Oxygen should be warmed and humidified

Oxygen concentration should be monitored hourly

The objective of continuous positive airway pressure (CPAP) is to apply enough pressure to open and keep open most of the alveoli and yet avoid overextending the already expanded alveoli

Infant receiving assisted or controlled ventilation is subject to problems associated with therapy

If oxygen saturation of blood cannot be maintained satisfactorily, infant will require controlled ventilation, usually positive end respiratory pressure (PEEP)

Removal of secretions can be facilitated by routine suctioning methods and application of percussion and vibration to the thoracic wall

Provide guides to management of shocklike state that may occur

Umbilical catheter may also be used for monitoring arterial blood gases and infusing fluids if necessary

production and, therefore, O_2 consumption

e. To maintain adequate nutrition and hydration

    i. Provide IV therapy to avoid dehydration due to water loss from tachypnea and diuresis and to maintain caloric intake

Parenteral fluids should be given through superficial vein in an extremity

    ii. Frequently monitor IV supplementation of glucose, electrolytes, and calcium as indicated

    iii. Monitor intake and output

Weigh diapers to accurately determine output

f. To preserve family unit

    i. Provide explanations of illness, treatment, and prognosis

    ii. Provide mother with pictures of infant if she is unable to visit

    iii. Encourage phone calls to nursing unit to discuss management, care, and progress of infant

    iv. Encourage and facilitate father's involvement with transport of infant when indicated

    v. Transfer mother with infant if feasible

DISCHARGE PLANNING/TEACHING

Teaching should begin at the time crisis is identified.

1. Diagnosis, treatment, and prognosis should be explained to parents and discussed openly with them
2. Involve parents in treatment plan as appropriate
3. Assist parents and encourage their interaction with infant, providing information as to why infant response might be restricted
4. Answer questions openly and honestly with support and reassurance

——————————— MECONIUM ASPIRATION ———————————

The presence of meconium in the amniotic fluid must be regarded as abnormal and appropriate individuals alerted to the possibility of fetal or neonatal complications. Meconium aspiration is an aspiration pneumonia with a significant mortality—up to 50 per cent.

DIAGNOSIS

Meconium aspiration in the infant having respiratory distress is determined from a history of meconium stained amniotic fluid, meconium in the trachea at birth, and an abnormal roentgenogram with a hyperinflated picture similar to that of respiratory distress syndrome.

1. **Incidence**
   a. Meconium stained amniotic fluid occurs in 10–20 per cent of all births
   b. Meconium aspiration occurs in approximately 20 per cent of infants with meconium staining

2. **Predisposing factors**
   a. Perinatal asphyxia
   b. Breech delivery
   c. Term or post-term infant
   d. Meconium stained amniotic fluid
   e. Prolonged or difficult delivery

ETIOLOGY

Infants often attempt to breathe in utero during prolonged or difficult delivery. This is a result of interference with the supply of oxygen via the placenta. Under these circumstances the infant aspirates amniotic fluid containing meconium. The meconium debris blocks the smallest airways and interferes with alveolar exchange of oxygen and carbon dioxide.

ASSESSMENT

1. **Clinical presentation**
   a. Signs and symptoms
      i. Meconium stained amniotic fluid
      ii. Nails, cords, and skin stained yellowish
      iii. Cord appears thin and dry
      iv. Vernix may be absent
      v. AP diameter of the chest increased; the chest barrel shaped
      vi. Breathing shallow and rapid
      vii. Rales and rhonchi common
      viii. Hypoxia often severe

2. **Biopsychosocial assessment**
   a. Vital signs: TPR; blood pressure
   b. Parents' understanding and reactions to infant's illness
   c. Support mechanisms: intrinsic and extrinsic
   d. Transport of infant to perinatal center will add stress of separation to family unit
   e. Observe separation of mother and father from infant and its impact on process of bonding

3. **Diagnostic data**
   a. Chest roentgenogram

i.   AP diameter increased
ii. Diaphragm flat
iii. Tendency for ribs to be elevated
iv. Some bulging in the intercostal spaces
b. Blood culture

PROBLEMS AND COMPLICATIONS

1. Aspiration pneumonia
2. Pneumothorax
3. Infant needs to be watched for pneumomediastinum and pulmonary interstitial air, which may progress to pneumothorax
4. Meconium aspiration is often complicated by an episode of asphyxia with resultant seizures, bleeding diathesis, cardiomyopathy, and renal failure
5. Neonatal death

PATIENT CARE MANAGEMENT

1. **Goals**

COMMENTS/TIPS/
CAUTIONS

a. To prevent meconium aspiration due to fetal distress
   i.   Initiate continuous FHR monitoring
   ii. Assign a qualified health professional, who can resuscitate a newborn, to attend the delivery

Can be a neonatologist, pediatrician, or neonatal nurse clinician

b. To maintain a patent airway at time of delivery
   i.   Suction infant's oropharynx and hypopharynx carefully after head is delivered either vaginally or by cesarean section and prior to delivery of thorax

If this cannot be done because of precipitous or breech delivery, it must be done prior to onset of breathing

   ii. Visualize cord, and suction trachea directly through endotracheal tube if meconium present
c. To monitor and observe for increased respiratory distress
   i.   Chest roentgenogram to confirm presence of pneumothorax
   ii. Aspiration of accumulated air or insertion of catheter into pleural space and use of water seal drainage

   d. To maintain physiological equilibrium
      i. Provide neutral thermal environment to maintain temperature within normal range with minimal heat production and, therefore, O_2 consumption
   e. To maintain adequate nutrition and hydration
      i. Provide IV therapy to avoid dehydration due to water loss from tachypnea and diuresis and to maintain caloric intake

Parenteral fluids should be given through superficial vein in an extremity

      ii. Monitor intake and output

Weigh diapers to accurately determine output

   f. To support vital functions
      i. Monitor vital signs: TPR, blood pressure
      ii. Monitor arterial blood gases as indicated by degree of respiratory distress
   g. To preserve family unit
      i. Provide explanations of illness, treatment, and prognosis
      ii. Provide mother with pictures of infant if she is unable to visit
      iii. Encourage phone calls to nursing unit to discuss management, care, and progress of infant
      iv. Encourage and facilitate father's involvement with transport of infant when indicated
      v. Transfer mother with infant if feasible

DISCHARGE PLANNING/TEACHING

Teaching should begin at the time crisis is identified.

1. Diagnosis, treatment, and prognosis should be explained to parents and discussed openly with them
2. Involve parents in treatment plan as appropriate

3. Assist parents and encourage their interaction with infant, providing information as to why infant response might be restricted
4. Answer questions openly and honestly with support and reassurance

_____ TRANSIENT TACHYPNEA OF THE NEWBORN _____

Transient tachypnea of the newborn usually occurs in the term or near term infant and has many similarities to respiratory distress syndrome. However, the cause of transient tachypnea is quite different and the outlook much better.

DIAGNOSIS

Transient tachypnea is characterized mainly by an increased respiratory rate soon after birth and usually lasts between 24 and 36 hours. It is particularly associated with cesarean deliveries.

1. **Predisposing factors**
   a. Cesarean section
   b. Asphyxia
   c. Thermal stress in the delivery room
2. Air exchange good
3. No cyanosis or acidosis

ETIOLOGY

X-ray examination of the chest may reveal central peripheral streaking and fluid in the interlobar fissures, suggesting that the syndrome is secondary to slow absorption of lung fluid.

ASSESSMENT

1. **Clinical presentation**
   a. Signs and symptoms
      i. Tachypnea (respiratory rate greater than 80)
      ii. Minimal grunting and retractions
      iii. Good air exchange
      iv. Minimal or no cyanosis
2. **Biopsychosocial assessment**
   a. Vital signs: TPR; blood pressure
   b. Prenatal and delivery history
      i. Apgar score
      ii. Type of delivery: vaginal or cesarean
   c. Parents' understanding and reactions to infant's illness
   d. Support mechanisms: intrinsic and extrinsic
   e. Observe separation of mother and father from infant and its impact on process of bonding
3. **Diagnostic data**
   a. Chest roentgenogram

   i. Central peripheral streaking
   ii. Fluid in the interlobar fissures
   iii. Slight bulging of the pleura seen between ribs
   iv. AP diameter increased
   v. Tendency for diaphragm to be flat
  b. Arterial blood gas (within normal limits)
   i. Hypoxemia: PO_2 less than 60 in 100 per cent FiO_2
   ii. PCO_2
   iii. Acidemia: pH less than 7.30
  c. Serum glucose (Dextrostix) decrease due to utilization during stress.
  d. Hematocrit: Hyperviscosity can cause or contribute to pulmonary blood flow

PROBLEMS AND COMPLICATIONS

In some infants who have a clinical picture similar to that of transient tachypnea, the condition may progress to severe persistent fetal circulation.

PATIENT CARE MANAGEMENT

1. Goals

  a. To provide supportive care during the period of tachypnea to achieve physiological equilibrium

   i. Maintain in neutral thermal environment

    This will avoid thermal stress and minimize need for additional oxygen

   ii. Monitor vital signs: TPR, blood pressure

   iii. Provide additional oxygen to relieve hypoxia and maintain arterial blood gases

    The PO_2 should be maintained between 50 and 70 mm Hg, pH between 7.25 and 7.40, and the PCO_2 at less than 50–55 mm Hg

   iv. Withhold oral feedings until respiratory rate decreased

    IV fluids may need to be administered to adequately maintain fluid and nutritional needs when oral feedings are being withheld

   v. Monitor intake and output

  b. To preserve family unit

   i. Provide explanations of illness, treatment, and prognosis

    Weigh diapers to accurately determine output

   ii. Provide mother with pictures of infant if she is unable to visit

   iii. Encourage phone calls to nursing unit to discuss management, care, and progress of infant

COMMENTS/TIPS/CAUTIONS

DISCHARGE PLANNING/TEACHING

Teaching should begin at the time crisis is identified.

1. Diagnosis, treatment, and prognosis should be explained to parents and discussed openly with them
2. Involve parents in treatment plan as appropriate
3. Assist parents and encourage their interaction with infant, providing information as to why infant response might be restricted
4. Answer questions openly and honestly with support and reassurance

_____ **APNEIC EPISODES** _____

Apnea is a symptom of some other condition that, when not treated, can result in hypoxia. Such hypoxia may result in electroencephalographic (EEG) changes, hypotonia, and permanent central nervous system (CNS) damage. Apnea, when left untreated, is thought to be a major cause of cerebral palsy and mental retardation in premature infants.

DIAGNOSIS

Apnea is cessation of breathing for more than 20 seconds or cessation of breathing with concomitant decrease in heart rate or the presence of cyanosis.

1. **Incidence**
   a. Occurs in 25 per cent of all infants less than 2500 gm
   b. Occurs in 80 per cent of all infants less than 1000 gm

ETIOLOGY

ASSESSMENT

1. **Clinical presentation**
   a. Signs and symptoms
      i. Apnea is a symptom or sign reflecting some other condition and not a disease in itself; the common causes of apnea are given in Table 15–3.
   b. History
      i. Maternal drugs
      ii. Maternal bleeding
      iii. Fetal distress
      iv. Risk factors for infection (maternal fever, prolonged rupture of membranes, amnionitis)
      v. Meconium staining
      vi. Indications of a difficult delivery
      vii. Low Apgar scores
      viii. Temperature instability
         (a) Patient
         (b) Environment

TABLE 15-3. COMMON CAUSES OF APNEA

Temperature instability
Infant—Increased or decreased temperature
Environment—Increased or decreased temperature

Sepsis
Apnea during the first 24 hours of life is always considered secondary to sepsis until proved otherwise.

Metabolic disorders
Decreased calcium
Decreased glucose
Decreased magnesium
Decreased sodium
Other (inborn errors of metabolism)

Cardiorespiratory disorders
Hypoxia
Acidosis
Patent ductus arteriosus
Hypotension
Anemia
Upper airway obstruction (flexed hand, phototherapy masks)
Pneumonia
Respiratory distress syndrome

Central nervous system disorders
Congenital malformation
Seizures
Asphyxia
Drugs (maternal narcotics, analgesics, "caine" drugs, anesthesia)
Intracranial hemorrhage
Meningitis

Reflexes
Posterior pharyngeal
Laryngeal

Necrotizing entercolitis

Reprinted with permission from Schreiner, R.L.: Care of the Newborn. New York, Raven Press, 1981.

ix. Association of apnea with feeding, defecation, suctioning
x. Respiratory distress
xi. Heart disease (patent ductus arteriosus)
xii. Congenital malformations
xiii. Upper airway obstruction (choanal atresia)
xiv. Generalized petechiae or purpura (sepsis, coagulation disorder)
xv. Neonatal seizures
xvi. Hepatomegaly (suggesting heart failure or congenital infection)
xvii. Distention (possibly indicative of necrotizing enterocolitis or bowel obstruction)

2. **Biopsychosocial assessment**
   a. Parents' understanding and reactions to infant's illness
   b. Support mechanisms: intrinsic and extrinsic

c. Transport of infant when indicated to perinatal center will add stress of separation to family unit

d. Observe separation of mother and father from infant and its impact on process of bonding

3. Diagnostic data

These assessments are for infants who have not responded to therapy and there is cause to suspect an inborn error of metabolism, hyperammonemia, drug toxicity, or a CNS disorder.

a. Laboratory work-up when apnea present during first 24 hours of life
    i. Hematocrit
    ii. Glucose, calcium, sodium
    iii. Arterial pH, PCO_2, PO_2
    iv. Blood culture
    v. Spinal tap
    vi. Suprapubic bladder tap

b. Laboratory work-up when apnea persists
    i. Urinalysis for detection of metabolic disorder (amino acids, organic acids)
    ii. Serum ammonia level
    iii. Magnesium
    iv. Serum for determination of "caine" drug level
    v. EEG
    vi. Computerized axial tomography (CAT scan)
    vii. Ultrasound

PROBLEMS AND COMPLICATIONS

1. Changes in EEG indicating permanent brain damage
2. Hypotonia
3. Permanent CNS damage

PATIENT CARE MANAGEMENT

1. Goal

a. To identify underlying cause of apnea
    i. Treat accordingly such possibilities as sepsis, hypoglycemia, shock, patent ductus arteriosus, neonatal depression from maternal drugs, seizures, and temperature instability

b. To ensure temperature stability
    i. Maintain neutral thermal environment
    ii. Decrease heat loss in small infant

COMMENTS/TIPS/CAUTIONS

Use plexiglass shield, line incubator with aluminum foil, and place incubator away from cold windows and air conditioning

Use stocking cap to fit over the top of infant's head

c. To avoid triggering reflexes
  i. Execute with caution such procedures as placement of orogastric tube and nasotracheal suctioning
  ii. Tube feed instead of nipple
  iii. Avoid hyperinflation during ventilation with bag
  iv. Avoid cold stimulus to face
d. To support vital functions
  i. Monitor vital signs: TPR, blood pressure
  ii. Monitor hematocrit
  iii. Monitor PO_2
e. To stimulate infant frequently
  i. Stimulate infant manually
  ii. Stimulate infant by use of an oscillating mattress or water bed
f. To improve oxygenation
  i. Stimulate nasopharyngeal area or decrease work of breathing by initiating CPAP
  ii. Maintain resuscitation bag and mask at infant's bed
  iii. Connect bag to an oxygen line equipped with an oxygen blender that provides approximately the same FiO_2 infant usually receives
  iv. Initiate bag and mask ventilation
g. To increase sensitivity of respiratory center to CO_2
  i. Administer theophylline and caffeine
h. To preserve family unit
  i. Provide explanations of illness, treatment, and prognosis
  ii. Provide mother with pictures of infant if she is unable to visit
  iii. Encourage phone calls to nursing unit to discuss

COMMENTS/TIPS/CAUTIONS

Maintain hematocrit greater than 40 per cent

Maintain PO_2 slightly high (70–80 mm Hg)

Avoid basing PO_2 determination on arterial blood gases obtained while stimulating infant

Transcutaneous monitoring ideal method to determine PO_2 for this purpose

A gentle but firm shake of infant will also result in spontaneous breathing

Mechanical ventilation may be indicated by infant's condition

               management, care, and progress of infant
- iv. Encourage and facilitate father's involvement with transport of infant when indicated
- v. Transfer mother with in-infant if feasible

DISCHARGE PLANNING/TEACHING

Teaching should begin at the time crisis is identified.

1. Diagnosis, treatment, and prognosis should be explained to parents and discussed openly with them
2. Involve parents in treatment plan as appropriate
3. Assist parents and encourage their interaction with infant, providing information as to why infant response might be restricted
4. Answer questions openly and honestly with support and reassurance

PNEUMOTHORAX

Pneumothorax can be life threatening in the neonate, particularly as a complication of positive pressure resuscitation, difficult delivery, cesarean section, or continuous positive airway pressure (CPAP).

DIAGNOSIS

Pneumothorax is a collection of air in the pleural cavity.

1. **Incidence**
   a. Spontaneous pneumothorax occurs in 0.5 to 2 per cent of all new-borns
   b. Occurs more frequently in infants with respiratory distress syndrome, with aspiration pneumonia, and after resuscitation

2. **Predisposing factors**
   a. Resuscitation
   b. Aspiration (blood, mucus, meconium)
   c. Continuous positive airway pressure
   d. Respiratory therapy
   e. Endotracheal tube down right main stem bronchus
   f. Respiratory distress syndrome
   g. Pneumonia
   h. Congenital lobar emphysema
   i. Hypoplastic lungs (e.g., diaphragmatic hernia)

ETIOLOGY

1. Pathophysiology of pneumothorax begins with hyperinflation of alveoli
2. Alveoli may rupture and allow air to escape under pressure gradient into interstitium advancing along perivascular spaces in lung

3. Air continues to dissect along perivascular spaces into mediastinum and through visceral pleura, resulting in pneumothorax

ASSESSMENT

1. Clinical presentation
   a. Signs and symptoms
      i. Tachypnea or apnea, retractions, grunting, cyanosis
      ii. Irritability
      iii. Tachycardia or bradycardia
      iv. Decreased PO_2, increased PCO_2
      v. Metabolic acidosis
      vi. Fighting the respirator
      vii. Increased ventilator inspiratory pressure with volume ventilator
      viii. Decreased breath sounds, shift or heart sounds, chest bulge
      ix. Hypotension

2. Biopsychosocial assessment
   a. Vital signs: TPR; blood pressure
   b. Check patency of airway
   c. Auscultation
   d. Transillumination of chest with high intensity fiberoptic light
   e. Assess color and peripheral perfusion
   f. Parents' understanding and reactions to infants' illness
   g. Support mechanisms: intrinsic and extrinsic
   h. Transport of infant to perinatal center will add stress of separation to family unit.
   i. Observe separation of mother and father from infant and its impact on process of bonding

3. Diagnostic data
   a. Chest roentgenogram (lateral)

PROBLEMS AND COMPLICATIONS

1. Increased lung compression and marked mediastinal shift can lead to deterioration and neonatal death
2. Pleural effusions, sterile or infected, may follow pneumothorax or its treatment
3. Pneumopericardium
4. Pneumoperitoneum

PATIENT CARE MANAGEMENT

1. Goals
   a. To monitor absorption of air
      i. Observe infant for increased signs and symptoms

COMMENTS/TIPS/CAUTIONS

Careful monitoring of infant's condition necessary

ii. Repeat chest x-ray study to determine amount of absorption

b. To hasten absorption of gas by washing out nitrogen from blood and tissues

  i. Administer 100 per cent oxygen as prescribed

c. To aspirate air with needle or chest tube

  i. Assist with aspiration of pneumothorax

  ii. Maintenance of catheter or chest tubes

d. To support vital functions

  i. Monitor vital signs: TPR; blood pressure

e. To maintain physiological equilibrium

  i. Provide neutral thermal environment to maintain the temperature within the normal range with minimal heat production and, therefore, O_2 consumption

f. To maintain adequate nutrition and hydration

  i. Provide IV therapy to avoid dehydration due to water loss from tachypnea and diuresis and to maintain caloric intake

  ii. Frequently monitor IV supplementation

  iii. Monitor intake and output

g. To preserve family unit

  i. Provide explanations of illness, treatment, and prognosis

  ii. Provide mother with pictures of infant is she is unable to visit

  iii. Encourage phone calls to nursing unit to discuss management, care, and progress of infant

  iv. Encourage and facilitate father's involvement with

COMMENTS/TIPS/CAUTIONS

Parenteral fluids should be given through superficial vein in an extremity

Weigh diapers to determine output accurately

transport of infant when indicated

v. Transfer mother with infant if feasible

DISCHARGE PLANNING/TEACHING

Teaching should begin at the time crisis is identified.

1. Diagnosis, treatment, and prognosis should be explained to parents and discussed openly with them
2. Involve parents in treatment plan as appropriate
3. Assist parents and encourage their interaction with infant, providing information as to why infant response might be restricted
4. Answer questions openly and honestly with support and reassurance

DIAPHRAGMATIC HERNIA

Congenital diaphragmatic herniation of abdominal contents into the thoracic cavity may be responsible for serious respiratory distress and usually constitutes a medical-surgical emergency in the immediate neonatal period.

DIAGNOSIS

Diaphragmatic hernia results from incomplete embryonic formation of the diaphragm, which allows abdominal contents to pass into the thoracic cavity.

1. **Incidence**
    a. 1 in 2200 births
    b. Boys more commonly affected than girls
    c. Defect on left side in 85 per cent of cases and on right side in 13 per cent; 1–2 per cent bilateral
    d. Mortality higher, 40–60 per cent, if symptoms occur early during perinatal period
    e. Mortality greater than 90 per cent in infants who present beyond 24 hours of age
    f. Most infants full term

ETIOLOGY

1. Alteration in processes of embryonic formation leads to a diaphragmatic hernia
    a. Diaphragm is formed between the eighth and tenth week of fetal life
    b. Ceolomic cavity then divided into its abdominal and thoracic components
    c. At this time the gastrointestinal tract returns to the abdominal cavity

2. All degrees of protrusion of abdominal viscera may occur through diaphragmatic opening into thoracic cavity

ASSESSMENT

1. **Clinical presentation**
   a. Signs and symptoms
      i. Symptoms of respiratory distress: dyspnea, tachypnea, retractions, cyanosis
      ii. Breath sounds diminished or absent
      iii. Barrel chest
      iv. Scyphoid abdomen
      v. Heart sounds heard in right side of chest (because of shift in mediastinum)

2. **Biopsychosocial assessment**
   a. Vital signs: TPR; blood pressure
   b. Auscultation
   c. Peripheral perfusion
   d. Parents' understanding and reactions to infant's illness
   e. Support mechanisms: intrinsic and extrinsic
   f. Transport of infant to perinatal center will add stress of separation to family unit
   g. Observe separation of mother and father from infant and its impact on process of bonding

3. **Diagnostic data**
   a. Chest x-ray examination
   b. Blood gases: for determination of hypoxemia and respiratory acidosis

PROBLEMS AND COMPLICATIONS

1. Circulatory problems secondary to the mediastinal shift
2. Pulmonary infections (also a major cause of death)
3. High incidence of associated anomalies, mainly malrotation
4. Pulmonary insufficiency (also a major cause of death)
5. Precipitation of anoxia and acidosis

PATIENT CARE MANAGEMENT

1. **Goals**

   COMMENTS/TIPS/CAUTIONS

   a. To maintain adequate oxygenation and ventilation
      i. Intubate the trachea and ventilate infant

      Avoid assisted ventilation with mask to face technique because it introduces a great deal of air into the gastrointestinal tract, leading to further respiratory distress by distortion of the bowel within the chest

   b. To empty stomach contents
      i. Insert nasogastric tube
   c. To support vital functions
      i. Monitor vital signs: TPR; blood pressure

      Avoid excessive pressures during ventilatory resuscitation because of risk of pneumothorax

      ii. Monitor blood pH, PO_2, and PCO_2 with serial blood gas values

TABLE 15-4. STANDARDS OF CARE FOR AN INFANT
BEING TREATED WITH A VENTILATOR

Special Needs/ Problems	Short Term Goals	Nursing Intervention
Adequate oxygenation	To maintain consistency in ventilator settings To assure full aeration of all lung fields	Vital signs with BP every 2 hr Report any bradycardia or increase or decrease in BP Observe ventilator every hour for proper settings of FiO_2, mode, rate, peak pressure, PEEP, and position of alarm switches Completely assess chest every hour to ascertain quality of aeration of lung fields by presence and equality of breath sounds Report any new wheezes, rales, rhonchi, or decreased breath sounds Observe correct placement of nasal prongs if CPAP is being used Suction and ventilate infant with bag if ventilator is not functioning properly
Endotracheal tube displacement	To maintain proper placement of endo-tracheal tube	Observe endotracheal tube for posi-tion and stabilization Support endotracheal tube and con-nections when moving infant Auscultate lung fields after changing infant's position Have extra endotracheal tube and laryngoscope at bedside Keep infant's head stabilized
Tension pneumo-thorax	To have nursing per-sonnel respond to an immediate and knowledgeable manner to alleviate a life threatening situation	Have the following equipment at bedside: Needle for aspiration (butterfly 23 g or 18 g intravenous catheter Syringe (at least 30 cc) 3-way stopcock Chest tube High powered light for trans-illumination "Ambu" bag with oxygen connected Recognize and report signs of pneumothorax: Sudden cyanosis Decreased breath sounds Increased respiratory difficulty Decrease in arterial pressure Diminished or displaced heart sounds Decrease in ECG QRS complex on monitor Bradycardia Hypotension
Hypotension with CPAP	To detect early abnormal BP in the infant	Check blood pressure every 2 hr and when CPAP is increased, reporting any hypotension to physician

TABLE 15-4. STANDARDS OF CARE FOR AN INFANT BEING TREATED WITH A VENTILATOR *(Continued)*

Special Needs/ Problems	Short Term Goals	Nursing Intervention
Ventilator malfunction	To detect/correct any malfunction in ventilator	Observe infant's activity for resistance to ventilation or CPAP Observe endotracheal tube for kinks Suction infant to clear possible airway obstruction and ventilate by bag if necessary Observe tubing for collection of water Check for patency of all connections of tubing, ventilator, and infant Notify respiratory therapy team of possible instrument malfunction
Secretions	To maintain a clear airway for optimum aeration	Suction endotracheal tube, nares, and mouth as needed and as ordered, using sterile catheter and glove for endotreacheal tube Perform chest percussion and pulmonary toilet as needed
Gastric distention	To facilitate decompression of infant's stomach and prevent collection of secretions	Maintain patent orogastric tube by observing position and presence of drainage
Separation from parents	To promote uninterrupted process of infant-patent bonding	Explain to parents purpose and instrument involved in ventilation Encourage parents to visit infant as often as possible Encourage parents to touch/stroke infant Keep parents informed of progress of infant
Discomfort from immobility	To provide comforting measures with minimal disturbance	Reposition infant every 2 hr (side-back-abdomen) Suction mouth and free nares of excess secretions Give mouth care, using lemon-glycerin swabs
Use of transcutaneous PO_2 monitor	To be knowledgeable in use of instrument to facilitate management of sick infant	Follow guidelines for use of the transcutaneous PO_2 monitor Change electrode sites as outlined in the guidelines for use of the transcutaneous PO_2 monitor or more frequently when indicated by condition of infant's skin
Safety	To provide uncomplicated course of ventilation	Check ventilator settings every hour Check vital signs and BP every 2 hr Calibrate oxygen analyzer daily according to procedure Follow guidelines for use of the transcutaneous PO_2 monitor Report any sudden changes in infant's condition to physician Indicate height of QRS complex on the cardiorespiratory monitor by marking with tape initially and by re-marking each time electrodes are changed

Courtesy of Susan Synnott, R.N., Clinical Coordinator, Newborn/Intermediate Care Nursery, Memorial Hospital, Houston, Texas.

d. To maintain physiological equilibrium
   i. Provide neutral thermal environment to maintain temperature within normal range with minimal heat production and, therefore, O_2 consumption

e. To maintain adequate nutrition and hydration
   i. Provide IV therapy to avoid dehydration due to water loss from tachypnea and diuresis and to maintain caloric intake

    Parenteral fluids should be given through superficial vein in an extremity

   ii. Frequently monitor IV supplementation of glucose, electrolytes, and calcium
   iii. Monitor intake and output

    Weigh diapers to accurately determine output

f. To preserve family unit
   i. Provide explanations of illness, treatment, and prognosis
   ii. Provide mother with pictures of infant if she is unable to visit
   iii. Encourage phone calls to nursing unit to discuss management, care, and progress of infant
   iv. Encourage and facilitate father's involvement with transport of infant when indicated
   v. Transfer mother with infant if feasible

COMMENTS/TIPS/CAUTIONS

DISCHARGE PLANNING/TEACHING

Teaching should begin at the time crisis is identified.

1. Diagnosis, treatment, and prognosis should be explained to parents and discussed openly with them
2. Involve parents in treatment plan as appropriate
3. Assist parents and encourage their interaction with infant, providing information as to why infant response might be restricted
4. Answer questions openly and honestly with support and reassurance

_____ CHOANAL ATRESIA _____

Choanal atresia is the most common congenital abnormality of the nasal passages. When both nares are involved and the infant is unable to breathe through the mouth, it may quickly become cyanotic and die.

DIAGNOSIS

Choanal atresia is an upper airway obstruction resulting in inspiratory stridor, nasal flaring, and severe retractions with poor breath sounds on auscultation.

1. **Incidence**
   a. 1 in 5000 live births
   b. More common in females, with a ratio of 2:1
   c. Unilateral atresia more common than bilateral
   d. Unilateral atresia more frequent on right side

ETIOLOGY

1. This congenital abnormality of the nasal passage can be found in either one or in both sides; the nares are blocked by a membranous, cartilaginous, or bony septum

ASSESSMENT

1. **Clinical presentation**
   Infants with bilateral atresia are symptomatic immediately after birth.
   a. Signs and symptoms
       i.   Cyanosis, retractions, dyspnea
       ii. Diminished air exchange
       iii. Mouth breathing
2. **Biopsychosocial assessment**
   a. Vital signs: TPR, blood pressure
   b. Close the mouth and occlude first the right then the left nostril, feel for air, and auscultate expired nasal air with stethoscope
   c. Attempt to pass a soft but firm catheter through the nose into the pharynx
   d. Parents' understanding and reactions to infant's illness
   e. Support mechanisms: intrinsic and extrinsic
   f. Observe separation of mother and father from infant and its impact on the bonding process

PROBLEMS AND COMPLICATIONS

1. **Associated anomalies**
   a. In 60 per cent with bilateral atresia
   b. In 45 per cent with unilateral atresia
   c. Most common in cardiovascular system
2. **Neonatal death**

PATIENT CARE MANAGEMENT

1. **Goals**
   a. To establish a patent airway
      i. Insert oral airway
      ii. Place infant in prone position
      iii. Suction frequently as indicated

Secure airway before continuing management to ensure patent airway

If symptoms of respiratory distress not relieved, insert endotracheal tube

   b. To support vital functions
      i. Monitor vital signs: TPR, blood pressure
   c. To maintain physiological equilibrium
      i. Provide neutral thermal environment to maintain temperature within normal range with minimal heat production and, therefore, O_2 consumption
   d. To maintain adequate nutrition and hydration
      i. Intermittent gavage feeding
      ii. Pass feeding tube through oral cavity
      iii. Monitor intake and output

Weigh diapers to accurately determine output

   e. To preserve family unit
      i. Provide explanations of illness, treatment, and prognosis
      ii. Provide mother with pictures of infant if she is unable to visit
      iii. Encourage phone calls to nursing unit to discuss management, care, and progress of infant
      iv. Encourage and facilitate father's involvement with transport of infant when indicated
      v. Transfer mother with infant if feasible

DISCHARGE PLANNING/TEACHING

Teaching should begin at the time crisis is identified.

1. Diagnosis, treatment and prognosis should be explained to parents and discussed openly with them

2. Involve parents in the treatment plan as appropriate
3. Assist parents and encourage their interaction with infant, providing information as to why infant response might be restricted
4. Answer questions openly and honestly with support and reassurance

--------- CONCLUSIONS ---------

The primary responsibility of the respiratory system is to distribute air and exchange gases so that cells are supplied with oxygen for body metabolism. The product of the metabolism, carbon dioxide, is then removed. The organs of the respiratory system—the nose, pharynx, larynx, trachea, bronchi, and lungs—provide the means by which gases enter the body. The circulatory system distributes these gases to and from the cells throughout the body. The alveoli, or minute air sacs of the lung tissue, are where the gas exchange takes place. All of the other structures of the respiratory system function in air distribution.

Some of the most common problems in the neonate are related to disturbed respiratory function and disorders involving the respiratory tract. This disturbance can be caused by disease, trauma, or physical anomalies or can be seen as a manifestation of a disturbance in another organ or system, such as neurological disorders involving the respiratory center. Respiratory failure is the chief cause of morbidity in the newborn period. When these problems are anticipated, preparations for appropriate care can significantly reduce the incidence of neonatal mortality.

--------- REFERENCES ---------

1. Alden, E.R., et al.: Morbidity and mortality of infants weighing less than 1000 grams in an intensive care nursery. Pediatrics, *50*: 40, 1972.
2. Arnold, P., Hodson, A., and Cisher, R.: Hyaline membrane disease: A discussion. J. Pediatr., *80*:129, 1972.
3. Avery, G.B.: Neonatology, 2nd ed. Philadelphia, J.B. Lippincott Co., 1981.
4. Beard, A., et al.: Neonatal hypoglycemia. J. Pediatr., *79*:314, 1971.
5. Dibbris, A.W., and Wiener, E.S.: Morbidity from neonatal diaphragmatic hernia. J. Pediatr. Surg., *9*:653, 1974.
6. Drage, J.S., et al.: The Apgar score as an index of infant morbidity: A report from the Collaborative Study of Cerebral Palsy. Dev. Med. Child Neurol., *8*:141, 1966.
7. Driscoll, J.M., and Mellins, R.B.: Idiopathic respiratory distress syndrome of infancy. Respir. Care, *19*:298, 1974.
8. Fanaroff, A.A., et al.: Controlled trial of continuous negative external pressure in the treatment of severe respiratory distress syndrome. J. Pediatr., *82*:921, 1973.
9. Freeman, J.: Neonatal seizures—Diagnosis and management. J. Pediatr., *77*:701, 1970.
10. Goldsmith, J., and Karotkin, E.: Assisted Ventilation of the Neonate. Philadelphia, W.B. Saunders Co., 1981.
11. Gotof, S.P., and Behnman, R.: Neonatal septicemia. J. Pediatr., *76*:142, 1970.
12. Gregory, G.A., et al.: Meconium aspiration in infants: A prospective study. J. Pediatr., *85*:848, 1976.

13. Hall, R.T., and Rhodes, P.G.: Pneumothorax and pneumomediastinum in infants with idiopathic respiratory distress syndrome receiving continuous positive airway pressure. J. Pediatr., 55:193, 1975.

14. Kenpe, C.H., Silver, H.K., and O'Brien, D.: Current Pediatric Diagnosis and Treatment, 4th ed., Los Altos, Calif., Lange Medical Publications, 1976.

15. Marlow, D.: Textbook of Pediatric Nursing, 4th ed. Philadelphia, W.B. Saunders Co., 1977.

16. Raphaely, R.C., and Ganes, J.J.: Congenital diaphragmatic hernia: Predictions of survival. J. Pediatr. Surg., 8:815, 1973.

17. Schreiner, R.L.: Care of the Newborn. New York, Raven Press, 1981.

18. Vaughan, V.C., McKay, R.J., and Behrman, R.E.: Nelson Textbook of Pediatrics, 11th ed. Philadelphia, W.B. Saunders Co., 1979.

19. Whaley, L., and Wong, D.: Nursing Care of Infants and Children. St. Louis, C.V. Mosby Co., 1979.

CHAPTER 16

CARDIOVASCULAR AND HEMATOLOGICAL CRISES IN NEONATES

Sheila Southwell, R.N., M.S.

OBJECTIVES

Upon completion of this chapter the reader will be able to accomplish the following:

1. Describe the physiology of the fetal and neonatal cardiovascular system
2. Describe the infant at risk for persistent fetal circulation syndrome and describe the clinical presentation of the syndrome
3. Describe the main clinical features of congenital heart disease in the neonate
4. List the five groups of heart defects presenting in the neonatal period
5. List the main causes of congestive heart failure in the neonate
6. Describe the clinical presentation and treatment of congestive heart failure in the neonate
7. Describe the risk factors for hypovolemia in the neonate and its clinical presentation
8. Describe the infant at risk for hyperviscosity syndrome and describe its clinical presentation
9. Describe the treatment and complications of hyperviscosity syndrome
10. Describe the main goals in the diagnosis and treatment of the bleeding neonate
11. Describe the infant at risk for hyperbilirubinemia
12. Name the main complication of hyperbilirubinemia and its prevention

The immediate neonatal period is one of transition for the infant from a completely dependent organism to a separate independent being. In no other organ system is this transition more immediately and dramatically evident than in the cardiovascular-hematological system.

The body of the infant must take over the complex functions involved in transport of oxygen, glucose, and waste products that have previously been managed through the placenta. These functions require vast changes in hemodynamics during the first minutes, hours, and days after birth. Blood of the right composition must be pumped to the right place at the right time to diffuse oxygen and glucose into the blood, carry them to the proper place, and pick up and transport waste products to the proper organs for excretion.

Just as this transition is most evident in the cardiovascular-hematological system, so are the effects of any malfunctions in the transition. The infant whose body cannot oxygenate blood or cannot carry that blood to the organs is often in immediate acute distress and is in danger of irreversible damage or death.

Many conditions during pregnancy or in the immediate perinatal period can lead to these malfunctions. Persistent fetal circulation, congenital heart disease, congestive heart failure, hyperviscosity syndrome, coagulopathies, hyperbilirubinemia, and hypovolemia all cause disturbances in the normal functioning of the cardiovascular-hematological system. Sometimes their effects are minor, sometimes major, and early recognition for prompt intervention can often reverse the condition or at least lead to its improvement.

The presentation of these conditions can be subtle and gradual or sudden and precipitous and is often unexpected. The nurse, together with the parents, is the most constant observer of the infant during the perinatal period and is often the first to perceive, or be told by the parents, that something is wrong. Therefore it is important for every nurse who comes into contact with the newborn infant—from the obstetrical nurse to the nursery nurse—to be aware of the difficulties that can arise during this transition so that early recognition and prompt intervention can maximize the positive outcome of every perinatal experience.

PERSISTENT FETAL CIRCULATION

Persistent fetal circulation (PFC) is an acute life threatening condition in the immediate neonatal period that requires intervention to prevent a downward spiral of hypoxemia, acidemia, and increasing pulmonary vasoconstriction.

DIAGNOSIS

Persistent fetal circulation is a syndrome of respiratory distress, hypoxemia, and acidemia caused by failure of the pulmonary vasculature to dilate at birth. This leads to maintenance of high pumonary vascular resistance causing the persistence of fetal circulatory pathways (foramen ovale, ductus arteriosus) (Figs. 16–1 and 16–2).

Pulmonary blood vessels are very reactive to changes in PO_2 and pH during fetal life and the neonatal period.

1. Increased PO_2 and pH cause dilation.
2. Decreased PO_2 and pH cause constriction.

Normal transition of fetal to neonatal circulation is as follows:

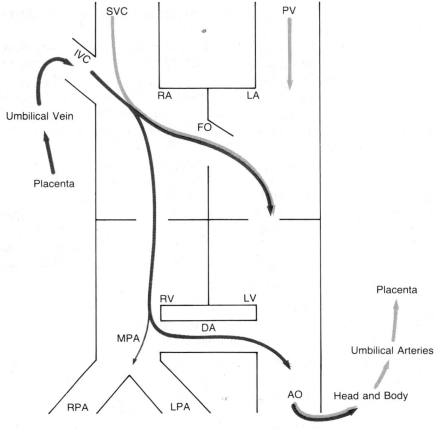

Figure 16-1. Fetal circulation. Key to Figures 16-1 to 16-10: SVC, superior vena cava; IVC, inferior vena cava; RA, right atrium; LA, left atrium; RV, right ventricle; LV, left ventricle; MPA, main pulmonary artery; LPA, left pulmonary artery; RPA, right pulmonary artery; PV, pulmonary veins; AO, aorta; DA, ductus arteriosus; FO, foramen ovale; TOF, tetralogy of Fallot; TGA, transposition of the great arteries; PS, pulmonary stenosis; PA, pulmonary atresia; VSD, ventricular septal defect; ECCD, endocardial cushion defect; TA, truncus arteriosus; AS, aortic stenosis; TAPVR, total anomalous pulmonary venous return; darker lines, direction of oxygenated blood flow; lighter lines, direction of unoxygenated blood flow.

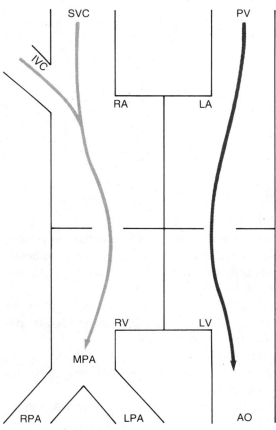

Figure 16-2. Neonatal circulation.

1. Fetus: PO_2 of 20 to 30 results in pulmonary vasoconstriction and increased pulmonary vascular resistance, increased pressure in the right side of the heart, and right to left shunting through fetal pathways

2. First breath: the pulmonary blood vessels dilate in response to increased alveolar PO_2 causing decreased pulmonary vascular resistance, increased pulmonary blood flow, and decreased pressure in the right side of the heart.

3. Increased PO_2, decreased pressure in the right side of the heart, plus increased pressure and volume in the left side of the heart after removal of the placenta result in closure of fetal shunts.

Failure of pulmonary blood vessels to dilate results in increased pulmonary vascular resistance and decreased pulmonary blood flow. This causes an increase in pressure in the right side of the heart and a decrease in Po_2 and pH, thus causing persistence of fetal shunts, hypoxia, and acidosis. These then result in further pulmonary vasoconstriction.

1. **Incidence**
   a. 1 in 1500 live births, with survival of 50 to 80 per cent[52]
   b. Occurs in term infants

2. **Predisposing factors[58]**
   a. Hypoxia and acidosis
   b. Hyperviscosity of blood
   c. Space occupying lesions of chest
   d. Pulmonary hypoplasia
   e. Pneumonia
   f. Aspiration syndromes

3. **Contributing factors[58]**
   a. Hypothermia
   b. Hypoglycemia
   c. Hypocalcemia
   d. Hypomagnesemia

ETIOLOGY

1. **Classification[49]**
   a. Normal pulmonary vascular development
      i. Acute pulmonary vasoconstriction (airway obstruction from meconium aspiration, atelectasis) results in hypoxia, acidosis, or both, and further pulmonary vasoconstriction (acidemia enhances the response to hypoxia)
      ii. Hyperviscosity (usually results from hematocrit of 65 per cent or greater), which causes sludging in pulmonary vessels, decreased pulmonary blood flow and hypoxia
   b. Increased pulmonary vascular development
      i. Smooth muscle layer of pulmonary arterioles normally decreases during first week of life
      ii. In these infants, the smooth muscle layer not only was hypertrophied in utero but it does not decrease after birth

      iii. Prognosis for survival is poor; infants are often not reactive to therapy

      iv. Examples

          (a) Chronic intrauterine hypoxia: placental insufficiency (intrauterine growth retardation, infant of diabetic mother)

          (b) Prenatal pulmonary hypertension: constriction of ductus arteriosus

          (c) Congenital heart disease in which pulmonary and systemic pressures are equal (aortic arch interruption)

  c. Decreased cross-sectional area of pulmonary vascular bed

      i. A decrease in the number of vessels to accommodate same amount of cardiac output leads to pulmonary hypertension, increased pulmonary vascular resistance, and decreased pulmonary blood flow, which ultimately results in hypoxia

      ii. Examples

          (a) Space occupying lesions of chest: diaphragmatic hernia, lung cysts

          (b) Lung hypoplasia: Potter's syndrome, oligohydramnios

          (c) Interference with vessel growth: drugs?, intrauterine infections?

ASSESSMENT

1. **Clinical presentation**

    PFC is present at birth or within first few hours.

  a. Signs and symptoms

      Signs and symptoms may be indistinguishable from those of congenital heart disease.

      i. Central cyanosis

      ii. Respiratory distress: usually only tachypnea

      iii. Systolic murmur (flow through foreman ovale, ductus arteriosus, or both)

      iv. Poor perfusion (capillary filling time greater than 3 seconds, pulses 1+ or less): decreased cardiac output due to myocardial ischemia

        Some infants require echocardiogram and cardiac catheterization.

2. **Biopsychosocial assessment**

  a. Vital signs and blood pressure

  b. Pregnancy and delivery history

  c. Parents' understanding and reactions to infant's illness

  d. Support mechanisms: intrinsic and extrinsic

  e. Remember that in most cases this is a life threatening emergency in an infant who was expected to be well; shock and disbelief (first state of grieving process), fear, and bewilderment are normal reactions; transport of the infant to a perinatal center will add the stress of separation of the family unit

3. **Diagnostic data**
   a. Arterial blood gas
      i. Hypoxemia: Po_2 less than 60 in 100 per cent oxygen
      ii. Acidemia: pH less than 7.30
      iii. Simultaneous right radial artery and umbilical artery (abdominal aorta) blood gases: PO_2 high in right radial artery (pre-ductus arteriosus blood); PO_2 much lower in umbilical artery (post-ductal shunt blood). Evidence of right to left shunt is one means to distinguish PFC from congenital heart disease.
   b. Chest roentgenogram: normal cardiac anatomy and normal lungs
   c. Serum glucose (Dextrostix reading will suffice), calcium, and magnesium
      i. Decreased because of utilization during stress
      ii. Decrease contributes to further decrease in pulmonary blood flow by reducing myocardial performance
   d. Hematocrit: hyperviscosity can cause or contribute to decrease in pulmonary blood flow

PROBLEMS AND COMPLICATIONS

1. Death from rapidly worsening cycle of hypoxemia, acidemia, and further vasoconstriction
2. Hypotension and shock
3. Neurological sequelae (varied) from hypoxia, acidosis, and hypotension
4. Necrotizing enterocolitis from hypoperfusion of gut during acute illness
5. Acute tubular necrosis of kidneys due to hypoperfusion and acidosis
6. Late pulmonary vascular disease? (not established)

PATIENT CARE MANAGEMENT
(At hospital of birth)

1. **Goals**
   a. To identify infant at risk
      i. Preparation for resuscitation at birth for infants in above risk groups
         (a) Intubation and hand ventilation systems
         (b) Umbilical artery catheterization
      ii. Observation of infant at risk in nursery for signs of decompensation
   b. To stabilize condition of and transport sick infant to perinatal center if condition warrants

COMMENTS/TIPS/CAUTIONS

May require regular periodic in-service for personnel if not used frequently

i. Administration of oxygen and ventilation to maximize pulmonary vasodilatation

ii. Monitor arterial blood gases at frequent intervals (every 1 hour or more often)

iii. Monitor glucose (Dextrostix), serum calcium, and magnesium; IV support as needed

iv. Maintain neutral thermal environment

c. To preserve family unit

i. Repeated detailed explanations of illness, treatment, prognosis

ii. Picture of infant, any booklets or brochures from perinatal center for mother if she remains in home hospital

iii. Facilitation of father's accompanying infant if desired: arrange to ride with transport team, arrange housing near center

iv. Transfer of mother with infant if feasible

(At perinatal center)

d. To relieve hypoxemia and acidemia

i. Hyperventilation by mechanical ventilator to produce hyperoxia and alkalosis

ii. IV infusions of vasodilators (tolazoline)

iii. Smooth muscle relaxants to decrease oxygen consumption and maximize ventilation (curare, pancuronium [Pavulon])

iv. Frequent arterial blood gas determinations

e. To support vital functions

i. Continuous cardiorespira-

COMMENTS/TIPS/CAUTIONS

Pulmonary vasculature dilates with hyperoxia (PO_2 100) and alkalosis (pH 7.45-7.55)

Levels may be low and contribute to further deterioration

Hypothermia can contribute to pulmonary vasoconstriction. Stable temperature can decrease O_2 consumption

If pneumothorax is produced, treat with chest tube insertion

Such drugs have many dangerous side effects (see Appendix B); may require infusions of other drugs (dopamine, isoproterenol (Isuprel) to support circulation

    tory monitoring with BP; may have transcutaneous PO_2, pulmonary artery catheters

  ii. Support circulation with volume expanders (whole blood, fresh frozen plasma) or drug infusions (dopamine, isoproterenol [Isuprel]) if hypotension or shock occurs

  iii. Frequent monitoring and IV supplementation of glucose, electrolytes, calcium

DISCHARGE PLANNING/TEACHING

Teaching should begin from the time a problem is noted.

1. Detailed and repeated explanations of diagnosis, treatment, and prognosis
2. Involvement of parents in treatment plan as appropriate
3. Reassurance that their giving tender, loving care to the infant is still important although infant's ability to respond may be restricted
4. Emphasize need for follow-up for their reassurance and early detection of any sequelae

CONGENITAL HEART DEFECTS

Congenital heart defects can produce a life threatening crisis in oxygenation to the newborn infant, yet many defects are improved or corrected by early recognition and appropriate medical and surgical treatment. However, since most infants with heart defects are the product of a normal pregnancy and delivery and the signs and symptoms of such defects are often masked by the normal changes in hemodynamics after birth, signs of even serious defects may be subtle until sudden deterioration occurs. The nurse and the parents, as joint close observers of neonatal behavior, are often the first to realize that a baby is not "quite right."

DIAGNOSIS

Congenital heart defects are structural defects of the heart that interfere with normal hemodynamics or oxygenation of the blood after birth.

The fetal heart is completely formed in the first 8 weeks of gestation by a complex series of transformations.

Infants with cardiac defects are usually from normal term pregnancy and often born at community hospitals without facilities for cardiac diagnosis and treatment. Early recognition is necessary to allow for transfer to regional center *before* a life threatening situation occurs.

Defects are often difficult to recognize at first because signs and symptoms are often masked by normal changes from fetal to neonatal circulation. They are also difficult to distinguish from those of PFC or septic shock.

Oxygenation and perfusion are often dependent on fetal shunts (foramen ovale, ductus arteriosus) remaining open.

1. **Incidence**
   a. 1 per cent of all live births

2. **Predisposing factors**[15,50]
   a. Chromosomal defects
      i. Down's syndrome (trisomy 21): endocardial cushion defect most common defect
      ii. Trisomy 13 and 18: multiple anomalies, including heart defects
      iii. Turner's syndrome (XO): coarctation of the aorta most common defect
   b. Other developmental anomalies
      i. Omphalocele
      ii. VATER association: a collection of anomalies including *ver*tebral defects, imperforate *a*nus, *t*racheoesophageal fistula, *r*enal defects
   c. Infant of diabetic mother: transposition of the great arteries or ventricular septal defect most common defect
   d. Previous child with congenital heart defect increases risk from 1 to 2 or 3 per cent
   e. Maternal viral disease in first trimester
      (a) Predominantly with rubella: pulmonary stenosis most common
   f. Maternal alcohol ingestion: fetal alcohol syndrome, a collection of defects including heart disease and mental retardation
   g. Environmental toxins: association unknown but have been implicated in cases of radiation, pesticide exposure in first trimester

ETIOLOGY

1. Predominantly in term infants
   a. Fetal oxygenation carried out by placenta
   b. Not a factor in fetal distress or preterm labor
2. Predominantly with normal pregnancy and delivery
3. Multifactorial occurrence
   a. Genetic component plus environmental factors
   b. Environmental or inheritance factors unknown
4. Circulatory changes from fetus to neonate
   a. *At birth* transition from fetal *parallel* circuits to neonatal *series* circuit
   b. Fetal shunts (foramen ovale and ductus arteriosus) close and pulmonary vessels dilate as PO_2 rises from 20–30 to 80–100 mm Hg
   c. Pulmonary circuit changes from a low flow/high resistance/high pressure circuit to a normal flow/low resistance/low pressure circuit

as result of dilation of the pulmonary vasculature and decreased pulmonary vascular resistance

d. Systemic circuit changes from a low pressure to a high pressure circuit because of removal of the placenta

ASSESSMENT

1. **Clinical presentation[46]**
   a. Signs and symptoms
      i. Central cyanosis: often increased with stress (feeding or crying)
      ii. Respiratory distress
         (a) Inadequate oxygenation
         (b) Pulmonary edema (congestive heart failure)
      iii. Lethargy, poor feeding, sweating
         (a) Often reported by parents
         (b) Due to hypoxia or congestive heart failure
      iv. Murmur
         (a) Extra heart sound, *turbulence* in blood flow
         (b) Defect itself (i.e., blood traveling through septal defect or stenotic valve) or fetal shunts
      v. Poor perfusion with or without cyanosis
         (a) Mottled skin
         (b) Capillary filling time on blanching greater than 3 seconds
         (c) Pulses 1+ or less; may not be present or equal in all four extremities
      vi. Hepatomegaly

2. **Most common defects noted in neonatal period grouped by type of lesion or type of clinical presentation[48]**

   Laws governing hemodynamics of lesions are as follows: (1) Blood follows the path of least resistance (pressure). (2) If enough blood did not flow through a structure during fetal life, that structure did not grow and will be either atretic (undeveloped) or hypoplastic (underdeveloped) at birth.
   a. Right ventricular outflow obstruction (Fig. 16–3)
      i. Obstruction of normal blood flow from right ventricle to lungs
      ii. Unoxygenated blood shunts from right to left through open fetal shunt (foramen ovale) or associated defect (atrial septal [ASD] or ventricular septal [VSD]) then left to right through ductus arteriosus into lungs
      iii. Shunts must remain open for the infant to live
      iv. Mixing of oxygenated and unoxygenated blood results in cyanosis
      v. Includes pulmonary valvular stenosis; tetralogy of Fallot with severe pulmonary stenosis (PS) (Fig. 16–4); transposition of the great arteries with PS; pulmonary valve atresia; and tricuspid valve atresia
      vi. Noted very early (first 12 to 24 hours of life) with the following:

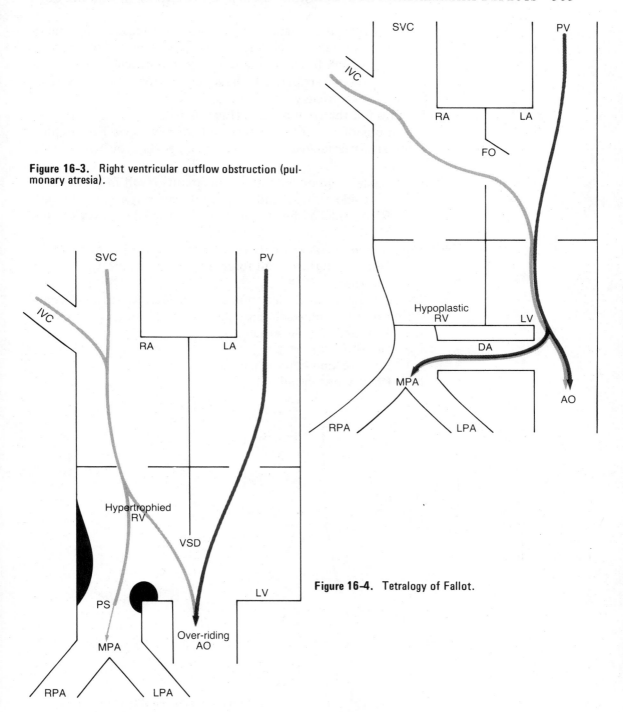

Figure 16-3. Right ventricular outflow obstruction (pulmonary atresia).

Figure 16-4. Tetralogy of Fallot.

(a)   Cyanosis

(b)   Hypoxemia: PO_2 less than 30 mm Hg, often less than 20

(c)   Acidemia often present: pH less than 7.30

(d)   Sometimes right heart failure

(e)   Systolic murmur from stenotic pulmonary valve or infundibulum or patent ductus arteriosus

(f) Roentgenogram: may show decreased pulmonary vascularity (severe pulmonary stenosis or atresia), small heart (hypoplastic right ventricle with pulmonary atresia), or large heart (hypertrophied right ventricle with tetralogy of Fallot)

b. Transposition of the great arteries (Fig. 16–5)
   i. Locations of pulmonary artery and aorta are switched: pulmonary artery attached to left ventricle, aorta attached to right ventricle
   ii. Two separate, noncommunicating circuits result in cyanosis
      (a) Left side of heart and lung recirculate oxygenated blood
      (b) Right side of heart and body recirculate unoxygenated blood
   iii. Connection must exist between the circuits for infant to live
      (a) Ductus arteriosus and foramen ovale remain open
      (d) Associated VSD
   iv. Usually present at 2 days of age when fetal shunts close; condition of infant may suddenly deteriorate when this occurs
      (a) Cyanosis: PO_2 less than 30 mm Hg
      (b) Usually not acidotic
      (c) Loud second heart sound
      (d) Usually not in failure

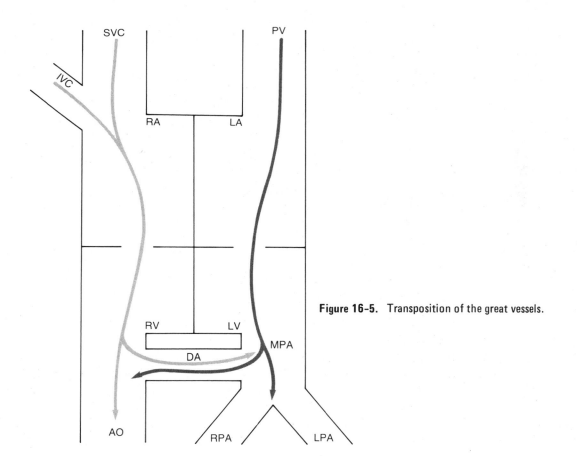

Figure 16-5. Transposition of the great vessels.

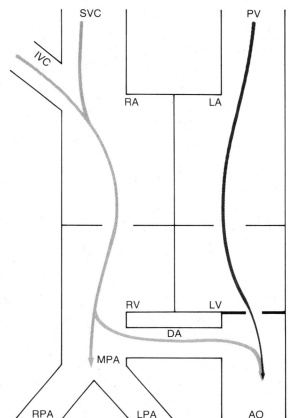

Figure 16-6. Left ventricular outflow obstruction (aortic stenosis).

      (e)   Roentgenogram: heart looks like egg on side

      (f)   Predominantly in males, often large for gestational age

  c. Left ventricular outflow obstruction (Fig. 16–6)

      i. Obstruction to flow out of left ventricle, causing decrease in cardiac output and congestive heart failure

     ii. Includes aortic stenosis, aortic arch interruption, coarctation of the aorta, hypoplastic left heart syndrome

   iii. Occurs at 2 to 3 days of life (may be later in some cases of coarctation) when fetal shunts close

      (a) Mild or no cyanosis

      (b) May be acidotic

      (c) Congestive heart failure

      (d) Decrease in cardiac output may be severe enough for infant to appear to be in shock

         (1) Decreased capillary filling time

         (2) Decreased pulses or no pulses (with coarctation: pulses will be stronger in upper extremities, decreased or absent in lower extremities)

         (3) Skin pale, ashen, cold, and clammy

         (4) Diaphoresis

  d. Left to right shunts and biventricular mixing lesions

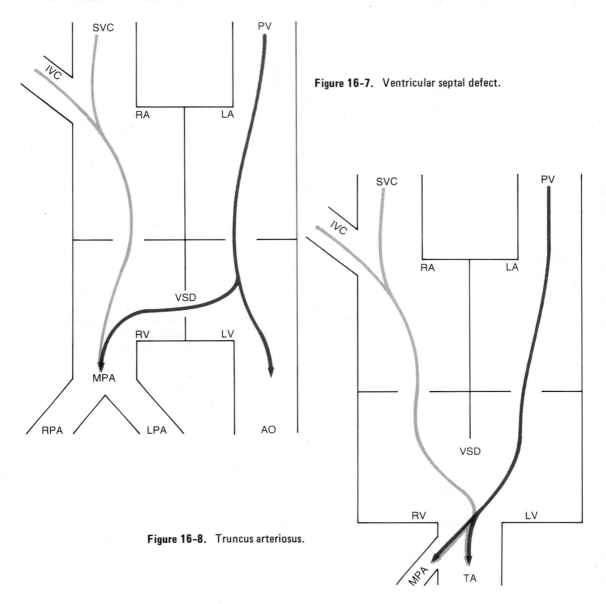

Figure 16-7. Ventricular septal defect.

Figure 16-8. Truncus arteriosus.

   i. Mixing of oxygenated and unoxygenated blood through VSD with or without associated lesions (Fig. 16–7)

  ii. Persistent truncus arteriosus: failure of fetal truncus to divide into aorta and main pulmonary artery, resulting in large midline vessel overriding VSD, from which pulmonary arteries later take off (Fig. 16–8)

 iii. Endocardial cushion defect: failure of endocardial cushions, which divide four chambers, to develop in middle of heart, and as a result all four chambers connect (Fig. 16–9)

 iv. Patent ductus arteriosus: primarily in premature infants

  v. Direction and degree of shunting through VSD, cyanosis, and congestive heart failure vary according to

     (a) Degree of pulmonary vascular resistance: falls rapidly at birth, reaches 0 at 6 weeks of age

     (b) Pressures within the heart: depend on type of lesion

        (1) Isolated VSD: because pressure on left side greater, shunt predominantly left to right after 6 weeks of age

        (2) Endocardial cushion defect: all four chambers communicate; shunts in all directions

        (3) Truncus arteriosus: large VSD communicates with single great artery; bidirectional shunting

  vi. Time of presentation varies with degree of failure; little cyanosis

e. Total anomalous pulmonary venous return (Fig. 16–10)

  i. Failure of pulmonary veins to implant normally into left atrium; instead, return to another area, usually into right side

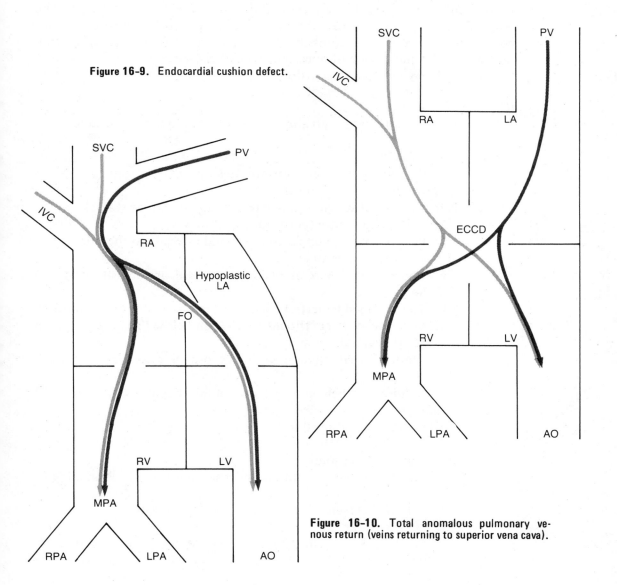

Figure 16-9. Endocardial cushion defect.

Figure 16-10. Total anomalous pulmonary venous return (veins returning to superior vena cava).

of heart (right atrium, superior or inferior vena cava, coronary sinus) or into portal system ("total veins below the diaphragm")

    ii. May be total (all pulmonary veins) or partial (some implant normally, others do not)

    iii. Congestive heart failure due to pulmonary venous obstruction

    iv. Time of presentation varies with onset of failure: may be 2 to 3 weeks of age or earlier. In total veins below the diaphragm, obstruction, and thus congestive heart failure, tend to be earlier. Mild cyanosis is present.

3. Biopsychosocial assessment

(On admission)

A diagnosis of heart disease in the neonate is usually an unforeseen one. Since few of these infants are born in cardiac centers, transport and the separation of the family unit are the rule rather than the exception. Instead of a healthy infant the parents are faced with a seriously ill infant who may die either from the defect or from the corrective surgery. When the defect is not correctable but palliation is possible the parents are left to deal with an infant with a chronic disease of uncertain prognosis.

  a. Delivery and neonatal history

    i. Timing and type of symptoms

(Cardiac examination)

  b. Inspection (what observation alone reveals about cardiac status)

    i. Color

    ii. Activity

    iii. Precordial (area on chest over heart) activity

    iv. Respiratory rate and character

  c. Palpation (what touching alone reveals about cardiac status)

    i. Skin temperature (perfusion)

    ii. Pulses: compare upper to lower and one side to the other

    iii. Capillary filling time

    iv. Location of point of maximal impulse or intensity (PMI) of heart

    v. Thrill: palpable part of a murmur, felt as a vibration on chest

    vi. Location of liver: should be 2–3 cm below right costal margin at midclavicular line

  d. Auscultation (what listening with stethoscope reveals about cardiac status)

Stethoscope: bell, low-pitched sound; diaphragm, high-pitched sounds

    i. Heart rate and rhythm

    ii. Location of PMI

    iii. Normal heart sounds

      (a) S_1: closing of mitral and tricuspid valves — beginning of systole

      (b) S_2: closing of aortic and pulmonary valves, beginning of diastole

      (c) S_2 is normally "split" (two sounds close together) in newborn infant because of high pulmonary vascular resistance, and pulmonary valve closes slightly after aortic valve

    iv. Extra heart sounds: murmurs
       (a) Timing in cardiac cycle: systolic or diastolic
       (b) Location on chest in relation to right or left sternal borders, upper and lower portions of chest
       (c) Radiation: transmission of sound from loudest point to aortic area (upper right sternal border at second intercostal space); pulmonic area (upper left sternal border at second to third intercostal space); apex or base of heart (difficult in small heart of infant); axilla or back
       (d) Intensity (Grades): I, barely audible; II, soft; III, moderately loud, radiates; IV, loud, palpable thrill (in all grades IV and above); V, louder (heard even when stethoscope not in complete contact with chest); VI, louder (heard when stethoscope off chest)
       (e) Pitch: high or low frequency of sound
       (f) Quality: rough (vibrations); blowing (no vibrations)
       (g) Contour (change in intensity):
          Increase (crescendo) or decrease (decrescendo) in intensity, characteristic of *systolic ejection murmur* through stenotic valves
          Plateau types, even in intensity, characteristic of *holosystolic murmur* through septal defects

  e. Vital signs and BP in all four extremities

4. Diagnostic data

  a. Blood glucose (Dextrostix)
    i. Infants with cardiac defect under stress, often are hypoglycemic; myocardium needs glucose

  b. Serum calcium
    i. Increased utilization under stress
    ii. Parathyroid glands (stimulate reabsorption of Ca in kidney), from same embryological origin as some cardiac structures, may be malformed, malfunctioning, or absent
    iii. Cardiac function may be compromised by hypocalcemia

  c. Arterial blood gases
    i. State of oxygenation, acidosis
    ii. Hyperoxia test may distinguish cardiac from pulmonary disease
       (a) ABG in 21 per cent forced inspiratory oxygen (FiO_2) (room air)
       (b) ABG after 5 to 10 minutes of ventilation with 100 per cent FiO_2
       (c) In infant with pulmonary disease PO_2 will increase as alveolar PO_2 rises
       (d) In infant with structural heart disease PO_2 cannot increase

  d. Chest roentgenogram
    i. Heart size

   ii. Cardiac silhouette
   iii. Pulmonary vascularity
   e. ECG
   i. Axis (direction of greatest force)
   ii. Dominant ventricle
   f. Echocardiogram if facilities available
   i. Sonogram of heart to detect presence, absence, or malposition of structures
   ii. Can now be done in utero in certain centers
   g. Cardiac catheterization if facilities available and indicated by examination
   i. Oxygenation and pressures in various structures of heart
   ii. Angiograms (dye studies) to determine hemodynamic status

PROBLEMS AND COMPLICATIONS

1. Death if minimally adequate oxygenation not present
2. Neurological sequelae from hypoxia and acidosis
3. Hypoglycemia and hypocalcemia both result in myocardial compromise, seizures
4. Polycythemia: attempt of body to increase O_2 carrying capacity leads to cerebrovascular accident
5. Bacterial endocarditis
6. Limitations on growth and development in uncorrected lesions
7. Pulmonary vascular disease due to increased pulmonary blood flow in some lesions
8. Pulmonary hypertension due to hypoxia in cyanotic lesions

PATIENT CARE MANAGEMENT
(At home hospital)

1. **Goals**
   a. To recognize possibility of defect early
      i. Close observation of infant who is "not right" or who has subtle signs of difficulty
      ii. Increased index of suspicion of any infant with predisposing factors
   b. To stabilize the condition and transport infant to cardiac center[14]
      i. History
      ii. Arterial blood gas, hematocrit, glucose (Dextrostix), calcium determinations. Supplement dextrose and calcium as needed

   iii. Oxygen not administered without consulting with cardiac center

   iv. Vital signs, BP, cardiorespiratory monitoring

   v. Chest roentgenogram

   vi. ECG

 c. To preserve family unit

   i. Repeated detailed explanations of diagnosis, treatment, prognosis

   ii. Picture of infant, any booklets or brochures from cardiac center for mother if she remains in home hospital

   iii. Facilitation of father's accompanying infant if desired: arrange to ride with transport team, arrange housing near center

   iv. Transfer of mother with infant if feasible

(At cardiac center)

 d. To accurately diagnose defect

   i. Admission assessment and tests as outlined

   ii. Administration of PGE_1 to keep ductal shunt open if necessary

 e. To treat defect as appropriate

   i. Corrective surgery; parents' consent for correctable lesion in which immediate surgery is indicated

   ii. Surgical palliation of defects that are life threatening but not correctable either because of age or nature of lesion

   iii. Treatment of infant awaiting surgery varies, depending on condition of infant, but usually consists of

    (a) Monitoring of vital signs, arterial blood gases, laboratory tests

    (b) Observation and assessment of changes

COMMENTS/TIPS/CAUTIONS

Oxygen will not help in most cyanotic defects and may worsen them by promoting closure of ductal shunt

This is a controlled drug available only in certain centers (see Appendix B)

Timing of correction varies from infant to infant and center to center; optimal time is usually judgment of cardiologist and surgeon

This decision is a difficult one and should be made carefully with all medical personnel and parents contributing; considerations are:
1. Infant's cardiac anatomy and how it might change with time
2. Possible future surgery
3. Infant's physical condition after surgery and what care would be at home
4. Parents' ability and desire to care for chronically ill infant

Some infants remain in the center for some weeks awaiting surgery (usually to permit growth); these infants require supportive therapy that cannot be given at home

in cardiorespiratory condition

(c) Gavage feeding to decrease O_2 consumption

(d) Parenteral alimentation may be necessary

(e) Drug and other therapy for congestive heart failure (see next section, Congestive Heart Failure)

(f) PGE_1 infusion

DISCHARGE PLANNING/TEACHING

Infant whose defect is surgically corrected

1. Education about defect, surgery, postoperative care and course, effects of defect and surgery on growth and development, short and long term complications of surgery
2. Mobilization of resources and support mechanisms (intrinsic and extrinsic): public health nurse referral, support groups, family
3. Plans for follow-up

Infant in whom operation was only palliative; infant with correctable lesion who is sent home to await optimal time for surgery

1. Education about defect, effects of surgery, prognosis, signs and symptoms of deterioration and complications and when to bring infant in for further treatment; effects of defect on growth and development; medication: method, dosage, side effects, symptoms of need for reevaluation of dosage
2. Mobilization of resources and support mechanisms: referral of public health nurse, support group, appropriate family community services (i.e., crippled children's services)
3. Planning for follow-up

CONGESTIVE HEART FAILURE

Congestive heart failure (CHF) in the neonate impairs oxygenation and perfusion of the tissues. It has long term effects on growth, on the heart, on the lungs, and on the pulmonary vasculature, inflicting irreversible damage. If not controlled or corrected, the infant can literally drown in the pulmonary edema that is a cardinal feature of neonatal heart failure. However, nursing and pharmacological measures can control or alleviate CHF in all but the most severe cases.

DIAGNOSIS

Congestive heart failure is failure of the heart to maintain the output necessary for the demands of the body.

1. **Predisposing factors**
   a. Congenital heart disease
   b. Overtransfusion
   c. Excessive tachycardia
   d. Intrauterine viral disease
   e. Hypoxia
   f. Metabolic disturbances
   g. Anemia

ETIOLOGY[1]

1. In neonate, heart can only increase output (CO) by increasing rate (HR); lacks sarcomeres to increase stroke volume (SV) (HR $\times$ SV = CO)
2. Inability to compensate for excessive demands on heart for increased output
3. Failure to maintain cardiac output will result in the following:
   a. Increased diastolic volume and pressure in left ventricle (LV)
   b. Increased pulmonary venous volume and pressure resulting in pulmonary edema
   c. Decreased systemic blood flow
4. Right ventricle affected by cause of LV failure or pulmonary hypertension, heart fails as a whole
5. Heart dilates and HR increases: attempt to compensate (sympathetic nervous system) results in increased O_2 consumption
6. Pulmonary edema leads to increased PCO_2, decreased pH and tachypnea, which result in increased O_2 consumption
7. Fluid retention due to decreased kidney perfusion and secondary hyperaldosteronism may in turn lead to dilutional hyponatremia
8. Hyperkalemia from increased cellular release due to decreased perfusion
9. Fatigue and failure to thrive due to decreased intake secondary to tachypnea and liver congestion, and increased O_2 and caloric consumption due to increased work of breathing
10. Main causes of LV failure[27]
    a. Volume overload
       i. Placental transfusion, late cord clamping
       ii. Twin to twin transfusion
       iii. Iatrogenic fluid overload
       iv. Left to right shunt lesions in congenital heart disease
          (a) VSD
          (b) Endocardial cushion defect
          (c) Patent ductus arteriosus (premature infant)
          (d) Truncus arteriosus
    b. Pressure overload
       i. LV outflow obstruction
    c. Myocardial damage or disease

       i. Viral myocarditis
      ii. Congenital cardiomyopathy
    iii. Hypoxic damage (birth asphyxia)
    iv. Hypoglycemia
     v. Infant of diabetic mother

  d. Rhythm disorders
      i. Supraventricular tachycardia

ASSESSMENT

1. Clinical presentation[8,27,46]

  a. Signs and symptoms

      i. Respiratory distress (primarily tachypnea: greater than 60 breaths/minute)

     ii. Tachycardia and gallop rhythm, active precordium

    iii. Hepatomegaly (liver more than 3 cm below costal margin at midclavicular line) from congestion

    iv. Cardiomegaly on roentgenogram

     v. Rales

    vi. Pulses: decreased in CHF with decreased CO and shock (LV outflow obstruction); may be increased in "high output failure" states (truncus arteriosus, patent ductus arteriosus, hypervolemia)

   vii. Decreased peripheral perfusion (pale, grayish, mottled cold skin; decreased urinary output) due to decreased CO and shunting of blood to brain and heart

  viii. Diaphoresis (increased sympathetic activity)

    ix. Fatigue and failure to thrive

  b. Causes

  Preterm infant

      i. Hypoxia: myocardial damage

     ii. Anemia: tachycardia

    iii. Hypoglycemia: myocardial compromise

    iv. Patent ductus arteriosus: volume overload

  In early days of life

      i. Hypoplastic left heart syndrome: pressure overload and myocardial incompetence

     ii. Obstructed total anomalous pulmonary venous return: volume and pressure overload

    iii. Paroxysmal atrial tachycardia: rhythm disorder

    iv. Myocarditis: myocardial damage

     v. Cerebral arteriovenous malformation: volume overload

    vi. Iatrogenic fluid overload

  In early weeks of life

      i. Coarctation of aorta: pressure overload

     ii. Truncus arteriosus: volume overload

    iii. Paroxysmal atrial tachycardia: rhythm disorder

    iv. Myocarditis: myocardial damage

  In early months of life

      i. VSD: volume overload

      ii. Transportation of great arteries with VSD: volume overload

      iii. Unobstructed total anomalous pulmonary venous return: volume overload

      iv. Patent ductus arteriosus: volume overload

  c. History

      i. Time of onset

      ii. Symptoms

      iii. To determine etiology

2. Biopsychosocial assessment

  a. Vital signs, BP, weight

  b. Chest examination

      i. Inspection: color, respiratory rate and character, precordial activity, whether distress is decreased with raising head of bed, diaphoresis, activity

      ii. Palpation: precordium, liver, temperature, perfusion of skin (capillary filling time)

      iii. Auscultation: heart rate and rhythm, murmurs, breath sounds and rates

  c. Assess parents' understanding of underlying disease and cause

  d. Assess parents' understanding of treatment and prognosis

  e. Parents' support mechanisms

  f. Parents' coping mechanisms (guilt for cause or fear of inadequate care as parents may be a factor)

3. Diagnostic data

  a. Chest x-ray examination: heart size and contour, pulmonary vascularity and fluid

  b. Urinary output, specific gravity

  c. ECG: to rule out arrhythmia; baseline for digitalization

  d. Blood: hematocrit, hemoglobin, electrolytes, calcium, arterial blood gas

PROBLEMS AND COMPLICATIONS

1. Death from single or combined effects of intractable (unresponsive to to treatment) failure, side effects of therapy, underlying illness
2. Cardiac rhythm disturbances from CHF or therapy
3. Failure to thrive
4. Apnea (primarily preterm infants with patent ductus arteriosus)
5. Pulmonary vascular disease in chronic CHF

PATIENT CARE MANAGEMENT

1. Goals

  a. To control CHF

      i. Digoxin (see Appendix B)

        (a) Cardiorespiratory monitor

        (b) Monitor vital signs

electrolytes, urinary output, specific gravity, ECG changes, signs and symptoms of toxicity

ii. Diuretics (see Furosemide in Appendix B)
    (a) Monitor potassium levels
    (b) Potassium supplement may be needed
    (c) Monitor urinary output, specific gravity, weight

iii. Decrease O_2 demands
    (a) Decrease activity; gavage feedings
    (b) Raise head of bed
    (c) Small, frequent feeding
    (d) Neutral thermal environment
    (e) O_2 therapy as ordered

iv. Frequent assessment
    (a) Respiratory pattern
    (b) Breath sounds
    (c) Liver

b. To diagnose and treat cause
    i. Admission assessment as above
    ii. Treat cause if possible

DISCHARGE PLANNING/TEACHING

1. Education about
    a. Etiology, physiology, and signs and symptoms of CHF
    b. Effects of CHF
    c. Treatment of CHF: giving of medications, side effects
    d. Follow-up care

HYPOVOLEMIA

Hypovolemia in the newborn causes hypoperfusion of vital organs and leads to ischemic damage from lack of oxygen. If significant, it can lead to shock and death.

DIAGNOSIS

Hypovolemia in the neonate consists of reduction in circulating blood volume to the point at which profusion of vital organs is inadequate for

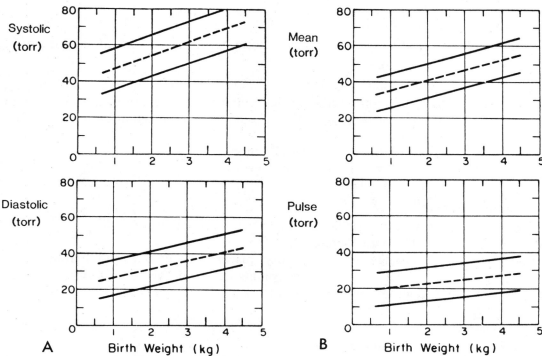

Figure 16-11. *A*, Linear regressions (*broken lines*) and 95 per cent confidence limits (*solid lines*) of systolic (*top*) and diastolic (*bottom*) aortic blood pressures on birth weight in 61 healthy newborn infants during the first 12 hours after birth. For systolic pressure, $y = 7.13X + 40.45$; $r = 0.79$. For diastolic pressure, $y = 4.81x + 22.18$; $r = 0.71$. For both, $n = 413$ and $P < 0.001$. *B*, Linear regressions (*broken lines*) and 95 per cent confidence limits (*solid lines*) of mean pressure (*top*) and pulse pressure (systolic-diastolic pressure amplitude) (*bottom*) on birth weight in 61 healthy newborn infants during the first 12 hours after birth. For mean pressure, $y = 5.16x + 29.80$; $n = 443$; $r = 0.80$. For pulse pressure, $y = 2.31x + 18.27$; $n = 413$; $r = 0.45$. For both, $P < 0.001$. (Reprinted with permission from Versmold, H.T., et al.: Aortic blood pressure during the first 12 hours of life in infants with birth weight of 610 to 4220 grams. Pediatrics, *67*:611, 1981. Copyright American Academy of Pediatrics 1981.)

normal metabolism and function. Average blood volume in newborn is 85 cc/kg. Normal newborn blood pressure is shown in Figure 16–11.

1. **Predisposing factors**[7,9]
   a. Intrapartum asphyxia
   b. Maternal bleeding
   c. Prematurity
   d. Maternal infection
   e. Breech delivery
   f. Ruptured umbilical or placental vessel
   g. Twins
   h. Early cord clamping
   i. Infant held higher than placenta when cord still pulsating
   j. Neonatal hemorrhage
   k. Neonatal infection

ETIOLOGY[7,9]

1. Asphyxia (vasoconstriction, vasodilatation and intravascular to extra-vascular fluid shift from damaged capillaries, and hypotension)
   a. Difficult breech delivery

      b. Prematurity

      c. Maternal infection

      d. Placental insufficiency in intrauterine growth retardation, infant of diabetic mother

2. Acute blood loss (hypovolemia/shock, inadequate cardiac output, hypoperfusion of vital organs, compensatory shunting of blood to brain and heart with peripheral vasoconstriction [gut, kidneys, skin] to maintain BP)

      a. Abruptio placentae or placenta previa

      b. Torn umbilical or placental vessel

      c. Neonatal hemorrhage

      d. Donor twin in twin to twin transfusion

3. Placental or umbilical hypoperfusion and transfusion

      a. Early cord clamping

      b. Holding infant higher than placenta when cord still pulsating (up to 55 per cent of blood volume can be delivered by uterine contractions in first minute of life, dependent on gravity)[41]

ASSESSMENT

1. Clinical presentation

      a. Signs and symptoms

         i. Apgar scores may be low

        ii. In 10 per cent blood loss

           (a) Mild hypotension

           (b) Slightly decreased urinary output

       iii. In 20 per cent blood loss

           (a) Pallor; cold skin

           (b) Increased capillary filling time: 4+ seconds

           (c) Decreased pulses: 1+ or absent

           (d) Tachypnea

           (e) Heart rate variable: tachycardia if blood loss mild or gradual, bradycardia if sudden and acute

           (f) Hypotension

           (g) Metabolic acidosis

           (h) Hypoglycemia

           (i) Decreased urinary output less than 1 cc/kg/hour

           (j) Disseminated intravascular coagulation if shock severe

           (k) Anemia: variable

2. Biopsychosocial assessment/diagnostic data

      a. Vital signs and BP (cuff in perfusion fair to good; intravascular if shock present)

      b. Color

      c. Pulses

      d. Capillary filling time

      e. Central venous pressure if possible

      f. Blood: hematocrit, arterial blood gas

      g. Often an acute, emergency event that is unexpected and shocking to parents; their perception of event is important

h. Support mechanisms
i. Coping mechanisms

PROBLEMS AND COMPLICATIONS

1. Death if blood loss is significant and shock is present
2. Necrotizing enterocolitis due to hypoperfusion of gut
3. Acute tubular necrosis and renal failure due to hypoperfusion of kidneys

PATIENT CARE MANAGEMENT

1. **Goals**
   a. To identify infant at risk
       i. Attendance of nursery personnel at delivery of infant with predisposing factors
       ii. Check and assess color, pulses, perfusion, arterial blood gases, vital signs, BP at birth and every 2 hours, or every 8 hours as needed if asymptomatic; continue if symptoms occur
       iii. Cardiorespiratory monitoring
   b. To correct shock
       i. Transfuse with 10 ml/kg whole blood, fresh frozen plasma, albumin, human plasma protein fraction (Plasmanate), Ringer's lactate, or normal saline (decreasing order of preference)

       COMMENTS/TIPS/CAUTIONS

       Choice of product varies with availability, time constraints, and hematocrit

   c. To prevent or treat complications
       i. Necrotizing enterocolitis
           (a) Nothing orally for 5–7 days in infants in shock or if 5 minute Apgar score is 6 or less
           (b) Measure abdominal girth on every shift
           (c) Test all stools for blood
       ii. Acute tubular necrosis
           (a) Measure intake and output

      (b) Check weight every 12–24 hours
      (c) Check specific gravity of urine with Labstix after each voiding

DISCHARGE PLANNING/TEACHING

1. Explanation of
   a. Diagnosis and prognosis
   b. Complications
   c. Follow-up

HYPERVISCOSITY SYNDROME

Hyperviscosity syndrome is a condition that has potentially damaging consequences for the newborn but that is easily treated. The nurse's immediate observation and assessment can identify the infant at risk, make the diagnosis, and initiate treatment.

DIAGNOSIS

Hyperviscosity syndrome is a serious complication due to sludging of the blood in small capillaries. It is often associated with polycythemia (hematocrit 65 per cent or greater). The sludging and obstruction of capillaries can cause neurological sequelae, necrotizing enterocolitis, cyanosis, respiratory distress, and renal problems.

1. **Incidence**
   a. 2.9 per cent at sea level, 5 per cent at high altitudes[61]
   b. Occurs only in term or near term infants
   c. Occurs within first 48 hours of life

2. **Predisposing factors**
   a. Late cord clamping, milking of cord
   b. Holding infant down while cord still pulsating
   c. Placental anastomosis of monochorionic diamnionic twins
   d. Chronic intrauterine hypoxia
   e. Preeclampsia
   f. Intrauterine growth retardation
   g. Postmaturity
   h. Diabetic pregnancy
   i. Down's syndrome
   j. High altitudes
   k. Twin pregnancy
   l. Chromosomal abnormalities
   m. Hypothermia
   n. Hypoxia
   o. Acidosis
   p. Hypoglycemia

ETIOLOGY

1. Three factors contribute to hyperviscosity[53,60]
   a. Increased number of erythrocytes: most significant in neonates
      i. Infants born at high altitudes
      ii. Chronic intrauterine hypoxia for placental dysfunction
         (a) Preeclampsia
         (b) Intrauterine growth retardation
         (c) Postmaturity
      iii. Infant of diabetic mother
      iv. Down's syndrome
      v. Placental transfusion
         (a) Late cord clamping
         (b) Milking of cord
         (c) Holding infant down while cord still pulsating
         (d) Placental anastomosis of monochorionic diamnionic twins
   b. Increased plasma viscosity: not very important in neonates
      i. Infants of diabetic mothers
   c. Impaired deformability of red blood cell membrane
      i. Newborn RBC membrane
      ii. When polycythemia occurs, newborn RBCs less able to fit together, resulting in greater viscosity at lower hematocrit values
      iii. Contributing conditions
         (a) Hypothermia
         (b) Hypoxia
         (c) Acidosis
         (d) Hypoglycemia
2. High viscosity causes sludging of blood flowing in small capillaries (brain, lungs, gut, and kidneys)

ASSESSMENT

1. **Clinical presentation**
   a. Signs and symptoms (in order of frequency)
      i. Plethora
(Of decreased cerebral blood flow)
      ii. Lethargy, hypotonia, difficult arousal
      iii. Tremors, seizures
      iv. Weak sucking, vomiting
(Of decreased pulmonary blood flow)
      v. Cyanosis
      vi. Respiratory distress
      vii. Congestive heart failure, cardiomegaly, metabolic derangements (increased work of heart with viscous blood)
      viii. Hypoglycemia
      ix. Hypocalcemia
(Hematological)
      x. Hyperbilirubinemia

      xi. Thrombocytopenia

(Of thrombosis)

      xii. Necrotizing enterocolitis

      xiii. Oliguria due to renal vein thrombosis

2. Biopsychosocial assessment

  a. Vital signs; character of respirations

  b. Neurological assessment

  c. Color

  d. Parents' understanding of syndrome, its short and long term effects

  e. Parents' understanding of treatment, its effects

3. Diagnostic data

  a. Hematocrit (venous hematocrit of 65 per cent or more is diagnostic; between 60 and 64 per cent may indicate hyperviscosity and blood should be tested with a microviscometer)

  b. Glucose (Dextrostix)

  c. Calcium

  d. Bilirubin

  e. Platelet count

PROBLEMS AND COMPLICATIONS

1. Cerebral vascular accident
2. Intraventricular hemorrhage
3. Neurological deficits
  a. Developmental delays
  b. Learning disorders, slowness
  c. Fine motor and speech abnormalities
  d. Spastic diplegia
  e. Paresis
4. Necrotizing enterocolitis
5. Renal vein thrombosis
6. Hyperbilirubinemia
7. Hypoglycemia

PATIENT CARE MANAGEMENT

1. Goals

  a. To identify infant at risk

    i. Obtain blood by heel stick for hematocrit determination at 3 hours of age in predisposed infant; determine venous hematocrit if value 65 per cent or greater

    ii. Glucose determination (Dextrostix) at birth and at 3 hours in predisposed infant

    iii. Close observation for signs and symptoms of complications

b. To prevent sequelae
    i. Partial exchange transfusion in infant with venous hematocrit of 65 per cent or greater, using 5 per cent albuminated saline to replace blood removed (see Appendix B)
    ii. Check viscosity of infant with venous hematocrit between 60 and 64. Exchange transfusion if hyperviscosity present

c. To identify and treat complications
    i. Close observation in nursery of infant at risk
    ii. Follow-up care

COMMENTS/TIPS/
CAUTIONS

By the time neurological symptoms occur, the damage is already done

Blood removed must be replaced to maintain blood volume; phlebotomy only increases viscosity by decreasing the flow of blood

DISCHARGE PLANNING/TEACHING

1. Education about syndrome, treatment, short and long term complications, and need for follow-up

—————————— NEONATAL COAGULOPATHIES ——————————

The bleeding newborn is at risk not only for death due to sudden or slow exsanguination but also for damage due to hemorrhages into vital organs such as brain, lungs, gut adrenals, and kidneys. Early signs of these coagulopathies in either the well or the already ill newborn can be as subtle as prolonged oozing from injection or puncture sites, most likely to be observed by the infant's nurse.

DIAGNOSIS

Neonatal coagulopathies are disturbances in the normal blood clotting mechanism caused either by congenital defects in that mechanism or by acute perinatal events that alter that mechanism.

1. **Predisposing factors**
    a. Acute perinatal hypoxia or asphyxia
    b. Infection
    c. Maternal disease
    d. Neonatal disease
    e. History of hereditary clotting disorder

Well infants
1. Immune-mediated thrombocytopenia
2. Nonimmune thrombocytopenia
3. Hemorrhagic disease of the newborn
4. Clotting factor deficiencies
5. Trauma

Sick infants

1. Disseminated intravascular coagulation (DIC)
2. Platelet consumption
3. Liver disease
4. Organ system hemorrhages

Site and character of bleeding

1. Generalized petechiae, small superficial ecchymoses, and mucosal bleeding indicate platelet abnormality
2. Larger ecchymoses, localized bleeding (cephalhematomas, umbilical cord bleeding, gastrointestinal bleeding), and diffuse bleeding from several sites (puncture sites, mucous membranes) indicate a generalized coagulation problem such as hemorrhagic disease of the newborn, DIC, or liver disease

ETIOLOGY

1. **Normal newborn clotting**[18,24]
   a. Interaction of platelet plug and fibrin clot formed from plasma proteins (Table 16-1)
   b. Proteins occur in "cascade" effect in which tissue injury initiates a series of reactions; one factor activates the next, which activates the next
   c. Cascade begins with factor XII and works backward to factor I
   d. Divided into two pathways (Fig. 16-12)
      i. Intrinsic pathway, measured by PTT, factors I, II, V, VIII, IX, X, XI, XII
      ii. Extrinsic pathway, measured by PT, factors I, II, V, VII, X
   e. Deficiencies in clotting in normal newborn
      i. Platelets: normal number, transient abnormal function
      ii. Vitamin K dependent factors (II, VII, IX, X) reduced at birth and further reduced within first few days
         (a) Prevented by prophylactic administration of vitamin K

TABLE 16-1. CLOTTING FACTORS

I.	Fibrinogen
II.	Prothrombin
III.	Tissue thromboplastin
IV.	Calcium
V.	Proaccelerin
VII.	Proconvertin
VIII.	Antihemophilic factor A
IX.	Antihemophilic factor B, Christmas factor
X.	Stuart
XI.	Plasma thromboplastin antecedent
XII.	Hageman factor
XIII.	Fibrin stabilizing factor

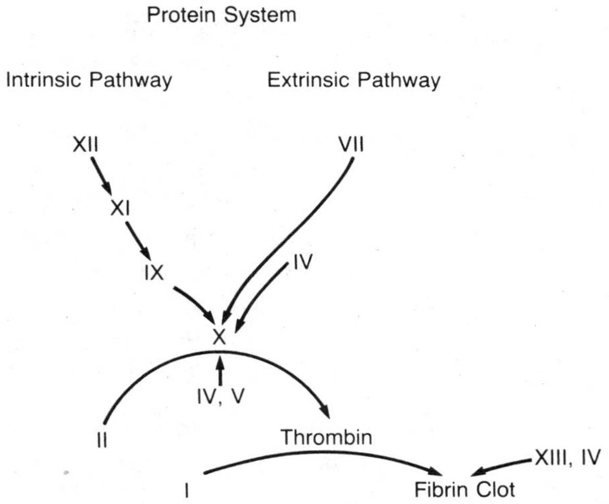

Protein System

Intrinsic Pathway   Extrinsic Pathway

XII   VII

XI

Figure 16-12. Protein system in normal clotting.

IX   IV

X

IV, V

II   Thrombin

XIII, IV

I   Fibrin Clot

        (b)   Transient hepatic immaturity in premature results in poor response to vitamin K
     iii. Factors I, V, VIII: normal levels
     iv. Factors XI, XII, XIII: mildly reduced
  f. Maternal clotting factors do not cross placenta because of large molecular size

2. Coagulopathies in well infant[18]
  a. Immune thrombocytopenia occurs secondary to transfer to maternal IgG antibody across placenta → coats infant's platelets → premature destruction
      i. Isoimmune thrombocytopenia: Infant's platelets contain antigen that mother lacks; leakage of fetal platelets across placenta stimulates maternal antibody production and antibodies enter fetal circulation
        (a) Little significant bleeding, occasional hemorrhage
        (b) Usually occurs in first born, with 85 per cent recurrence rate
     ii. Immune thrombocytopenia secondary to maternal disease: differs in that antibody directed at antigen common to *all* platelets
        (a) Maternal thrombocytopenia
        (b) No significant bleeding beyond first few days
  b. Nonimmune thrombocytopenia
      i. Due to platelets being used up
        (a) Occult infection
        (b) Localized thrombosis
     ii. Due to decreased platelet production, rare
        (a) Bone marrow hypoplasia (leukemia, aplastic anemia)
        (b) Hereditary defects in production
  c. Hemorrhagic disease of newborn (HDN), vitamin K deficiency
      i. Occurs when vitamin K not given or mother receiving medication that impairs function (coumarin, hydantoin)
     ii. Well infant unless significant blood loss occurs

      iii. Occurs more often in breast fed infant, who is deficient in intestinal bacteria on which production of vitamin K is dependent

  d. Hereditary clotting factor deficiencies (hemophilia A and B, von Willebrand's disease)

      i. 99 per cent of all factor deficiencies

      ii. Bleeding rare in neonates

  e. Local vascular factors

      i. Birth trauma: bruises, petechiae

      ii. Gastrointestinal hemorrhage: swallowed maternal blood, stress ulcer

3. Coagulopathies in sick infant[18]

  a. Disseminated intravascular coagulation (DIC, consumption coagulopathy)

      i. History: trigger event (Table 16–2) causes inappropriate activation of clotting and consumption of clotting factors and platelets[10,44]

TABLE 16–2. TRIGGER EVENTS FOR DIC

Hypoxia and acidosis due to neonatal disease
  Hyaline membrane disease
  Necrotizing enterocolitis
  Shock
  Birth asphyxia
  Severe Rh disease

Infection

Maternal factors
  Abruptio placentae
  Dead twin
  Eclampsia

      ii. Consumption of clotting factors and platelets results in diffuse bleeding, localized hemorrhage, and thrombosis

  b. Platelet consumptive disorders

      i. Bacterial septicemia

      ii. Thrombosis

      iii. Intrauterine infection

  c. Liver disease

      i. Almost all clotting factors synthesized in liver

      ii. Liver disease results in decreased production of clotting factors and generalized hemorrhage

      iii. Hepatitis or cirrhosis

        (a) Intrauterine infection

        (b) Metabolic disorders (galactosemia)

        (c) Alpha$_1$-antitrypsin deficiency (rare)

  d. Organ hemorrhage

      i. More frequent in prematures

      ii. Local factors plus normal newborn deficiencies

        (a) Hypoxia and acidosis
        (b) Hyperosmolarity
        (c) Delivery trauma
     iii. Mostly pulmonary or CNS

ASSESSMENT

1. **Clinical presentation**
   a. Signs and symptoms
      i. Immune thrombocytopenia
         (a) Well infant
         (b) Bleeding rare
      ii. Nonimmune thrombocytopenia
         (a) Well infant
         (b) Possibly localized thrombosis or occult infection
         (c) Thrombocytopenia; other tests normal
      iii. HDN
         (a) Well infant: but history of vitamin K_2 never given after birth
         (b) Occurs at 2 to 4 days of age
         (c) Cutaneous, umbilical, gastrointestinal, CNS hemorrhage
      iv. Hereditary clotting disorders
         (a) Well infant, usually male
         (b) Bleeding uncommon; can follow circumcision
      v. Local vascular factors
         (a) Well infant
         (b) Bruises, petechiae
         (c) Screening tests normal
      vi. DIC
         (a) Sick infant
         (b) History of triggering event
         (c) Diffuse bleeding at puncture sites, mucous membranes
         (d) Localized gastrointestinal or umbilical hemorrhage, or localized thrombosis, or both
      vii. Platelet consumption
         (a) Sick infant
      viii. Liver disease
         (a) Sick infant
         (b) Jaundice (increased direct bilirubin)
         (c) Hepatomegaly
         (d) Liver function tests abnormal
      ix. Organ hemorrhages
         (a) Sick premature infant
         (b) Tests normal
         (c) Pulmonary or CNS hemorrhage
         (d) Bradycardia and hypotension with significant blood loss
2. **Biopsychosocial assessment**
   a. Well or sick infant
   b. History of bleeding: timing, character, location
   c. Vital signs, BP

TABLE 16–3. SCREENING TESTS FOR COAGULOPATHIES*

Tests	Normal Term	Normal Premature	HDN	Inherited Defects	DIC	Immune ↓ plts	Liver Disease	Plt Consump
Plt count (per cu mm)	150–400,000	150–400,000	N	N	↓	↓	N	↓
PT (sec)	≤18	≤21	↑	N	↑	N	↑	N
PTT (sec)	≤55	≤65	↑	↑	↑	N	↑	N
Fibrinogen (mg/100 ml)	200–300	130–400	N	N	↓	N	↓	N
FSP (µg/ml)	<7	<10	N	N	↑	N	↑	↑

*Values may vary in different laboratories.
HDN, hemolytic disease of newborn; DIC, disseminated intravascular coagulation; plt, platelets; PT, prothrombin time; PTT, partial thromboplastin time; FSP, fibrin split products; N, normal.

    d. Parents' understanding of diagnosis, treatment, prognosis
    e. Support mechanisms
    f. Coping mechanisms

3. Diagnostic data
    a. Primary laboratory clotting studies
       i. Platelet count, prothrombin time (PT), partial thromboplastin time (PTT)
      ii. Secondary tests, depending on above results and clinical condition fibrinogen, fibrin degradation products (fibrin split products [FSP], assays of various clotting factors

PROBLEMS AND COMPLICATIONS

1. Death from coagulopathy or underlying disease; rate can be as high as 60–80 per cent in DIC
2. Damage from organ hemorrhages
    a. Intracranial: neurologic sequelae
    b. Pulmonary: require mechanical ventilation
    c. Gastrointestinal: require parenteral alimentation
    d. Renal: oliguria and ischemic damage from thrombosis
    e. Adrenal

PATIENT CARE MANAGEMENT

1. Goals

COMMENTS/TIPS/ CAUTIONS

    a. To identify infant at risk
       i. Close observation of infants with risk factors for any prolonged bleeding
      ii. Primary screening tests if prolonged bleeding occurs
    b. To treat disorder when diagnosed
       i. Isoimmune thrombocytopenia
         (a) Transfusion with antigen-free platelets

Platelet transfusion is not helpful since antibody is directed toward antigen common to all platelets

if count less than 30,000

ii. Immune thrombocytopenia
   (a) Steroids (prednisone 2 mg/kg/day) if count 10,000 or less or bleeding

iii. Nonimmune thrombocytopenia
   (a) Treatment of underlying disease

iv. HDN
   (a) Vitamin K
   (b) Fresh frozen plasma 10–15 ml/kg transfusion every 8–24 hours for severe bleeding

v. Hereditary disorders
   (a) Minimal bleeding: local pressure, fresh frozen plasma as above
   (b) Severe bleeding: transfusion of factor concentrate (amount depends on severity of bleeding)

vi. Local factors
   (a) No treatment needed

vii. DIC
   (a) Treatment of underlying disease
   (b) Repeated platelet transfusions (1 unit every 12 to 24 hours) and fresh frozen plasma transfusions (10 to 15 ml/kg every 12 to 24 hours)
   (c) Heparin (see Appendix B)
   (d) Exchange transfusion with fresh whole blood for infant who continues to bleed

viii. Platelet consumption
   (a) Treatment of underlying disease

COMMENTS/TIPS/CAUTIONS

Controversy exists as to accepted treatment; some believe platelets or plasma given without heparin to arrest consumptive process will only add to the disease, but experience does not bear this out; use of heparin is very controversial, since dosage and effects are difficult to monitor and control, and it has not been shown to increase survival; it is used in those infants with DIC who also have localized thrombosis

Supplies clotting factors and platelets while removing toxins and FSP; adult RBCs have lesser affinity for oxygen and may deliver O_2 to tissues better and reduce tissue damage

    (b) Platelet transfusion for bleeding or count of 10,000 or less

  ix. Liver disease

    (a) Treatment of underlying disease

    (b) Vitamin K

    (c) Transfusion with fresh frozen plasma

  x. Organ hemorrhage

    (a) Treatment for volume loss

    (b) Treatment of underlying cause

DISCHARGE PLANNING/TEACHING

1. Education about diagnosis, treatment, prognosis, and need for follow-up

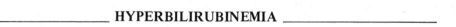

HYPERBILIRUBINEMIA

Hyperbilirubinemia in the newborn carries the risk of kernicterus, a serious condition causing serious neurological impairment. Early diagnosis and appropriate treatment can virtually eliminate this risk.

DIAGNOSIS

Hyperbilirubinemia is an increase in unconjugated serum bilirubin caused by either overproduction of bilirubin or deficiency in its conjugation.

1. **Incidence**
   a. Occurs in 50 per cent of term infants, 80 per cent of preterm[44]

2. **Predisposing factors**
   a. Blood group incompatibility with mother
   b. Prematurity
   c. Infection
   d. Birth trauma
   e. Polycythemia
   f. Maternal or neonatal metabolic or endocrine disorders
   g. Malfunction of gastrointestinal tract

ETIOLOGY

1. **Conjugation and excretion of bilirubin**
   a. Hemoglobin in cells of the reticuloendothelial system is broken down into biliverdin, which is converted to bilirubin, which is released into the circulation where it combines with albumin (unconjugated [indirect] bilirubin)

    b. In the liver (endoplasmic reticulum): this bilirubin-albumin complex is dissociated and carried to the hepatocyte by y-protein, where it reacts with UDPGA and glucuronyl transferase (in presence of glucose and O_2), to become conjugated (direct) bilirubin and moves into the bile ducts and gallbladder

    c. From bile ducts and gallbladder, the direct bilirubin is transferred to gastrointestinal system

    d. In the intestines, there are two pathways

        i. Reconverted to unconjugated bilirubin and either reabsorbed across intestinal mucosa (recirculated via enterohepatic circulation) or excreted in stool

        ii. Bacterial action forms urobilinogen, which is either excreted in stool or reabsorbed by the liver or kidney and excreted in the urine

2. **Common causes**[43,31]

    a. Overproduction of bilirubin

        i. Physiological jaundice (normal)

            (a) Increased RBCs

            (b) Decreased life span of RBCs

            (c) Increased enterohepatic circulation

            (d) Defective uptake

            (e) Defective conjugation

            (f) Reduction of hepatic blood supply during transitional circulation

        ii. Hemolytic anemias

            (a) Congenital defects of RBCs—glucose-6-phosphate dehydrogenase (G6PD), sickle cell

            (b) Acquired defects—blood group incompatibilities, drugs

        iii. Infection

        iv. Extravascular blood

        v. Polycythemia

        vi. Gastrointestinal obstruction

    b. Deficient conjugation

        i. Congenital defects in glucuronyl transferase

        ii. Breast milk jaundice

    c. Undefined mechanism

        i. Maternal diabetes

        ii. Neonatal hypothyroidism

        iii. Galactosemia

        iv. Down's syndrome

ASSESSMENT

1. **Clinical presentation**

    a. Signs and symptoms

        i. Jaundice prior to 36 hours of age or persisting after 8 days

        ii. Total bilirubin 12 mg/100 ml or more, rising by more than 5 mg/24 hours

        iii. Lethargy, poor feeding

        iv. Hydrops fetalis

      (a) Generalized edema, including ascites, pleural effusion, pulmonary edema

      (b) Hemolysis leads to decreased intravascular colloid osmotic pressure cause fluid shift to extravascular space

      (c) Severe hemolytic anemias

b. First day of life
  i. Blood group incompatibility
  ii. Very large hematomas
  iii. Severe infection

d. On second or third day of life
  i. Mild blood group incompatibility
  ii. Polycythemia
  iii. Infection
  iv. Congenital RBC defects
  v. Enclosed hemorrhage
  vi. Physiological jaundice

d. On third through seventh day
  i. Breast feeding
  ii. Maternal drugs
  iii. Congenital conjugation defects

e. In second week
  i. Hepatitis
  ii. Biliary tract obstruction
  iii. Biliary atresia
  iv. Galactosemia
  v. Hypothyroidism
  vi. Infection

f. History
  i. This pregnancy, delivery
  ii. Hyperbilirubinemia of previous children, treatment
  iii. Neonatal: time of onset, symptoms, rate of rise (mg per hour)

2. **Biopsychosocial assessment**
  a. Jaundice: severity, extent
  b. Liver size
  c. Neurological examination
  d. Weight, vital signs
  e. The parents' anxiety and their ability to cope with this illness depend not only on their usual coping methods and their support systems but also on
    i. Severity of jaundice or underlying illness (i.e., whether due to breast feeding or severe Rh disease)
    ii. Previous experience with this disease
    iii. Treatment
    iv. Degree of separation of family unit caused by illness and treatment

3. **Diagnostic data**
  a. Maternal screening tests
    i. Indirect Coombs'

      ii. Blood and Rh type
     iii. VDRL (Venereal Disease Research Laboratory)
  b. Infant screening tests
      i. Direct Coombs'
      ii. Blood and Rh type; CBC; platelets and reticulocyte counts
     iii. Total and direct bilirubin (difference = indirect)
     iv. Albumin or total protein
      v. Glucose (Dextrostix)
     vi. pH
    vii. Cultures if sepsis indicated as cause

PROBLEMS AND COMPLICATIONS

1. Kernicterus (deposit of unconjugated bilirubin primarily with neurons, but also renal tubular cells, intestinal mucosa, and pancreatic cells, causing interference with metabolic activities and necrosis)
  a. Caused by unconjugated bilirubin not bound to albumin ("free bilirubin"): bilirubin-albumin complex too large a molecule to pass through blood-brain barrier
  b. Degree of bilirubin bound to albumin influenced by
      i. Reductions in albumin pool
        (a) Prematurity
        (b) Hypoproteinemia
      ii. Agents binding albumin and displacing bilirubin
        (a) Free fatty acids and bile acids
        (b) Drugs (sulfonamides, salicylates, furosemide, cephalothin, heparin)
        (c) Conjugated bilirubin
     iii. Respiratory or metabolic acidosis: displaces bilirubin
     iv. Asphyxia
  c. *Phase I:* hypotonia, vomiting, lethargy, high-pitched cry, poor sucking, decreased Moro reflex
  d. *Phase II:* spasticity, opisthotonos, hyperpyrexia
  e. *Phase III:* decreased spasticity, sunsetting eyes, convulsions; 75 per cent succumb with gastric, pulmonary, or CNS hemorrhage
  f. *Phase IV:* survivors have athetoid cerebral palsy, deafness, mental retardation, loss of vertical gaze, visual and motor incoordination

PATIENT CARE MANAGEMENT

1. Goals
  a. To recognize infant at risk
      i. Close observation of infant with predisposing factors
      ii. Bilirubin testing at birth every 6 hours in infants with known hemolytic anemia

Serum Bilirubin mg/100 ml	Birth weight	<24 hrs	24-48 hrs	49-72 hrs	>72 hrs
<5	ALL				
5-9	ALL	PHOTO-THERAPY IF HEMOLYSIS			
10-14	<2500Gm	EXCHANGE IF HEMOLYSIS	PHOTOTHERAPY		
	>2500Gm			INVESTIGATE IF BILIRUBIN >12 mg	
15-19	<2500Gm	EXCHANGE		CONSIDER EXCHANGE	
	>2500Gm		PHOTOTHERAPY		
20 and+	ALL		EXCHANGE		

Figure 16-13. Guidelines for the management of hyperbilirubinemia. (Reprinted with permission from Avery, G.: Neonatology, 2nd ed. Philadelphia, J.B. Lippincott Co., 1981, p. 511.)

☐ Observe   ▨ Investigate Jaundice

Use phototherapy after any exchange

In presence of:
1. Perinatal asphyxia
2. Respiratory distress
3. Metabolic acidosis (pH 7.25 or below)
4. Hypothermia (temp below 35° C)
5. Low serum protein (5g/100 ml or less)
6. Birth weight <1500 Gm
7. Signs of clinical or CNS deterioration

} Treat as in next higher bilirubin category

iii. Screening tests as above in infants with jaundice in first 36 hours of life

iv. Bilirubin testing in infant jaundiced after 36 hours or after 8 days; testing as indicated by level and rate of rise

b. To prevent kernicterus (Fig. 16-13)
    i. Phototherapy
      (a) Infant unclothed in incubator or radiant warmer
      (b) Eyes covered
      (c) Head covered
      (d) Bank of cool white fluorescent lamps changed after 2000 hours; plexiglass cover

COMMENTS/TIPS/CAUTIONS

Normal physiological jaundice occurs after 36 hours

Test further infant with total bilirubin greater than 12 mg/100 ml or rate of rise greater than 5 mg/24 hours[9]

Free bilirubin absorbs light energy and transfers it to oxygen causing oxidation of bilirubin; may be used prophylactically in severely bruised small premature infant or infant with hemolytic disease awaiting exchange

Protection from retinal damage

Reports of hypocalcemia

Plexiglass cover provides protection from breakage and ultraviolet light

(e) Monitor intake and output, urinary specific gravity, water loss from loose stools, daily weight, skin turgor, fontanel depression, sagittal suture approximation; temperature every 4 hours; bilirubin at least every 12 hours. After phototherapy discontinued monitor bilirubin for rebound

ii. Exchange transfusion (see Appendix B)

COMMENTS/TIPS/CAUTIONS

Phototherapy causes increased insensible water loss; state of hydration must be monitored and fluids increased as needed, dehydration will increase bilirubin level

Phototherapy causes hyperthermia

DISCHARGE PLANNING/TEACHING

1. **Education about:**
   a. Etiology and physiology of hyperbilirubinemia
   b. Effects of hyperbilirubinemia
   c. Rationale and procedure for treatment
   d. Possible separation of family unit during treatment
   e. Difficulties anticipated after discharge
   f. Need for follow-up

CONCLUSIONS

The birth of an infant is usually an eagerly anticipated, joyful, family event. Malfunction of the cardiovascular-hematological systems due to a structural abnormality or a perinatal difficulty can change this happy time into a stressful crisis.

Each of the problems discussed in this chapter can be life threatening or cause serious sequelae. However, early recognition and prompt treatment based on both identification of the infant at risk and understanding the pathophysiology and rationale of treatment can prevent death and decrease complications in many cases.

Every nurse involved with the birth process has a responsibility to be aware of these problems in order that treatment can be initiated before irreversible complications occur. Such prompt nursing action helps give every infant the maximum opportunity to survive these crises and become the normal, healthy infant the family expected.

REFERENCES

1. Agarwala, B., and Baffes, T.: Congestive heart failure in the infant. Heart Lung, 5(1):62–70, 1976.
2. Alexander, M.M., and Brown, M.S.: Pediatric History Taking and Physical Diagnosis for Nurses. New York, McGraw-Hill Book Co., 1979.

3. Allen, J.P., and Chilcote, R.: Transient erythrocytosis during the neonatal period: Possible neurologic complications. South. Med. J., *72*:681–683, 1979.
4. Amanullah, A.: Neonatal jaundice. Am. J. Dis. Child., *130*:1274–1280, 1976.
5. Amit, M., and Camfield, P.R.: Neonatal polycythemia causing multiple cerebral infarcts. Arch. Neurol., *37*:109–110, 1980.
6. Anthony, C.L., Arnon, R.G., and Fitch, C.W.: Pediatric Cardiology. Garden City, N.Y. Medical Examination Publishing Company, 1979.
7. Avery, G.B.: Neonatology, 2nd ed. Philadelphia, J.B. Lippincott Co., 1981.
8. Buchanan, G.P.: Neonatal coagulation: Normal physiology and pathophysiology. Clin. Haematol., *7*:85–109, 1978.
9. Cloherty, J.P., and Startk, A.R.: Manual of Neonatal Care. Boston, Little, Brown & Co., 1980.
10. Corrigan, J.J.: Activation of coagulation and disseminated intravascular coagulation in the newborn. Am. J. Pediatr. Hematol./Oncol., *1*:245–249, 1979.
11. Drummond, W.H., Gregory, G.A., Heyman, M.A., and Phibbs, R.A.: The independent effects of hyperventilation, tolazoline, and dopamine on infants with persistent pulmonary hypertension. J. Pediatr., *98*:603–611, 1981.
12. Drummond, W.H., Peckham, G.J., and Fox, W.W.: The clinical profile of the newborn with persistent pulmonary hypertension. Clin. Pediatr., *16*:335–341, 1977.
13. Engel, M.A.: Cyanotic congenital heart disease. Am. Cardiol., *37*:283–308, 1976.
14. Ferrera, A., and Hardin, A.: Emergency Transfer of the High Risk Neonate. St. Louis, C.V. Mosby Co., 1980.
15. Fink, B.: Congenital Heart Disease: A Deductive Approach to Its Diagnosis. Chicago, Yearbook Medical Publishers, 1975.
16. Fox, W.W., Gerwitz, M., Dinwiddie, R., Drummond, W.H., and Peckham, G.J.: Pulmonary hypertension in the perinatal aspiration syndromes. Pediatrics, *59*:205–211, 1977.
17. Gersony, W.M., Duc, G.V., and Sinclair, J.C.: PFC syndrome (persistence of the fetal circulation). Circulation, *40*(Suppl. 3):87, 1969.
18. Glader, B.E., and Buchanan, G.R.: The bleeding neonate. Pediatrics, *58*:548–555, 1976.
19. Glider, J.H., Sacksteder, S., Sutton, P., Kreuz, J., and Quirk, T.R.: Congenital heart defects: Pre- and post-operative nursing care. Am. J. Nurs., *78*:273–278, 1978.
20. Goetzman, B.W., Sunshine, P., Johnson, J., Wennberg, R., Hackel, A., Merten, D., Bartoletti, A., and Silverman, N.: Neonatal hypoxia and pulmonary vasospasm: Response to tolazoline. J. Pediatr., *89*:617–621, 1976.
21. Gross, G.P., Hathaway, W.E., and McGaughey, H.R.: Hypervisosity in the neonate. J. Pediatr., *82*:1004–1012, 1973.
22. Guneroth, W.G.: Initial evaluation of the child for heart disease. Pediatr. Clin. North Am., *25*:657–675, 1978.
23. Gupta, J.M. Neonatal jaundice. Med. J. Austr., *1*:745–747, 1977.
24. Guyton, A.C.: Textbook of Medical Physiology, 6th ed. Philadelphia, W.B. Saunders Co., 1981.
25. Hakanson, D.O., and Oh, W.: Necrotizing enterocolitis and hyperviscosity in the newborn infant. J. Pediatr., *90*:458–461, 1977.
26. Hathaway, W.E.: The bleeding newborn. Clin. Perinatol., *1*:83–97, 1975.
27. Hawker, R.E.: Cardiac failure in infancy and childhood. Med. J. Austr., *1*:408–410, 1977.
28. Haworth, S.G.: Normal structural and functional adaptation to extrauterine life. J. Pediatr., *98*:915–918, 1981.
29. Haworth, S.G., and Reid, L.: Persistent fetal circulation: Newly recognized structural features. J. Pediatr., *88*:614–620, 1976.
30. Hoffman, J.I., and Christianson, R.: Congenital heart disease in a cohort of 19,502 births with long-term follow-up. Am. J. Cardiol., *42*:641–647, 1978.
31. Lanzkowsky, P.: Erythroblastosis fetalis. Pediatric Ann., 3(2): 7–34, 1974.
32. Leake, R.D., Thanopoulis, B., and Nieberg, R.: Hyperviscosity syndrome associated with necrotizing enterocolitis. Am. J. Dis. Child., *129*:1192–1194, 1975.

33. Levin, D.L., Cates, L., Newfeld, E.A., Muster, A.J., and Paul, M.A.: Persistence of the fetal cardiopulmonary circulatory pathway: Survival of an infant after a prolonged course. Pediatrics, 56:58–64, 1975.
34. Levin, D.L., Heymann, M.A., Kitterman, J.A., Gregory, G.A., Phibbs, R.A., and Rudolph, A.M.: Persistent pulmonary hypertension of the newborn infant. J. Pediatr., 89:626–630, 1976.
35. Levin, D.L., Hyman, A.I., Heymann, M.A., and Rudolph, A.M.: Fetal hypertension and the development of increased pulmonary vascular smooth muscle: A possible mechanism for persistent pulmonary hypertension of the newborn infant. J. Pediatr., 92:265–269, 1978.
36. Levin, D.L., Mills, L.J., and Weinberg, A.G.: Hemodynamic, pulmonary, vascular and myocardial abnormalities secondary to pharmacologic constriction of the fetal ductus arteriosus. Circulation, 60:360–364, 1979.
37. Mentzer, W.C.: Polycythaemia and the hyperviscosity syndrome in newborn infants. Clin. Haematol., 7(1):63–74, 1978.
38. Mercer, R.T.: Nursing Care for Parents at Risk. Thorofare, N.J., Charles B. Slack, 1977.
39. Miller, G.M., Black, V.D., and Lubchenco, L.O.: Intracerebral hemorrhage in a term newborn with hyperviscosity. Am. J. Dis. Child., 135:377–378, 1981.
40. Murphy, J.D., Rabinovitch, M., Goldstein, J.D., and Reid, L.M.: The structural basis of persistent pulmonary hypertension of the newborn infant. J. Pediatr., 98(6):962–967, 1981.
41. Paxson, C.L.: Neonatal shock in the first postnatal day. Am. J. Dis. Child., 132:509–514, 1978.
42. Peckham, G.J., and Fox, W.W.: Physiologic factors affecting pulmonary artery pressure in infants with persistent pulmonary hypertension. J. Pediatr., 93:1005–1010, 1978.
43. Peevy, K.J., Landaw, S.A., and Gross, S.S.: Hyperbilirubinemia in infants of diabetic mothers. Pediatrics, 66:417–419, 1980.
44. Perez, R.H.: Protocols for Perinatal Nursing Practice, St. Louis, C.V. Mosby Co., 1981.
45. Roberts, N.K., Child, J.S., and Cabeen, W.R.: Congestive cardiac failure in a twenty-day-old infant. West. J. Med., 133:91–94, 1980.
46. Rowe, R.D., Freedam, R.M., Mehrizi, A., and Bloom, K.: The Neonate with Congenital Heart Disease, 2nd ed. Philadelphia, W.B. Saunders Co., 1981.
47. Riemenschneider, T., Nielsen, H., Ruttenberg, H., and Jaffe, R.: Disturbances of the transitional circulation: Spectrum of pulmonary hypertension and myocardial dysfunction. J. Pediatr., 89:622–625, 1976.
48. Rudolph, A.M.: Congenital Diseases of the Heart. Chicago, Year Book Medical Publishers, 1974.
49. Rudolph, A.M., High pulmonary vascular resistance after birth. Clin. Pediatr., 19:585–589, 1980.
50. Sacksteder, S.: Congenital heart defects: Embryology and fetal circulation. Am. J. Nurs., 78:262–265, 1978.
51. Sacksteder, S., Gildea, J.H., and Dassy, C.: Common congenital heart defects. Am. J. Nurs., 78:266–272, 1978.
52. Saucier, P.H.: Persistent fetal circulation. J. Obstet. Gynecol. Neonat. Nurs., 9:50–53, 1980.
53. Sheftel, D.N.: Neonatal polycythemia and the hyperviscosity syndrome. Wis. Med. J., 80(2):39–40, 1981.
54. Shor, V.Z.: Congenital heart defects: Assessment and case-finding. Am. J. Nurs., 78:256–261, 1978.
55. Siassi, B., Goldberg, S.J., Emmanouilides, G., Higashino, S., and Lewis, E.: Persistent pulmonary vascular obstruction in newborn infants. J. Pediatr., 78:610–615, 1971.
56. Stevens, K., and Wirth, F.: Incidence of neonatal hyperviscosity at sea level. J. Pediatr., 97:118–119, 1980.

57. Thaler, M.M.: Jaundice in early infancy. Pediatr. Ann., *6:*286-297, 1977.
58. Tudehope, D.I.: Persistent pulmonary hypertension of the newborn. M. J. Aust., *1*:13-15, 1979.
59. Turner, T.L.: Neonatal coagulation defects. Clin. Endocrinol. Metab., *5*:89-106, 1976.
60. Wesenberg, R.: Neonatal thick blood syndrome. Hosp. Pract., *13*(5):139-140, 145, 1978.
61. Wirth, F.H., Goldberg, K.E., and Lubchemco, L.O.: Neonatal hyperviscosity: I. Incidence. Pediatrics, *63*:833-836, 1979.
62. Woods, W.G., Luban, N.L.C., Hilartner, M.W., and Miller, D.: Disseminated intravascular coagulation in the newborn. Am. J. Dis. Child., *133*:44-46, 1979.

CHAPTER 17

NEUROLOGICAL CRISES

Kathy A. Hausman, R.N., M.S., C.C.R.N.

OBJECTIVES

Upon completion of this chapter the reader will be able to accomplish the following:

1. Define spina bifida cystica, meningocele, and myelomeningocele
2. State three nursing care modalities in the postoperative care of the child with myelomeningocele
3. Define seizure
4. State at least five items that must be charted after a seizure is observed
5. Define hydrocephalus
6. List three complications that may occur after insertion of a shunt for hydrocephalus
7. List the two major causative organisms of neonatal meningitis
8. List six signs and symptoms of neonatal meningitis
9. Distinguish between asphyxia and hypoxic ischemic encephalopathy
10. List two reasons for close observation of the infant's cardiovascular status after asphyxia
11. Define intracranial hemorrhage and list three types
12. List three nursing goals in the care of the infant with an intracranial hemorrhage

The brain is one of the most complex organs of the human body. At birth the full term infant's brain weighs approximately 330 gm and has its full complement of brain cells. The neonate's brain is highly susceptible to insult, and once damaged the cells do not recover. Factors such as asphyxia, metabolic dysfunction, radiation, maternal illness, or infection often lead to permanent neurological dysfunction. The neurological defects may be extensive, involving the brain, spinal cord, and surrounding bone and skin, or relatively minor, with a gradually improving neurological status.

The first step in treating the neonate with a neurological problem is to stabilize the condition; particular attention is paid to establishing an airway, obtaining appropriate laboratory work, and treating the underlying cause of dysfunction, if known. As soon as possible a detailed history is obtained from the infant's mother, father,and significant others as indicated. Attention is focused on prenatal and perinatal events. Information about events that occurred during the third to fifth week of gestation are important because that was the period of neural tube development. Disruption of normal neural development may lead to multiple defects such as spina bifida or anencephaly. Details of events that occurred during labor and delivery are significant and often provide valuable clues to the baby's problem. Traumatic injuries and asphyxia and hypoxia are often associated with difficult delivery; prolonged labor or premature rupture of the membranes may lead to sepsis.

The neonate's gestational age is estimated by the pediatrician or neonatologist in the standard format. This provides information concerning the etiology, diagnosis, and methods of treatment. The infant is observed at rest for signs of gross abnormalities, abnormal positioning, or movements, as well as for signs of trauma. Particular attention is paid to the head. The circumference is measured and plotted on the appropriate graph. The size of the anterior fontannel is noted, as well as placement of the metopic and coronal sutures. The neonate's level of consciousness is observed for appropriateness to gestational age. Finally, the infant's cranial nerves, reflexes, and muscle tone are tested. The examination is concluded by transillumination of the head, if feasible.

Once the history and examination of the infant are completed a more thorough diagnostic work-up and treatment plan can be initiated. Additional laboratory work may be obtained or special x-ray examination ordered such as computerized axial tomography. Other diagnostic tests include electroencephalography or echography. More invasive tests such as a lumbar puncture or cerebral angiography may be necessary.

The role of the nurse throughout this initial diagnostic period as well as throughout the infant's hospitalization cannot be underemphasized. Nursing observations are crucial in recognizing potential problems as well as for accurately recording the infant's response to the various treatments. The nurse's role is not limited to providing care for the infant. The family looks to the professional for support, guidance, and education as they await their infant's homecoming.

This chapter will present the major neurological defects commonly encountered by the neonatal nurse. These dysfunctions include asphyxia and hypoxia, intracranial hemorrhage, seizures, hydrocephalus, meningitis, and myelomeningocele. Particular emphasis is placed on clinical observations. Nursing management is presented in global terms that will be useful to nurses in a variety of health care settings.

MYELOMENINGOCELE

Myelomeningocele is a defect of the central nervous system that requires prompt surgical intervention to prevent infection and worsening of the neurological condition. In the past, these defects were not treated. The infant was given supportive care, and usually died within a few months. Now, however, as a result of advances in medical, surgical, and nursing techniques, the defect is repaired and the associated problems are managed. The nurse plays an instrumental role in supporting the parents in their decision to treat or not to treat the child. Further, if surgical intervention is carried out, the nurse must give direct care to the infant and provide the teaching necessary for the parents to care for the infant at home.

If multiple anomalies are present, the physician may recommend only supportive care of the infant. This may be the case if the neonate has complete paralysis below L-1, hydrocephalus at birth, rachischisis, and multiple anomalies involving other major organs.

DIAGNOSIS

Distinction must be made between myelomeningocele and meningocele. These defects are collectively referred to as spina bifida cystica as they both include an open posterior vertebral arch through which the meninges herniate. In addition, myelomeningocele includes herniation of the spinal cord parenchyma as well as spinal nerve roots.

Meningocele is generally covered by skin, meninges, or dura and usually there is no motor, sensory, reflex, or sphincter loss.

Myelomeningocele (Fig. 17–1) is covered by thin membrane, which may tear and leak cerebrospinal fluid. Neurological dysfunction is present and based on the level of the lesion (Table 17–1).

1. **Incidence**
   a. 1 to 2 per 1000 live births
   b. 10 per cent meningocele, 80 per cent myelomeningocele
   c. Most lesions in the lumbar sacral area
   d. Occurs slightly more often in females

ETIOLOGY

1. Results from failure of fusion at the mid or caudal tube at 26 to 28 days' gestation
2. Exact cause unknown
   a. Genetic factors

TABLE 17-1. NEUROLOGICAL DYSFUNCTION AND LEVEL OF LESION IN MYELOMENINGOCELE

Level of Lesion	Reflex	Motor	Bowel/Bladder
Above L-3		Complete paraplegia	Incontinent
L-4	Knee	Ambulatory with crutches, braces	Incontinent; may be taught intermittent catheterization
L5-S1	Ankle	Ambulatory with little assistance; wide based gait	Variable, may be continent
S-3 and below	Anal wink	Normal motor	Variable, may be continent

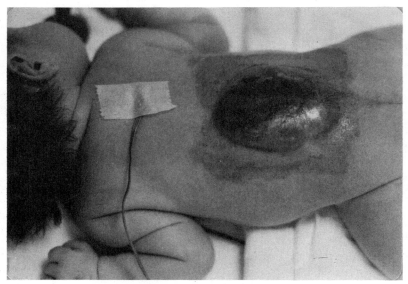

Figure 17-1. Myelomeningocele.

       i. Familial incidence: 5 to 8 times greater chance of subsequent sibling having spina bifida or other central nervous system dysfunction[14]

  b. Environmental factors implicated

       i. Radiation

      ii. Viral

3. Associated defects

  a. Hydrocephalus

  b. Orthopedic

  c. Urological

ASSESSMENT

1. Clinical presentation

  a. Signs and symptoms

       i. Saclike protrusion at any point along the spinal canal

      ii. Motor and sensory dysfunction

     iii. Orthopedic defects

     iv. Head may be large for gestational age

  b. History

       i. Defect occurs in first 28 days of gestation

      ii. Mother often did not realize she was pregnant and cannot recall any unusual events during that time

     iii. Defect can be detected by amniocentesis

2. Biopsychosocial assessment

  a. Sac partially epithelialized, oozes combination of cerebrospinal fluid and serum

  b. Spinal and peripheral nerve roots may be seen within sac

  c. Motor and sensory dysfunction below level of lesion

  d. Orthopedic defects may include

       i. Clubfoot

   ii. Dislocated hips

   iii. Arthrogryposis

   iv. Scoliosis

  e. Urological dysfunction may include

   i. Dribbling, atony, reflex

   ii. Malformation, hydronephrosis

  f. Hydrocephalus may be present at birth, but it usually occurs after surgical repair of the myelomeningocele

   i. Enlarged head: may be only sign

   ii. Tense, full fontannel

   iii. Sunset eyes

   iv. Distended scalp veins

  g. If myelomeningocele is the only problem, infant appears healthy, robust

  h. Determine what information has been given to the parents and their reaction

  i. Assess family dynamics: supportive, blaming each other, guilt, grief, anxiety, apathy

  j. Assess father's or significant other's reaction to infant or ability to talk to or touch baby

  k. Assess parents' comprehension of neonate's condition

   i. Awareness of immediate and long term needs

   ii. Awareness of alternatives: no treatment, treatment, foster care, adoption

  l. Assess parents' cultural mores regarding handicapped and deformed infants

3. Diagnostic data

  a. Appearance of lesion

  b. History and physical examination

  c. Spinal roentgenograms

  d. CT scan: size of ventricles, position of lesion (Fig. 17–2), extent of cerebral disorder

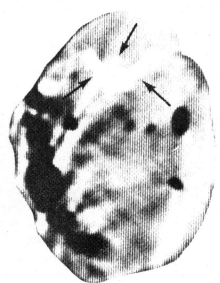

Figure 17–2. Spinal dysraphic lesion demonstrated by CT scan. Body scan in 1 day old male with thoracolumbar myelomeningocele. (Reprinted with permission from Hammock, M.K., and Milhorat, T.H.: Cranial Computed Tomography in Infancy and Childhood. Baltimore, Copyright © Williams & Wilkins, 1981.)

PROBLEMS AND COMPLICATIONS

1. Hydrocephalus with Arnold-Chiari type 2 malformation, which consists of elongation of cerebellar vermis and subsequent herniation through the foramen magnum, often compressing the fourth ventricle (Fig. 17–3)
2. Orthopedic defects
3. Urinary defects, urinary tract infection
4. Bowel incontinence and oozing
5. Motor and sensory dysfunction
6. Spinal cord abnormalities that may be associated
   a. Hydromyelia
   b. Syringomyelia
   c. Diastematomyelia
7. Meningitis if sac ruptures
8. Skin breakdown

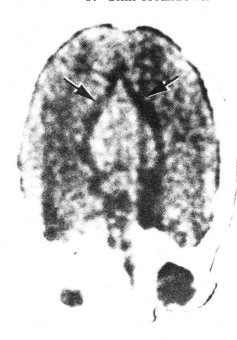

Figure 17–3. CT scan, axial plane, in newborn infant with lumbar myelomeningocele and associated hydrocephalus. *Arrows* indicate Arnold-Chiari malformation. (Reprinted with permission from Hammock, M.K., and Milhorat, T.H.: Cranial Computer Tomography in Infancy and Childhood. Baltimore, Williams & Wilkins, Copyright ©, 1981.)

PATIENT CARE MANAGEMENT

1. **Goals**
   a. To maintain integrity of myelo-meningocele
      i. Position infant prone
      ii. Place small roll under abdomen to prevent stress on sac

      COMMENTS/TIPS/CAUTIONS

      Reposition infant frequently for comfort; do *not* place on side or hold unless physician writes specific order

   b. To prevent infection of sac
      i. Apply sterile dressing; more physicians prefer dressing to be kept moist with antibiotic or povidone-iodine (Betadine) solution

      Use strict sterile technique; keep dressing moist, do not remove if dry; moisten until easily removed; report any leaks or tear in sac to physician

ii. Keep stool and urine away from sac

iii. Begin antibiotic IV as ordered

c. To prevent further deterioration in neurological status

   i. Neurological checks with particular emphasis on head circumference, motor status

d. To support family in their decision to treat or not to treat the infant

   i. Answer questions or refer to appropriate person

   ii. Enlist the support of the social worker, clinical specialist, family's religious leader

   iii. If decision is to *not* correct the lesion, let the family know infant will receive supportive care

     (a) Feedings as appropriate

     (b) Kept clean and dry

     (c) Kept warm

     (d) Will be held when crying, and the like

   iv. If decision is to correct the lesion, prepare family

     (a) Explain when and by whom surgery will be done

e. To prepare the infant for surgical repair of defect and later for treatment of hydrocephalus

   i. Obtain blood (umbilical artery) for laboratory work: CBC, type, and cross-match

   ii. Be sure infant has identification bracelet

   iii. Obtain roentgenograms; be sure they are ready in time for surgery

   iv. Be sure operating room permit is signed

   v. Transport infant to OR in incubator for warmth

COMMENTS/TIPS/CAUTIONS

Do not use diaper or fold away from sac; face mask often provides sufficient substitute

Note any dribbling of urine or oozing of stool

Ensure dosage correct for weight of infant

Watch for signs of increased intracranial pressure secondary to hydrocephalus

Describe sac and its condition if leakage present

Be especially attentive to charting motor function and level of consciousness

Some families are not able to accept or adjust to a handicapped child; they need to be aware of alternatives of foster care or adoption

Generally, if the infant has rachischisis (severe defect with other multiple defects) the recommendation is not to treat

Early closure prevents meningitis and further deterioration of neurological status

Be alert for signs of hydrocephalus

Keep infant prone; do not position on side or hold until physician approves

Because of motor and sensory defects reposition every hour

f. To provide postoperative care (see also b, c above)
  i. Vital signs
  ii. Neurological checks
  iii. Head circumference
  iv. Dressing checks
  v. IVs and antibiotics
  vi. Skin care

g. To collaborate with the primary physicians for referrals to other health team members

  i. Rehabilitation medicine, physical therapy, electro-myelography

  ii. Orthopedics
  iii. Urology
  iv. Social worker
  v. Genetic counselor

These baseline data are useful in beginning a long term rehabilitation program and determining progress

Infant will need long term management of any orthopedic defect

May request intravenous pyelogram or cystometrogram to evaluate renal function and as baseline data

Important to ensure family obtains financial assistance if needed; can also refer family to an appropriate infant stimulation program when medical condition permits; refer family to clinic for handicapped children

Evidence indicates a familial tendency; genetic counseling important for understanding dysfunction and potential risk to subsequent offspring

DISCHARGE PLANNING/TEACHING

1. Educate parent or care giver about myelomeningocele; define myelomeningocele in terms family is able to understand and use pictures and charts
2. Reinforce information given by primary physician and consultants
3. Provide literature or refer parents to Spina Bifida Association

_____ HYDROCEPHALUS _____

Hydrocephalus, a neurological disorder, may be congenital in origin, or it may be acquired, secondary to inflammation or hemorrhage. Left untreated it may lead to atrophy of the white matter of the brain as well as to "spongy edema of the brain surrounding the ventricles".[17] These processes result in severe neurological dysfunction.

DIAGNOSIS

Hydrocephalus is an abnormal collection of cerebrospinal fluid (CSF) within the ventricular system and its pathways[9] (Fig. 17–4).

1. Incidence
  a. 1 to 1.5 per 1000 live births
2. Predisposing factors
  a. Maternal malnutrition

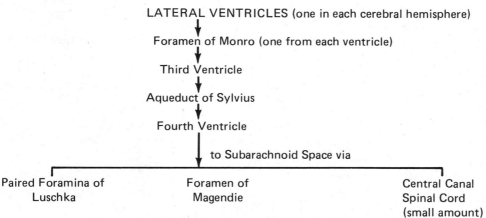

Figure 17-4. Cerebrospinal fluid circulation.

   b. Toxins
   c. Radiation exposure
   d. Cytomegalovirus infection
   e. Increased risk with first pregnancy and advanced maternal age
3. Suspected if infant's head is large for gestational age with respect to body
4. Excessive rate of head growth

ETIOLOGY

1. Classification

Hydrocephalus may be classified in a variety of ways to emphasize the characteristic elements. In general

   a. *Communicating:* obstruction in the flow of CSF at the subarachnoid space; flow to the subarachnoid space from the ventricle is normal
   b. *Noncommunicating:* obstruction within the ventricular system itself preventing free flow of CSF to the subarachnoid space
2. Exact cause unknown
3. Excessive production of CSF by the choroid plexus (groups of cells located in the lateral ventricles)
4. Abnormal absorption of CSF. Although not clinically proven, it is theorized that if the cephalic venous pressure is sufficient, increased back pressure on the arachnoid villi may cause hydrocephalus[17]
5. Obstruction in CSF flow
6. Congenital hydrocephalus most often related to
   a. Aqueductal stenosis
   b. Arnold-Chiari malformation type 2
   c. Dandy-Walker cyst
7. Acquired hydrocephalus related to
   a. Meningitis
   b. Intracranial bleeding
   c. Inflammation
   d. Infection
   e. Trauma

ASSESSMENT

1. **Clinical presentation**
   a. Signs and symptoms
      i. Head circumference large for gestational age, disproportionate to chest
      ii. Sutures widened, often palpable
      iii. Frontal bossing (prominent forehead)
      iv. In severe hydrocephalus
         (a) Distended scalp veins
         (b) Setting sun eyes: eyeballs displaced downward
      v. Irritability

2. **Biopsychosocial assessment**
   a. Anterior fontanel may be tense and full when infant at rest or upright
   b. Skull: cranium large with respect to face; suture split and excessively wide for age; head percusses like a melon
   c. Transillumination abnormal if cerebral mantle 1.0 cm or less in thickness (Fig. 17–5)
   d. Paralysis of one or both sixth cranial nerves
   e. Nystagmus
   f. Poor feeding, vomiting
   g. Motor disintegration
   h. Spastic extremities
   i. Possible seizures
   j. Altered level of consciousness
   k. Determine what information has been given to family
   l. Reinforce physician's explanation: answer questions, correct misinformation

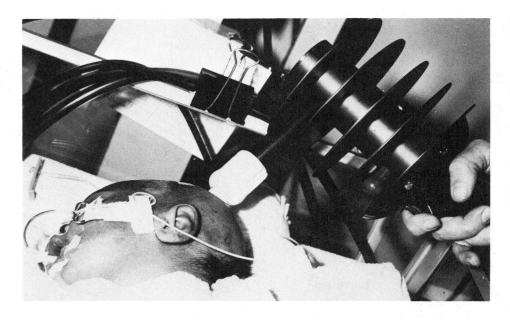

Figure 17-5. Transillumination.

m. Family's preparation for surgical intervention
n. Family's knowledge of handling infant
o. Assess family's ability to cope with grief, anxiety over infant's condition

3. **Diagnostic data**
   a. History and physical examination
   b. CT scan will show enlarged ventricles or possible cause of obstruction if related to hemorrhage or the like
   c. Isotope cisternography and ventriculography provide information about CSF flow and dynamics

PROBLEMS AND COMPLICATIONS

1. Increased intracranial pressure (Table 17–2)
2. Postoperative complications
   a. Infection: of wound, septicemia, peritonitis
   b. Shunt malfunction: blockage, disconnection
   c. Subdural hemotomas
   d. Paralytic ileus

TABLE 17–2.
SIGNS AND SYMPTOMS OF INCREASED INTRACRANIAL PRESSURE

Head large with respect to body size	Sixth cranial nerve(s) dysfunction
Growth of head accelerated	Random eye movement, nystagmus
Frontal prominence or bossing	Vomiting, poor feeding
Scalp thin and shiny	Irritability
Scalp vein distention	Seizures
Anterior fontanel tense, full	Irregular respirations
Cranial sutures separated and palpable	Spasticity of extremities
Cracked pot sound to head percussion	Change in level of consciousness
Setting sun eyes	

PATIENT CARE MANAGEMENT

1. **Goals**
   a. To maintain the infant's physiological integrity
      i. Total physical assessment of the infant; ensure adequate airway; weight
   b. To monitor neurological function
      i. Neurological checks per hospital routine and physician's and nursing orders
      ii. Measure head circumference at least twice a day and record

COMMENTS/TIPS/CAUTIONS

Hydrocephalus may be secondary to infection such as meningitis; therefore attention must be given to total condition of the neonate

Data should be recorded in a systematic manner for future comparison

Neurological flow sheet should be used, observe pupillary function closely

Normally head circumference will increase about 0.5 cm/month

iii. Observe for signs of increased intracranial pressure

iv. Elevate head of bed

Be especially observant of infant's level of alertness; have equipment nearby for bedside emergency ventriculostomy

c. To maintain nutritional status

i. Ensure adequate intake either intravenously or through routine feedings

Infant will require surgical procedure to treat hydrocephalus; state of poor nutrition and hydration increases surgical risk

ii. Monitor intake and output; maintain fluid restriction if ordered

Neonate at risk for fluid overload, which could also lead to cerebral edema

d. To maintain skin integrity

i. Position at least every half hour

Keep infant clean and dry to prevent rash from developing, which would postpone shunt insertion

Provide frequent touch, affection, tender loving care

ii. Check head, especially ears, for signs of pressure areas developing

Talk to infant

Use lamb's wool pad

e. To prepare infant and family for surgery

i. Obtain needed laboratory work

Preoperative check list helpful to ensure that all preparation is done

ii. Ensure diagnostic test results on chart or readily available

iii. Ensure identification bracelet in place

iv. Reinforcement of physician's explanation of surgical procedure; explain where incisions will be and type of dressing (Fig. 17–6)

If family is fully informed their anxiety often decreases

v. Tell family where the infant will go after surgery and anticipated time for return to room

Help family cope with grief, anxiety over infant's condition

f. To provide postoperative care

i. Monitor vital signs

ii. Monitor neurological status

iii. Maintain IV fluids. Begin oral administration of fluids when indicated; measure intake and output

Observe for signs of increased intracranial pressure secondary to shunt obstruction or subdural hematoma; *never* pump and push on shunt valve unless physician specifically so orders

Oral administration of fluids not started until bowel sounds present (usually 24 hours postoperatively); be observant for potential complication of paralytic ileus

g. To prevent infection

i. Inspect dressing and wound site

If meningitis, ventriculitis, or wound infection occurs it may be necessary to remove shunt and begin external drainage until CSF is sterile and cell count is 15 to 20 per cu mm

ii. Keep diaper off if abdominal incision

iii. Keep dressing clean and dry

Peritonitis could develop; watch for distended abdomen, inflammation, tenderness

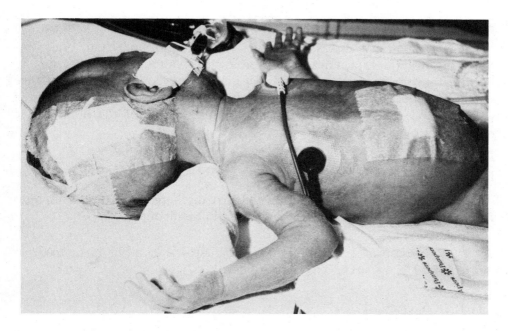

Figure 17-6. Appearance of infant's dressings and site after insertion of shunt device for treating hydrocephalus.

	COMMENTS/TIPS/CAUTIONS
h. To assist infant to adjust to shunt	
i. Position head frequently	Do not position directly on shunt valve; move head carefully to prevent strain on tubing and discomfort
ii. Increase head of bed as ordered	If ventricle particularly enlarged, head of bed may be flat to prevent rapid decompression of ventricles and subsequent development of subdural hematomas

DISCHARGE PLANNING/TEACHING

1. Prepare infant and family for discharge
2. Ensure that family is aware of dynamics of hydrocephalus
3. Teach family how to care for infant and observe family giving the care
4. Instruct family how to care for shunt, emphasizing strongly that they should never pump the shunt bubble/valve unless instructed by physician; many families will push on the valve to see how it feels or when they think the shunt is not working and this may lead to shunt obstruction
5. Teach family the signs and symptoms of shunt failure and what they should do
6. Make follow-up appointments
7. Provide number for family to call if they have questions. During the infant's first few months at home many families feel that any time the baby is sick or irritable the shunt has failed; they are reassured when they know they have someone to call; the number could be that of the physician's office, the clinical specialist or nurse practitioner, or the nurse on the unit where the infant was hospitalized.
Emphasize the need for routine well child care

SEIZURES

Seizures are not a disease but rather a symptom of underlying brain dysfunction—structural, chemical, or physiological. Although they are generally not life threatening, it is estimated that half of the neonates who experience seizures are left with neurological dysfunction. If seizures are associated with asphyxia and hypoxia, only 10 to 20 per cent of the infants have normal neurological development.

DIAGNOSIS

Seizures consist of abnormal or excessive discharge of electrical impulses from the brain. They are not well organized in the neonate.

1. **Incidence**
   a. Ranges from 1.5 per 1000 in the first 4 days after birth to 3 per 1000 in the first 30 days after birth

ETIOLOGY (Table 17–3)

1. **Classification**
   There are five groupings of neonatal seizures.
   a. *Subtle:* horizontal deviation of the eyes that may be accompanied by repetitive blinking or fluttering of the eyelids; drooling, sucking movements; abnormal posturing of extremities; respiratory irregularities; apnea; this type must be distinguished from jitteriness
   b. *Multifocal clonic:* associated with generalized brain injury or hypoxic-ischemic episodes; clonic movements in one extremity that progress to other body areas in a migratory, nonordered fashion
   c. *Focal clonic:* well localized clonic activity; no loss of consciousness; may be followed by Todd's paralysis of affected areas; focal clonic

TABLE 17–3. ETIOLOGY OF SEIZURES

Perinatal complications
Asphyxia
Hypoxia
Intracranial hemorrhage
Traumatic labor and delivery
Maternal health disorders

Metabolic
Hypoglycemia
Hypocalcemia
Hyponatremia
Hyperbilirubinemia

Infectious processes
Meningitis
Encephalitis
Sepsis

Developmental disorders
Cortical atrophy
Porencephaly
Hydrocephalus

seizures are often associated with bilateral cerebral or metabolic disturbances

    d. *Tonic:* similar to decerebrate-decorticate posturing; body stiffening; tonic movements and clonic movements; irregular respirations; this group is seen in association with intraventricular hemorrhage

    e. *Myoclonic:* synchronous jerking of upper or lower extremities or both; uncommon in newborns; myoclonic seizures are indicative of diffuse brain damage

2. Idiopathic: 90 per cent due to birth complications
3. Perinatal complications: hypoxic ischemic encephalopathy, cerebral contusion, intracranial hemorrhage
4. Metabolic dysfunction
5. Infection
6. Developmental disorders
7. Difficult to distinguish from normal random neonatal motor activity
8. Seizure activity most often confined to brain stem because of absence of correctly formed pathways for cortical propagation
9. Seizure results from an unstable cell cavity membrane that causes an ionic imbalance; the cell cannot handle the impulse and becomes bombarded, resulting in excessive discharge

ASSESSMENT

1. **Clinical presentation**
   a. Signs and symptoms
        i. Seizure activity as described under Etiology
   b. History
        i. Sepsis, metabolic derangement, hypoxic episode during first days of life
        ii. Sepsis after first week

2. **Biopsychosocial assessment**
   a. Observe susceptible infants for seizure activity
   b. Seizure pattern
   c. Vital signs
   d. Neurological status
   e. Respiratory status
   f. Reinforce physician's explanation of disorder: answer questions, correct any misconceptions
   g. Assess potential family feelings of "social stigma"
   h. Observe and support the family as they visit the infant
   i. Assess family's knowledge of how to hold, touch, talk to, and care (as appropriate) for the infant

3. **Diagnostic data**
   a. History and physical examination
   b. Urine and blood studies: CBC, differential count, electrolytes, blood urea nitrogen, glucose, calcium, phosphorus
   c. Roentgenograms of skull and spine
   d. CT scan to rule out congenital lesions, edema, hemorrhage, dilated ventricles

e. EEG to confirm diagnosis, localize lesion if one present
f. Lumbar puncture to determine if infection present; obtain CSF for diagnostic studies

PROBLEMS AND COMPLICATIONS

1. Status epilepticus
2. Often difficult to treat with anticonvulsants

PATIENT CARE MANAGEMENT

1. Goals

a. To recognize and initiate prompt intervention during seizure activity
   i. Initiate seizure precautions
   ii. Monitor infant's condition during seizure
      (a) Respiratory status
      (b) Vital signs
      (c) Pupil reaction
   iii. Record seizure events carefully (Table 17–4)
b. To assist physician in determining cause of seizures
   i. Coordinate scheduling of diagnostic procedures in a timely manner without overtiring or overstressing the infant
   ii. Coordinate laboratory studies to avoid multiple venous puncture or finger or heel sticks
c. To maintain therapeutic blood levels of prescribed medications
   i. Give medications on time
   ii. Weigh infant and recognize need for periodic medication adjustment
   iii. Be alert for signs of medication toxicity
d. To maintain infant's physiological status and prevent deterioration in neurological function
   i. Complete physical assessment at least once during every shift
   ii. Monitor vital and neurological signs

COMMENTS/TIPS/CAUTIONS

Do not force anything into the infant's mouth or restrain extremities; protect from injury and turn head to side if feasible

TABLE 17–4. SEIZURE RECORDING

Time seizure began
Body parts involved
Motor movement
Level of consciousness
  Before
  During
  After
Color
Respiratory difficulty
Head deviation
Eye deviation
Pupil reaction
Time seizure ended
Postictal status

Be sure infant gets all the medication. Check with the physician regarding preferences if infant does not take all of oral medications

e. To provide prompt intervention in status epilepticus

COMMENTS/TIPS/ CAUTIONS

   i. Notify physician

   ii. Be prepared to draw blood for laboratory studies: glucose, calcium, sodium, magnesium

May be related to altered P_{O_2}

   iii. Dextrostix

   iv. Oxygen as indicated

   v. Medications as ordered; may start IV

May need intubation; if diazepam (Valium) is given, watch for respiratory depression

   vi. Frequent monitoring of vital and neurological signs

DISCHARGE PLANNING/TEACHING

1. Prepare infant and family for discharge
2. Teach family how to care for infant and observe family providing the care
3. Teach family about the nature of the disorder, medications, what to do in event of a seizure
4. Be sure family is aware of the importance of the infant's getting all the medication and on time; be sure blood levels are determined periodically
5. Refer family to local epilepsy society
6. Provide support, guidance, and education for other significant family members and friends

NEONATAL MENINGITIS

Bacterial meningitis occurring in the first month of life is referred to as neonatal meningitis. Prompt recognition, diagnosis, and aggressive intervention are necessary to prevent serious neurological sequelae or death.

DIAGNOSIS

Neonatal meningitis is an inflammation of the meninges of the brain. Either *Escherichia coli* or group B Streptococcus is usually the responsible organism.

1. **Incidence**
   a. Reported to be responsible for 1 to 4 per cent of all neonatal deaths[15]
   b. Occurs more often in males
2. **Predisposing factors**
   a. Maternal infection
   b. Premature rupture of membranes
   c. Prolonged labor
   d. Excessive manipulation during delivery
   e. Low birth weight
3. Early onset meningitis occurs within first week

      a. Associated with complications during labor and delivery
      b. High mortality

4. Late onset meningitis occurs after first week
      a. Infection after delivery
      b. Lower mortality

ETIOLOGY

1. **Causative organisms**[15]
      a. *E. coli* K_1 and group B streptococcus responsible for 70 per cent
      b. *Listeria monocytogenes* responsible for 5 per cent
      c. Gram negative organisms, cause of 25 per cent
      d. *Citrobacter* infection is being identified more frequently and is very difficult to treat

2. Premature infant is particularly susceptible because of immature immunological system
3. When organism enters subarachnoid space the process can easily spread over the convexity of the brain and within the ventricular system and may lead to cerebral edema, ventriculitis, and rupture or thrombosis of the blood vessels
4. Bacteria may attack the meninges
      a. Secondary to infections of the respiratory or intestinal tract, umbilical cord, skin
      b. After catheterization of the umbilical artery
      c. After insertion of arterial, venous, or central lines
      d. After exposure to contaminated equipment: resuscitation, Isolette or incubator, suction catheters, linens

ASSESSMENT

1. **Clinical presentation**
      a. Signs and symptoms
         i. Variable, similar to those of septicemia
         ii. Vomiting, diarrhea
         iii. Jaundice
         iv. Irritability, lethargy
         v. Pyoderma
         vi. Petechiae
         vii. Purpura
         viii. Convulsions
         ix. Respiratory distress
      b. History
         i. Infant infected with bacterial agent before, during, or after delivery
         ii. Complications during labor and delivery coupled with low birth weight (increase susceptibility)

2. **Biopsychosocial assessment**
      a. Infant refuses feedings

b. Bulging, tense fontanel (seen infrequently)
c. High pitched cry
d. Decreased level of consciousness
e. Vacant stare, seizures (seen often)
f. Fever, wide fluctuation in body temperature
g. Abdominal distention
h. Shock
i. Nuchal rigidity (seen infrequently)
j. Tachypnea
k. Determine what information has been given to family
l. Reinforce physician's explanation: answer questions, correct any misconceptions
m. Assess family's knowledge of how to touch and hold infant as condition permits

3. **Diagnostic data**
   a. Lumbar puncture: CSF pressure; protein (increased); glucose (decreased); cell count (normal to increased)
   b. Blood and urine cultures to rule out sepsis and diagnose causative organism

PROBLEMS AND COMPLICATIONS

1. Hydrocephalus
2. Seizures
3. Learning disabilities
4. Subdural effusions (usually seen in older infant [more than 3 months)] (Fig. 17–7)
5. Water intoxication
6. Hypoglycemia
7. Hypocalcemia
8. Hyperbilirubinemia

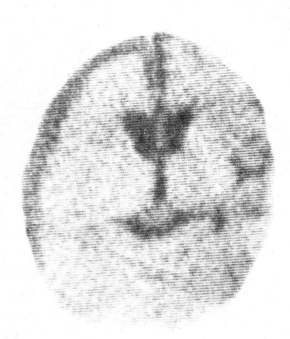

Figure 17-7. CT scan without contrast enhancement in an infant with *Hemophilis influenzae* meningitis showing development of spontaneously resolving ventriculomegaly following subdural effusions. (Reprinted with permission from Hammock, M.K., and Milhorat, T.H.: Cranial Computed Tomography in Infancy and Childhood. Baltimore, Williams & Wilkins, Copyright ©, 1981.)

PATIENT CARE MANAGEMENT

1. **Goals**
    a. To monitor neurological status
        i. Vital signs and neurological checks at least every 1 to 2 hours
        ii. Strict intake and output
        iii. Fluid restriction if indicated
        iv. Elevate head of bed
        v. Initiate seizure precautions
        vi. Record seizure events
        vii. Measure head circumference
    b. To monitor fluid and electrolytes
        i. Laboratory work as indicated: serum and urine
        ii. Intake and output
        iii. IV fluids as ordered, with attention to electrolytes
    c. To prevent development of hypoxia
        i. Monitor arterial blood gases
        ii. Position infant to maximize airway
    d. To maintain physiological integrity of infant
        i. Complete physical assessment at least every 8 hours
        ii. Maintain skin integrity by frequent positioning
        iii. Use strict sterile technique for all dressing changes, venous puncture, and the like
        iv. Isolation precautions
    e. To give medications on time to maintain therapeutic blood levels
        i. Give medications on time: steroids, antibiotics
        ii. Record response to medications
        iii. Laboratory work as indicated re specific medication
        iv. If ordered, have antibiotics for intrathecal or intraventricular administration available for physician to give on rounds

Disease process may lead to significant intracranial hypertension and cerebral edema

See Table 17–4 for seizure recording

Infant susceptible to hypoglycemia, hypocalcemia, hyperbilirubinemia

Weigh diapers

Infant prone to inappropriate secretion of antidiuretic hormone

Ventilatory assistance often needed

Need to be alert for process that predisposes infant to meningitis and attentive to technique during any invasive procedure

Maintain until infant has received antibiotics for 24 hours

Antibiotic therapy will continue for at least 2 weeks after sterilization of CSF cultures if causative organism is gram positive and for 3 weeks if gram negative

Gentamicin given intrathecally or intraventricularly for gram negative organism; strict technique for injection

f. To maintain hemopoietic state

    i. Monitor other laboratory values such as hemoglobin, hematocrit, platelet count, prothrombin time

    ii. Be prepared to assist with exchange transfusion

g. To be alert for signs of complications

    i. Observe infant for signs of increased intracranial pressure

    ii. Be attentive to visual difficulties

    iii. Observe for signs of mental retardation

h. To provide support for family

    i. Allow frequent visits by family

    ii. Be honest with family regarding infant's condition

    iii. If appropriate, alert family to potential problems, e.g., hydrocephalus

    iv. Refer to social worker, pastoral counseling

COMMENTS/TIPS/CAUTIONS

Infection may exacerbate anemia; bleeding diathesis may occur

May be needed to treat hyperbilirubinemia; may also increase infant's resistance

Hydrocephalus and subdural effusions are complications

Blindness may result from meningitis; observe infant's response to faces, lights, moving objects

30 to 50 per cent of infants who survive have neurological damage[15]

DISCHARGE PLANNING/TEACHING

1. Prepare family for infant's discharge
2. Stress importance of follow-up medical care
3. Refer family to infant stimulation program because many infants eventually have mental retardation even though they appear normal at discharge

ASPHYXIA

Asphyxia, an interference with respirations, leading to hypoxic ischemic encephalopathy is the single most important cause of neurological dysfunction in the neonatal period. It may lead to seizures, spasticity, ataxia, and mental retardation.[23]

DIAGNOSIS

Asphyxia is the condition due to lack of oxygen caused by interference with respiration. Hypoxic ischemic encephalopathy is the injury to the brain tissue itself, due to decreased cerebral oxygenation, which results in death of the nerve cells, edema, and ischemia.

ETIOLOGY

1. **Classification**
   a. *Mild injury:* signs and symptoms are more severe in first 24 hours, then diminish
   b. *Moderate injury:* level of consciousness steadily deteriorates over first 48 hours
   c. *Severe injury:* infant is comatose; the condition worsens over 24 hours

2. Neuropathology varies with gestational age, nature of insult, type of intervention
3. Infant susceptible to ischemic injury as a result of impaired vascular autoregulation; when perfusion pressure falls, autoregulation does not maintain cerebral profusion
4. Widespread neuron necrosis due to oxygen deprivation occurs especially at the cerebral cortex, diencephalon, midbrain[24]
5. Strong evidence indicates relationship between fetal bradycardia, which begins during a uterine contraction and reaches a peak 30 to 60 seconds after the contraction, and asphyxia with subsequent hypoxic ischemic incident

ASSESSMENT

1. **Clinical presentation**
   a. Signs and symptoms
      i. May change over 72 hour period
      ii. Altered level of consciousness; lethargy; comatose
      iii. Irregular respiratory status
      iv. Jitteriness
   b. History
      i. Umbilical cord may be compressed during labor, or wrapped around infant's neck
      ii. Placenta may separate prematurely causing decreased blood flow to infant
      iii. Severe maternal hypotension may cause inadequate placental profusion
      iv. Infant's lungs may not inflate properly

2. **Biopsychosocial assessment**
(On admission)
   a. Stupor or coma
   b. Periodic breathing; apnea
   c. Weakness
   d. Seizures, which increase after first 12 hours
(Appearance of severe insult)
   e. Tense bulging fontanel
   f. Split cranial sutures
   g. Brain stem signs, ocular bobbing, cranial nerve dysfunction
   h. Absence of extraocular movements (doll's eyes)
   i. Pupils dilated, do not respond to light

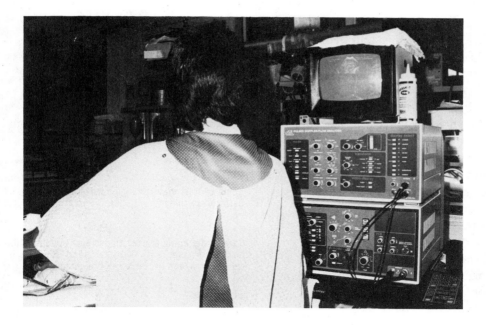

Figure 17-8. Infant in intensive care unit having diagnostic portable brain scan.

j. Assess need for support of mother, who may not have seen infant after birth

k. Reinforce physician's explanation; answer questions

l. Assess family's potential to handle questions posed by extended family

3. **Diagnostic data**

a. Arterial blood gas: low PO_2 bicarbonate pH; high PCO_2

b. Cerebral blood flow (flow of blood to brain) decreased

c. CT scan: edema, ischemia

d. EEG indicative of severity of injury

e. Brain scan indicative of cerebral profusion (Fig. 17–8)

PROBLEMS AND COMPLICATIONS

1. Intraventricular hemorrhage
2. Seizures
3. Altered electrolyte balance
4. Increased intracranial pressure
5. Altered temperature control
6. Long term: mental retardation, motor disturbances, spasticity, choreoathetosis, ataxia

PATIENT CARE MANAGEMENT

1. **Goals**

a. To prevent further decrease in respiratory status

    i. Monitor arteral blood gases

COMMENTS/TIPS/
CAUTIONS

Record amount of blood removed for study; infant may need replacement if volume loss too high

ii. Ventilatory support

iii. Note color of lips, nail beds

iv. Observe for signs of increased respiratory distress

b. To prevent further deterioration in neurological status

i. Neurological checks at least every hour

ii. Measure cerebral perfusion pressure

iii. Measure head circumference

iv. Observe for seizures, treat as indicated

v. Maintain unit procedure if intracranial pressure monitoring initiated (see Intraventricular Drain Insertion in Appendix B)

c. To maintain infant's cardiovascular status

i. Monitor and record vital signs at least every hour

d. To monitor laboratory values

i. Be alert to altered blood volume due to asphyxia; be aware that signs and symptoms are similar in asphyxia and hypovolemia

ii. Be alert for hypoglycemia, hyperkalemia, and hypocalcemia

e. To maintain infant's physiological status

i. Complete nursing assessment every 8 hours

ii. Maintain warmth; prevent hypothermia

iii. Maintain IV fluids at correct rate; accurately record intake and output

iv. Provide skin care with attention to sites of tape for intubation stabilization

v. Reposition frequently

f. To provide support to family

i. If mother unable to visit, picture of infant may be reassuring

ii. Answer questions, offer explanations, reassurance

COMMENTS/TIPS/CAUTIONS

Mild asphyxia may progressively worsen; periodic asphyxic episodes may occur, all of which have a cumulative effect

Be alert for signs and symptoms of increased intracranial pressure

Fluid restrictions

Some centers may use high dose glucocorticoids or barbiturate coma

Barbiturate coma is used to decrease metabolic demands of cerebrum, increase blood flow to ischemic area, and decrease cerebral edema

Hypertension and bradycardia may indicate myocardial failure secondary to decreased energy supplies. Blood flow to the brain will be decreased with further increase of ischemia

Blood volume may be increased if asphyxia occurred during labor; it may be lowered secondary to cord compression, hemorrhage, maternal hypotension[23]

Hypoglycemia would occur secondary to depletion of glucose reserves during initial insult; disturbance of calcium can lead to myocardial failure

If radiant heater used, utilize temperature probe and keep monitor alarms on

Mother may not have seen infant after delivery because of resuscitation efforts

Be sure infant's appearance is explained by a professional prior to mother's seeing it

———————————— INTRACRANIAL HEMORRHAGE ————————————

Intracranial hemorrhage is one of the most frequent neurological problems in the neonatal nursery.

DIAGNOSIS

Intracranial hemorrhage is bleeding within the cranial cavity.

1. **Incidence**
   a. About one half of all premature infants have periventricular-intraventricular hemorrhage.[23]
2. **Predisposing factors**
   a. Trauma (subdural hemorrhage)
   b. Asphyxia (intraventricular hemorrhage)
   c. Trauma and asphyxia (subarachnoid hemorrhage)
   d. Prematurity
   e. Delivery by cesarean section
   f. Breech births
   g. Toxicity in mothers
3. **Major steps in recognizing hemorrhage**
   a. Identify predisposing factors
   b. Define abnormal clinical features
   c. Examine cerebrospinal fluid
   d. Visualize site and extent of hemorrhage[23]

ETIOLOGY

1. **Classification**
   a. *Subdural hemorrhage:* hemorrhage under the dura
   b. *Primary subarachnoid hemorrhage:* bleeding occurring in the subarachnoid space that is not secondary to subdural hemorrhage or intraventricular hemorrhage
   c. *Intraventricular hemorrhage:* bleeding within the ventricles
   d. *Intracerebellar hemorrhage:* hemorrhage within the cerebellar hemispheres
2. **Source of bleeding**
   a. *Subdural hematoma:* tentorial laceration, e.g., sinus, infratentorial vein; tear of superficial cerebral veins; laceration of the falx, e.g., inferior sagittal sinus
   b. *Intraventricular hemorrhage* (Fig. 17–9) (more descriptive term is periventricular-intraventricular hemorrhage): capillaries surrounding the ventricles; hemorrhage then extends into ventricles, although in a small number of cases bleeding confined to area around ventricles
   c. *Primary subarachnoid hemorrhage:* presumed to be small veins of leptomeninges or bridging veins within the subarachnoid space
   d. *Intracerebellar hemorrhage* (occurs in premature infants, but rarely after 32 weeks[23]): may be tear or rupture of the major veins or occipital sinus, or may also be extension of an intraventricular or subarachnoid hemorrhage

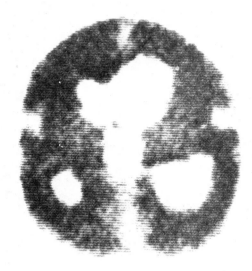

Figure 17-9. CT scan without contrast enhancement in a premature infant with an intraventricular hemorrhage grade 3. (Reprinted with permission from Hammock, M.K., and Milhorat, T.H.: Cranial Computed Tomography in Infancy and Childhood. Baltimore, Williams & Wilkins, Copyright ©, 1981.)

ASSESSMENT

1. **Clinical presentation**
   a. Signs and symptoms
      i. Subdural hematoma
         (a) Stupor or coma
         (b) Pupils sluggish in reaction to light or dilated and fixed
         (c) Full, tense fontannel
         (d) Irregular respirations
      ii. Intraventricular hemorrhage (premature infants less than 1500 g particularly sensitive to development)
         (a) Stupor or coma
         (b) Pupils may be dilated and fixed
         (c) Irregular respiration
      iii. Primary subarachnoid hemorrhage (usually not of major clinical importance[23])
         (a) Signs and symptoms of increased intracranial pressure uncommon
         (b) Seizures or respiratory distress in severe cases
      iv. Intracerebellar hematoma (seen more often in small premature infants, before 32 weeks' gestation[23])
         (a) Brain stem signs in 40 to 50 per cent of premature infants[23]

2. **Biopsychosocial assessment**
   a. Subdural hemorrhage
      i. Depressed at birth
      ii. Pupils unequal with little reaction to light
      iii. Bradycardia
      iv. Ocular bobbing
      v. Irregular respirations: ataxic
      vi. Seizures
      vii. Hemiparesis
      viii. Eye deviation

       ix. Stupor to coma as condition progresses

        x. Transillumination abnormal

  b. Intraventricular hemorrhage

Signs and symptoms depend on magnitude of hemorrhage

        i. Stupor to coma

       ii. Flaccid quadriparesis

      iii. Seizures

      iv. Bulging anterior fontanel

       v. Increased intracranial pressure

      vi. Pupils unreactive to light

     vii. Irregular respirations

      ix. Decerebrate posturing

       x. Alteration in vital signs

  c. Primary subarachnoid hemorrhage

There may be no symptoms

        i. Baby appears well but exhibits seizure activity on the second day of life

       ii. If severe, may be respiratory distress, hydrocephalus, increased intracranial pressure

  d. Intracerebellar hemorrhage

        i. Bradycardia

       ii. Apnea

      iii. Ocular bobbing

      iv. Eye deviation

       v. Decreased hematocrit

      vi. Cerebellar signs

  e. Assess family understanding of disorder

  f. Reinforce physician's explanation: answer questions

  g. Since infant critically ill and may die, assess family's need for support during this time (when possible provide a room for family to be alone)

3. Diagnostic data

  a. CT scan

  b. Cerebral echogram

  c. Brain scan

  d. EEG

  e. Lumbar puncture (with extreme caution)

PROBLEMS AND COMPLICATIONS

1. Hydrocephalus
2. Permanent neurological dysfunction
3. Subdural effusions

PATIENT CARE MANAGEMENT

1. Goals

  a. To prevent further deterioration in neurological status

i. Vital signs every hour, more frequently if necessary

ii. Neurological check every hour; more often if indicated

iii. Measure head circumference every shift

iv. Routine care for intracranial pressure monitoring devices or intraventricular drains (see Appendix B)

b. To prevent or treat hypoxia and asphyxia

i. Assess color of lips and nail beds

ii. Monitor arterial blood gases

iii. Check ventilator or other respiratory devices to ensure correct settings

c. To prepare infant and family for diagnostic tests

i. Be sure infant's condition is stabilized if transport necessary

ii. When test will be done notify department of infant's condition; ensure that equipment needed for infant care is there and in working order

iii. Explain purpose and procedure of test to family

d. To prevent development of infection

i. Care for IV site per hospital procedure

ii. Strict sterile technique in caring for external subdural or intraventricular drains (see Appendix B)

iii. Observe sites of subdural taps or injection sites for irritation or infection

e. To assist physician with treatment

i. Have necessary equipment ready; be sure to include extra needles

COMMENTS/TIPS/CAUTIONS

Be especially alert for signs of hemorrhagic shock

Space nursing procedures to allow periods of rest; be attentive to effects of nursing care on intracranial pressure[17]

Be alert for signs of infection

Ensure equipment needed for transport is available and working, e.g., O_2 tank filled, cardiac monitor battery fully charged

Check that permits are signed if indicated

Immune system not fully developed; infant prone to development of meningitis

See procedure on Subdural Tap in Appendix B.

	COMMENTS/TIPS/ CAUTIONS
ii. Ensure that everyone involved in procedure uses strict sterile techniques throughout	
iii. Prepare infant and family for surgical intervention	Surgery indicated for subdural or intracerebellar hematomas
f. To maintain physiological status of infant	
i. Monitor hematocrit and hemoglobin	Large volume of blood may be lost to the hemorrhage area
ii. Monitor arterial blood gases	
iii. Provide adequate nutrition via IVs, hyperalimentation, or gastric feedings	
iv. Strict measurement and recording of intake and output	Weigh diapers; if using pediatric collection device be attentive to skin care
v. Turn and position infant and give skin care at least every hour	

DISCHARGE PLANNING/TEACHING

1. Initiate referrals per institution policy, e.g., social worker, chaplain, nurse specialist

REFERENCES

1. Ahmann, P.A., Lazzara, A., Dykes, F.D., Schwartz, J.F., and Brann, A.W.: Intraventricular hemorrhage: Incidence and outcome. Ann. Neurol., 4:186, 1978.
2. American Association of Neurosurgical Nurses: Core Curriculum for Neurosurgical Nursing. Chicago, AANN, 1977.
3. Brawn, J.K.: Convulsions in the newborn period. Dev. Med. Child Neurol., 15:823-846, 1976.
4. Chee, C.M.: Seizure disorders. Nurs. Clin. North Am., 15:71-82, 1980.
5. Conway, B.L.: Pediatric Neurologic Nursing. St. Louis, C.V. Mosby Co., 1977.
6. Feign, R.D.: Bacterial meningitis in the newborn infant. Clin. Perinatol., 4:103-116, 1977.
7. Feinchel, G.M.: Neonatal Neurology. New York, Churchill Livingstone, 1980.
8. Gilles, F.H., Jammes, J.L., and Berenberg, W.: Neonatal meningitis. Arch. Neurol., 34:560-562, 1977.
9. Hausman, K.A.: Nursing care of the patient with hydrocephalus. J. Neurosurg. Nurs., 13:326-332, 1981.
10. Hausman, K.A.: Nursing care of the patient with a myelomeningocele. Proceedings of the 3rd International Congress of the World Federation of Neurosurgical Nurse. In press.
11. Holden, K.R., and Freeman, J.M.: Neonatal seizures and their treatment. Clin. Perinatol., 2:3-13, 1975.
12. Leech, R.W., and Alvord, E.C.: Anoxic-ischemic encephalopathy in the human neonatal period: The significance of brain stem involvement. Arch. Neurol., 34:109-113, 1977.

13. Lenichel, G.M.: Neonatal Neurology. New York, Churchill Livingstone, 1980.
14. Matson, D.D.: Neurosurgery of Infancy and Childhood. Springfield, Ill., Charles C Thomas, 1969.
15. McCracken, G.H.: Bacterial and viral infections of the newborn. *In* Avery, G.B. (ed.) Neonatology: Pathophysiology and Management of the Newborn. Philadelphia, J.B. Lippincott Co., 1981.
16. McLaughlin, J.F., and Shurtleff, D.B.: Management of the newborn with myelodysplasia. Clin. Pediatr., *18*:463-475, 1979.
17. Milhorat, T.H.: Pediatric Neurosurgery. Philadelphia, F.A. Davis Co., 1978.
18. Mitchell, P.H., and Mauss, N.K.: Relationship of patient-nurse activity to intracranial pressure variation: A pilot study. Nurs. Res., *27*:4-10, 1980.
19. O'Donohue, N.V.: Epilepsies of Childhood. London: Buttersworth and Co., 1979.
20. Overall, J.C.: Neonatal bacterial meningitis. J. Pediatr., *76*:499-511, 1970.
21. Pressman, S.D.: Myelomeningocele: A multidisciplinary approach. J. Neurosurg. Nurs., *13*:333-336, 1981.
22. Volpe, J.J.: Cerebral blood flow in the newborn infant: Relation to hypoxic-ischemic brain injury and periventricular hemorrhage. J. Pediatr., *94*:170-173, 1979.
23. Volpe, J.J.: Neurology of the Newborn. Philadelphia, W.B. Saunders Co., 1981.
24. Volpe, J.J., and Koeningsberger, R.: Neurologic disorders. *In* Avery, G.B. (ed.): Neonatology: Pathophysiology and Management of the Newborn. Philadelphia, J.B. Lippincott Co., 1981.

CHAPTER 18

RENAL AND METABOLIC CRISES

Jane Bliss-Holtz, R.N., M.S.N.

OBJECTIVES

Upon completion of this chapter the reader will be able to accomplish the following:

1. Recognize predisposing factors that may lead to serum glucose, calcium, and magnesium imbalances in the neonate

2. Identify the signs and symptoms of serum glucose, calcium, and magnesium imbalances in the neonate

3. List the nursing goals appropriate to the care of the infant with serum glucose, calcium, and magnesium imbalances

4. Develop a nursing care plan that will include nursing actions toward the nursing goals in caring for a neonate with serum glucose, calcium, or magnesium imbalances

5. Define prerenal, renal, and postrenal causes of acute renal failure

6. Recognize the signs and symptoms of acute renal failure

7. List the major nursing goals in the care of the infant with acute renal failure

8. Develop a nursing care plan that will include nursing actions toward the major nursing goals in caring for an infant with acute renal failure

---

This chapter will focus on metabolic disorders in the neonate associated with glucose, calcium, and magnesium, and pathological conditions of the neonatal renal system.

Glucose is used as an energy source by the brain, which needs a constantly circulating supply of this substrate to survive. Calcium and magnesium share similar physiological and biochemical functions, particularly in the central nervous system, and because of this, when either calcium or magnesium is in imbalance, signs and symptoms will be similar. Although these ions are discussed separately, it must be kept in mind that a serum alteration in one often results in a serum imbalance of the other. All of the above substrates play a vital role in maintaining life. Nurses need to be cognizant of predisposing factors that may lead to serum imbalances. The monitoring of an identified high risk population of neonates is a primary factor in preventing serum alterations of glucose, calcium, or magnesium.

In this discussion of the neonatal renal system the primary emphasis will be placed on nursing management of acute renal failure. In caring for the neonate who has experienced difficulty in the first days of life, the nurse must recognize the complications that can result from these problems. The nurse caring for the neonate who has experienced intrauterine asphyxia, hypotensive episodes, hypovolemia, or congestive heart failure must be aware that acute renal failure may follow.

SERUM GLUCOSE IMBALANCES

Abnormal serum levels of glucose can have life threatening implications for the neonate. Since the brain is dependent upon a constantly circulating supply of glucose, neurological impairment may occur if hypoglycemia is left untreated. Hyperglycemia can produce cerebral tissue swelling and subsequent damage. The nurse needs to be aware of the factors that may precipitate serum glucose imbalances and to be alert for early signs and symptoms.

DIAGNOSIS

Hypoglycemia during the first 72 hours of life in the term infant is defined as a serum glucose level equal to or below 35 mg/100 ml, or in the low birth weight infant as equal to or below 25 mg/100 ml. After the first 72 hours, hypoglycemia is a serum glucose level less than 45 mg/100 ml.

Hyperglycemia is a serum glucose level over 125 mg/100 ml.

1. Incidence

Hypoglycemia
  a. In full term, appropriate for gestational age (AGA) infants: approximately 10 per cent
  b. In full term, small for gestational age (SGA) infants: approximately 25 per cent
  c. In preterm (under 38 weeks) SGA infants: approximately 67 per cent

Hyperglycemia
  a. Evident in 20 to 80 per cent of very low birth weight infants (less than 1200 gm)

2. Predisposing factors

Hypoglycemia
  a. Placental dysfunction
  b. Infants of mothers with eclampsia
  c. Multiple births
  d. Neonatal asphyxia
  e. Respiratory distress syndrome (RDS)
  f. Neonatal hypothermia
  g. Erythroblastosis fetalis
  h. Infants of diabetic mothers

Hyperglycemia
  a. Prematurity
  b. Severe shock

        i. Sepsis
      ii. Intracranial hemorrhage
  c. Rapid parenteral infusion of dextrose

ETIOLOGY

Hypoglycemia

1. Under normal conditions, the concentration of serum glucose declines during the first 24 hours after birth with the lowest level usually reached 2 hours after delivery, followed by a subsequent rise
   a. Per kilogram of body weight the glocuse requirement of the neonate is twice that of the adult
   b. Ability to produce glucose from glycogen or from alternate substrates (gluconeogenesis) is limited
2. Pathogenesis may involve one or both of these mechanisms
   a. Decreased source of serum glucose
      i. Insufficient glycogen stores
      ii. Insufficient fat stores
      iii. Insufficient glucose infusion
   b. Increased rate of serum glucose removal
      i. Neonatal asphyxia, hypoxia
      ii. Hypothermia
      iii. Respiratory distress syndrome
      iv. Hypermetabolism (SGA infant with increased cell numbers per unit of weight)
      v. Temporary hyperinsulinism in infants of diabetic mothers or with erythroblastosis fetalis

Hyperglycemia

1. Usually a transient condition
2. Associated with birth asphyxia and intracranial hemorrhage; relationship between these not fully understood
3. Hyperglycemia of the premature appears to be a result of deficient insulin secretion or production of a biologically inactive form of insulin
4. 10 per cent glucose rapidly infused to combat insensible water loss may not be metabolized by the immature infant

ASSESSMENT

Hypoglycemia

1. Clinical presentation
   a. Signs and symptoms
      i. Irritability, jitteriness, tremors
      ii. Eye rolling, convulsions, localized seizures
      iii. Irregular respirations, tachypnea, apnea, cyanosis in absence of pulmonary complications
      iv. Listlessness; poor feeding
      v. High pitched, weak cry
      vi. Decrease in muscle tone

       vii. Inability to regulate temperature
     viii. Tachycardia
       ix. Diaphoresis
        x. Hypothermia
  b. History
        i. Maternal history of diabetes, eclampsia, use of oral hypoglycemic agents
       ii. Infant small for gestational age history
      iii. Prolonged gestation (postmaturity)
      iv. Prematurity
       v. Asphyxia or hypoxia at birth
      vi. Large for gestational age
     vii. Smaller of twins
    viii. Infant cold stressed

2. Biopsychosocial assessment
  a. Reflex response: hyperactivity may be apparent
  b. Muscle tone: decrease in tone
  c. Temperature: hypothermia due to decreased thermal regulation
  d. Change in quality of pitch of cry
  e. Change in feeding habits or poor feeding
  f. Respiratory rate and quality
  g. Color: cyanotic or gray shocklike appearance
  h. Heart rate: tachycardia

3. Diagnostic data
  a. Serial screening by peroxidase reagent strips (Dextrostix) in first hours of life
  b. Quantitative blood glucose levels when Dextrostix reading is below 40 to 45 mg/100 ml

Hyperglycemia

1. Clinical presentation (severe prolonged cases)
  a. Signs and symptoms
      i. Lethargy
     ii. Vomiting
    iii. Tachypnea caused by metabolic acidosis
    iv. Profound hypotonia with depression of consciousness

2. Biopsychosocial assessment
  a. Check for diminished muscle tone and hyporeflexia
  b. Respiratory rate and quality

3. Diagnostic data
  a. Urine glucose monitored every 4 to 8 hours with Clinitest or Clinistix
  b. If urine glucose 1+ or more, Dextrostix reading should be obtained or quantitative serum glucose level should be determined

PROBLEMS AND COMPLICATIONS

Hypoglycemia

1. If hypoglycemia is left undetected and untreated, severe and irreversible neurological sequelae may result

2. There is a 50 per cent incidence of permanent and serious neurological sequelae in newborns who exhibit seizures due to hypoglycemia

Hyperglycemia
1. In every low birth weight infant (under 1200 gm), the urinary glucose threshold may be lower (spillage may occur at a serum glucose level of 80 to 100 mg/100 ml) with resultant osmotic diuresis; potential exists for significant free water loss and dehydration
2. Glucose enters the brain easily; the potential for generalized cerebral tissue swelling and damage is recognized

PATIENT CARE MANAGEMENT
1. Goals

COMMENTS/TIPS/CAUTIONS

a. To prevent abnormal serum glucose levels
  i. Identification of population at high risk for hypoglycemia

Information regarding maternal conditions (diabetes, eclampsia) that can predispose the infant to serum glucose imbalances, or infant conditions such as birth anoxia, can be retrieved from the prenatal and intrapartal records; in those infants identified as at risk, serum glucose levels are then monitored carefully

    (a) Neonates in whom source of serum glucose is decreased because of reduced liver glycogen store
      (1) Premature (less than 37 weeks' gestation)
      (2) Postmature (over 42 weeks' gestation)
      (3) SGA
    (b) Neonates in whom serum glucose removal is increased (see Etiology: Hypoglycemia)
  ii. Identification of population at high risk for hyperglycemia (see Diagnosis: Predisposing factors)

Signs of hypoglycemia may be very subtle or attributed to other causes; most signs will be seen within the first 48 to 72 hours of life; they may be persistent or may occur periodically

  iii. Assess for signs and symptoms (see Assessment: Hypoglycemia; Assessment: Hyperglycemia)
  iv. Laboratory monitoring of serum glucose

Since some of the signs and symptoms of hypoglycemia and hyperglycemia are similar, it is often the laboratory results that will differentiate the cause of the symptoms

Hypoglycemia
    (a) Blood glucose levels should be

Dextrostix readings under 40 to 45 mg/100 ml warrant alerting the physician and

determined hourly with peroxidase reagent strips (Dextrostix) for the first 3 hours of life, then every 4 to 6 hours thereafter.

COMMENTS/TIPS/CAUTIONS

drawing blood for determination of serum glucose levels; serum specimens should be placed in ice until processed, or false readings may occur

Hyperglycemia

(a) Urine should be tested for glucose every 4 to 8 hours with Clinitest or Clinistix

If urinary glucose is 1+ or more, a Dextrostix reading should be obtained or a blood glucose drawn

v. Glucose replacement in hypoglycemia

(a) Asymptomatic infants at risk may be fed by bottle or gavage with 10 per cent dextrose (5 mg/kg body weight) at 1 hour of age

In infants weighing less than 2 kg, parenteral administration of dextrose should be started immediately

(b) By the time the infant is 12 hours of age a formula containing 20 calories/ounce may be started, with extra dextrose if needed

Forced feedings should be avoided, since this could result in regurgitation with aspiration

b. To treat serum glucose imbalance

i. Hypoglycemia

(a) Intramuscular or subcutaneous administration of crystalline glucagon (300 μg/kg to maximum dose of 1.0 mg) may be used as initial treatment in infant with adequate glycogen stores

Glucagon administration will be less successful in SGA or premature infants with decreased glycogen stores; resultant rise in serum glucose may last 2 to 3 hours

(b) Intravenous injection of 5–10 ml/kg of 10 per cent solution

Glucose infusion must be maintained at steady rate to avoid serum glucose rebound

(c) Infusions of 10–15 per cent glucose solution should be given at a rate of 4 ml/kg/hour

Serum glucose must be monitored carefully, since hyperglycemia with resultant osmotic diuresis and dehydration may occur

Urinary output and specific gravity should be monitored carefully; urine glucose should be checked every 4 to 6 hours

(d) Hydrocortisone 5 mg/kg or ACTH 4 units every 12 hours may be given if the glucose

Weight should be checked every 12 hours to avoid fluid overload

levels fail to rise above 30 mg/100 ml after 6 hours

ii. Hyperglycemia

  (a) Amount of dextrose infusion should be reduced by

    (1) Decreasing the rate of the infusion

    (2) Decreasing the concentration of dextrose

COMMENTS/TIPS/CAUTIONS

Parenteral dextrose should not be discontinued abruptly, since this may result in rebound hypoglycemia

The effect of hyperglycemia on serum osmolality has not been established

Concentration of the infusion should not be reduced to the point of hypotonicity; this increases the risk of intravascular hemolysis

SERUM CALCIUM IMBALANCES

Calcium metabolism is regulated through four processes: levels of intake; intestinal absorption; renal excretion; and actions of parathormone, calcitonin, and vitamin D metabolites. The parathyroids, liver, kidneys, bones, and intestines all affect calcium equilibrium in the body. Sudden swings of serum calcium levels outside the normal limits can result in neuromuscular changes that can be life threatening.

DIAGNOSIS

Hypocalcemia is a serum calcium level less than 7.0 mg/100 ml (3.5 mEq/liter).

Hypercalcemia is a serum calcium level more than 10 mg/100 ml (5 mEq/liter) in the first 72 hours of life.

1. Incidence

Hypocalcemia

a. One third of infants under 36 weeks' gestational age are hypocalcemic

b. One third of infants who experience birth asphyxia are hypocalcemic

c. One half of infants whose mothers are insulin dependent diabetics are hypocalcemic

2. Predisposing factors

Hypocalcemia

a. Maternal diabetes, eclampsia, or hyperparathyroidism

b. Maternal calcium deficiency

c. Prematurity

d. Neonatal asphyxia or hypoxia

e. Shock

f. Sepsis

g. Metabolic acidosis treated with bicarbonate

h. RDS

i. Administration of citrated blood

Hypercalcemia

a. Dehydration

b. Maternal hypoparathyroidism
c. Hypersensitivity to vitamin D (idiopathic hypercalcemia)

ETIOLOGY

Hypocalcemia

1. Before the first 3 days of life

a. Parathormone and vitamin D metabolites. Hypocalcemia may be due to maternal deficiency of calcium or to hyperparathyroidism with resultant suppression of fetal parathyroids

2. After the first 3 days of life

a. *Levels of intake:* hypocalcemia may result from a high phosphate diet (whole cow's milk) or magnesium deficiency
b. *Intestinal absorption:* hypocalcemia may be due to intestinal malabsorption of calcium and magnesium
c. *Renal excretion:* the kidney may not respond to parathormone, or tubular disease may prevent calcium reabsorption

3. Not dependent on age

a. Blood products containing acid citrate dextrose (ACD) or citrate phosphate dextrose (CPD) can produce the citrate complex with calcium, resulting in a decrease in ionized calcium
b. Alkalosis from bicarbonate or hyperventilation from respirators may result in shifts of calcium from ionized to protein-bound states

Hypercalcemia

1. Levels of intake

a. Administration of calcium gluconate as a treatment of hyperkalemia or hypocalcemia or as an adjunct to resuscitation attempts may result in hypercalcemia if serum levels are not carefully monitored or dosages are not accurately calculated or administered

2. Parathormone and vitamin D metabolites

a. Maternal hypoparathyroidism during pregnancy can result in compensatory fetal hyperparathyroidism and hypercalcemia
b. High maternal intake of vitamin D may result in idiopathic hypercalcemia in some infants who are hypersensitive to vitamin D

ASSESSMENT

Hypocalcemia

1. Clinical presentation

a. Signs and symptoms
   i. Tremor, irritability, jitteriness, high pitched cry
   ii. Seizures
   iii. Classic Chvostek sign and carpopedal spasms may be present
b. History
   i. Maternal diabetes, eclampsia, calcium deficiency, hyperparathyroidism
   ii. Infant hypoxia, asphyxia; prematurity; shock; sepsis; RDS; metabolic acidosis treated with bicarbonate; administration of citrated blood

2. **Biopsychosocial assessment**
   a. Chvostek sign
   b. Trousseau sign
3. **Diagnostic data**
   a. Total serum calcium level under 7.0 mg/100 ml or ionized calcium level under 4.0 mg/100 ml.
   b. ECG
       i. Q–T interval, corrected for heart rate, over 0.4 seconds
       ii. Beginning of Q interval to beginning of T, corrected for rate, over 0.2 seconds

Hypercalcemia

1. **Clinical presentation**
   a. Signs and symptoms
       i.   Poor feeding with vomiting
       ii. Irritability
       iii. Lethargy
       iv. Decreased reflex response
       v.   Bradycardia
   b. History
       i. Maternal history of hypoparathyroidism, high intake of vitamin D
       ii. Infant history of resuscitation attempts; hyperkalemia or hypocalcemia with use of calcium gluconate treatment
2. **Biopsychosocial assessment**
   a. Heart rate: may be decreased
   b. Reflexes: may be decreased
   c. Reflex irritability
3. **Diagnostic data**
   a. Serum calcium levels over 10 mg/100 ml
   b. Shortening of Q-T interval on ECG

PROBLEMS AND COMPLICATIONS
Hypocalcemia
1. Cardiac and respiratory arrest may result from rapid lowering of the serum calcium level

Hypercalcemia
1. Most serious effect is kidney insult, reflected in loss of concentrating ability and polyuria; if not corrected, renal damage with loss of glomerular function can be permanent
2. Cardiac arrest may occur in undetected, severe cases

PATIENT CARE MANAGEMENT
1. **Goals**
    a. To prevent abnormal serum calcium levels
        i. Identification of population at high risk for hypocalcemia (see Diagnosis: Predisposing factors)

COMMENTS/TIPS/
CAUTIONS

Infants identified as at risk for hypocalcemia should be monitored for sudden alteration in neuromuscular functioning

The presence of Trousseau and Chvostek signs may be significant; their absence, however, does not rule out hypocalcemia

    ii. Identification of population at high risk for hypercalcemia (see Diagnosis: Hypercalcemia)

    iii. Dietary prevention of hypocalcemia

        (a) Oral calcium supplementation at a dose of 75 mg elemental calcium/kg/day has been effective

b. To treat abnormal serum calcium levels

Hypocalcemia

    i. Oral calcium therapy

        (a) Elemental calcium dosage

            (1) 75 mg/kg/day for first 24 hours

            (2) 37.5 mg/kg/day for second 24 hours

            (3) 18.75 mg/kg/day for third 24 hours

            (1 ml 10 per cent calcium gluconate = 100 mg calcium gluconate = 9 mg elemental calcium)

        (b) Parenteral preparations of 10 per cent calcium gluconate are well tolerated orally. Daily doses can be given at 4 to 6 hour intervals.

    ii. Intravenous calcium therapy

        (a) Treatment of acute symptoms (seizures)

            (1) Bolus IV dose of 1–2 ml/kg 10 per cent calcium gluconate

                (i) Maximum dose: 5 ml for premature infants; 10 ml

---

COMMENTS/TIPS/
CAUTIONS

Infants identified as at risk for hypercalcemia should be monitored for bradycardia and shortening of Q-T intervals on ECG; diagnosis of hypercalcemia sometimes based only on total serum calcium levels

Serum calcium levels should be determined daily to verify that they are within normal range

Serum calcium levels should be determined daily

Hypertonic solutions should be avoided because of the uncertainty of the role they play in precipitating necrotizing enterocolitis

Bowel movements will increase in frequency

IV administration of calcium must be *slow* (10 per cent calcium gluconate should be given at a rate not greater than 2 ml/kg/10 minutes); ECG monitoring should be used during IV administration of calcium

Rapidly infused calcium may cause bradycardia and arrhythmias; rapid calcium infusion into the aorta via umbilical artery catheter has caused blanching of the bowel in laboratory animals; extravasation of calcium can cause severe tissue necrosis; calcium can cause liver necrosis if it is administered through an umbilical vein catheter that does not reach the inferior vena cava

Calcium cannot be mixed with sodium bicarbonate; the two form a precipitate of calcium carbonate; separate IV lines should be utilized if these are being administered, or the lines should be flushed between usage

for full term infants

(b) Treatment of asymptomatic hypocalcemia
(1) 75 mg/kg/day of elemental calcium given over 48 hours

Hypercalcemia

i. If total serum calcium is less than 13 mg/100 ml
(a) Force fluids orally or intravenously
(b) Reduce calcium intake
(c) Stop intake of vitamin D

ii. If total serum calcium is 13 to 15 mg/100 ml
(a) Oral phosphates, dexamethasone, IM intravenous saline, and IM furosemide have been used.
(b) Calcitonin (1 to 5 units/kg/day) has been used.

iii. If total serum calcium is more than 15 mg/100 ml
(a) Peritoneal dialysis may be considered
(b) EDTA can be used intravenously in glucose or saline at a concentration of less than 7 mg/ml in a dose of 50 mg/kg (1.5 g/sq m) over a 3 to 4 hour period.

COMMENTS/TIPS/CAUTIONS

If IV fluid load is increased, signs of congestive heart failure should be watched for, including rales and edema, and intake and output and weight should be determined daily

EDTA may lower the calcium level rapidly, causing cardiac and respiratory arrest; calcium gluconate should be available as an antagonist

SERUM MAGNESIUM IMBALANCES

Magnesium homeostasis and calcium homeostasis are intimately related. Hypermagnesemia commonly results in hypocalcemia. Hypermagnesemia may result in profound central nervous system depression in the neonate.

DIAGNOSIS

Hypomagnesemia is a serum magnesium level less than 1 mEq/liter.

Hypermagnesemia is a serum magnesium level more than 3.5 mEq/liter.

1. **Incidence**
   a. Hypomagnesemia and hypermagnesemia are relatively infrequent,

but reports of tetany from hypomagnesemia have increased within the past few years

2. Predisposing factors

Hypomagnesemia

    a. Maternal diabetes, hyperparathyroidism

    b. Maternal magnesium deficiency

    c. Infant SGA

    d. Idiopathic intestinal malabsorption of magnesium in infant

    e. Neonatal intestinal surgery with extensive resection or fistulas or increased intestinal losses through drainage

    f. Exchange transfusion

    g. Congenital biliary atresia

    h. Hepatitis in infant

Hypermagnesemia

    a. Treatment of maternal eclampsia with magnesium sulfate

    b. Prematurity

    c. Birth asphyxia

ETIOLOGY

Hypomagnesemia

1. Decreased magnesium availability

    a. Maternal magnesium deficiency: relation to poor maternal nutritional intake is suspected; SGA infants commonly have hypomagnesemia; hypomagnesemia frequently occurs in infants of young primiparous mothers who develop eclampsia

    b. Infants of diabetic mothers may develop hypomagnesemia that is directly related in severity to the diabetes; since diabetes is associated with hypomagnesemia, neonatal hypomagnesemia may reflect maternal magnesium deficiency

    c. Idiopathic intestinal malabsorption of magnesium has been reported in neonates

    d. Intestinal surgery

        i. Drastic resection

        ii. Procedure resulting in increased intestinal transit time

2. Magnesium loss

    a. Exchange transfusion utilizing citrated blood can result in magnesium forming a complex with citrate

    b. Defects in renal tubular reabsorption may lead to magnesium loss

    c. Intestinal surgery resulting in ileostomy or draining fistulas may produce magnesium loss

Hypermagnesemia

1. Increased magnesium availability

    a. Maternal treatment of preeclampsia with magnesium sulfate can result in neonatal hypermagnesemia

        i. Maternal serum magnesium levels of 1.3–7.0 mEq/liter have resulted in umbilical cord serum levels of 1.0–5.75 mEq/liter (normal cord values are 0.9–2.6 mEq/liter)

2. **Decreased magnesium clearance**
    a. Decreased renal excretion of magnesium has been associated with
        i. Birth asphyxia
        ii. Prematurity

ASSESSMENT

Hypomagnesemia

1. **Clinical presentation**
    a. Signs and symptoms
        i. Irritability
        ii. Eye rolling
        iii. Muscle twitching
        iv. Convulsions
    b. History
        i. Maternal diabetes, hyperparathyroidism, or magnesium deficiency
        ii. SGA, intestinal surgery, exchange transfusion, congenital biliary atresia, hepatitis
2. **Biopsychosocial assessment**
    a. Check for hyperactive reflexes
3. **Diagnostic data**
    a. Low serum calcium levels with normal phosphorus levels suspicious of hypomagnesemia
    b. Serum magnesium level less than 1 mEq/liter

Hypermagnesemia

1. **Clinical presentation**
    a. Signs and symptoms
        i. Hypotension
        ii. Urinary retention
        iii. Central nervous system depression
        iv. Hypotonia and hyporeflexia
        v. Increased atrioventricular and ventricular conduction
        vi. Severe respiratory depression with apnea and cyanosis
        vii. Cardiac arrest
    b. History
        i. Maternal eclampsia treated with magnesium sulfate
        ii. Prematurity
        iii. Birth asphyxia
2. **Biopsychosocial assessment**
    a. BP, heart rate, respiratory rate
    b. Check reflexes for hyporeflexia
    c. Check for bladder distention
3. **Diagnostic data**
    a. Serum magnesium level over 3.5 mEq/liter

PROBLEMS AND COMPLICATIONS

Hypomagnesemia

1. Since hypomagnesemia is related to hypocalcemia, the sequelae related

to the latter condition, i.e., cardiac and respiratory arrest, may result from untreated hypomagnesemia

Hypermagnesemia

1. Untreated hypermagnesemia may result in profound central nervous system depression with possible neurological sequelae

PATIENT CARE MANAGEMENT

1. Goals

    a. To prevent abnormal serum magnesium levels

        i. Identification of population at high risk for hypomagnesemia (see Diagnosis: Predisposing factors)

        ii. Identification of population at high risk for hypermagnesemia (see Diagnosis: Predisposing factors)

        iii. Dietary prevention of hypomagnesemia

            (a) In asymptomatic, at-risk infants, 50 per cent magnesium sulfate can be given orally in a dosage of 0.1 ml/kg/day; this should be diluted fivefold before administration

            (b) In specific magnesium malabsorption cases, daily oral dosage of 1 ml/kg/day of 50 per cent magnesium sulfate may be required

    b. To treat abnormal serum magnesium levels

Hypomagnesemia

        i. In symptomatic hypomagnesemia (seizures)

            (a) 50 per cent magnesium sulfate in a dose of 0.1–0.3 ml/kg given IM or IV

            (b) Dose may be repeated every 8 to 12 hours

Hypermagnesemia

        i. Asymptomatic hypermagnesemia is usually not treated

        ii. In severely depressed neo-

COMMENTS/TIPS/CAUTIONS

Careful assessment of maternal prenatal and delivery history is essential in identifying high risk population

Serum magnesium levels should be determined daily

IV administration of magnesium should be accompanied by
1. BP monitoring for hypotension
2. ECG monitoring for
    a. Prolonged atrioventricular conduction time
    b. Sinoatrial block
    c. Atrioventricular block

nate, exchange transfusion with citrated blood has been effective

Citrated blood is utilized because the complex formed between citrate and magnesium expedites magnesium removal

Respiratory assistance may be necessary for the depressed infant until magnesium levels decrease

ACUTE RENAL FAILURE

Acute renal failure is characterized by alterations in fluid and electrolyte balance, acid-base disturbances, increased BUN and serum creatinine, and oliguria. Most neonates with renal failure are included in one of two classifications; those who are anuric at birth and those in whom postnatal renal function shows deterioration.[7]

In a healthy newborn, 16–44 ml of urine may be retained in the bladder at birth;[20] 92 per cent of all infants void within the first 24 hours of life, while a full 99 per cent void within 48 hours. In the newborn still anuric 48 hours after delivery, one or more of the conditions listed in Table 18–1 may be present.

Acute renal failure (ARF) in the newborn is a life threatening event that can occur as a complication of preexisting conditions or as a result of congenital malformations. Survival of the neonate depends, in part, on early recognition of oliguria and abnormal hematological values.

DIAGNOSIS

Acute renal failure of prerenal origin is the type most likely to be a complication in neonates in intensive care settings, since this classification includes renal hypoperfusion.

1. **Incidence**
   a. Depends upon etiology
2. **Predisposing factors**
   a. Dehydration
   b. Prenatal or neonatal hemorrhage or asphyxia
   c. Nephrotoxic medication

ETIOLOGY

Approximately 70 per cent of instances of renal failure occur in the first year of life; 20 per cent of cases in newborns are secondary to renal hypoperfusion. In addition to those secondary to renal hypoperfusion, conditions responsible for the remaining cases include renal agenesis (Potter's syndrome), renal dysplasia, and obstructive uropathies.

1. **Classification of origin**
   a. Prerenal ARF
      i. Associated with inadequate kidney perfusion; may follow
         (a) Hypovolemia
         (b) Hypotension
         (c) Congestive heart failure
      ii. Oliguria is functional, and no actual damage is evident; oliguria lasts only 2–3 days or until the underlying cause is corrected
      iii. Usually reversible if underlying cause promptly treated

TABLE 18–1. CONDITIONS ASSOCIATED WITH RENAL FAILURE IN THE NEONATE

Condition	Incidence	Cause	Associated Abnormalities	Treatment	Expected Outcome
Potter's syndrome	1 in 3000 births; 75% of affected are male; 40% stillborn	Often associated with oligohydramnios; resultant fetal compression possible factor in development[22]	Wide set eyes, parrot beak nose, low set ears, receding chin (Potter facies); pulmonary hypoplasia, lower urinary tract or genital defects, especially in female infants[24]		Most live born infants die before several weeks of age from renal failure or pulmonary problems
Renal dysplasia	Unilateral multicystic kidney most common renal disorder in infants and most common cause of unilateral abdominal mass in newborn	Developmental defect in nephrogenic tissue generation; may involve both kidneys	When seen with cystic formation, known as multicystic kidney	Surgical removal and exploration	
Childhood type multicystic kidneys		Autosomal recessive disorder affecting liver and kidneys; associated with oligohydramnios	Kidneys grossly enlarged; contain radially arranged fusiform cysts	Dialysis or transplantation	When clinical manifestations apparent in early infancy, death within weeks to months without treatment; diagnosis at autopsy in 75% of cases
Obstructive lesions of urinary tract: VATER association			Five associated defects: *vertebral* defects, *anal* atresia, *tracheoesophageal* fistula with esophageal atresia, *renal* defects, radial dysplasia	Repair defects if possible	

Prune belly syndrome (Engle-Barrett syndrome)	Deficiency of anterior abdominal wall musculature, cryptorchidism, abnormalities of urinary tract	Abdominal wall defect may range from virtual absence of contractile muscle in front of the abdominal line to small patch of wrinkled skin overlying muscle defect; urinary tract defects include megaloureters, megalocystis, or urethral obstruction, cystic renal dysplasia (pinpoint meatal stenosis or atresia of urethra).	Straighten most affected ureter, reimplant into bladder; vesicostomy	Most deaths occur within the first 3 months
Tubular/cortical necrosis (diminution of superficial cortical blood flow)	Severe fetal asphyxia; if ischemia severe enough, tissue death may result in renal cortical necrosis. Suspect if oliguria is present.	Cortical calcification may develop within few weeks as result of cortical necrosis.	Dialysis	Extensive necrosis may result in irreversible renal failure if dialysis is not initiated
Renovascular accidents (renal vein thrombosis)	Hemoconcentration due to dehydration	When extensive thrombosis occurs, there is renal enlargement, hematuria, and hematological evidence of intravascular coagulation (platelets decrease, fibrin split products increase)	Careful regulations of fluids	In most cases some renal tissue is uninvolved, thus sparing the infant from permanent damage

    b. Renal ARF
        i. Associated with renal damage of permanent nature
            (a) Potter's syndrome
            (b) Severe renal dysplasia or hypoplasia
            (c) Tubular and cortical necrosis
        ii. Oliguria is associated with actual renal damage or deformity
    c. Postrenal ARF
        i. Associated with congenital malformations and obstructive lesions of the urinary tract
            (a) VATER group of congenital defects
            (b) Prune belly syndrome
            (c) Neurogenic bladder

ASSESSMENT

1. **Clinical presentation**
    a. Signs and symptoms
        i. Oliguria (less than 0.6 ml/kg/hour of urine)
        ii. Edema
        iii. Pulmonary edema
    b. History
        i. Congestive heart failure
        ii. Dehydration
        iii. Prenatal or neonatal hemorrhage or asphyxia
        iv. Nephrotoxic medications
        v. Genetic predisposition
        vi. Oligohydramnios
        vii. Dystocia

2. **Biopsychosocial assessment**
    a. Gentle palpation for abdominal masses
    b. Temperature, pulse, respiration
    c. Pulmonary auscultation (especially in advanced cases)

3. **Diagnostic data**
Laboratory studies may vary slightly with the underlying cause of ARF.
    a. Prerenal ARF
        i. Rise in serum BUN out of proportion to the comparable increase in serum creatinine
        ii. Increase in urine osmolality and urinary urea levels
        iii. Decrease in urinary sodium
        iv. Ratio of urine to plasma urea more than 4:8
    b. Renal ARF
        i. Serum BUN and serum creatinine levels increase proportionally
        ii. Low urine osmolality
        iii. Urinary sodium levels of more than 40 mEq/liter
        iv. Ratio of urine to plasma urea less than 4:8
    c. In *all* cases of ARF, laboratory values reflect:
        i. Elevated level of serum BUN, with peak occurring at 4 to 5 days
        ii. Low or normal level of serum potassium at onset with rise beginning in 2 to 3 days
        iii. Low serum CO_2 level and pH with elevated chloride level (these findings are indicative of metabolic acidosis)

iv. Urinalysis: may indicate hematuria, proteinuria, and cylindruria. Specific gravity usually 1.010 or less; pH above 6.0. Creatinine and urea excretion low; urine sodium level usually elevated

v. Hypocalcemia; hyperphosphatemia; hypomagnesemia

d. Contrast dye roentgenogram may be used to outline renal or urinary tract deformities

PROBLEMS AND COMPLICATIONS

1. If underlying conditions are not quickly diagnosed and treated
   a. Fluid and electrolyte imbalances may develop
   b. Permanent renal damage may occur (especially in cases of prerenal ARF)
2. Sepsis is prime reason for mortality in ARF

PATIENT CARE MANAGEMENT

1. Goals

COMMENTS/TIPS/ CAUTIONS

a. To maintain fluid balance
   i. Keep accurate records of intake

Intake in ARF usually restricted to replacement of insensible water loss plus loss through renal and nonrenal means

Changes in feeding habits may herald sepsis or metabolic acidosis

If infant is not fed orally, the need to suck should not be ignored; use a pacifier if not contraindicated

   (a) Oral, nasogastric, gastrostomy feedings
   (b) IV therapy
   (c) Parenteral alimentation
   (d) Blood products

   ii. Keep accurate records of output

Weighing diapers on a gram scale before placement under infant allows closer calculation of urinary output (1 gm = 1 ml urine)

   (a) Urine
   (b) Stool
   (c) Drainage
   (d) Blood loss, including from specimens
   (e) Insensible water loss
       (1) 0.7 to 1.0 ml/kg/ hour in term infants for first 3 days
       (2) Add 15 to 20 ml/ kg/24 hours if radiant warmer or phototherapy used

   iii. Weigh infant every morning to detect accumulation of body fluid
   iv. Frequent assessment for edema and pulmonary edema

In early stages of formation of pulmonary transudate, fine rales usually heard at lung bases

b. To maintain acid base and electrolyte balance

i. Be alert for tachypnea; in absence of rales or lung disease, this may be the first symptom of increase in serum hydrogen ions
   (a) Sodium bicarbonate may be used for partial correction of severe metabolic acidosis
ii. Monitor heart rate; assess ECG for
   (a) Hyperkalemia—if the serum level is increased to 8 mEq/L or above, the following changes may occur:
      (1) Peaked T waves
      (2) Widened QRS complexes
      (3) ST depressions
      (4) Prolonged P–R intervals
      (5) Flattened P waves

Alert physician if the preceding signs appear

   (b) Have IV calcium gluconate (10 per cent solution) available; usual dose 0.5 to 1 ml/kg over 2 to 4 minutes
   (c) Sodium polystyrene (a calcium exchange resin) may be used
iii. Frequent assessment for neurological symptoms
   (a) Twitching of extremities
   (b) Jitteriness
   (c) High pitched cry
   (d) Seizures

If the above signs are present, serum calcium and magnesium should be checked

iv. Dietary management usually includes use of human breast milk
v. Peritoneal dialysis may be necessary to combat conditions such as congestive

The renal mechanism is one of three primary systems that regulate acid-base balance; kidneys retain hydrogen ions and excrete bicarbonate ions in alkalosis, and retain bicarbonate loss and excrete hydrogen ions in acidosis

If sodium bicarbonate is used to correct acidosis, watch for signs and symptoms of congestive heart failure, intraventricular hemorrhage (sudden apnea, poor peripheral perfusion, falling hematocrit, seizures), or tetany

Hyperkalemia results from kidney's inability to excrete potassium as well as increased cellular potassium release in metabolic acidosis

Infant should always have ECG monitoring during calcium gluconate administration

These may indicate hypocalcemia (serum level less than 3.5 mEq/liter or hypomagnesemia (serum level less than 1 mEq/liter)

Human breast milk provides a smaller sodium, potassium, calcium, chloride, and phosphorus load than does standard cow's milk formula; since it is higher in carbohydrate and lower in protein than cow's milk formulas, beast milk provides more calories with less urea production

The word *dialysis* refers to passage of ions from an area of high concentration to an area of lower concentration across a semipermeable membrane, such as the peritoneal membrane

heart failure, severe hyper-kalemia, metabolic acidosis, and extreme overhydration with pulmonary edema

COMMENTS/TIPS/ CAUTIONS

(a) Weigh infant before and after procedure to ensure accuracy in calculating fluid loss

(b) Infant sized catheter inserted percutaneously

Since infection is a prime reason for mortality in ARF, insertion of catheter and introduction of dialysate must be a sterile procedure

(c) Dialysate introduced into peritoneal cavity by gravity and 15 to 20 minutes allowed for equilibration

(d) Vital signs and BP monitored frequently

Hypotension may occur if excessive sodium and water are removed

(e) Old dialysate drained and fresh dialysate introduced

Dialysate should be warmed to body temperature

(f) Keep accurate record of dialysate inflow and outflow

Excessive retention should be reported to the physician

 (1) Time introduced
 (2) Time drained
 (3) Total amount of dialysate used

(g) Process continues until electrolyte balance is within normal limits and toxic substances removed (10 to 12 hours)

(h) Sample of outflow dialysate drawn for routine culture and sensitivity determination

Call physician if feces, urine, or blood appears in dialysate; this may indicate perforation of bowel, bladder, or a blood vessel

_____ CONCLUSIONS _____

In most cases, ARF is of prerenal origin and is treated and corrected by the time of the neonate's discharge. There are, however, conditions that will necessitate parental teaching to assure optimum home management of the infant's condition.

Those infants who have been discharged with unilateral multicystic kidney disease, for example, usually have good renal function in the remaining kidney. If an infant has only one kidney or one that is not functioning, the parents should be told to report this to their family physician and to report it any time the infant is hospitalized for conditions not associated with the renal problem. Since some medications, especially antibiotics, are cleared through renal mechanisms, it is important that those who are treating the child be made aware of the possibility of lesser drug clearance. It may be suggested that, when older, the child wear a Medic Alert bracelet with this information.

If the infant is discharged while still convalescing from ARF, the parents should be taught the signs and symptoms of degenerating renal function:

1. A change in feeding patterns or increasing refusal to feed
2. A decrease in output: the parents should be made aware of how much the infant usually has been voiding and should also be aware that output must be viewed in relation to intake; if the infant has been taking feedings as usual and the output is lowered, then there may be cause for concern, especially if this corresponds with an appreciable weight gain; if the environment is hot, however, then the urine output may be somewhat less without being regarded as abnormal
3. Dark or blood-tinged urine
4. Edema
5. Tachypnea at rest: again, the parents should be taught what is normal for their infant, so a standard for comparison is prepared
6. Wheezing
7. Poor general growth pattern

If breast feeding is to be continued, the mother will need encouragement and teaching in regard to breast care throughout her infant's hospitalization. If the infant was too sick for breast feeding initially, it is the nurse's responsibility to give the mother instructions on pumping her breasts to keep her milk supply adequate. The mother should also be taught safe storage of her breast milk if it is to be used to feed her hospitalized infant. Breast pumping often can be a tedious and seemingly unrewarding procedure for the mother awaiting her infant's recovery. The nurse needs to spend time with the mother to allow expression of any problems the mother has been experiencing and any feeling she has regarding the procedure. The infant should not be discharged until feeding well at the breast and the mother feels comfortable with the procedure. Alternative formulas should be discussed with the parents should the success of long term breast feeding be questionable.

Arrangements for the infant's follow-up care should be made prior to discharge. After assessment of the parents' financial, emotional, and intellectual resources, referrals to the appropriate agencies can be made. The nurse should take time to evaluate the parents' knowledge of their infant's care and reemphasize any important points that may be needed. Individual written instructions are helpful, especially if given to the parents a few days prior to the infant's discharge. This will allow time for questions to be generated. The parents should leave the hospital with telephone numbers of whom to call in an emergency and also whom to contact with questions of routine care.

REFERENCES

1. Avery, G.: Neonatology: Pathophysiology and Management of the Newborn, 2nd ed. Philadelphia, J.B. Lippincott Co., 1981.
2. Babson, G., Pernoll, M., and Benda, G.: Diagnosis and Management of the Fetus and Neonate at Risk: A Guide for Team Care, 4th ed. St. Louis, C.V. Mosby Co., 1980.
3. Behrman, R.: Neonatal-Perinatal Medicine: Disease of the Fetus and Infant, 2nd ed. St. Louis, C.V. Mosby Co., 1977.
4. Bloom, D., and Brosman, J.: The multicystic kidney. J. Urol., *120*:211–215, 1978.
5. Cloherty, J., and Epstein, M.: Maternal diabetes. *In* Cloherty, J., and Stark, A. (eds.): Manual of Neonatal Care. Boston, Little, Brown & Co., 1980.
6. Dulock, H., and Swendsen, L.: Hypoglycemia in the Newborn. *In* Duxbury, M. (ed.): A Staff Development Program in Perinatal Nursing Care. New York, National Foundation/March of Dimes, 1977.
7. Jain, R.: Acute renal failure in the neonate. Pediatr. Clin. North Am., *24*:605–618, 1977.
8. James, J.A.: Renal Disease in Childhood. St. Louis, C.V. Mosby Co., 1976.
9. Jeffs, R.D., Comisarow, R.H., and Hanna, M.K.: The early assessment for individualized treatment in the prune belly syndrome. *In* Bergsma, D., and Duckett, J. (eds.): Urinary System Malformations in Children. New York, National Foundation/March of Dimes, 1977.
10. Kagan, L.: Renal Disease: A Manual of Patient Care. New York, McGraw-Hill Book Co., 1979.
11. Korones, S.: High-Risk Newborn Infants: The Basis for Intensive Care Nursing. St. Louis, C.V. Mosby Co., 1981.
12. Lemons, J.: Neonatal glucose metabolism and the infant of the diabetic mother. Crit. Care Q., *4*(1):59–69, 1981.
13. Lerch, C., and Bliss, V.J.: Maternity Nursing. St. Louis, C.V. Mosby Co., 1978.
14. Lubchenco, L., and Bard, H.: Incidence of hypoglycemia in newborn infants classified by birth weight and gestational age. Pediatrics, *47*:831, 1971.
15. McCrory, W.: Renal failure in the newborn. Contrib. Nephrol., *15*:10–20, 1979.
16. Mitcheson, H.D., Williams, G., and Castro, J.E.: Clinical aspects of polycystic disease of the kidneys. Br. Med. J., *1*:1196–1198, 1977.
17. Philip, A.: Neonatology: A Practical Guide. New York, Medical Examination Publishing Co., 1977.
18. Pramanik, A., Altshuler, G., Light, I., and Sutherland, J.: Prune belly syndrome associated with Potter (renal nonfunction) syndrome. Am. J. Dis. Child., *131*:672–674, 1977.
19. Quan, L., and Smith, D.: The VATER association. J. Pediatr., *82*:104–107, 1973.
20. Rodriguez-Soriano, J.: Developmental aspects of renal function. Paediatrician, *4*:4–15, 1975.
21. Sharer, J.: Reviewing acid-base balance. Am. J. Nurs., *6*:980–983, 1975.
22. Symchych, P., and Winchester, P.: Potter's syndrome. Am. J. Pathol., *90*:779–782, 1978.
23. Trompeter, R., Chantler, C., and Haycock, G.: Tolazoline and acute renal failure in the newborn. Lancet, *2*:1219, 1981.
24. Vaughan, V., McKay, J., and Behrman, R.E. (eds.): Nelson Textbook of Pediatrics, 11th ed. Philadelphia, W.B. Saunders Co., 1979.
25. Volpe, J.: Neurology of the Newborn. Philadelphia, W.B. Saunders Co., 1981.

CHAPTER 19

GASTROINTESTINAL CRISES AND NUTRITIONAL SUPPORT

Jane Pohodich, R.N., M.S.

OBJECTIVES

Upon completion of this chapter the reader will be able to accomplish the following:

1. State the basic daily nutritional requirements for and function of the following in a term neonate:
   a. Calories
   b. Fluids
   c. Protein, fats, carbohydrates
   d. Vitamins and minerals

2. Identify factors that alter nutritional requirements for the following:
   a. Preterm infants
   b. Intrauterine growth retarded neonate
   c. Infant of diabetic mother

3. Contrast the following nutritional sources on the basis of purpose and rationale as well as special precautions and considerations:
   a. Basic proprietary formulas
   b. Modular formulas
   c. Special formulas

4. State etiology, prognosis, and usual treatment of the following neonatal gastrointestinal crises:
   a. Omphalocele
   b. Gastroschisis
   c. Atresia
   d. Stenosis
   e. Necrotizing enterocolitis

5. Design plans of nursing care for infants with gastrointestinal and nutritional problems that reflect assessment and evaluation parameters

6. Plan nursing management of infants receiving parenteral or special enteral feedings

7. Recount basic factors to be considered when implementing and maintaining the following specialized care:
   a. Peripheral IVs
   b. Central venous catheters
   c. Parenteral alimentation
   d. Tube feedings

The gastrointestinal system of the neonate is immature in both size and function. Thus even the normal term infant is susceptible to problems. Successful functioning of the gastrointestinal tract is a prime requisite for survival after birth. Prior to that time, the main source of nutrition is via the mother and the placenta. What little activity there is in the gastrointestinal system consists of swallowing and digesting amniotic fluid, resulting in production of meconium. Failure of the system to perform this function usually results in polyhydramnios and indicates a potential for a neonatal gastrointestinal crisis.

With birth, the neonate's natural total parenteral nutrition source—the mother—is lost. It is essential for survival that the infant begin ingestion, digestion, and elimination. Three major sources for problems in the establishment of extrauterine function are as follows:

1. Immaturity of the gastrointestinal system, which results in inadequate digestion and absorption capabilities

2. Anatomical or structural life threatening anomalies, such as omphalocele, gastroschisis, and diaphragmatic hernia, that interfere with optimal gastrointestinal tract function

3. Neonatal complications such as necrotizing enterocolitis result in both altered digestion and absorption, which may necessitate emergency surgical intervention

Only several of the most frequently encountered gastrointestinal crises or those most threatening to the neonate's survival will be discussed. Likewise, discussion of maturational difficulties will be limited to information the nurse will need for initial assessment of the infant's status and emergency stabilization and then for planning, implementing, and evaluating the ongoing care of the neonate.

Failure of the neonate to maintain adequate nutrition results in one or more of the following: growth retardation due to diminished tissue and enzyme production or function; increased risk of infection; mental retardation or death if uncorrected.

Neonatal nutritional requirements are greater than adult requirements primarily as a result of the following:

1. Large body surface area predisposing to heat and energy loss; the neonate's only mechanism for heat production is through an increased metabolic rate, which requires additional caloric intake to provide the fuel to sustain it.

2. Growth rate, which requires large amounts of nutrients for the tremendous body growth that continues to take place after birth.

Inadequate nutritional support results when:

1. Physiological ability to ingest and digest nutrients is limited: weak sucking and limited stomach capacity and stamina all contribute to diminished intake; bowel ability to utilize ingested nutrients may be inefficient or absent; foods with high fat content, complex proteins, or sugars all compromise stomach capacity and retard gastric emptying time and bowel transit time. These factors in turn may alter the frequency, amount, and route employed to feed the infant.

2. Health care providers frequently continue to employ outdated or dangerous ideas regarding infant feeding: the still common practice of withhold-

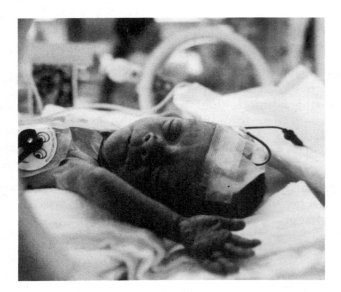

Figure 19-1. The premature infant is more vulnerable than the term neonate to the consequences of nutritional deprivation. (Courtesy of Hermann Hospital, Houston, Texas.)

ing formula feedings from normal neonates until 12 to 24 hours after birth predisposes them to hypoglycemia. If the infant is sick or premature this practice can be particularly hazardous unless an alternate nutritional support mechanism such as parenteral feeding is employed.

The sick or premature infant is more vulnerable to nutritional deprivation than the term neonate. It is therefore the responsibility of the health care team to apply knowledge of nutritional requirements in assessment and then to utilize appropriate techniques accurately and safely to provide adequate nutritional support. If this responsibility is to be met it is essential that the nurse be knowledgeable in basic fluid and nutritional requirements, possess the ability to assess adequacy of current intake, and recognize problems and obstacles that may interfere with adequate nutrition and modify care accordingly. In addition, specialized skills will frequently need to be employed to support the neonate's nutritional state. These skills include assisting the mother with breast or bottle feeding; establishing alternate enteral feeding methods, such as gavage or nasojejunal infusions; and starting peripheral IVs and maintaining central venous or arterial lines. Survival of the neonate with a gastrointestinal crisis very often depends on the nurse's early recognition of problems and meticulous nursing care of the critically ill infant.

NUTRITIONAL REQUIREMENTS

Maintenance of adequate nutritional support is essential for growth and development of a healthy neonate. Failure to provide adequate fluids, calories (from appropriate protein, carbohydrate, and fat sources), vitamins, and minerals can and does result in life threatening situations either as a direct result of their absence or indirectly through improper tissue development or repair and/or impaired metabolic states.

FACTORS INCREASING BASIC REQUIREMENTS

1. **Caloric requirements when temperatures are outside neutral thermal range (Table 19-1)**
   b. Respiratory distress
   c. Increased cardiac output
   d. Infection
   e. Gestational age

2. **Fluid requirements**
   a. Gestational age at birth: the more premature the greater the total body water (85 per cent at 28 weeks' gestation, 70 per cent at term) and the greater the risk
   b. Low environmental humidity: increases insensible water loss (environmental humidity less than 40 to 60 per cent)
   c. Respiratory distress increases insensible water loss; normally one third of all insensible water loss (IWL) is respiratory—infants receiving ventilatory support via ventilators with heated nebulization may have less IWL via the respiratory tract, which must be considered when fluid needs are calculated. Fluid overload is a potential hazard.
   d. Use of phototherapy and radiant warmers: increases insensible water loss (by as much as 50 to 100 per cent)
   e. Disease processes: vomiting, diarrhea, acute tubular necrosis, glycosuria, inappropriate ADH secretion

3. **Vitamin requirements**
   a. Gestational age: most infants whose formula intake is less than 1 quart/day will require supplementation to achieve minimal daily requirements
   b. Malabsorptive syndromes

4. **Requirements for mineral and trace elements**
   a. Gestational age: most minerals, including iron, are not deposited until the last 2 months of gestation

TABLE 19-1. BASIC CALORIC REQUIREMENTS IN THE NORMAL NEONATE

Calorie Use	Cal/Kg/Day	Average Cal/Kg/Day Requirement
Basal metabolic rate*	50	
Activity*	10	To maintain body weight: 80–90
Environmental temperature stress*	10	To provide growth: 120
Digestive losses	10	
Fecal losses	10	
Body growth	30	

*Infants maintained in a neutral thermal environment with minimal handling and stress have been known to gain weight on 80 cal/kg/day, but this is not the ideal state.

    b. Prolonged IV therapy without supplementation increases risk for trace element deficiency

ASSESSMENT

This includes recognition of the infant's ability and readiness to feed as well as identification of nutritional and fluid deficiencies.

1. **Factors influencing ability and readiness to feed**
   a. Reflex Activity: gestational age less than 32 to 34 weeks is *not* compatible with oral feeding because of poorly coordinated suck-swallow mechanism; oral feeding prior to establishment of suck-swallow activity predisposes infant to aspiration
   b. Suck-Swallow Pattern
      i. Sucking pattern is influenced by nipple flow and type of food (infants suck more vigorously when fed formula than when fed glucose)
      ii. "Mature" suck-swallow pattern consists of prolonged sucking bursts with multiple swallows *in conjunction* with sucking activity
      iii. "Immature" suck-swallow pattern consists of short sucking bursts *preceded* or *followed* by swallowing
   c. Lower esophageal sphincter: during the perinatal period incomplete development may result in vomiting. In premature infants altered respiratory rate, periodic breathing, and apnea may be associated with feeding, most frequently within the first 15 minutes.
   d. Gastric Capacity, Emptying, and Function
      i. Gastric capacity at birth is approximately 6 ml/kg of body weight[24]
      ii. Gastric emptying is mediated by the pylorus
         (a) Volume sensitive receptors in the stomach are stimulated as distention occurs, triggering pyloric relaxation; these receptors are more sensitive to liquid than to solid foods
         (b) In the duodenum receptors sensitive to the content of food leaving the stomach inhibit pyloric relaxation; these receptors are particularly sensitive to fat content, acidity, and amino acid content[30]
      iii. Gastric emptying time is approximately 5 to 8 hours in a normal term infant; in a premature infant receiving glucose or water stomach emptying is usually less than 5 hours, and formula ingestion results in delay of complete emptying until 7 to 8 hours.
      iv. Gastric emptying is delayed
         (a) In respiratory distress
         (b) In infants receiving supplemental medium chain triglycerides
      v. Gastric emptying is enhanced
         (a) In infants receiving glucagon
         (b) If infant in prone or right lateral position following feeding[32]

TABLE 19-2. DAILY NUTRITIONAL AND VITAMIN REQUIREMENTS*

Total Nutrients	Per Kg	Vitamins	Total/Day†
Calories	100–140	A	1500–2500 IU
Water	130–200 ml‡	Thiamine	0.4 mg
Protein	3–4 gm (10–15%)	Riboflavin	0–5 mg
Carbohydrate	10–15 gm (45–55%)	Pyridoxine	0.25 mg
Fat	5–7 gm (30–45%)	B_{12}	1.0 μg
Sodium	2–4 mEq	C	30–50 mg
Chloride	0.5–2 mEq	D	400 IU
Potassium	0.5–2 mEq	C	5–100 IU
Calcium	4–6 mEq	Niacin	6.0 mg
Phosphorus	2–4 mEq	Panthenol	
Magnesium	0.5–1 mEq	Folic acid	0.35 mg
		K	1.5 mg
Iron	6 mg/day		

*Table of Basic Requirements is provided; all these requirements can be and frequently are revised upward, depending on the presence of the factors listed in A to D.
From Klaus, M.H., and Fanaroff, A.A.: Care of the High-Risk Neonate, 2nd ed. Philadelphia, W.B. Saunders Co., 1979, p. 120.
†Start vitamin supplementation between 5th and 10th day of life.
‡Adequate to maintain normal urine output of 1 to 3 ml/kg/hr.

    (c)   With tube feedings
    (d)   In those receiving breast milk

2. Nutritional and fluid deficiencies
  a. Assessment of Fluid and Caloric Requirements (Table 19–2)
     i. Done weekly on all long term hospitalized infants
    ii. Calculated by[17]
      Weight in kilograms (rounded to nearest 0.1 kg) multiplied by fluid and calorie requirement
      Example: 1847 gm infant = 1.8 kg
      Calorie needs: 1.8 kg x 120 cal/kg/day = 216 cal/day
      Fluid needs: 1.8 kg x 150 ml/kg/day = 270 ml/day

   iii. Adequacy of fluid and calorie intake determined by[17]
    (a)   Weight gain
       less than 28 weeks — 16.8 gm/day
       28 to 32 weeks — 23.9 gm/day
       32 to 36 weeks — 30.7 gm/day
       36 to 42 weeks — 27.1 gm/day
    (b)   Initial weight loss (first 4 days) not to exceed 10 per cent of body weight
    (c)   Urine output greater than 30 ml/kg/day
    (d)   Specific gravity of urine: 1.008 to 1.012 (maximal urinary concentration prior to 1 to 2 months of age is 1.018 to 1.021)

  iv. Factors increasing fluid and caloric requirements
   (a) Ambient temperature outside neutral thermal range
   (b) Muscular activity
   (c) Respiratory distress
   (d) Cardiac output
   (e) Infection
   (f) SGA infant
  v. Factors increasing fluid losses
   (a) High skin permeability in premature infant
   (b) Use of phototherapy and radiant warmers
   (c) Vomiting and diarrhea
   (d) Acute tubular necrosis
   (e) Glycosuria
   (f) Inappropriate ADH secretion
   (g) Respiratory distress syndrome
  vi. Consequences of fluid overload
   (a) Shunting and cardiac decompensation
   (b) Bronchopulmonary dysplasia in ventilated infants
  vii. General considerations for management
   Achievement of recommended caloric intake orally in a sick or premature infant may require 7–10 days minimum because
   (a) Physical capacity of stomach limits volume and calories
   (b) Circulatory load is generally limited to 150 ml/kg/day and is not achievable until about 4 days of age. Prior to that time fluids in the neonate may be limited to 80 to 100 ml/kg/day to allow for stabilization of the extracellular fluid levels.
  viii. Parameters for monitoring parenteral nutrition therapy (Table 19–3)
 b. Assessment of Nutrients. See Tables 19–4 through 19–7; normal requirements are in Table 19–2.

3. Biopsychosocial assessment
 a. The critically ill infant and the very premature infant may be unable to experience breast feeding by the mother for an extended period. This delay in essential care giving by the mother is associated with increased incidence of child abuse, neglect, and failure to thrive.
 b. Special care must be taken to involve the family in all aspects of the infant's care. This is particularly critical with regard to feeding, as it is one key role of the primary care giver.
 c. The nurse must exercise caution not to be viewed as being in competition with the mother as "expert care giver" but rather must encourage and support the mother's self-confidence as care giver.

PATIENT CARE MANAGEMENT

1. Sources of nutritional support: see Table 19–8
2. Suggested feeding regimens based on weight and age at birth: see Table 19–9
3. Types of formula available and indications for use: see Table 19–10

TABLE 19-3. MONITORING PARENTERAL NUTRITION THERAPY

	Suggested Frequency
Weight	Daily
Intake and output	Every 8 hr
Urine specific gravity	Every 4–8 hr (every voiding first 24 hr of therapy)
Urine protein, glucose, ketone, pH	Every 4–8 hr (every voiding first 24 hr of therapy)
Serum for hyperlipidemia	8 hr after fat infusion
Triglycerides, free fatty acids	Weekly
Serum electrolytes	3 ×/wk
BUN, Ca, P, pH	2 ×/wk
Mg, total protein and albumin (serum)	Weekly
Liver function studies (creatinine, SGOT, SGPT, bilirubin)	Weekly
Blood glucose	Daily
Serum zinc, copper	Monthly
Serum amino acids	Biweekly
X-ray long bones	As indicated

Adapted from Palma, P.A., et al.: TPN for the Neonate. II: Major minerals and micronutrients. Nutritional Support Services, 2(Jan):1, 1982, p. 9.

4. Nurses's responsibility in management of parenteral therapy: see Tables 19–11 and 19–12
5. Guidelines for hyperalimentation: see Table 19–13
6. Metabolic problems associated with parenteral hyperalimentation: see Table 19–14
7. Fluid and caloric assessment record (Fig. 19–2)

NECROTIZING ENTEROCOLITIS

Necrotizing enterocolitis has become one of the most serious problems in neonatal services. Early recognition and prompt and vigorous therapy are essential if the infant is to survive. Delayed recognition increases the infant's risk for serious complications and death.

Necrotizing enterocolitis is an acute inflammation of bowel mucosa with formation of pseudomembranous plaques overlying an area of superficial ulceration; pseudomembranous material is passed in the feces. The disease often seems to be precipitated by early feedings.

Diagnosis is based on x-ray confirmation of gas in the bowel mucosal wall (pneumatosis intestinalis) and portal venous gas. X-ray findings of free abdominal air indicates bowel perforation and is an ominous sign.

1. **Incidence**
   a. Occurs in 2 to 15 per cent of all admissions to neonatal intensive care units

Text continues on page 489.

TABLE 19-4. ASSESSMENT OF CARBOHYDRATE, PROTEIN, AND FATS IN THE NEONATE

Nutritional Substance and Function	Normal Blood Values	Causes of Disorder or Infants at Risk	Symptoms	Sequelae	Therapy	Comments
Carbohydrates (glucose) Primary energy source for all cellular activity	Preterm 30–80 mg/100 ml Term 40–100 mg/100 ml	*Hypoglycemia* Infant of diabetic mother Infant of alcoholic mother Premature SGA infant Erythroblastosis fetalis Exchange transfusion Asphyxia/sepsis Beckwith syndrome Transposition of great vessels *Iatrogenic Causes* Hypothermia Rapid or abrupt discontinuation of parenteral alimentation or IV fluids with high glucose level	Irritability Lethargy Limpness High pitched cry Difficulty feeding Sweating Apnea/cyanosis Tremors/convulsions	Survivors of symptomatic transient neonatal hypoglycemia show 30–50% incidence of neurological impairment and 10% incidence of recurrence of hypoglycemia[17]	*Prophylactic* Identify at risk infant Initiate early feedings if not contraindicated by condition 10% glucose IV* <24 hr old: 70–80 ml/kg/day >24 hr: 100–120 ml/kg/day *Maintain rate of 6–8 mg glucose/kg/min *Example* 1 kg infant receiving 10% glucose = 10 gm glucose/ 100 ml or 100 mg/ml Determine requirement 6 mg/kg/min = 6 mg × 1 kg × 60 min = 360 mg/hr Determine rate 100 mg: 1 ml = 360: X ml 100 X = 360 X = 3.6 ml/hr of 10% glucose infusion *Symptomatic Hypoglycemia* (Blood glucose < 30 mg/100 ml)	Screen for hypoglycemia with Dextrostix; values outside 45–120 mg/ 100 ml should be verified by laboratory analysis Failure to warm the heel prior to blood collection or allowing blood to remain at room temperature for long periods of time prior to test measurement may result in falsely low readings

			Hyperglycemia Blood levels > 125 mg/100 ml Immaturity 30 wk gestation < 1100 gm at birth Insults to CNS (hemorrhage, birth asphyxia)	Osmotic diuresis Elevated blood glucose level 3+ glucose in urine	Blood glucose levels > 200 mg/100 ml have been associated with hemorrhage because of hyperosmolarity Dehydration with electrolyte imbalance	50% glucose immediately diluted 1:1 with sterile water 1–2 ml/kg Continuous infusion of 7–8 mg/kg/min Reduce energy needs Monitor hourly with Dextrostix until condition stable
			Iatrogenic Causes IV therapy—rate in excess of 7 mg/kg/min of glucose in very small infants Hyperalimentation			Reduce glucose load by reducing rate of IV infusion or glucose concentration Avoid peripheral IV concentration > 12.5% Monitor blood levels with Dextrostix Insulin may be administered if caloric intake must be maintained
						Causes venous sclerosis and is hyperosmolar
Amino acids	Positive nitrogen balance for synthesis of proteins, body tissues, enzymes, and hormones	**Ammonia** Newborn 90–150 µg/100 ml 0–2 wk 70–129 µg/100 ml **SGOT** 1–3 days 16–74 IU/liter 6 mo 20–43 IU/liter	**Natural Causes** Genetic metabolic disorders Phenylketonuria Maple syrup urine disease Tyrosinemia Cystinuria Premature/sick infants unable	**Inadequate Intake** Poor weight gain Low serum albumin level with edema Decreased brain DNA **Excessive Intake** (from TPN administration)	Long term excessive intake from TPN may result in decreased intelligence Long term effects of excessive oral protein intake include increased incidence of febrile states, lethargy, poor feeding, and pos-	**Hyperalimentation** Initially 0.5 gm/kg/day gradually increased to 2–3 gm/kg/day Premature infants receiving TPN may need a source of essential amino acids *cystine, taurine,* and *ty-* See Table 19-3 for guidelines for monitoring serum values in infants receiving TPN Sick preterm infants can be maintained in positive nitro-positive nitro-

Table continues on following page.

TABLE 19-4. ASSESSMENT OF CARBOHYDRATE, PROTEIN, AND FATS IN THE NEONATE – *Continued*

Nutritional Substance and Function	Normal Blood Values	Causes of Disorder or Infants at Risk	Symptoms	Sequelae	Therapy	Comments
	SGPT up to 54 IU/liter	to consume adequate nutrients orally	Metabolic acidosis Hyperammonemia	sibly apnea Protein intake of 6 gm/kg/day has been associated with strabismus and lowered IQ	*rosine* as they may lack capacity to create them from amino acids Oral formulas that maintain a whey:casein ratio of 60:40 result in fewer metabolic derangements in infants	gen balance with as little as 60 cal/kg/day when 10 cal/kg/day is in form of protein
	BUN Premature 1st week 9.3 ± 5.2 mg/100 ml Term 6–23 mg/100 ml	*Iatrogenic Causes* Failure to provide 2–4 gm/kg/day				
	Total Protein Preterm 4.3–7.6 gm/100 ml Term 4.6–7.4 gm/100 ml					
	Alkaline Phosphatase Preterm 100–250 IU/liter Term 200–800 IU/liter					
	Creatinine 0.3–1.0 mg/100 ml					
	Serum Albumin Preterm 2.8–3.9 gm/100 ml Term 2.3–5.1 gm/100 ml					
Lipids–Fat Fuel, high energy storage, transport for fat soluble	*Cholesterol* Term 50–120 mg/100 ml	*Natural Causes* Metabolic/hereditary malabsorption Inadequate endo-	Essential fatty acid deficiency Scaliness of skin Thrombocytopenia Poor wound healing	*IV Lipids* Allergic reaction Hepatomegaly Shock Eosinophilia	Provision of medium chain triglycerides in formula *Intravenous Lipids* Initial	Improves fat absorption, weight gain, enhances calcium absorption and nitro-

vitamins, enhance calcium absorption and protein retention

Fatty Acids—Free
1627 μg/ml
±155 μg/ml

Total Fat—Lipids
170–440 mg/100 ml

crine pancreatic function
Defective reabsorption of intestinal bile acid

Iatrogenic Causes
Failure to provide 40–50% of total calories as fat
Hyperlipidemia occurring after infusion of IV fat emulsions

Alopecia
Growth retardation
Liver and kidney changes

Blood hypercoagulability
Decreased platelet adhesions
Interference with bilirubin binding
Interference with pulmonary diffusion of gases

0.4–0.5 gm/kg/day with gradual increase to 2–4 gm/kg/day
Infusion rate AGA and >33 wk gestation 0.3 gm/kg/hr SGA and <33 wk gestation 0.16 gm/kg/hr

gen retention
IV lipids contraindicated in infant with severe respiratory distress or deranged liver function

TABLE 19-5. ASSESSMENT OF BASIC ELECTROLYTES IN THE NEONATE

Nutritional Substance and Function	Normal Blood Values	Causes of Disorder or Infants at Risk	Symptoms	Sequelae	Therapy	Comments
Calcium Bone mineralization Blood clotting Regulates cell membrane permeability Exerts control over neuromuscular excitability Body intake: Absorbed through active transport in upper small bowel Requires vitamin D and parathormone for adequate uptake Absorption reduced by dietary constituents that form insoluble complexes in the gut	*Total Calcium* Preterm 4.7 ± 0.4 mEq/liter or 7–10 mg/100 ml Term 3.7–6.0 mEq/liter or 7.3–12 mg/100 ml *Unbound Calcium* About 50% of total calcium level *Ionized Calcium* 4.4–5.4 mg/100 ml	Inadequate intake; oral or failure to provide Ca++ for infants receiving IV therapy and nothing orally Malabsorption: Rapid transit through bowel Vitamin D deficiency Excessive loss: renal insufficiency *Hypocalcemia* Preterm and SGA infant with low serum albumin level Infant of diabetic mother Infant with respiratory or metabolic problems producing hypoxia or rapid pH changes Associated hypomagnesemia After asphyxia Exchange transfusion	*Hypocalcemia* (total serum Ca++ <7 mg/100 ml) Irritability High pitched cry Tremors/twitching Convulsions Apnea Cyanosis Hypotonia/hypertonia Vomiting Laryngospasm Blood clotting disorder Bone demineralization Prolonged Q-T interval on ECG greater than 0.19 sec in term infant or 2.0 sec in preterm	Death Rickets	*Mild/Asymptomatic* Calcium replacement of 24–35 mg/kg/24 hr per intravenous infusion *Moderate/Severe* IV administration 10% calcium gluconate 0.5–1 ml/kg calcium gluceptate 0.5 ml/kg Initial IV administration not to exceed 3 ml/kg of calcium gluconate *Slow* IV infusion of at least 1 ml/min with continuous *cardiac monitoring.* Halt if bradycardia occurs Continued therapy: Parenteral 50–60 mg/kg/24 hr Internal	Decrease in ionized calcium is responsible for signs and symptoms Calcium potentiates digitalis effect IV infiltrate will result in severe damage and sloughing Serum potassium levels may be diminished during calcium administration Other calcium sources: Calcium gluceptate = 18 mg calcium per ml 10% calcium gluconate = 9 mg (calcium per ml) Neo-Calglucon = 23 mg calcium per ml

Function	Normal value	Cause	Signs and symptoms	Result	Treatment	Remarks
		Hyperparathyroidism in mother Associated with administration of alkali buffers Renal failure Intracranial trauma			Interal calcuim lactate, calcium gluconate, and calcium glubionate, to provide 35–70 mg calcium per 100 ml of feeding	Neo-Calglucon has high osmolality and should be used with caution in infant's susceptible to necrotizing enterocolitis
		Hypercalcemia Iatrogenic Improper administration Laboatoy error Hypervitaminosis D Massive subcutaneous fat necrosis Idiopathic Hyperparathyroidism *Infants at risk* Severe cold stress with fat necrosis After exchange transfusion	Constipation Anorexia Muscle hypotonicity Premature ventricular contractions, ventricular tachycardia Prolonged P-R interval, QRS duration, and/or AV heart block Shortened Q-T interval due to decreased ST segment	Failure to thrive Severe iatrogenic cause may result in death		
Potassium Muscle contraction Nerve impulse conduction Intracellular osmotic pressure and fluid balance	Preterm 4.5–7.2 mEq/liter or 18–28 mg/100 ml Term 3.7–5.2 mEq/100 ml or 15–21 mg/100 ml	**Hypokalemia** Iatrogenic Inappropriate or excessive IV therapy Laboratory error Excessive losses from body Renal losses, metabolic or respiratory	Weakness or paralysis of skeletal muscles Abdominal distention, ileus Bradycardia Tachycardia Diminished reflexes Prolonged Q-T interval	Cardiac irritability Heart block Cardiac arrest	2 mEq/kg/24 hr per IV Correct concurrent hyponatremia	*Do not administer K+ unless infant is voiding*

Table continues on following page.

TABLE 19-5. ASSESSMENT OF BASIC ELECTROLYTES IN THE NEONATE – *Continued*

Nutritional Substance and Function	Normal Blood Values	Causes of Disorder or Infants at Risk	Symptoms	Sequelae	Therapy	Comments
Maintenance of cardiac rhythm		alkalosis Hypernatremia GI losses from vomiting/diarrhea *Infants at risk* Infant receiving diuretic/steroids Infant undergoing long term IV therapy Congenital Cushing disease or aldosteronism	Broad, flat T wave Depressed S-T segment Prolonged P-R interval Prominent P wave			
		Hyperkalemia Iatrogenic Laboratory error Exchange transfusion with bank blood Excessive administration of K⁺ IV or orally Tissue damage with cellular death, releasing intracellular K⁺ Acidosis Shock and hypoxia with failure of sodium po-	*ECG* "Tended" T waves Widened QRS Flattened P waves Ectopic rhythms Ventricular block Muscle weakness, flaccid paralysis Twitching Oliguria Apnea, respiratory arrest	Arrhythmias Death	Discontinue exogenous K⁺ administration Administer sequentially or concurrently 100–300 mg/kg calcium gluconate IV over 5–10 min 1–2 mEq/kg NaHCO₃ IV over 5–10 min 1–2 gm/kg glucose with 0.3 units regular insulin per gram of glucose IV over 2 hr Kayexalate 1–2 gm/kg/day oral, or as retention enema	Toxic effects are enhanced by sodium or calcium depletion Monitor for bradycardia when giving calcium IV line must be flushed between administration of calcium gluconate and NaHCO₃, as they are incompatible Kayexalate 1 gm/kg body weight should lower serum K⁺ 1 mEq/liter

Sodium						
Predominantly extracellular electrolyte	Preterm 130–140 mEq/liter	tassium pump mechanism			IV maintenance 0–48 hr of age: no added sodium >48 hr of age: 1/8 to 1/4 normal saline added to dextrose 5% or 10%	Check for other electrolyte imbalances; chloride and potassium may both be abnormal if sodium level is abnormal
Regulates osmotic pressure	Term 135–145 mEq/liter	Acute renal failure				
Maintains water balance		Hypoadrenalism				
Regulates muscle and nerve irritability		*Infants at risk*				
		Rh-ABO incompatibility with exchange transfusion				
		Severe respiratory distress or sepsis with massive tissue hypoxia and acidosis				
		Hyponatremia	Convulsions	CNS damage due to increase in brain volume	Specific therapy for hyponatremia: correct deficit when serum sodium <125 mEq/liter	
		Iatrogenic	Irritability		Calculate Na^+ replacement by subtracting actual Na^+ level from 135 and multiplying remainder by infant weight $\times$ 0.6 (extracellular volume)	
		Laboratory error	Lethargy			
		Inappropriate IV fluid therapy	Shock			
		Overhydration orally	Apnea		Example: Wt. 2 kg. Na^+ 120 mEq/liter 135–120 = 15	
		Excessive diuretic therapy				
		Increased environmental humidity causing decreased IWL				
		Inappropriate ADH secretion (due to asphyxia, stress, CNS injury)				

Table continues on following page.

467

TABLE 19–5. ASSESSMENT OF BASIC ELECTROLYTES IN THE NEONATE – *Continued*

Nutritional Substance and Function	Normal Blood Values	Causes of Disorder or Infants at Risk	Symptoms	Sequelae	Therapy	Comments
		Congestive heart failure GI losses (vomiting, diarrhea, nasogastric drainage) Potassium deficiency Hypoxia and shock (failure of Na$^+$ pump mechanism) Sepsis *Infants at risk* Infant receiving ventilator support Infant for whom nebulizers being used Infant receiving parenteral fluids Infant with GI obstruction/vomiting/diarrhea Infant with CNS insult Asphyxiated infant			15 mEq/liter $\times$ 2 $\times$ 0.6 = 1.8 mEq for replacement over 12–24 hr Recheck serum sodium levels Limit fluid intake if inappropriate ADH is suspected	

		Etiology	Clinical Manifestations	Pathophysiology	Treatment	Comments
		Hypernatremia	Lethargy	Hypernatremia causes a shift of water away from the brain, leading to pressure differences within the system and causing dilation and possible rupture of capillaries in the brain	1. Reduce serum sodium levels over 24–48 hr	Fluid deficit is significant if there is 10% loss of body weight
		Iatrogenic	Extreme irritability		2. Replace fluid deficit in addition to maintenance with 5% glucose with 4 mEq/kg NaCl in 24 hr	Plain glucose will only increase cerebral edema and cerebrovascular problems
		Laboratory error	Convulsions			
		Excessive buffering with NaHCO₃	Cardiac failure			
		Inappropriate parenteral or oral fluid therapy	Concurrent hypokalemia, hypocalcemia, acidosis	Occasionally acute tubular necrosis		
		Steroid therapy				
		GI losses of free water				
		↑IWL				
		Renal losses of free water				
		Congenital aldosteronism				
Magnesium	1.5–2.33 mEq/liter	*Hypomagnesemia*	Weakness	Laxative effect with oral magnesium therapy	0.2 ml/kg 50% magnesium sulfate solution IM q 8–12 hr	Suspect when serum calcium levels are low but phosphorus levels are normal
Essential for carbohydrate, protein, and energy metabolism		Chronic diarrhea or intestinal malabsorption	Poor feeding			
necessary for muscle contractions		Renal tubular disease	Failure to thrive			
		Inadequate dietary intake	Paralytic ileus			
		Associated hypocalcemia	Calcium resistant tetany			
		Infants at risk				
		Infant undergoing exchange transfusion				
		Infant or diabetic mothers				
		Small for gestational age infant				
		Infant receiving hyperalimentation				

Table continues on following page.

469

TABLE 19-5. ASSESSMENT OF BASIC ELECTROLYTES IN THE NEONATE – *Continued*

Nutritional Substance and Function	Normal Blood Values	Causes of Disorder or Infants at Risk	Symptoms	Sequelae	Therapy	Comments
		Hypermagnesmia Iatrogenic overdose in hyperalimentation Maternal magnesium sulfate treatment for toxemia *Infants at risk* Infant of mother with preeclampsia or eclampsia Infant receiving hyperalimentation Infant receiving exchange transfusion	7 mEq/liter: drowsiness hypotension, bradycardia 10 mEq/liter: absence of deep tendon reflexes, coma 15 mEq/liter: respiratory failure 24 mEq/liter: cardiac arrest	Apnea in toxic levels	Replacement therapy for calcium losses Ventilatory support if necessary IV fluids as indicated Supportive therapy is generally sufficient if severe toxic levels are reached. Exchange transfusion may be required	Magnesium is excreted by kidney; infants with poor renal function can have toxic effects at lower serum levels
Chloride Regulates osmotic pressure Essential element in gastric juices Participates in acid base balance	Preterm 95–110 mEq/liter Term 96–116 mEq/liter	*Hypochloremia* Iatrogenic a. Laboratory error b. Inappropriate fluid therapy Metabolic alkalosis Hyponatremia Respiratory acidosis GI losses *Infants at risk* Infant receiving IV fluids	Found in association with sodium depletion		Corrected as sodium levels are corrected with administration of normal saline solution	

Infant receiving diuretic therapy

Hyperchloremia

Iatrogenic

Laboratory error

Inappropriate fluid therapy

Metabolic acidosis

Respiratory alkalosis

Infants at risk

Infant receiving ventilatory support

Hypoxic infant

Infant with renal failure

Infant with starvation

Found in association with sodium excess

Corrected as fluid levels are corrected, as with hypernatremia

Data from Biller, J.A., and Yeager, A.M. (eds.): Harriet Lane Handbook, 9th ed. Chicago, Year Book Medical Publishers, 1981; Silver, H.K., Kempe, C.H., and Bruyn, H.B.: Handbook of Pediatrics, 13th ed. Los Altos, Calif., Lange Medical Publications, 1980; Klaus, M.H., and Fanaroff, A.A.: Care of the High-Risk Neonate, 2nd ed. Philadelphia, W.B. Saunders Co., 1979; Harper, R.G., and Yoon, J.J.: Handbook of Neonatology. Chicago, Year Book Medical Publishers, 1974.

TABLE 19-6. SOME TRACE ELEMENTS AND THEIR DEFICIENCIES

Element	Minimum Level Recommended	Human Milk	Neonatal Values in Human Plasma	Some Effects of Deficiency
Chromium		11.6 ng/ml	5–17.5 ng/ml (serum)	Impaired glucose tolerance, poor growth
Copper	(60–90 μg/100 kcal)	(60–90 μg/100 kcal)	Newborn: 0.7 μg/ml	Neutropenia-anemia, osteoporosis
Iodine	(5 μg/100 kcal)	(4–9 μg/100 kcal)	0.053–0.2 μg/ml	Endemic goiter, hypothyroidism
Iron	(1.0 mg/100 kcal)	(0.1 mg/100 kcal)	Newborn: 1.1–2.7 μg/ml	Anemia, impaired learning ability?
Manganese	(5 μg/100 kcal)	(1.5 μg/100 kcal)		In animals only: growth retardation, ataxia of newborn, bone changes
Selenium		13–50 μg/ml	Newborn: 1 wk 80 ng/ml 2 wk 60 ng/ml 3 wk 40 ng/ml 4 wk 40 ng/ml 5 wk 35 ng/ml	Increased fragility of red cells
Zinc	(0.5 mg/100 kcal)	(0.5 mg/100 kcal)	Newborn: 1.0 μg/ml	Impaired appetite, impaired taste, growth retardation, acrodermatitis enteropathica

From Klaus, M.H., and Fanaroff, A.A.: Care of the High-Risk Neonate, 2nd ed. Philadelphia, W.B. Saunders Co., 1979; modified from Hambridge, M.: The importance of trace elements in infant nutrition. Curr. Med. Res. Opin., 4(1):44, 1976.

TABLE 19-7. VITAMIN DEFICIENCIES AND EXCESSES

Vitamin	Normal Blood Level*	Deficiency	Excess
A	15–46 μg/100 ml	Growth failure Mental retardation Apathy Dry skin	Anorexia Irritability Intracranial pressure Desquamation of skin Loss of hair
D	0.8–2.5 ng/100 ml	Tetany Rickets	Hypercalcemia Anorexia Constipation Azotemia Failure to thrive Mental retardation
C	0.4–1.5 mg/100 ml	Scurvy Petechial hemorrhage Fatigue Irritability Tenderness of lower extremities Joint swelling	Unknown—excess is excreted
E	Preterm 0.05–0.35 mg/100 ml Term 0.1–0.35 mg/100 ml	Oxidative damage to cells; retinal vessels of eyes most vulnerable Edema of legs and eye- lids Hemolytic anemia	
K		Clotting disorders	Hemolytic anemia Abnormal albumin binding of bilirubin
Thiamine	5.5–9.5 μg/100 ml	Anorexia Irritability Fatigue Constipation Peripheral neuropathy	
Niacin		Diarrhea Dermatitis CNS symptoms	
Pyridoxine		Irritability Convulsions Weakness Dermatitis Anemia	
B_{12}	330–1025 μg/100 ml	Pernicious anemia	
Folic Acid	5–21 ng/liter	Malabsorptive states Megaloblastic anemia GI disturbances	

Adapted from Fomon, S.: Infant Nutrition. Philadelphia, W.B. Saunders Co. 1974. *Other sources: Biller, J.A., and Yeager, A.M. (eds.): Harriet Lane Handbook, 9th ed. Chicago, Year Book Medical Publishers, 1981; Silver, H.K., Kempe, C.H., and Bruyn, H.B.: Handbook of Pediatrics, 13th ed. Los Altos, Calif., Lange Medical Publications, 1980.

TABLE 19-8. SOURCES OF NUTRITIONAL SUPPORT

Route	Indications	Advantages	Disadvantages	Nursing Care Considerations
Oral, intermittent	Preferred when infant has adequate suck/swallow ability and stomach capacity	Physiological/psychological meeting of oral girate function growth and development	Respiratory distress frequently makes this route hazardous	Infant with respiratory rate greater than 60/min, infant less than 32–34 wk (who lacks maturational ability to suck/swallow effectively), and any distressed infant *are not* candidates for oral feeding because of above normal stress
Nasogastric or orogastric	Infants with poorly developed suck/swallow ability or for whom oral feeding is too stressful	Minimizes infant energy expenditure; allows for ingestion of nutritional substances even in distressed infant *Nasogastric*, usually indwelling, reduces trauma of repeated tube insertion *Orogastric*, usually intermittent insertion	*Nasogastric*, usually indwelling, interferes with respiratory ability, as infants are obligatory nose breathers *Orogastric*, difficult to secure and more prone to dislodging, predisposes infant to vagal stimulation and bradycardia with insertion	Nasogastric, indwelling Observe for pressure on nasal septum with possible ulceration/erosion; above normal mucus formation with potential nasal obstruction Requires reconfirmation of placement prior to each instillation of substance through tube Orogastric, intermittent Observe for vagal stimulation with insertion General: fluids should flow by gravity *not* by push. Check for gastric residual prior to each instillation; record amount/content, e.g., 1 cc partially digested formula, 1 cc thick mucus Size selection by weight Less than 1000 gm: 3 or 5 F 1000–1500 gm: 5 or 8 F Greater than 1500 gm: 8 F

Nasojejunal, indwelling	Very small premature infant Any infant who retains large volumes or regurgitates frequently	Allows for continuous feeding: reduces incidence of regurgitation and overdistention associated with intermittent feeding	Use of polyvinylchloride tubing can result in stiffness after long term placement with associated bowel perforations, infection, necrotizing enterocolitis, and intussusception, regurgitation, aspiration Requires 1–4 hr after insertion before passage through pylorus into jejunum	Prior to actual use of nasojejunal tube, placement should be checked; alkaline pH (5–7) signifies placement in bowel; acid pH (less than 5) indicates placement in stomach Radiopaque tube and weighted tube are preferred to aid in accurate placement
Intravenous	Infant too sick to tolerate any form of gastric feeding			
Peripheral	Short term supplementation of fluids/nutrition: usually less than 2 weeks	Decreased incidence of septicemia when administering parenteral alimentation solution	Generally limited to glucose concentrations less than 12% because of osmolarity Frequent infiltration, difficulty in obtaining adequate venous sites	Preferred infusion site: scalp (avoid hands and feet, as infiltration in these areas may result in significant tissue hypoxia accompanied by necrosis) (see Peripheral Cannulation in Appendix B)
Central	Infant requiring maintenance longer than 2 wk		Difficulty in meeting full caloric and nutritional requirements because of fluid concentration restrictions	Requires strict practice of asepsis with dressing change observe urine and blood glucose carefully because of risk of hyperosmolar diuresis associated with hyperglycemia

TABLE 19-9.   SUGGESTED FEEDING REGIMENS BASED ON WEIGHT AND AGE AT BIRTH

Type of Feeding	Less than 1250 gm	1250-1500 gm	1501-2000 gm	Greater than 2000 gm	SGA Infant
Intravenous fluids	First 24-48 hr, nothing by mouth; IV fluids only $D_{10}W$ 80-100 cc/kg/24 hr* >24 hr D_{10}, with Na^+ and K^+ added, 100 cc/kg/day	Same*	Same if needed*	Same if needed*	Only if clinical hypoglycemia develops
Oral feedings	After 48 hr begin oral feedings as condition permits; 1st feeding 1 cc 5% glucose water	1st feeding 3 cc 5% or 10% glucose 2nd feeding 5 cc glucose water	1st feeding 5 cc 5-10% glucose 2nd feeding 2-3 hr later 8 cc 5% glucose × 1	Initial feeding 15 cc 5% glucose every 3 hr × 2	Soon after birth 10-15 cc with rapid advance to frequent formula feeding Monitor blood glucose every 2 hr × 6 and institute IV therapy if lower blood sugar level persists despite oral feeding
Glucose water	Feed every hr as tolerated 1 cc × 2 2 cc × 1 3 cc × 2				

Formula/Breast Milk	Then begin formula feedings at 3 cc/hr; increase slowly to 6 cc/hr and maintain until *at least* 6 days of age Less than 1100 gm maintain at 5–6 cc/hr for 6–10 days (many will require this level until 14 days of age) When tolerating hourly feedings with difficulty increase to 8 cc/hr then switch to feedings every 2 hr as follows: hr 1 9 cc hr 2 7 cc hr 3 10 cc hr 4 6 cc If feeding not tolerated or if marked residual present, return to next lower volume	Feed every 2–3 hr Begin with 5 cc and increase by 1 cc every other feeding until 10–14 cc volume achieved; maintain for 3 days	Feed every 2–3 hr Begin with 8 cc and increase by 1 cc every other feeding to maximum of 14 cc, then increase 2–4 cc *daily* until calculated caloric requirements are met	Feed every 3 hr Begin with 15 cc and increase by 5 cc every other feeding until 30 cc maximum obtained

*Parenteral fluid intake *plus* oral intake should not exceed total daily fluid requirement. IV intake should be decreased as oral intake increases. IV fluids should be discontinued when oral feedings reach 100–200 cal/kg/day.
Data from Klaus, M.H., and Fanaroff, A.A.: Care of the High Risk Neonate, 2nd ed. Philadelphia, W.B. Saunders Co., 1979.

TABLE 19-10.   COMPONENTS, EFFECTS, AND INDICATIONS FOR MAJOR INFANT FORMULAS

Formula	Company	Carbohydrate	Protein	Fat	Stool Characteristics	Explanations
Milk-based						
Enfamil	Mead Johnson	Lactose	Nonfat milk	Soy and coconut oils	Formed, greenish brown, with very little free water around the stool	Milk formulas are similar and interchangeable; an iron-supplemented formula provides the daily requirement for iron
Similac	Ross	Lactose	Nonfat milk	Soy, coconut, and corn oils		
SMA	Wyeth	Lactose	Electrodialized whey, nonfat milk	Oleo, coconut, oleic (safflower), and soybean oils	Similar to breast milk stool; small volume, pasty, yellow, with some free water	SMA has a relatively low renal solute load. (Renal solute load refers to the amounts of ingested protein and minerals that must be excreted by the kidneys in the form of urea and mineral salts. Fluid intake must be adequate for this excretion to take place). It is low in sodium but supplies the daily requirement and so is used for normal babies. (See Similac PM 60/40 for uses.)
Soy-based						
Isomil	Ross	Sucrose, corn starch, corn syrup solids	Soy protein isolate	Soy, coconut, corn oils	Mushy, yellow-green with more free water than cow's milk stools	Soy formulas are based on soy products. Since they do not contain milk protein or lactose, they are interchangeable in their use for milk protein hypersensitivity
Neo-Mull-Soy	Syntex	Sucrose	Soy protein isolate	Soy oil		

Formula	Manufacturer	Carbohydrate	Protein	Fat	Stool Characteristics	Comments
Nursoy	Wyeth	Sucrose, corn syrup solids	Soy protein isolate	Oleo, coconut, oleic (safflower), and soybean oils		or lactose intolerance. (Lactose intolerance may be due to a temporary lactase deficiency following diarrhea.)
ProSobee	Mead Johnson	Sucrose, corn syrup solids	Soy protein isolate	Soy oil		
Lofenalac	Mead Johnson	Corn syrup solids, tapioca starch	*Special* Specially processed hydrolyzed casein	Corn oil	Similar to cow's milk formula; formed, greenish brown with very little free water around the stool	Infants with phenylketonuria are unable to convert phenylalanine to tyrosine. Unused phenylalanine accumulates in the blood causing irreversible central nervous system damage. Lofenalac is used to provide enough phenylalanine for growth while preventing excessively high levels in the blood.
Lonalac	Mead Johnson	Lactose	Casein	Coconut oil	Similar to cow's milk formula stools	Lonalac is essentially sodium free and may be used in severe renal disease or heart failure. Due to its low sodium content, it is not recommended for long-term use without sodium supplement.
Similac PM 60/40	Ross	Lactose	Partially demineralized whey and nonfat milk	Coconut and corn oils	Similar to cow's milk formula stools	This is a cow's milk base formula with a low renal solute load. It is low sodium yet supplies the daily requirements of this essential

Table continues on following page.

TABLE 19-10.   COMPONENTS, EFFECTS, AND INDICATIONS FOR MAJOR INFANT FORMULAS – *Continued*

Formula	Company	Carbohydrate	Protein	Fat	Stool Characteristics	Explanations
						nutrient. It is used in long term management of renal or heart disease.
Portagen	Mead Johnson	Sucrose, corn syrup solids	Sodium caseinate	Fractionated coconut oil (MCT), corn oil (trace)	Similar to cow's milk formula stools	Pancreatic or liver disease causes interference in fat absorption. Long chain triglycerides are absorbed through the lymphatic system and require a certain amount of bile and pancreatic enzymes. Medium chain triglycerides (MCT) are absorbed directly into the portal circulation and do not require bile and pancreatic enzymes. Portagen contains MCT oil as its major fat source and is indicated for an infant with pancreatic or liver disease.
Special						
Nutramigen	Mead Johnson	Sucrose, tapioca starch	Enzymically hydrolyzed 8 casein	Corn oil	Low volume, green stool with some mucus	Nutramigen provides protein in the form of hydrolyzed casein. Protein hypersensitivity is a rare disease process where intact proteins are not tolerated. Hydrolyzation breaks the protein structure into

						amino acids and polypeptides.
Pregestimil	Mead Johnson	Dextrose, tapioca starch	Enzymically hydrolyzed 8 casein	Fractionated coconut oil (MCT), corn oil (trace)	Low volume, green mucus stool	Pregestimil is composed of simple structures which are easily absorbed: glucose, MCT oil, and hydrolyzed casein. It is used in some cases of fat or carbohydrate malabsorption. It is important to remember that Pregestimil has a high intestinal osmotic load. It may draw more fluid into the intestine than is desired, resulting in diarrhea. To avoid this, Pregestimil should be started at half strength and gradually increased to full strength. Presumably this method allows the intestine to accommodate the increased osmotic load.
Cho-Free	Syntex	None	Soy protein isolate	Soy oil	Similar to soy formula stools	Cho-Free is a carbohydrate-free soy formula. Prepared without added carbohydrate, it provides only 12 calories per ounce. (Standard formulas provide 20 calories per ounce.) Additional calories may be supplied by intravenous fluids until carbohydrates can be

Table continues on following page.

TABLE 19-10.   COMPONENTS, EFFECTS, AND INDICATIONS FOR MAJOR INFANT FORMULAS — *Continued*

Formula	Company	Carbohydrate	Protein	Fat	Stool Characteristics	Explanations
						added to the feeding in sufficient amounts. Cho-Free is used in short-term carbohydrate intolerance.
Modular formula	Ross	None	Calcium-sodium caseinate	None	Green curds with loss of free water	Modular formula is composed of a core of proteins and minerals to which carbohydrates and fats are added in increasing amounts. It is used as a method of allowing the intestine to gradually recover absorptive capacity without introducing components the gut is not able to handle. It may also be used to identify a specific intolerance or it may be used following a long period of total parenteral nutrition.

Reproduced with permission from Stokan, R.: The right formula for the right infant: Making sense of infant nutrition. MCN, (Mar-Apr) 2:102, 1977. Copyright, the American Journal of Nursing Company. Components were obtained from product can labels, indications from the literature, and stool characteristics from clinical observations.

GENERAL CONSIDERATIONS

INSENSIBLE WATER LOSS VALUES

Phototherapy & Radient Warmers
40 ml/Kg/day

Ambient Temperature >NTE 3-4
fold increase   37.5 degree C

Elevated body temperature 3-4
fold increase > 37.5 degree C

Immaturity <1250gms c̄ heat-
shield 40 ml/Kg/day s̄ heat-
shield 80 ml/KG/day

Basal Values IWL=17-34 ml/Kg/day

URINE VALUES

Output: Preterm 15-40 cc/day
        Term   15-60 cc/day
        3-5 days 100-300 cc/day

Specific gravity: 1.001-1.020
        (1.008 - 1.012 avg) ph: 5-7

BASE FLUID/CALORIE REQUIREMENTS

Calories: 100-120 cal/Kg/day

Fluids:

1-3 days of age - 100 ml/Kg/day
4 days of age -120-150 ml/Kg/day

CALORIC VALUES OF SELECTES
SUBSTANCES

Formula: 20 cal/oz=0.66 cal/ml
         24 cal/oz=0.8 cal/ml
         30 cal/oz=1.0 cal/ml

IV Solutions:

  5% Dextrose = 0.2 cal/ml
7.5% Dextrose = 0.3 cal/ml
 10% Dextrose = 0.4 cal/ml
 12% Dextrose = 0.48 cal/ml

FLUID/CALORIC ASSESSMENT RECORD

INFANT BIRTH WEIGHT: _____ Kg. GESTATIONAL AGE: _____ Wks.

DATE	AGE	WT(Kg)	CALCULATED FLUID REQUIRED	ACTUAL INTAKE Oral	ACTUAL INTAKE IV	CALCULATED CALORIC REQUIRED	ACTUAL INTAKE Oral	ACTUAL INTAKE IV	FLUID LOSSES URINE	FLUID LOSSES GI VOMIT/DIARRHEA	EST IWL

Figure 19-2. Fluid and caloric assessment record.

TABLE 19–11. NURSE'S ROLE IN PARENTERAL THERAPY: PHYSICAL ACTIONS IN ADMINISTERING THERAPY

Clinical Considerations	Nursing Interventions	Rationale
Solution for IV fluid	Use solutions at room temperature and not cold from refrigerator	Solutions given at room temperature are rapidly absorbed by patient Very cold solution can result in vasoconstriction Fluid given slowly will mix with blood or fluid tissue spaces and will be quickly brought to body temperature
Flow rate	Check types of solutions patients are receiving	Knowledge of tonicity (osmolality) of fluids will aid in determining rate of flow; rate of hyperosmolar solutions should be slower than that of iso-osmolar solutions
	Utilize infusion pump on all neonates	Regulation of IV fluids is important in prevention of overhydration
	Check rate every 30 min. with hyperalimentation solutions	Rapid flow of high sugar (glucose) concentration can cause hyperglycemia and glycosuria; slow rate will cause insufficient nutrients; with hyperalimentation solutions, if behind, never try to catch up
Injection site	Choose distal portion of arm for IV therapy; scalp veins are preferred site in neonates	Distal portion of arm is preferred to elbow to avoid necessity for immobilizing elbow and to avoid possibility of infiltration into interstitial spaces Veins in lower extremities will develop phlebitis more rapidly than those in upper extremities
	Observe injection site for infiltration	Injection site should be checked for infiltration into interstitial spaces as well as for swelling and soreness; damage to surrounding tissues can be prevented
	Observe injection site for phlebitis	Red, swollen, hard, and warm to touch are signs of phlebitis; injection site needs to be changed
Intake and output	Keep accurate intake and output record	Accurate intake and output records will indicate fluid and electrolyte balance or imbalance; it will determine degree of fluid

Table continues on opposite page.

Clinical Considerations	Nursing Interventions	Rationale
		retention and ensure that losses do not exceed replacement
	Check that patient is not becoming overloaded with liquids—orally and parenterally	An hourly check on output can help in correction of fluid and electrolyte imbalance before it becomes irreversible
	Test urine at least every 6 hr for sugar when using hyperalimentation solutions	Glycosuria occurs with rapid flow rates, since body cannot utilize sugar
IV needles	Note when parenteral therapy began and type of needle used	IV needles should not be left in site for periods longer than 24–48 hr, since they may produce local inflammatory reaction or painful thrombophlebitis
	Change injection site every 24–48 hr when using 20–21 gauge needle; every 48–72 hr when using polyethylene tubing	
	23–25 gauge butterfly needles can be inserted into scalp veins of the smallest infants and 22 gauge over the needle catheters can be used for brachial, cephalic, external jugular, and saphenous veins as well as the dorsum of the hand	
		If polyethylene tubing (Intracath) is used in vein, it should not remain longer than 3 days, since it may produce phlebitis or thrombophlebitis
		Scalp-vein needles are less irritating to veins, since they are small in length and lumen
Vital signs	Check patient's BP, temperature, pulse, and respiration for any adverse reaction while patient is receiving parenteral therapy	Identification of abnormal vital signs can eliminate complications
	Identify adverse reactions according to kind of parenteral therapy used	Any adverse reaction during IV therapy can change vital signs, e.g., in blood transfusion; rise in temperature and pulse rate can indicate incompatibility

From Kee, J.L.: Fluids and Electrolytes with Clinical Application. A Programmed Approach, 2nd ed.,
pp. 276–278. Copyright 1978, John Wiley & Sons, Inc., New York. Reprinted by permission.

TABLE 19-12. NURSE'S ROLE IN PARENTERAL THERAPY: SIDE EFFECTS OF THERAPY

Clinical Considerations	Adverse Reactions	Nursing Interventions
Varying flow rate according to specific solutions:		
Hydrating solutions	Large quantities of hydrating solutions can result in overhydration	Note that hydrating solutions are mainly iso-osmolar and aid in restoring urinary output
		Note that iso-osmolar solutions can replace fluid loss quickly, since they do not increase osmotic pressure
		Regulate rate of hydrating solutions to run fast at first and then at slower rate thereafter, unless overhydration is present
		Identify symptoms of overhydration, e.g., dyspnea, coughing, and cyanosis
Proteins solutions, also known as amino acid solutions	Reactions to amino acid solutions frequently occur from administering solution too fast; these reactions include nausea, feeling of warmth, and flushing	Note these solutions are helpful in combating hypoproteinemia and conditions due to malnutrition
		Regulate rate of amino acid solutions to run slowly at first and later to run faster if patient can tolerate solution
		Observe and identify adverse reactions to amino acid solutions
Dextrose solutions	Iso-osmolar dextrose can cause rise in CNS fluid pressure; symptoms of increased pressure, also referred to as cerebral edema, include slow pulse rate, high BP, and headaches	Note that dextrose cannot be metabolized more rapidly than 1 g/kg or 4.5 g/10 lb of body weight per hr
		Regulate rate of flow not to exceed metabolizing rate, especially for patients who are very sick or have head injuries
		Observe if patients exhibit symptoms of increased CNS fluid pressure or cerebral edema, especially patients with head injuries
Hyperosmolar solutions	When administered too fast hyperosmolar solutions can cause sclerosis of recipient's vein or can cause thrombophlebitis	Note which IV fluids are hyperosmolar
		Regulate rate of hyperosmolar solutions to run no faster than 3–4 ml/min

486

Table continues on opposite page.

Clinical Considerations	Adverse Reactions	Nursing Interventions
	Hyperosmolar solutions can pull fluid from body cells, causing dehydration; symptoms are those similar to shock, namely, rapid pulse rate, low BP, and restlessness	Observe patient for symptoms of shock; frequently hyperosmolar solutions are used in treating cerebral edema—if too much is administered, dehydration or loss of water occurs followed by shock
Whole blood and RBCs (packed cells)	"Old" whole blood has higher concentration of potassium; it may lose platelets and undergo hemolysis	Check date of whole blood, patient's serum potassium, and urinary output
	Very cold blood given rapidly can cause ventricular fibrillation	Permit blood to reach room temperature before administering
	Citrate in blood bottles will lower serum ionized calcium	Note patient's serum calcium level: with infusion or exchange transfusion cardiac arrhythmias may occur; cardiac monitoring is recommended, and calcium gluconate may be needed
	Blood transfusion reaction: chills, fever, dyspnea, rash, cyanosis, and shock-like symptoms (pulse up, BP down)	Check patient's blood type with transfusion and observe reaction symptoms; check temperature and pulse before and during transfusion—if reaction occurs, stop transfusion
	A unit of packed RBCs flows slowly owing to lack of fluid	Administer saline before and after unit of RBCs to aid in cell dilution and prevention of clot formation. This may not be appropriate in the tiny infant whose blood volume is approximately 85 ml/kg and overhydration is a risk
		Infusion of packed RBCs in the neonate may require the use of an infusion pump
		With RBCs there is drop in potassium levels, transfusion reaction, and overhydration than with whole blood
IV tubing and bags	Tubing and bags may harbor bacteria	Change IV tubing every 24 hr with new liter of fluids; a 250 ml bag is suggested for use with keep vein open (KVO)

Table continues on following page.

487

Clinical Considerations	Adverse Reactions	Nursing Interventions
Overhydration by parenteral therapy	Increase in respiratory rate, onset of coughing, and development of cyanosis suggest overhydration of patient's circulation with transudation of fluid from blood into alveoli of lungs, thus resulting in pulmonary edema	Note clinical diagnosis and physical changes of patient receiving parenteral therapy Observe changes in rate and depth of respiration; dyspnea accompanies pulmonary edema or fluid Observe for constant and irritated cough, which can result from pulmonary fluid Observe for signs of cyanosis, resulting from lack of pulmonary ventilation, depriving tissues of O_2 Observe individuals with cardiac, renal, or liver diseases receiving parenteral therapy for signs of overhydration, including edema Regulate flow rate according to patient's clinical condition and solution used Discontinue injection when discovering adverse signs
Increased fluid intake	Patients receiving large quantities of oral fluid along with large quantities of IV fluid can overload intravascular system	Monitor fluid intake—oral and parenteral—on postoperative patients of 1 day, the very sick, the cardiac, and patients with chronic renal and liver diseases, all neonates
Inadequate urinary output	Patients with poor urinary output and receiving potassium may experience cardiac arrest	Check patient's urinary output before and during administration of parenteral fluid containing potassium
Electrolyte imbalance:		
Sodium retention	Sodium solutions given in excess quantities can result in edema due to retention of sodium and fluid; tachycardia with fall or rise in BP can indicate hypernatremia	Observe signs and symptoms of developing edema
Potassium deficit	Potassium deficit can result from surgery, trauma, injury, stress, dehydration, diarrhea, vomiting, anorexia,	Observe signs and symptoms of potassium deficit or hypokalemia

Table continues on opposite page.

TABLE 19-12. NURSE'S ROLE IN PARENTERAL THERAPY:
SIDE EFFECTS OF THERAPY – *Continued*

Clinical Considerations	Adverse Reactions	Nursing Interventions
	and so on, along with dilution due to excessive parenteral fluids; dizziness, muscular weakness, and arrhythmia can indicate hypokalemia	
Potassium excess	Potassium excess can be most hazardous, leading to cardiac arrest; concentration of potassium in 1000 ml of fluid exceeding 40 mEq/liter or more than 3 mEq/kg/24 hr may result in potassium intoxication leading to death	Note "safe" range for using concentrated potassium salts. Nurses preparing concentrate KC1 ampules to be diluted in IV solution should be cognizant of this responsibility and realize that an error in dilution can be fatal
	Nausea, abdominal cramps, and tachycardia followed by bradycardia can indicate hyperkalemia	Determine that concentration of potassium does not exceed 40 mEq/1000 ml; 30 mEq/liter is preferred to avoid potassium intoxication
		Observe for signs and symptoms of potassium excess or hyperkalemia

From Kee, J.L.: Fluids and Electrolytes with Clinical Application: A Programmed Approach, 2nd ed., pp. 276–278. Copyright 1978, John Wiley & Sons, Inc., New York. Reprinted by permission.

    b. Survival is 75 per cent with prompt recognition and treatment

2. Predisposing factors
    a. Preterm AGA infant
    b. Asphyxiation or RDS
    c. Sepsis
    d. Polycythemia
    e. Patent ductus arteriosus

ETIOLOGY

The cause is unknown. Current hypotheses include the following:

1. Diving seal reflex, which is felt to occur in response to asphyxia; this mechanism shunts blood away from the gut *to* the brain, heart, and kidneys to protect them during an asphyxial episode

2. Other possible causes (see Fig. 19-3)
    a. Infection: *Klebsiella* and *Escherichia coli* most often associated
    b. Hyperosmolar feedings
    c. Polycythemia (hematocrit more than 65 per cent)
    d. Lack of maternal milk
    e. Umbilical catheterization
    f. Ductus steal: in patent ductus arteriosus blood flow to intestinal circulation decreased

Text continues on page 498.

TABLE 19-13.   GUIDELINES FOR HYPERALIMENTATION

Nursing Practice	Outcome	Rationale
Explain therapy (including all procedures) to patient and family, encouraging dialogue that includes questions and answers	Insures understanding of patient and family	This is a basic patient right
Establish and maintain a nursing care plan	Clarifies nursing approach	Initiates working basis for continuity of care
Actively assist physician and patient during catheterization	Insures sterile catheter placement and reassures patient	A catheter contaminated during insertion is unclean
Hang isotonic infusion until central catheter-tip location verified	Prevents infusion into incorrect location and may decrease severity of complications	Hypertonic solutions sclerose small veins
Remain alert for signs and symptoms of catheterization complications, particularly bleeding and respiratory distress	Arrests acute problem in early stage and allows for prompt treatment	
Document cather-tip location in patient's record before instituting TPN* infusion	Clarifies communication	Enables verification of proper placement
Examine solution for precipitate or turbidity	Prevents infection	May indicate contamination
Scrutinize bottle or bag for cracks or holes	Prevents infection	Cracks or holes mean container is contaminated
Begin hypertonic solutions at slow rates and increase increments gradually	Prevents hyperglycemia	Allows for physiologic insulin level adaptation
When infusing solutions by gravity; double clamp the IV tubing, time-tape solution container, recheck flow rate every 30 min, use measured IV fluid chamber and 50 cc bottle as maximum size	Prevents "runaway IV," which could cause congestive heart failure, pulmonary edema, hyperglycemia, hyperosmolar dehydration and coma	Pediatric patients (especially low birth-weight neonates) are very susceptible to both glucose and fluid overload. Stressed or septic patients may also demonstrate intolerance to glucose overload
Always make sure that the drops per minute are appropriate to deliver the volume per hour that is ordered	Delivers correct amount of fluid	Drip calibration varies with commercial IV sets. Drop size may change (drops become smaller as hypertonic solution narrows IV dropper)

Use infusion apparatus to administer TPN solution whenever possible; always use infusion apparatus for infants	Maintains constant rate of flow	Hypertonic solutions raise the challenge of maintaining a constant flow rate; a crying infant is performing Valsalva's maneuver. This causes blood backup, which could clot the line
Carefully record intake and output	Provides accurate fluid intake and output profile	Indicates fluid balance and calories received
Measure urinary sugar and acetone every 6 hr (measure every voiding of infant)	Obtains urinary sugar profile	Indicates glucose tolerance
Use Tes-Tape® if patient is receiving Keflin® or Keflex®	Prevents inaccurate urinary sugar test	Keflin® and Keflex® cause "false positive" results with Clinitest® tablets
Report glycosuria and anticipate serum glucose evaluation when glycosuria exceeds 2+	Establishes individual patient's renal threshold	Transient glycosuria is usual during adaptation phase but greater than 2+ may indicate serious hyperglycemia
		It is impossible to know patient's serum glucose by urinary sugar levels until renal threshold has been established; premature neonates with under-developed renal tubules may require serum glucose measurements for reliable evaluation
Observe, record, and report signs and symptoms of peripheral edema or respiratory distress	Recognizes fluid overload	This is a possible side-effect of IV therapy, especially when hypertonic solutions are infused
Weigh patient ever 24 hours at same time on same scale—do this before AM feeding if patient not NPO†	Obtains accurate weight profile	Indicates weight gain (or loss), fluid balance, caloric requirements
Measure head circumference of infant (especially neonate) daily	Obtains accurate head size profile	Indicates growth and helps define caloric requirement
Measure length of infant at least weekly	Obtains accurate length profile	Indicates growth and helps define caloric requirement
Change dressing every 48–72 hr and PRN‡	Prevents infection	Inhibits growth of bacteria; dressing should be changed when leakage or drainage noted
Change IV tubing and filter every 24 hr	Prevents infection	Center for Disease Control recommends that IV tubing and filters be changed every 24 hr

Table continues on following page.

TABLE 19-13.   GUIDELINES FOR HYPERALIMENTATION – *Continued*

Nursing Practice	Outcome	Rationale
Connect IV tubing, employing aseptic technique	Prevents infection	Manual dexterity here is essential and often overlooked; painting all junctions with iodophor solution may enhance asepsis
Change tubing and filter at institution of new daily solution	Prevents infection	Avoids additional break in system; avoids placing old tubing in new bottle
Have patient perform Valsalva's maneuver when catheter junction is open to air (at catheter insertion time and during IV tubing–change time)	Prevents air embolus	Valsalva's maneuver is forced exhalation with a closed glottis; negative pressure in a central vein can cause air to be drawn in
When patient unable to perform Valsalva's maneuver, simulate it by compressing the abdomen or maintaining the inspiratory phase of a breathing bag during tubing change	Prevents air embolus	Remember that initial inspiration causes negative pressure in central veins so that, if using the breathing bag technique, wait about 3–5 sec before disconnecting tubing
When changing infant's tubing that has an exposed catheter or adult's tubing that has an exposed extension tubing not to be changed, merely pinch the exposed end back on itself before and after tubing change	Prevents air embolus	Using this technique, catheter will never be open to air
Maintain inviolate catheter system; do not withdraw blood, measure CVPs, § administer IV bolus drugs, or piggyback infusions through the lifeline	Prevents infection	Maintains closed system
Monitor temperature at least every 6 hr and report elevation immediately	Prevents infection	Temperature elevation often indicates catheter sepsis
Be aware of unexplained glycosuria or leukocytosis	Prevents infection	Often indicators of catheter sepsis; may be only indicators in neonates whose temperature is artificially controlled
Check peripheral IV sites frequently for early signs and symptoms of phlebitis: erythema, edema, warmth, and pain	Prevents extensive phlebitis and may detect infection in early stages	Peripheral sites easily become phlebitic when hypertonic solutions are infused

Observe, record, and report violations of catheters if they deviate from hospital policy or safe standards of practice	Protects patient	These data may influence catheter removal or change in therapy (to a safer method); this action, of course, safeguards the patient and may prevent a catastrophe
Practice continuity of care; document this care plan	Prevents infection	Rigid protocol necessary; documentation facilitates continuity
Protect the IV site from mishandling, pressure, or stress	Prevents dislodgment of IV system and interference with infusion delivery	Padding and anchoring IV tubing or shield around the site maintains this objective
Check infusion site for infiltration	Prevents extensive tissue damage	Lines may dislodge and infuse into tissue
Wean patient gradually from concentrated dextrose solutions by decreasing flow rate in increments	Prevents rebound hypoglycemia	Abrupt cessation of IV glucose may cause a hypoglycemic shock if serum insulin levels remain elevated
Observe, record, and report signs and symptoms of electrolyte deficit or excess	Aids physician in determining patient's nutritional IV requirements and provides clinical output (as well as the lab data)	These upsets arise when the IV diet is insufficient or excessive; early detection of signs is as necessary as careful serum monitoring to prevent serious upsets
Include oral examination as part of daily nursing care and implement consistent, successful mouth care	Provides patient comfort and prevents side-effects, such as edema, dryness, or parotitis	NPO† patients require careful consideration
Encourage active exercise if possible and provide passive exercise if it is not	Prevents muscle atrophy and other side-effects of prolonged bed rest	In addition to the considerations always mentioned in nursing texts (e.g., decubitus, phlebitis) remember that inactive muscle will break down and, therefore, increase catabolism
When using Intralipid® 10% or Liposyn®: Refrigerate Intralipid® (4°–8°C) until infused Place no additives	Maintains stability of emulsion	Additive incompatibility could break the emulsion
Check each bottle before hanging; observe emulsion for "oiling out" or "frothiness;" never use if this phenomenon is seen	Prevents infusion of unstable emulsion	Instability of this emulsion is usually not visible to the naked eye; however, this phenomenon would display a cracked emulsion

Table continues on following page.

TABLE 19-13.   GUIDELINES FOR HYPERALIMENTATION – *Concluded*

Nursing Practice	Outcome	Rationale
Use appropriate IV tubing Never filter	Follows company recommendation Maintains stability of emulsion	Read package insert Company recommendations
Infuse fat solution as solo IV if possible	Prevents emulsion instability	Could occur if not run separately from other IV solutions
If infusing by means of a y-connector located near infusion site, read company information booklet and follow instructions exactly	Prevents emulsion instability and floating of Intralipid® upstream into other IV tubing	See company literature
Initial rate of pediatric infusion is 0.1 cc/min for the first 15–30 min	Prevents severe reaction from large amount and allows early detection of acute reaction	These drugs are new to the American market and patients should be watched carefully for side-effects; review company literature
Monitor temperature and vital signs 30 min after infusion begins and then every 6 hr; stop infusion if febrile reaction, respiratory distress, or colloid-type allergy occurs	Prevents extension of allergic response	Same as above
Do not store partially used bottle—it must not be reused	Prevents infection	Intralipid® supports bacterial growth when contaminated

Reproduced with permission from Colley, R., Wilson, J., and Wilhem, M.P.: Intravenous nutrition—nursing considerations. Issues Compr. Pediatr. Nurs., *1*:74, 1977. Copyright © 1977. Reproduced by permission of McGraw-Hill Book Co.
*TPN, total parenteral nutrition.
†NPO, nothing by mouth
‡PRN, whenever necessary.
§CVP, central venous pressure.

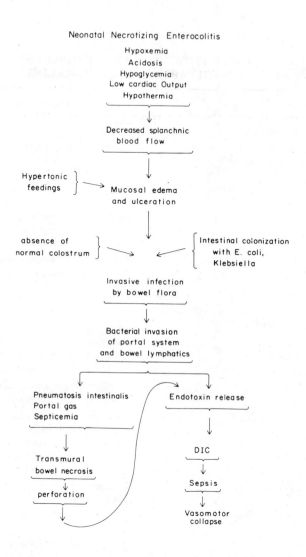

Figure 19-3. Possible factors in etiology and outcome of neonatal necrotizing enterocolitis. (From Burrington, J.D.: Necrotizing enterocolitis in the newborn infant. Clin. Perinatol., *5*:30, 1978.)

TABLE 19–14. METABOLIC PROBLEMS
ASSOCIATED WITH PARENTERAL HYPERALIMENTATION

Problems	Possible Etiology
I. Glucose metabolism	
A. Hyperglycemia, glycosuria, osmotic diuresis, hyperosmolar nonketotic dehydration, and coma	Excessive total dose or rate of infusion of glucose; inadequate endogenous insulin
B. Ketoacidosis in diabetic mellitus	Inadequate endogenous insulin response; inadequate exogenous insulin therapy
C. Postinfusion hypoglycemia	Persistence of endogenous insulin production secondary to prolonged stimulation of islet cells by high carbohydrate infusion
II. Amino acid metabolism	
A. Hyperchloremic metabolic acidosis	Excessive chloride and monohydrochloride content of crystalline amino acid solutions
B. Serum amino acid imbalances	Unphysiologic amino acid profile of the nutrient solution
C. Hyperammonemia	Excessive ammonia in protein hydrolysate solutions; arginine, ornithine, aspartic acid and glutamic acid deficiency in amino acid solutions; primary hepatic disorder
D. Prerenal azotemia	Excessive protein hydrolysate or amino acid infusion
III. Calcium and phosphorus metabolism	

A. Hypophosphatemia
     1. Decreased erythrocyte 2,3-diphosphoglycerate
     2. Increased affinity of hemoglobin for oxygen
     3. Aberrations of erythrocyte intermediary metabolites
	Inadequate phosphorus administration, redistribution of serum phosphorus into cells and bone

Table continues on opposite page.

**TABLE 19-14. METABOLIC PROBLEMS
ASSOCIATED WITH PARENTERAL HYPERALIMENTATION** – *Continued*

Problems	Possible Etiology
B. Hypocalcemia	Inadequate calcium administration; reciprocal response to phosphorus repletion without simultaneous calcium infusion
C. Hypercalcemia	Excessive calcium administration with or without high doses of albumin
D. Vitamin D deficiency; Hypervitaminosis D	Inadequate or excessive vitamin D administration
IV. Essential fatty acid metabolism	
A. Serum deficiencies of phospholipid linoleic and arachidonic acids; serum elevation of Δ 5,8,11-eicosatrieonic acid	Inadequate essential fatty acid administration; inadequate vitamin E administration
V. Miscellaneous	
A. Hypokalemia	Inadequate potassium intake relative to increased requirements for protein anabolism
B. Hyperkalemia	Excessive potassium administration especially in metabolic acidosis
C. Hypomagnesemia	Inadequate magnesium administration relative to increased requirements for protein anabolism
D. Anemia	Iron deficiency; folic acid deficiency; vitamin B_{12} deficiency; copper deficiency
E. Bleeding	Vitamin K deficiency
F. Hypervitaminosis A	Excessive vitamin A administration
G. Elevations in SGOT, SGPT, and serum alkaline phosphatase	Enzyme induction secondary to accelerated glucose metabolism, possible hepatotoxicity secondary to amino acid imbalance; excessive glycogen and fat deposition in the liver

Reprinted with permission from Dudrick, S., McFayden, B., Van Buren, C., et al.: Parenteral hyperalimentation. Metabolic problems and solutions. Ann. Surg., *176:*260, 1972.

ASSESSMENT
1. **Clinical presentation**
   a. Signs and symptoms
      i. Gastric retention
      ii. Vomiting
      iii. Abdominal distention
      iv. Bloody stools
      v. Signs of sepsis: lethargy, hypothermia, hypotension
   b. History
      i. Onset usually 3 to 5 days after birth or after initial feedings of formula or breast milk
2. **Biopsychosocial assessment**
   a. Thermoregulation: inability to maintain stable body temperature in neutral thermal environment
   b. Abdominal inspection: erythema at umbilicus; increase in abdominal girth
   c. Abdominal auscultation: bowel sound faint, hypoactive, or absent
   d. Abdominal palpation: distended loops of bowel, hepatosplenomegaly
   e. Character and frequency of vomiting
   f. Gastric residual: bile stained, coffee ground appearance
   g. Gastric drainage
   h. Blood in gastric aspirate and stools
   i. Renal: intake and output
   j. Heart rate
   k. Blood pressure
   l. Respiratory rate
   m. Tissue perfusion, poor capillary filling
   n. Vasodilation or vasoconstriction of skin
   o. Patent ductus arteriosus with murmur common
   p. Parents' knowledge and understanding of disease process
   q. Parents' feelings of guilt, anger, denial (grief process)
   r. Crisis state in parents resulting in inability to realistically focus on, comprehend, or retain information given
3. **Diagnostic data**
   a. Hematological
      i. Determination of hemoglobin, hematocrit, leukocyte, and platelet values every 12 hours during disease process; CBC generally reveals an increase in white cells; development of low platelet count or abnormal prothrombin time and partial thromboplastin time may indicate development of clotting problems associated with disseminated intravascular coagulation (DIC)
      ii. Blood gases: infant characteristically acidotic, but PaO_2 and $PaCO_2$ within normal limits
      iii. Sepsis work-up of blood, stool, and CSF may reveal causative organism
   b. Roentgenographic
      i. Distended loops of bowel
      ii. Ascites
      iii. Thickened bowel walls

PROBLEMS AND COMPLICATIONS

1. Perforation of bowel, peritonitis
2. Surgery for bowel resection
3. Death
4. Bowel strictures after initial recovery from disease process
5. Malabsorption syndrome; short gut syndrome

PATIENT CARE MANAGEMENT

1. Goals

COMMENTS/TIPS/
CAUTIONS

   a. To restore normal level of wellness and reduce risk of further complications

      i. Observe for

         (a) Abdominal distention

Measure abdominal girth every 8 hours at or just above umbilicus; all measurements should be at same level; mark abdomen at level of measurement.

         (b) Vomiting

         (c) Diarrhea

Test all vomitus and stools for blood; note frank or old blood; blood tinged vomitus should receive Apt test to differentiate maternal from neonatal blood

         (d) Sepsis

      ii. Obtain vital signs and BP every hour if infant not attached to cardiorespiratory monitor

BP of 60/20 probably indicates shock

Dropping BP associated with wide pulse pressure, tachycardia, and warm extremities indicates "warm shock" and precedes the more familiar vasoconstrictive "cold shock"

Major cause of shock is transfer of intravascular fluids into abdomen in response to bowel inflammation and necrosis

      iii. Observe for apnea

Temperature less than 36.5°C in neutral thermal environment indicates hypothermia and is frequently associated with sepsis (rare for neonate to have elevated temperature with infection)

      iv. Do not give infant anything orally

      v. Insert 8 F feeding tube or Salem sump tube for abdominal distention and vomiting; attach to low intermittent suction for bowel decompression

Abdominal distention, vomiting or diarrhea may be associated with bowel obstruction or inflammation; giving infant nothing orally reduces risk of further stress to bowel

      vi. Administer parenteral fluids as indicated

Observe for signs of dehydration and electrolyte imbalance, which may occur as gastric secretions are removed

      vii. Keep strict record of intake and output

      viii. Monitor electrolyte values

Signs of dehydration include decreased urinary output, irritability, lethargy, dry skin (poor turgor), sunken fontanels, marked weight loss (more than 5 per cent of body weight in less than 48 hours)

      ix. Provide mouth care

Sterile water with cotton tipped applicators or prepackaged lemon and glycerin swabs may be used; lips dry and crust easily

   b. To facilitate parent-infant attachment and reduce parental stress and anxiety

      i. Observe for

         (a) Positive parenting behaviors

Willingness to touch, frequent calling, speaking of infant by name are all positive behaviors

         (b) Positive coping skills

Parents ask questions, participate in infant's care, realistically discuss infant's condition, have other support systems available

      ii. Explain all procedures, treatments, and condition to parents

      iii. Encourage parents to write down questions as they think of them

Parent-infant attachment is at risk whenever there is a perceived threat to the infant's survival; parents may experience anticipatory grief, guilt, or crisis as result of illness; crisis intervention may be necessary to aid family

	COMMENTS/TIPS/ CAUTIONS
iv. Encourage parents to participate in infant care	
v. Make referral to available parent support group or perinatal social worker	
vi. Employ primary care when possible to minimize the number of different staff members the parents must communicate with and to establish continuity of care and information	
vii. Always refer to infant by name and personalize infant and environment	Place infant's name on bed and encourage parents to bring special music box, toy, or clothes
viii. Take pictures of infant	Pictures may help parents reinforce infant's recovery but also may aid attachment to infant

OMPHALOCELE AND GASTROSCHISIS

Omphalocele and gastroschisis are both life threatening congenital anomalies. Prompt treatment is required if the infant is to survive.

DIAGNOSIS

Omphalocele consists of protrusion of bowel through a large central abdominal wall defect covered with a clear sac of peritoneum

Gastroschisis is an abdominal wall defect that results from failure of closure of a lateral fold and is usually accompanied by protrusion of small and part of large intestine.

1. **Incidence**
   a. Omphalocele
      i. 1 in 3000 to 5000 live births
      ii. Mortality 30 per cent with small defect; 73 per cent with defect larger than 8 cm and liver and bowel eviscerated; overall survival about 70 per cent with prompt management
   b. Gastroschisis
      i. 1 in 50,000 live births
      ii. Mortality 40 per cent

ETIOLOGY

Size may vary from several centimeters to many inches. The omphalocele sac may contain intestine and liver. Peritoneal cavity is not fully developed and in large defects prevents primary surgical repair. Bowel malrotation and atresia are common; cardiovascular and genitourinary anomalies are also common.
   a. Develops between 8 and 11 weeks of gestation
   b. Results from failure of the intestines to return to the abdominal cavity from the umbilical cord

2. Gastroschisis

Margins of defect are round and smooth. There is *no sac* covering eviscerated abdominal content. Exposed organs may extend from stomach to rectum. A green fibrous peel composed of fibrogelatinous membrane containing squamous cells and vernix covers the exposed organs. Peritonitis, midgut shortening, malrotation, and atresia may be present.

    a. Results from abdominal wall muscular defect, usually near the umbilicus but not involving umbilical cord

    b. Most often found on right side

    c. Measures 2.5–15.0 cm in diameter

ASSESSMENT

1. Clinical presentation

    a. Signs and symptoms

        i. Inspection of defect can differentiate between omphalocele and gastroschisis; neither may have a sac surrounding abdominal viscera, but gastroschisis *does not* involve umbilical cord

        ii. Infant frequently premature

        iii. Hypothermia resulting from heat loss from exposed viscera

2. Biopsychosocial assessment

    a. Vital signs, especially temperature and respiration

    b. Parents' response to obvious physical anomaly

    c. Parents' coping skills and support systems

3. Diagnostic data

    a. Laboratory determination of electrolyte and glucose levels to rule out Beckwith's syndrome

    b. Identify presence of other anomalies

PROBLEMS AND COMPLICATIONS

1. Respiratory distress: abdominal cavity not sufficiently large to accommodate bowel viscera; with attempts to reinsert viscera, respiratory distress may occur
2. Sepsis: absence of protective sac in gastroschisis or rupture of sac in omphalocele predisposes to infection
3. Ileus or intussusception
4. Necrosis and perforation
5. Malabsorption

PATIENT CARE MANAGEMENT

1. Goals

    a. To support stable metabolic state

        i. Reduce risk for hypothermia and insensible water loss

            (a) Wrap abdomen care-

COMMENTS/TIPS/CAUTIONS

Infant should be prepared for transport to level II institution

Reduces heat and fluid loss until defect is repaired
Do not place pressure on sac of omphalocele or try to replace eviscerated abdominal organs

fully with padded saline soaked gauze and plastic (Saran wrap) outer layer

(b) Start peripheral IV immediately; replacement requirements for fluids three to four times maintenance levels

(c) Place infant in Isolette with Servo control

Radiant warmers increase insensible water loss and should be used with caution in infant with exposed abdominal viscera

ii. Monitor

(a) Intake and output

(b) Electrolytes

(c) CBC for signs of hemoconcentration

Urine specific gravity greater than 1.012, sodium greater than 145 mEq/100 ml, hematocrit more than 65 per cent reflect fluid loss

b. To minimize risk of infection and sepsis

i. Maintain sterile dressing on sac or exposed viscera

Normal saline with antiseptic solution added

(a) Sac may be painted daily with one of the following until epithelialization occurs: 0.5 per cent silver chloride, 70 per cent alcohol, or 2 to 4 per cent merbromin

Mercury intoxication has been reported with of merbromin (Mercurochrome), and care sho be taken with its use

ii. Monitor temperature for instability or hypothermia

Early signs of infection

iii. Monitor for lethargy, hypotonia

c. To promote normal bowel function

i. Orogastric or nasogastric tube for bowel decompression

ii. Minimal handling of exposed bowel or sac

Handling traumatizes tissues and may contribute to ileus or perforation of bowel or rupture of sac

iii. Nothing given orally

iv. Support bowel in such a way as to avoid folding over edge of defect by wrapping it with several turns of soft roller gauze and girdling this around trunk in a figure of 8 fashion

v. If nonelastic synthetic material such as Teflon mesh or Silastic has been used to encase exposed viscera, *do not apply pressure* or manipulate prosthesis unnecessarily; observe suture sites for breakdown or infection

Because abdominal cavity is small, prosthesis may be sutured around defect to supply controlled intra-abdominal pressure; as size of abdominal cavity increases, size of prosthesis will be decreased

vi. Observe for signs of bowel function or nonfunction
  (a) Peristalsis
  (b) Bowel sounds
  (c) Abdominal distention
  (d) Bile in gastric aspirate
  (e) Passage of meconium (usually occurs 4–7 days after surgery to close defect)

Observe closely for signs of respiratory distress and poor venous return caused by pressure of viscera and diaphragm, abdominal aorta, and inferior vena cava

d. To maintain adequate nutritional state
  i. Peripheral or central hyperalimentation until normal bowel function established

Long term therapy may be necessary because prolonged postoperative ileus is not uncommon

e. To minimize stress to family unit and facilitate parent-infant attachment
  i. Keep parents fully informed; and explain all equipment and procedures fully
  ii. Encourage parental participation in infant's care
  iii. Utilize parent support group
  iv. "Personalize" infant for family
    (a) Call infant by name
    (b) Refer to particular infant characteristics or behavior
    (c) Take pictures when possible
  v. Encourage parents to come or call frequently
  vi. Utilize primary care whenever possible

Reduces number of different people parents must continually learn to relate to or seek out for information

f. To discuss genetic counseling for families of infants with omphalocele

Sixty-six per cent of infants with omphalocele have other anomalies that may be of genetic origin

GASTROINTESTINAL OBSTRUCTION

Early identification of gut anomalies and prompt medical intervention, either surgical or supportive, are required to sustain the infant and restore normal body function.

DIAGNOSIS

Obstruction occurs whenever there is interference with the transit of ingested material from the mouth through the anus. Actual diagnosis of a specific obstruction depends on type and location.

1. **Incidence (see also Table 19-16)**
   a. The frequency of anomalies of the gut varies from 1 in 3000 to 1 in 20,000 live births, and many are associated with obstruction.

ETIOLOGY
1. **Classification of obstruction**
   a. Mechanical
      i. Atresia: complete obstruction of lumen, ranging from webbing to complete absence of major section of bowel
      ii. Stenosis: narrowing that may involve the entire thickness of the bowel wall or be a partial web
      iii. Duplication: may range from cystlike projections to complete replication of gastrointestinal segment
   b. Functional (obstruction not associated with anatomical malformations)
      i. Achalasia
      ii. Pyloric stenosis
      iii. Aganglionic megacolon
      iv. Meconium plug
      v. Meconium ileus
2. **Location of obstruction (Table 19-15)**
   a. Stomach
   b. Small bowel
   c. Large bowel
3. Table 19-16 delineates the most common lesions, their incidence, etiology, pathogenesis, symptoms, diagnostic criteria, and possible treatment

ASSESSMENT
1. **Clinical presentation: Table 19-16**
   a. Signs and symptoms
2. **Biopsychosocial assessment**
   a. Palpation of abdomen for masses (volvulus): doughy intestinal loops (meconium ileus); and scaphoid abdomen (diaphragmatic hernia or esophageal atresia)
   b. Examination of anus with rectal tube or thermometer to rule out imperforate anus

TABLE 19-15.   LOCATIONS AND TYPES OF GASTROINTESTINAL OBSTRUCTION IN INFANCY

Stomach	Small Bowel	Large Bowel
Mechanical	Mechanical	Mechanical
Pyloric stenosis	Atresia or stenosis	Imperforate anus
Prepyloric or antral diaphragm	Hypertrophic stenosis of	Duplication cyst
Pyloric gastric duplication cyst	duodenum	Atresia or stenosis
Volvulus of the stomach	Duplication cysts	
	Annular pancreas	
	Malrotation	
	Volvulus	
	Nonrotation with fibrous bands	
	Incarcerated hernia	
	Congenital adhesions or bands	
	Preduodenal portal vein	
	Meconium ileus	
Acquired	Acquired	Acquired
Foreign body	Intussusception	Drug-induced meconium
Bezoar	Peritoneal adhesions	ileus equivalent
	Mesenteric thrombosis	Meconium plug syndrome
	Necrotizing enterocolitis	Inspissated stool or milk
	Neuroma	syndrome
	Tumor	Fecalith
	Polyp	Toxic dilatation of the colon
	Foreign body	Intussusception
Functional	Functional	Functional
Gastric atony	Total aganglionosis of	Hirschsprung's disease
	colon	
	Absence of musculature	
	Paralytic ileus	

From Gryboski, J.: Gastrointestinal Problems in the Infant. Philadelphia, W.B. Saunders Co., 1975.

TABLE 19-16.   ASSESSMENT AND MANAGEMENT OF GASTROINTESTINAL OBSTRUCTION

Lesions	Etiology/Pathogenesis	Symptoms	Diagnosis	Treatment and Complications
Atresia Esophageal 1:1000 to 1:4500 live births Associated conditions: Congenital heart disease Imperforate anus Genitourinary anomalies Intestinal atresia Prematurity LBW	*Esophageal atresia, fistula* Failure of septal development between trachea and esophagus during week 4 of gestation Types: Atresia without fistula 7.7% Atresia with proximal end TE* fistula 0.8% Atresia with distal and TE fistula 86.5% Atresia with TE fistula, both ends 0.7% TE fistula without atresia 4.2%	General findings with atresia Polyhydramnios Increased salivation, cyanosis, and choking with feedings Large gastric aspirate at birth (15–20 ml) Vomiting Abdominal distention No stool Specific findings with esophageal atresia, fistula Pneumonitis Atelectasis Scaphoid abdomen	Inability to pass 10–12 F catheter into newborn's stomach at least 10–13 cm Inability to obtain acid pH from nasogastric tube aspirate Radiographic studies define nasogastric tube placement† Gas patterns on x-ray abnormal or absent†	Surgery One stage end to end anastomosis in healthy infants Two stage for sick infants with gastrotomy tube placement until final reanastomosis Complications: anastomotic leaks 2–7 days after surgery, strictures, fistula
Duodenal 1:5000 births, higher incidence in females Down's syndrome Malrotation of bowel	Most likely due to persistence in the proliferative stage and defect in recanalization of gut between weeks 5 and 10 of gestation	Same as general findings with atresia (except 2) Bile stained vomitus, mild or no distention upper abdomen, lower abdomen scaphoid	"Double bubble" on x-ray (air in upper GI tract, airlessness beyond duodenum)	Surgery with resection of atretic segment and reanastomosis
Jejunal and ileal atresia 38% of affected infants have multiple atresias; 25%–56% are preterm infants	Believed to arise after insult to part of small bowel during fetal life Types Diaphragm obstruction	Abdominal distention Bile stained vomitus Abnormal passage of meconium—usually gray, green, or mucoid Jaundice Active peristalsis with	X-ray shows distended loops of bowel with air fluid levels Barium enema will show a microcolon in cases of distal ileal atresia	Surgery to remove atretic area and reanastomosis of ends Complications: meconium ileus, peritonitis

	Signs and Symptoms	Diagnosis	Treatment / Complications
Atretic areas form long cords Bowel ends in a sausage-like blind sac "Apple peel small bowel"	ladder-like appearance visible on abdominal wall		
Stenosis Pyloric, 4–5:1000 live births; most common in male infants Duodenal 10% of all cases of duodenal atresia		Persistent projectile vomiting diagnostic in pyloric stenosis X-ray findings demonstrate stenotic area	Correction of metabolic state Surgical correction of stenosis area Complications: dyspepsia, vomiting, epigastric heaviness, gastric ulcers
Pyloric stenosis Etiology unclear; most common theory, hypertrophy of circular muscle fibers of pyloric sphincter secondary to spasm of sphincter	Late onset at several weeks to 3 mo of age; then Poor feeding Intermittent vomiting (becoming projectile in pyloric stenosis) Failure to thrive Aspiration Visible peristaltic waves in left upper quadrant (pyloric stenosis) Metabolic alkalosis (pyloric stenosis)		
Duodenal stenosis Caused by intrinsic factor, annular pancreas, or congenital bands			
Malrotation Abnormal rotation of bowel			
Volvulus Twisting of gut (usually occurs with malrotation) Surgical emergencies produce strangulation of bowel arteries, causing rapid development of gangrene	Vomiting: bile stained contents Distention Sudden onset of vomiting in previously asymptomatic infant Shock	X-ray film of abdomen: Absence of air in gut Fluid filled distended loop of bowel Barium enema shows cecum in upper right or central abdomen	Surgical resection and release of strangulation Complications: peritonitis, gangrene
Meconium ileus High correlation with cystic fibrosis (can confirm CF with sweat chloride test) Abnormally thick, tenacious meconium that obstructs ileum with inspired dried meconium	Symptoms similar to ileal atresia Whitish meconium if any is expelled	Pasty feeling of abdomen (distended loops of bowel impacted with meconium) X-ray reveals soaplike bubbles of meconium	Surgical resection for ileus and nutritional support Complications: volvulus, gangrene, perforation

Table continues on following page.

TABLE 19-16.   ASSESSMENT AND MANAGEMENT OF GASTROINTESTINAL OBSTRUCTION — *Continued*

Lesions	Etiology/Pathogenesis	Symptoms	Diagnosis	Treatment and Complications
Imperforate anus Congenital anorectal malformation; 1:20,000 births	Failure of differentiation of urogenital sinus and cloaca during embryological development	Failure to pass meconium Absence of rectal opening General symptoms of obstruction Fistula Rectovaginal Rectourethral Rectoperineal	filled loops of bowel and no air/fluid levels Inability to pass catheter or thermometer through anal opening	Depends on distance from rectum to skin and whether innervation is present; complete repair, staged repair, or permanent colostomy, according to level of defect
Hirschsprung's disease 1:5000 births 4 X more frequent in males	Abnormal innervation of colon beginning with rectal sphincter and extending back up colon to varying degrees	General symptoms of obstruction Difficulty in passing meconium or stool	Rectal biopsy identifies absence of or reduction in ganglionic cells	Colostomy, resection or both Complications: shock, necrotizing enterotolitis

*TE, tracheoesophageal
†Use of radiopaque material for x-ray may be hazardous because of aspiration

    c. Passage of 10 to 12 F catheter and aspiration of stomach (15 to 20 ml of aspirant is significant and may indicate obstruction; failure to pass catheter may indicate esophageal atresia)

    d. Auscultation of abdomen and chest for bowel sounds (bowel sounds in chest may indicate diaphragmatic hernia)

    e. Observation of character of vomitus: whether bile stained, blood tinged, containing mucus or formula, whether clear fluid; whether vomiting was projectile or drooling

    f. Recording of timing of vomiting in relation to feeding

    g. Parents' response to obvious physical anomaly

    h. Parents' coping skills and support systems

    i. Parents' knowledge and understanding of condition

    j. Parents' feelings of guilt, anger, denial (grief process)

    k. Crisis state in parents resulting in inability to realistically focus on, comprehend, or retain information given

3. Diagnostic data: Table 19–16

**PROBLEMS AND COMPLICATIONS:
TABLE 19–16**

PATIENT CARE MANAGEMENT

1. Goals

    a. To reduce gastrointestinal distress and support normal body function

	COMMENTS/TIPS/CAUTIONS
i. Give infant nothing by mouth	Abdominal obstruction associated with distention, bowel sounds, and vomiting
ii. Insert 8 F feeding tube or Salem sump tube and attach to intermittent low suction	Bowel decompression essential to avoid impairment of respiratory function and possible ischemia to bowel
iii. Postoperatively maintain nasogastric drainage	
iv. Postoperatively observe for signs of peritonitis associated with leaks at bowel anastomosis site	Abdominal distention, abdominal tenderness Tissue breakdown with possible evisceration

    b. To promote adequate circulation and ventilation

i. Maintain bowel decompression	
ii. Position infant in manner that reduces risk of aspiration or pressure on diaphragm	Usually head-up prone, or right lateral position; until corrective surgery performed, infant with tracheoesophageal fistula kept prone with head of bed elevated to prevent gastric reflux into lungs
iii. Observe for signs of cardiac and respiratory distress	
(a) Assess breath sounds	Infant attached to continuous cardiorespiratory monitor
(b) Note signs of tachypnea, cyanosis, apnea,	

grunting, or retractions

   (c) Note signs of shock

c. To prevent hypothermia

    i. Keep infant protected from cold stress during transport for x-ray, ultrasound studies, or surgery

   ii. Keep infant on warmer or in Isolette with Servo control

d. To maintain normal fluid and electrolyte balance

    i. Keep strict record of intake and output

   ii. Maintain peripheral IV

  iii. Maintain central venous infusion line if long term parenteral administration of nutrition anticipated

   iv. Monitor electrolyte levels

    v. Provide mouth care with sterile water or lemon and glycerin swabs

e. To prevent postoperative infection

    i. Keep diaper below incision site

   ii. Change dressing when necessary

  iii. Maintain respiratory status with frequent changes of position and bronchopulmonary toilet

f. To prevent breakdown of skin postoperatively

    i. Use Montgomery straps to facilitate frequent dressing change

   ii. Protect skin around ostomy sites

g. To facilitate parent-infant attachment and reduce parental stress and anxiety

    i. Observe for positive parenting behavior

   ii. Observe coping skills; whether they are positive

  iii. Explain all procedures, treatments, and conditions to parents

COMMENTS/TIPS/CAUTIONS column:

Bradycardia, decrease in BP (less than 60/20)

Very premature infant can be wrapped in plastic (Saran) wrap to reduce heat and water loss

Continuous nasogastric suction, vomiting, or diarrhea predisposes infant to electrolyte imbalance

Obstructive disorders frequently require surgery; postoperatively the bowel will need time to heal or recover from ileus prior to establishment or resumption of oral feeding

An adhesive barrier drape or semipermeable adhesive drape may provide protection from fecal contamination, particularly if colostomy has been performed and its location prevents placement of stoma protector and bag until incision heals

Zinc oxide spray or powder skin preparations

Willingness to touch, frequent calling, speaking of infant by name

Asking appropriate questions, realistic discussion of infant's condition, availability of other support systems

iv. Encourage parents to write questions they want to ask so as not to forget them later when speaking with staff or physician

v. Encourage parents to participate in infant care
  (a) Early involvement in care of stoma in infant with ostomy
  (b) Special feeding techniques for infants with gastrostomy or esophageal fistula

vi. Referral to available parent support group or perinatal social worker

vii. Employ primary care whenever possible to minimize the number of different staff members the parents must communicate with and to establish continuity of care

viii. Refer to infant by name and personalize infant and environment

ix. Take pictures of infant

COMMENTS/TIPS/CAUTIONS

Place infant's name on bed; encourage parents to bring special music box, toy, or clothes

Picture may help parents reinforce infant's recovery and aid in attachment

DISCHARGE PLANNING/TEACHING

1. Establish written goals and objectives with parents regarding special care for infant and educational needs of parents

2. Periodic conferences with the parents and members of health care team may facilitate transition from hospital to home if infant requires
  a. Home hyperalimentation
  b. Staged surgery for correction of defect or obstruction

3. Initiate appropriate referrals
  a. Perinatal social worker
  b. Discharge planning nurse
  c. Public Health Nurse or Visiting Nurses Association
  d. Enterostomal therapist as appropriate

4. Provide minimum of 24–48 hours of continuous direct parent care to infant prior to discharge

CONCLUSIONS

Quality nursing care for any infant must include provision for adequate nutrition. Providing nutritional support to the healthy infant is frequently time consuming and frustrating and requires the nurse to employ extensive practical knowledge and patience to assist the parents with their infant. The knowledge, patience, and experience are even more critical when the infant is premature, sick, or suffering from conditions that compromise the gastrointestinal tract.

The neonatal nurse must be able to recognize the infant at risk, assess nutritional status and needs of the infant, and then develop and employ specialized feeding techniques in conjunction with medical requirements to meet those needs. Evaluating nutritional status and technique effectiveness is a continuous process. Fulfillment of all these expectations requires that the nurse have a broad knowledge base and in depth expertise. When one considers the consequences of failure to secure adequate nutritional support for the infant—mental retardation, growth retardation, infection, and death—the cost in time and commitment for nursing seems a small one.

REFERENCES

1. Avery, G.: Neonatology. Philadelphia, J.B. Lippincott Co., 1975.
2. Babson, S.G., Pernoll, M.L., and Benda, G.I.: Diagnosis and Management of the Fetus and Neonate at Risk, 4th ed. St. Louis, C.V. Mosby Co., 1980.
3. Barrington, J.D.: Necrotizing enterocolitis in the newborn infant. Clin. Perinatol., 5(1):30, 1978.
4. Biller, J.A., and Yeager, A.M. (eds.): The Harriet Lane Handbook, 9th ed. Chicago, Year Book Medical Publishers, 1981.
5. Boles, E.T.: Imperforate anus. Clin. Perinatol., 5(1):149, 1978.
6. Boley, S.J. Dinare, G., and Cohen, M.I.: Hirschsprung's disease in the newborn. Clin. Perinatol., 5(1):45, 1978.
7. Colley, R., Wilson, J., and Wilhem, M.P.: Intravenous nutrition—Nursing considerations. Issues Compr. Pediatr. Nurs. 1:74, 1977.
8. Daily, W., Klaus, M., and Meyer, B.: Apnea in premature infants—Monitoring, incidence, heartrate changes and the effects of temperature. Pediatrics, 43:510, 1969.
9. Denson, S.E., Palma, P.A., and Adcock, E.W.: TPN for the neonate. I. Macronutrients. Nutr. Supp. Serv. J. Pract. Application Clin. Nutr., 1(8):24, 1981.
10. Dudrick, S., MacFayden, B., Van Buren, C., et al.: Parenteral hyperalimentation, metabolic problems and solutions. Ann. Surg., 176:260, 1972.
11. Fonkalsrud, E.W.: Selective repair of neonatal gastroschisis. Ann. Surg., 191:139, 1980.
12. Fomon, S.: Infant Nutrition, 2nd ed. Philadelphia, W.B. Saunders Co., 1974.
13. Gryboski, J.: Gastrointestinal Problems in the Infant. Philadelphia, W.B. Saunders Co., 1975.
14. Harper, R.G., and Yoon, J.J.: Handbook of Neonatology. Chicago, Year Book Medical Publishers, 1974.
15. Kee, J.L.: Fluids and Electrolytes with Clinical Applications: A Programmed Approach, 2nd ed. New York, John Wiley & Sons, 1978.
16. Kerner, J.A., and Sunshine, P.: Parenteral alimentation. Semin. Perinatol., 3:417, 1979.
17. Klaus, M.H., and Fanaroff, A.A.: Care of the High-Risk Neonate, 2nd ed. Philadelphia, W.B. Saunders Co., 1979.

18. Klaus, M.H., and Kennell, J.H.: Maternal-Infant Bonding. St. Louis, C.V. Mosby Co., 1973.

19. Korones, S.B.: High-Risk Newborn Infants, 3rd ed. St. Louis, C.V. Mosby Co., 1981.

20. Mayer, T., Black, R., Matlak, M.E., and Johnson, D.G.: Gastroschisis and omphalocele: An eight-year review. Ann. Surg., *192:*783, 1980.

21. Oehler, J.M.: Family Centered Neonatal Nursing Care. Philadelphia, J.B. Lippincott Co., 1981.

22. Palma, P.A., Denson, S.E., and Adcock, E.W.: TPN for the neonate. II: Major minerals and micronutrients. Nutr. Supp. Serv. J. Pract. Application Clin. Nutr., *2*(1):8, 1982.

23. Perez, R.H.: Protocols for Perinatal Nursing Practice. St. Louis, C.V. Mosby Co., 1981.

24. Pierog, S.H., and Ferrara, A.: Medical Care of the Sick Newborn, 2nd ed. St. Louis, C.V. Mosby Co., 1976.

25. Seashore, J.: Congenital abdominal wall defects. Clin. Perinatol. *5*(1):61, 1978.

26. Stokan, R.: The right formula for the right infant: Making sense of infant nutrition. MCN, *2*(Mar-Apr):102, 1977.

27. Touloukian, R.J.: Intestinal atresia. Clin. Perinatol. *5*(1):3, 1978.

28. Vaughan, V.C., McKay, R.J., and Behrman, R.E.: Nelson Textbook of Pediatrics, 11th ed. Philadelphia, W.B. Saunders Co., 1979.

29. Vestal, K.W.: Pediatric Critical Care Nursing. New York, John Wiley & Sons, 1981.

30. Walker, W.A.: Development of gastrointestinal function and selected dysfunction. Selected Aspects of Perinatal Gastroenterology, Mead-Johnson Symposium on Perinatal Developmental Medicine, 1977.

31. Whaley, L.F., and Wong, D.L.: Nursing Care of Infants and Children. St. Louis, C.V. Mosby Co., 1979.

32. Yu, V.Y.H.: Effects of body positioning on gastric emptying in the neonate. Arch. Dis. Child., *50:*500, 1975.

CHAPTER 20

NEONATAL INFECTIONS

Madonna Cronin, R.N., M.S.

OBJECTIVES

Upon completion of this chapter the reader will be able to accomplish the following:

1. Identify common risk factors that make both the normal and sick neonate more vulnerable to infection
2. Cite common etiological factors predisposing the infant to infection
3. Recognize common pathogenic organisms causing neonatal infections
4. Relate the pathogenesis of specific bacteria, viral, and protozoan infections
5. Discuss methods used to make differential diagnosis
6. Describe the signs and symptoms of neonatal infection
7. Recall the type of antibiotic therapy used to combat specific infections
8. List five interventions employed to discourage the spread of infection in the nursery environment
9. Design a plan of care for the treatment of the infected infant
10. Describe the potential sequelae of each infection discussed

Fighting infection in the nursery is an ongoing and unrelenting battle. Normal defenses of babies are limited at best and they are extremely vulnerable to severe infection that can cause extensive tissue damage and death. Thus an obsession with the control and prevention of neonatal infection is warranted.

Defense against infection is directly related to exposure and experience with infectious agents. The fetus's immune system structures are seen as early as the 8th to 12th week of gestation.[1] Maturation of the lymphoid and hematopoietic systems is slow. The fetus has low levels of immunoglobulins because of the lack of antigenic stimulation. Active transport of immunoglobulin G (IgG) from the mother to the fetus occurs in utero. The neonate acquires immunoglobulin A (IgA) from the mother by ingestion of breast milk. The mother's experience with the defense against infection is passively acquired by the fetus or neonate. Fetal production of immunoglobulin A and M is unusual unless intrauterine infection has occurred.[9] IgA and IgM are particularly important for the newborn since they have a bactericidal effect on gram negative bacteria, a common cause of neonatal sepsis.

The neonate's inflammatory response is poor. The number of functional leukocytes is deficient in the first 24 hours of life. The infant's body is unable to localize infection effectively, and this is demonstrated in inability to identify infection sites selectively and dispatch appropriate cells for the defense of those areas. The result is the multiplication and spread of bacteria. In addition, the phagocytic capability of polymorphonuclear leukocytes is minimal.[6]

The sick infant has an even greater deficit for combating infection. In infants weighing less than 2000 gm phagocyte bactericidal properties are less than in normal newborns. The passive acquisition of immunoglobulins is directly related to time spent in utero. Thus the more premature the infant the fewer maternal antibodies there will be. Further, the more compromised an infant is by illness, as in congenital heart disease, the less capable the defense against infection.

It is important to remember that newborns will react differently from older children to infectious organisms. An infant's exposure to rubella can be fatal, whereas in an older child symptoms are usually mild. On the other

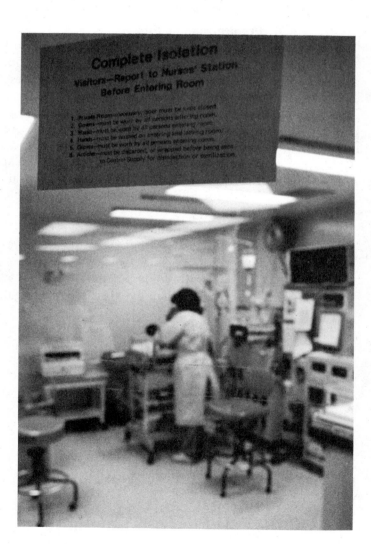

Figure 20-1. Isolation of an infant can create barrier to family-infant attachment. Facilitating visits by the family should be an important goal of the nurse. (Courtesy of Hermann Hospital, Houston, Texas.)

hand, severe disease caused by *Hemophilus influenzae* is rare in neonates but is common in older children.

Although all infants are at risk for infection, it is the sick neonate who requires greater scrutiny and protection.

INFECTION

Neonatal infection can be a major threat to the life and well-being of the fetus or newborn infant. The astute and informed nurse is better able to recognize the early, subtle signs of infection. Together the nurse's expertise and medical management are essential for the infant's recovery from the disease process with minimal limitations to future health.

DIAGNOSIS

Infection is the invasion and multiplication of microorganisms in the body; it may or may not be clinically apparent. All infants, especially sick or premature, are at risk for infection.

1. **Predisposing factors**

Fetal or Neonatal
   a. Prematurity, infant small for gestational age
   b. Prolonged rupture of membranes, maternal infection, forceps delivery, fetal distress
   c. Fetal monitoring and blood sampling
   d. Congenital malformations, e.g., omphalocele; congenital heart disease
   e. Resuscitation, asphyxia, meconium staining or aspiration
   f. Catheterization: umbilical, central venous line, cardiac, radial arterial line; venipuncture; arterial puncture
   g. Surgery
   h. Abrasions and lacerations
   i. Injections, IV and IV infiltration sites, blood transfusions

Nursery
   j. Respiratory equipment
   k. Personnel, family, visitors, other infants
   l. Milk, formula
   m. Equipment for invasive procedures, i.e., lumbar puncture trays, endotracheal tubes, exchange transfusion trays and tubing

ETIOLOGY

1. **Common bacterial causes of infection**
   a. Groups A, B, D streptococci
   b. *Escherichia coli*
   c. *Listeria monocytogenes*
   d. *Staphylococcus aureus*
   e. Pneumococcus
   f. Gonococcus
   g. Meningococcus

    h. *Pseudomonas*
    i. *Klebsiella*
    j. *Proteus*
    k. *Aerobacter*
    l. *Hemophilus influenzae*

2. **Causes of TORCH and other infections**
    a. *Toxoplasma gondii*
    b. Rubella virus
    c. Cytomegalovirus
    d. *Treponema pallidum*
    e. Herpes simplex virus
    f. Echovirus
    g. Coxsackie virus
    h. Adenovirus

SEPSIS NEONATORUM

DIAGNOSIS

Septicemia is the systemic invasion of pathogenic bacteria into the blood stream. In the newborn it is known as sepsis neonatorum.

1. **Incidence**
    a. 1 in 1000 live full term births
    b. 1 in 250 live premature births
    c. Twice as many males as females are affected

ETIOLOGY

1. **Common offending organisms**
    a. *Escherichia coli*
    b. Groups B and D hemolytic streptococci
    c. *Listeria*
    d. *Klebsiella*
    e. *Staphylococcus aureus*
    f. *Hemophilus influenzae*
    g. *Pseudomonas*

2. **Infective source and route of transmission**
    a. Transplacental assault
    b. Contact with infectious agent during descent through birth canal
    c. Aspiration of meconium
    d. Aspiration of infected amniotic fluid
    e. Nursery personnel or equipment
    f. Infected infants
3. Portal of entry may be nasopharynx, skin, eye, umbilicus
4. Infant's body unable to localize infection
5. Pathogenic bacteria multiply, infection spreads, and bacteria migrate into systemic circulation

ASSESSMENT

1. **Clinical presentation**
   a. Signs and symptoms
      i. Altered temperature (usually hypothermia)
      ii. Lethargy
      iii. Poor feeding
      iv. Apnea or tachypnea
      v. Cyanosis
      vi. Vomiting, diarrhea, abdominal distention
      vii. Weight loss
      viii. Hypoglycemia (common with gram negative bacteria)
      ix. Thrombocytopenia, leukopenia, disseminated intravascular coagulation (DIC)
      x. High IgM levels (greater than 20 mg/100 ml)
2. **Diagnostic data**
   a. Identification of organism through blood cultures (prior to antibiotic therapy): Ear canal, nasopharynx, skin, rectum, gastric aspirate, urine, spinal fluid, blood
   b. CBC with differential count
   c. Chest roentgenogram
   d. Spinal tap

SEPSIS DUE TO GROUP B β-HEMOLYTIC STREPTOCOCCUS AND TO LISTERIA MONOCYTOGENES

Disease processes associated with sepsis due to group B β-hemolytic streptococcus and with sepsis due to *Listeria monocytogenes* can be of early onset or late onset.

EARLY ONSET

ETIOLOGY

1. Maternal-fetal transmission
2. Portal of entry: aspiration of organism through airway. The lung is the usual primary site of infection, indicative of aspiration of infected amniotic fluid

ASSESSMENT

1. **Clinical presentation**
   a. Signs and symptoms
      i. Onset birth to 72 hours of age
      ii. Pneumonia
      iii. Skin eruptions
      iv. Early apnea: onset of apnea much earlier than that associated with RDS
      v. Meningitis (rare)
      vi. Hypotension
      vii. Thrombocytopenia, leukopenia, DIC

       viii. Low birth weight
        ix. Peculiar to *Listeria*
           (a)   Erythematous rash over trunk and extremities
           (b)   Hepatosplenomegaly
           (c)   Meconium staining of amniotic fluid
           (d)   Pulmonary hypertension
   b. History
         i. Maternal infection
        ii. Complicated delivery, premature delivery, premature rupture of membranes
      iii. Intrauterine catheterization
      iv. Fetal monitoring
       v. Low birth weight
      vi. Peculiar to *Listeria*
          (a)   Maternal flu-like symptoms 2 weeks prior to delivery

2. Diagnostic data

   a. Gram positive cocci in gastric aspirate
   b. Ventilatory support may require less peak pressures than commonly associated with hyaline membrane disease
   c. Blood cultures positive for β-hemolytic streptococcus or *Listeria*
   d. Peculiar to sepsis due to group B streptococcus: x-ray pattern similar to that of RDS
   e. Peculiar to sepsis due to *Listeria*: x-ray pattern similar to that of bronchopneumonia or aspiration pneumonitis rather than to that of RDS

PROBLEMS AND COMPLICATIONS

1. Neurological damage
2. Bronchopulmonary dysplasia
3. Death

TREATMENT

1. Antibiotics: penicillin and an aminoglycoside

—————————————— **LATE ONSET** ——————————————

ETIOLOGY

1. Nosocomial transmission, i.e., through nursery personnel
2. Portal of entry: blood, middle ear, meninges

1. Clinical presentation

   a. Signs and symptoms
         i. Onset 72 hours to 4 weeks of age (seen as late as 16 weeks of age)
        ii. Poor feeding
      iii. Fever
      iv. Focal infections: conjunctivitis, otitis media, facial cellulitis, septic arthritis, meningitis (predominant clinical presentation)
   b. History

      i. Uncomplicated labor
     ii. Birth weight appropriate for gestational age
2. Diagnostic data
   a. Spinal fluid cultures positive for gram positive organisms
   b. Blood and skin cultures may be negative

PROBLEMS AND COMPLICATIONS
1. Neurological damage
2. Hydrocephalus
3. Death

TREATMENT
1. Antibiotics
   a. Group B streptococcus: penicillin
   b. *Listeria:* an aminoglycoside and ampicillin

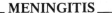

MENINGITIS

    Meningitis is due to invasion of the infecting organism into the meninges, which leads to inflammation, thus creating a collection of purulent exudate at the base of the brain.

DIAGNOSIS
1. Incidence
   a. 0.4 to 1 in 1000 live births
   b. More frequent in males than in females

ETIOLOGY
1. Common bacterial and viral causes of meningitis
   a. Group B β-hemolytic streptococcus
   b. *Escherichia coli*
   c. *Listeria*
   d. Coxsackie virus
   e. Echovirus
2. Transmission is frequently via personnel (labor and delivery, nursery) or equipment
3. Entry is by indirect invasion via blood stream (septicemia) from distant site of infection, i.e., omphalitis, or direct invasion of head, i.e., scalp electrode abscess, otitis media, myelomeningocele
4. Indirect or direct invasion of infecting organism into meninges
5. Inflammatory response causing irritation of meninges and underlying structures of brain
6. Destruction of brain cells
7. Accumulation of purulent exudate at base of brain
8. Interruption of CSF circulation
9. Cerebral edema
10. Increased intracranial pressure

11. Hydrocephalus
12. Further damage to brain cells

ASSESSMENT

1. **Clinical presentation**
   a. Signs and symptoms
      i. Lethargy, respiratory distress, hyporeflexia
      ii. High pitched cry
      iii. Increased irritability, jitteriness
      iv. Full, bulging anterior fontanelle
      v. Poor feeding
      vi. Vomiting, diarrhea, abdominal distention
      vii. Altered temperature
      viii. Bradycardia
      ix. Hypertension
      x. Seizures, tremors, coma
      xi. Petechiae
      xii. Setting sun eyes
      xiii. Peculiar to viral meningitis: erythematous maculopapular rash
   b. History
      i. Complicated pregnancy or delivery
      ii. Invasive fetal monitoring
      iii. Prematurity
      iv. Local infection
2. **Diagnostic data**
   a. Analysis of CSF
      i. WBC count greater than 32
      ii. Glucose less than 50 per cent (compared with serum glucose)
      iii. Cultures positive for pathogen
      iv. Elevated protein level
   b. Blood cultures
      i. Positive
      ii. Increased WBC, serum glucose and uric acid
   c. Inappropriate ADH
      i. Increased urinary sodium and specific gravity
      ii. Decreased serum sodium
   d. Peculiar to viral meningitis: absence of bacterial offenders on smears and cultures; incidence concomitant with community outbreak

PROBLEMS AND COMPLICATIONS

1. Fluid and electrolyte disturbances: hyponatremia, hypocalcemia, hypoglycemia, hyperbilirubinemia, anemia, DIC
2. Hydrocephalus
3. Blindness
4. Seizures
5. Retardation
6. Death

TABLE 20-1.   DOSAGE SCHEDULE FOR COMMONLY PRESCRIBED
ANTIBIOTICS IN NEWBORN INFANTS

Antibiotic	Usual Individual Dose	Daily Dosage and Intervals (Number of Divided Doses/24 hr)	
		0–7 Days of Age	> 7 Days of Age
Amikacin	7.5 mg/kg	15 mg/kg (2)	15 (?22.5) mg/kg (2 or ?3)†
Ampicillin			
Septicemia	25 mg/kg	50 mg/kg (2)	75–100 mg/kg/day (3 or 4)
Meningitis	100 mg/kg	200 mg/kg/day (2)	300 mg/kg/day (3)
Carbenicillin	100 mg/kg	200 mg/kg (2)	300–400 mg/kg (3 or 4)
Chloramphenicol	25 mg/kg	25 mg/kg (1)	50 mg/kg (2)
Gentamicin	2.5 mg/kg	5 mg/kg (2)	7.5 mg/kg (3)
Kanamycin	7.5–10 mg/kg	15–20 mg/kg (2)*	20–30 mg/kg (2 or 3)*
Methicillin			
Septicemia	25 mg/kg	50–75 mg/kg (2 or 3)	75–100 mg/kg (3 or 4)
Meningitis	50 mg/kg	100–150 mg/kg (2 or 3)	150–200 mg/kg (3 or 4)
Penicillin G			
Septicemia	25,000 U/kg	50,000 U/kg (2)	75,000 U/kg (3)
Meningitis	50,000 U/kg	100,000–150,000 U/kg (2 or 3)	150,000–250,000 U/kg (3 or 4)
Ticarcillin	75 mg/kg	150–225 mg/kg (2 or 3)*	225–300 mg/kg/day (3 or 4)*
Tobramycin	2 mg/kg	4 mg/kg (2)	4 (?6) mg/kg (2 or ?3)†
Vancomycin	15 mg/kg	30 mg/kg (2)	45 mg/kg (3)

Reprinted with permission from Avery, G.: Neonatology, Pathophysiology, and Management of the Newborn. Philadelphia, J.B. Lippincott Co., 1981, p 733.
*Smaller dose for infants <2000 gm; larger dose for infants >2000 gm
†Additional studies required before larger dose can be recommended

TREATMENT
1. **Antibiotics**
   a. Bacterial
       i. Initially penicillin, aminoglycoside, or cephalosporin
       ii. Chloramphenicol has been used against coliform bacilli
   b. Viral
       i. None available except treatment of symptoms and containment of infection

TORCH INFECTIONS

The TORCH infections consist of *t*oxoplasmosis, *r*ubella, syphilis, *c*ytomegalovirus disease, and *h*erpes.

TOXOPLASMOSIS

Adults with toxoplasmosis are often asymptomatic. Infants with the disease become profoundly ill; neurological damage, multiple anomalies, and sometimes death result.

DIAGNOSIS

Toxoplasmosis is a protozoan infection, caused by *Toxoplasma gondii*, that may be either congenital or acquired.

1. **Incidence**
   a.   1 to 4 in 1000 live births

ETIOLOGY

1. Maternal ingestion of cat feces or undercooked or raw meat (maternal infection)
2. Spread and replication of infective organism in placenta
3. Transmission of organism across placenta to fetus; fetal transmission is more likely in third trimester if maternal acquisition of infection occurs at this time; the earlier the gestation the less chance there is of fetal infection–early transmission, however, is more likely to cause a severe disease process
4. Rapid replication of parasite and spread to all fetal organ systems
5. Formation of tissue cysts
6. Interference in circulation and blood supply to cells
7. Interruption or slowing of cell growth and function, especially cerebral tissue

ASSESSMENT

1. **Clinical presentation**
   a.   Signs and symptoms appear at birth or several weeks thereafter
      i.   Hepatosplenomegaly, jaundice, increase in indirect bilirubin
      ii.   Abnormal bleeding, petechiae, ecchymoses, rash
      iii.   Anemia, pallor, thrombocytopenia
      iv.   Chorioretinitis, cataracts
      v.   Prematurity
      vi.   Abnormal CSF
      vii.   Intracranial calcifications, convulsions, hydrocephalus
      viii.   Lymphadenopathies
      ix.   Hypothermia, fever
      x.   Vomiting, diarrhea
   b.   History
      i.   Maternal exposure to infection
      ii.   *Toxoplasma* antibody in maternal serum
      iii.   Gestational age
2. **Diagnostic data**
   a.   Serological testing
      i.   Increase in IgM and IgG in cord
      ii.   Sabin-Feldman dye test
   b.   Spinal tap
      i.   Elevated protein levels
   c.   Skull films
      i.   Intracranial calcification

PROBLEMS AND COMPLICATIONS

1. Microcephaly

2. Hydrocephalus
3. Hearing and visual impairment
4. Psychomotor retardation
5. Death

TREATMENT
1. Avoidance of ingestion of raw meat and handling of cat feces during gestation is the primary means of prevention.

RUBELLA

Rubella infection is seasonal and pandemic, but it persists throughout the year at low levels. It can be transmitted to the fetus in utero, or it can be acquired postnatally by the infant.

DIAGNOSIS
Rubella is a viral, systemic infection.

ETIOLOGY
1. Rubella is transmitted to the fetus across the placenta, or from the maternal genital tract by viral ascent or during delivery
2. Postnatally it is transmitted from infected nursery population to the infant by direct or indirect contact with respiratory and conjunctival secretions, feces, and urine
3. Virus may be present throughout gestation, shed months or years later
4. Infection may spread to fetal organs, with vascular obstruction to fetal tissues, cellular necrosis, and arrest of cell development and tissue injury; cellular lesions evident in most organs, especially eye, ear, and heart

ASSESSMENT
1. **Clinical presentation**
   a. Signs and symptoms
      i. Prematurity
      ii. Thrombocytopenia, leukopenia, anemia
      iii. Petechiae, bluish red lesions over skin, purpura
      iv. Increase in direct bilirubin, hepatitis, enlargement of liver and spleen
      v. Intrauterine or extrauterine growth retardation
      vi. Retinopathy, cataracts (present at birth or may develop later)
      vii. Bony radiolucency
      viii. Encephalitis
      ix. Interstitial pneumonia
      x. Congenital heart disease
   b. History
      i. Prenatal: exposure of mother to virus, maternal rash
      ii. Postnatal: exposure of infant to others (other infants or nursery staff) with virus.
2. **Diagnostic data**
   a. Spinal tap

   i. Elevated protein level
   ii. Elevated white blood cell count
  b. Increased level of serum IgM
  c. Pharyngeal culture (pharynx optimal site for identification of virus)
  d. Ophthalmological examination
  e. X-ray study of bones
  f. Cardiac evaluation

PROBLEMS AND COMPLICATIONS

Infection in the first trimester is associated with a greater number of defects. During the last two trimesters it is likely that deafness will be the only defect.

1. Intrauterine death
2. Microcephaly, cerebral palsy, mental retardation
3. Congenital heart defects
4. Eye defects, cataracts
5. Deafness
6. Death

TREATMENT

1. Prevention by immunization of children and of women during child-bearing years with live rubella vaccine

SYPHILIS

Syphilis is a contagious venereal disease caused by the spirochete *Treponema pallidum*. When untreated in the mother, it can be transmitted to the fetus as congenital syphilis; severe neonatal pathological changes result.

ETIOLOGY

1. Transmission by sexual contact with infected person or in utero
2. Maternal spirochetemia
3. Transplacental migration
4. Dissemination of spirochete into fetal tissues
5. Inflammation of affected organs (organs particularly susceptible to disease include liver, spleen, kidney, pancreas, bone)
6. Cell and tissue destruction

ASSESSMENT

1. Clinical presentation
  a. Signs and symptoms
   i. Prematurity
   ii. Hepatitis, high direct bilirubin level, hepatosplenomegaly
   iii. Hemolytic anemia, DIC
   iv. Septicemia
   v. Abnormal CSF
   vi. Spasticity
   vii. Bulging fontanelle
   viii. Periostitis

    ix. Pneumonitis
    x. Petechiae, papulosquamous lesions, gray raised, flat moist
       lesions
  b. History
    i. Serological evidence of infectious syphilis in the mother
    ii. Prematurity
    iii. Premature labor and delivery
 2. Diagnostic data
  a. Elevated IgM level
  b. Prolonged positive VDRL (Venereal Disease Research Laboratory)
     reaction
  c. Radiological examination of long bones

TREATMENT

 1. Prevention in infant by early detection of maternal syphilis by means of
    VDRL test
 2. Treatment with penicillin or erythromycin

—————————— CYTOMEGALOVIRUS (CMV) INFECTION ——————————

Maternal infection with cytomegalovirus has a vast range of neonatal
effects. The infant may be asymptomatic or display a variety of clinical
symptoms, the worst of which is widespread tissue damage; death may
occur.

DIAGNOSIS

 1. Incidence
  a. 1 in 100 live births in mothers from a low socioeconomic popula-
     tion

ETIOLOGY

 1. Virus persists in the host indefinitely, with periods of reactivation with-
    out symptoms
 2. It can be transmitted via the placenta and contact with infected mater-
    nal cervical secretions
 3. Postnatally it can be transmitted by ingestion of breast milk, blood
    transfusion, and contact with infected urine or pharyngeal secretions
 4. Maternal viremia
 5. Invasion of tissues and multiple organs
 6. Cytolysis, necrosis, interference with cell production in affected organs
 7. Inflammation of infected tissues
 8. Fibrosis and calcification of brain
 9. Intrauterine or extrauterine growth retardation

ASSESSMENT

 1. Clinical presentation
  a. Signs and symptoms
    i. Jaundice, hyperbilirubinemia

      ii. Hemolytic anemia, thrombocytopenia, DIC
     iii. Growth retardation, prematurity
     iv. Hypoactivity
      v. Convulsions
     vi. Petechiae, ecchymoses
    vii. Apnea
   viii. Pneumonia (occasionally)
  b. History
      i. Maternal serological test positive for cell fixed antibody

2. Diagnostic data
  a. Increase in serum IgM and IgG
  b. Urine, stool, or throat cultures for CMV
  c. Skull x-ray study for brain calcifications
  d. CBC

PROBLEMS AND COMPLICATIONS
1. Mental and motor retardation
2. Microcephaly
3. Spastic diplegia
4. Blindness
5. Deafness
6. Neonatal death

──────────── HERPES SIMPLEX ────────────

Herpes simplex type 2 or genital herpes is categorized as a major venereal disease. When the fetus acquires this infection the potential for fetal or neonatal death is great. In the infant, herpes simplex type 1, which is usually associated with oral lesions in the adult, can be just as catastrophic, but it is less common than type 2.

DIAGNOSIS
Herpes simplex is an acute viral infection.

1. Incidence
  a. Estimated to be 1 in 1000 pregnancies

ETIOLOGY
1. Pathogenic organism is herpes simplex virus
2. Principally acquired during birth by
  a. Ascent of the infective organism through birth canal to fetus after rupture of membranes
  b. Direct fetal contact with herpes lesion or infected vaginal secretions during descent through birth canal
3. Placental transmission and cross-contamination via nursery personnel are thought to be rare
4. Neonatal contact with herpes virus

Local form

5. Infection may be localized at site of entry, such as eye, skin, mouth, CNS

Disseminated form

1. Infective organism enters mouth, eye, skin
2. Proliferation of virus into blood stream
3. Viremia
4. Systemic spread of virus
5. Visceral lesions form
6. Interference with blood supply to surrounding tissue
7. Tissue infarction and cytolysis
8. Target organs: liver, blood, lung, adrenals, brain

ASSESSMENT

1. **Clinical presentation**
    a. Signs and symptoms of localized form
        i. Meningitis, encephalitis, convulsions, coma, lethargy
        ii. Abnormal muscle tone
        iii. Bulging fontanelle
        iv. Keratitis, chorioretinitis, conjunctivitis
        v. Vesicular lesions on skin, maculopapular rash
    b. Signs and symptoms of disseminated form
        i. Respiratory distress
        ii. Fever
        iii. Hepatosplenomegaly, jaundice, hyperbilirubinemia, hepatitis
        iv. Petechiae, ecchymoses, abnormal bleeding
        v. Anemia, DIC
        vi. Irritability
        vii. Opisthotonus, seizures
        viii. Bulging fontanelle
    c. History
        i. Maternal genital herpes
        ii. Sexual partner with herpes
        iii. Exposure to herpes simplex type 1 via oral sexual relations in last trimester

2. **Diagnostic data**
    a. Mother
        i. Cultures of cervix and vaginal secretions for virus
    b. Neonate
        i. Cultures of lesion, if present, for virus: throat, skin, mouth, conjunctiva, CSF
        ii. Smear from specimen obtained at base of vesicular lesion (diagnosis difficult in absence of lesions)
        iii. Values abnormal: white blood cells and protein increased

PROBLEMS AND COMPLICATIONS

1. Visual disturbances
2. Psychomotor retardation

3. Microcephaly
4. Hydrocephaly
5. Death

TREATMENT

1. Prevention

a. Maternal cervical cultures beginning at 32 weeks of gestation; if positive in the last week of gestation, cesarean section highly recommended

b. If Papanicolaou smear prior to delivery is positive, infant should be closely monitored.

2. Ara-A antiviral agent given to the infected infant

PATIENT CARE MANAGEMENT

1. Goals

COMMENTS/TIPS/
CAUTIONS

a. To prevent, detect early, treat, or contain infection in the nursery

    i. When an infant is admitted to the nursery the history and physical appearance should be carefully assessed for the possibility of infection

If any predisposing factors exist (cited earlier in chapter), then appropriate precautions should be instituted immediately

    ii. Take appropriate precautions

      (a) Rigorous hand washing

      (b) Place infant in Isolette

      (c) Change Isolette weekly

      (d) Wipe Isolette daily with antiseptic cleaner

Hands should be considered the primary carriers of pathogens and scrupulously washed with antiseptic solution before and after contact with each infant and contaminated material

Isolette is one of primary defenses against the spread of infection

    iii. Use isolation precautions if the suspected infection is particularly communicable and dangerous to the patient population

      (a) Isolate infected infants

      (b) Use gloves, gown, mask when appropriate

      (c) Separate linen and trash. Double-bag, and label ISOLATION.

      (d) Use separate receptacle for disposal of

It is essential to be cognizant of how a particular infection is spread so that specific precautions can be instituted; e.g., the rubella virus is present in urine and stool so gloves must be used when handling the infant, and diapers should be double bagged and labeled

TABLE 20-2.   COMMON LOCAL INFECTIONS

Name of Infection and Primary Site of Pathogenic Invasion	Usual or Common Pathogen	Pathogenesis and Sequelae	Clinical Signs and Symptoms	Treatment
Urinary tract infection	*Escherichia coli*	Invasion of pathogen into urinary tract Inflammation of urinary tract Obstruction Bladder distention Hydronephrosis Urinary tract damage Systemic infection	Weight loss greater than 10% of body weight Cyanosis Lethargy Poor feeding Temperature instability Abdominal distention Diminished or weak urinary stream	Identification of pathogen: urine specimen via clean catch or suprapubic tap Containment of pathogen; good hand washing technique Parenteral antibiotic: kanamycin or gentamicin Repeat urine cultures 2 days after therapy
Eye: Neonatal ophthalmia	*Neisseria gonorrhoeae, Staphylococcus aureus, Pseudomonas aeruginosa, Chlamydia*	Gonorrhea Invasion of pathogen into conjunctiva via passage through birth canal and contact with infected maternal tissue Conjunctivitis Hyperemia Spread to cornea Corneal perforation Blindness	Symptoms noted 2nd to 5th day of life Watery eye discharge Copious thick, white, purulent discharge from eyes Conjunctival swelling and redness	Instillation of 1% silver nitrate into both eyes after delivery (after maternal-infant eye contact) Identification of pathogen by eye culture Administration of antibiotic; penicillin or cephalosporin Irrigate eyes with saline to remove purulent exudate Strict hand washing technque Isolate infant from other infants
		Invasion of *Chlamydia* into conjunctiva	Symptoms usually become apparent 3rd week of life	Identification of organism by eye culture

Infection	Pathology	Symptoms	Nursing interventions
	Possible endophthalmitis	Severe swelling and inflammation of eyelids Purulent discharge from eyes Pseudomembrane formation	Strict hand washing technique Cleanse eye of exudate with saline Administer antibiotic: sulfisoxazole or erythromycin
	Bacterial invasion of *Pseudomonas* and *S. aureus* into conjunctiva Possible endophthalmitis	Mild conjunctivitis Redness Swelling Purulent discharge Infection may spread to entire eye, causing increasing severity of symptoms	Identification of organism through eye culture Strict hand washing technique Antibiotic administration: carbenicillin, gentamicin, or methicillin
E. coli Gastrointestinal tract: Diarrheal disease	*E. coli* invasion Organism adheres to small bowel wall Production of enterotoxin Interference with transfer of Na, Cl, and H_2O in stool	Lethargy Poor feeding Weight loss 7–10 green watery stools a day Metabolic acidosis Dehydration Pallor Cyanosis Vomiting	Identification of infected infant through stool culture Strict isolation Strict hand washing technique Isolate infected infants Correct electrolyte and fluid disturbances Correct metabolic acidosis Antibiotic therapy *E. coli*: neomycin *Salmonella*: ampicillin
Shigella	Invasion of *Shigella* into bowel wall: pathologic changes as above	As above Stools contain blood, mucus, and pus	

Table continues on following page.

TABLE 20–2.   COMMON LOCAL INFECTIONS – *Continued*

Name of Infection and Primary Site of Pathogenic Invasion	Usual or Common Pathogen	Pathogenesis and Sequelae	Clinical Signs and Symptoms	Treatment
		In addition Destruction of intestinal mucosa		
	Salmonella	*Salmonella* invasion of bowel mucosa Pathologic changes as *E. coli* Organism does not destroy epithelial lining	Symptoms same as *E. coli*	
Umbilical stump: Omphalitis	Staphylococci or streptococci	Invasion of pathogen into umbilicus Abdominal wall cellulitis Spread to abdominal cavity Peritonitis Portain vein thrombosis Portal hypertension Septicemia	Umbilical redness Umbilical swelling Umbilical induration Purulent drainage from umbilicus	Identification of pathogen by umbilical culture Strict hand washing technique Local or systemic antibiotics
Cutaneous infections (frequently seen in diaper and umbilical areas)	*Staphylococcus aureus*	Invasion of organism into skin Appearance of lesion Spread of lesion If extensive, organism may enter blood stream Septicemia	Solitary clusters of pustules and furuncles	Identification of pathogen by culture of lesion Strict isolation and hand washing technique Antibiotic therapy
Scalded skin syndrome	Staphylococcus of phage group II	Invasion of organism into skin Exotoxin release into stratum granolosum epidermidis	General erythema Inflammation Desquamation Flaccid bullae	As above

needles and syringes marked ISOLATION

(e) Specimens sent to laboratory should be bagged and marked ISOLATION

(f) Maintain separate equipment for infant for whom isolation precautions are being used: BP, Doppler, stethoscope

Some infections, such as herpes simplex, are particularly virulent and are dangerous to the general nursery population; therefore, when possible, it is advisable that the nurse be assigned only that patient to avoid the chance of further infection in the nursery

(g) Nurse caring for infant should not care for other infants or infants particularly susceptible to infection

iv. Upon infant's admission, paint umbilical cord with triple dye

Triple dye is one of the most effective agents against severe infection of the umbilicus

v. Instill 1 per cent silver nitrate drops in eyes

Silver nitrate is prophylactically effective against gonococci and will protect the infant against corneal perforation and blindness; in the interests of maternal-infant bonding, it is recommended that the infant and mother be allowed to interact visually prior to instillation of silver nitrate, since the medication will temporarily interfere with the infant's vision

vi. Collect specimens for identification of the infectious disease process and specific pathogen: skin, gastric aspirate, ear, nasopharynx, stool, urine, blood, spinal fluid; CBC, Igm levels

Generally prophylactic treatment with wide spectrum antibiotics (such as ampicillin and gentamicin) is initiated whenever infection is suspected

Cultures must be obtained prior to initiation of antibiotic therapy to avoid interference with laboratory results; specific identification of infective agent is necessary to determine specific drug sensitivity and most effective antibiotic agent

vii. Administer antibiotic therapy as ordered

(a) Double check antibiotic dosage according to age, weight, condition being treated.

Drug administration always presents risks to the patient—therefore, careful scrutiny of medications administered is in order; for example, chloramphenicol, used to treat meningitis, will cause vascular collapse and gray baby syndrome when toxic levels are reached

(b) Be informed about drug, its actions, contraindications, incompatibilities, side effects, recommended route and dosage

Aminoglycosides, such as gentamicin, are nephrotoxic and ototoxic, so to avoid toxicity this drug should not be administered in less than 20 minutes; many infusion pumps will deliver the medication as a bolus when injected in IV tubing—therefore, it is advised that the medication be diluted in the Soluset or delivered by slow manual injection

viii. Restrict staff and visitors from contact with infant if the infant has any of the following conditions

(a) Fever

Since the infant is susceptible to infection, screening of all staff and visitors is recommended to avoid unnecessary contact with infection

(b)   Active febrile respiratory infection

(c)   Open draining lesions, e.g., herpes

(d)   Diarrhea

ix.   Restrict staff member from the care of infant with a TORCH infection if staff member is pregnant or susceptible to particular infection

A pregnant staff member risks abortion or serious damage to her unborn child if she is exposed to TORCH infections

All staff members working in the nursery should be tested for susceptibility to identified TORCH infections

b.   To maintain ventilation and oxygenation of tissues

i.   Frequently assess infant for increasing oxygen demand and respiratory failure

As the infant becomes more compromised by the infectious process, respiratory effort will become weakened and increasing amounts of oxygen will be required

(a)   Increasing cyanosis

(b)   Tachypnea

(c)   Apnea

(d)   Tachycardia

(e)   Bradycardia

(f)   Blood gas: PCO_2 increased, PO_2 decreased, and pH acidotic

(g)   Retractions

(h)   Nasal flaring

(i)   Grunting

ii.   Administer ordered amount of supplemental oxygen

(a)   Maintain airway by properly positioning infant

(b)   Suction oral, nasal and pharyngeal secretions; note amount, color, character

Always suction oral secretions prior to nasal suction to avoid gasping reflex and aspiration of secretions

(c)   Calibrate O_2 equipment as required

(d)   Analyze O_2 concentration frequently

(e)   Draw blood for gas determinations as ordered

(f)   Ensure proper humidity and change hu-

Oxygen administration without humidity will dry airway membranes; respiratory equipment will harbor *Pseudomonas* and other "water bugs"—changing water every 8 hours will decrease the threat of infection

midification reservoir every 8 hours

iii. Ventilator maintenance

    (a) Assist in intubation procedure

    (b) Maintain patent airway

        (1) Check breath sounds frequently

        (2) Frequently check endotracheal tube for kinking or secretions obstructing it

        (3) Suction, using sterile technique, every 2 hours or as necessary

        (4) Increase O_2

        (5) Perform chest percussion and vibration to all lung areas prior to suctioning

        (6) Change position every 2 hours

    (c) Evaluate blood gases

    (d) Check ventilator settings every hour

    (e) Ventilator tubing must be changed every 24 hours

    (f) Change water in humidity chamber every 8 hours

c. To maintain fluid and electrolyte balance

    i. Keep accurate records of intake and output

    (a) Report decrease in amount of urine

    (b) Report increase in specific gravity (greater than 1.015)

    (c) Report spilling of

COMMENTS/TIPS/CAUTIONS

Respiratory failure is a frequent complication of severe neonatal infection; nursing responsibilities are very often directed toward minimizing further insult through mechanical respiratory support

Evaluate infant's production of secretions to determine frequency of suctioning

Chest physiotherapy and changing position assist in evacuation of secretions from the lungs; the infant should be assessed for tolerance for the procedure, and the nurse's actions should be paced accordingly

When the infant's platelet count is less than 100,000 avoid vigorous percussion and use only mild vibration

Respiratory equipment is a prime reservoir for bacteria

Normal urine output for a neonates is 2–3 ml/h

protein, blood, and sugar in urine

ii. Administer IV fluids as ordered

(a) Check IV site every hour

(b) Record amount infused hourly

iii. Continually assess infant for signs and symptoms of electrolyte imbalance: hyponatremia, hypernatremia, hypokalemia, hyperkalemia

iv. Evaluate serum electrolytes and administer electrolytes parenterally as ordered

v. Weigh infant daily and alert physician to any abnormal weight gain or loss

vi. Monitor skin hydration

vii. Administer diuretics as ordered

d. To maintain normal body temperature

i. Check infant's axillary temperature at least every 2 hours

ii. Maintain infant in Isolette on Servo control

iii. Use heat lamp during procedures requiring infant to be out of Isolette

iv. Coordinate nursing care to minimize entries into Isolette and convective heat loss

v. Ensure that portholes have plastic sleeves

vi. Place a silver swaddler or aluminum foil inside and in the back of the Isolette

vii. Place skull cap on infant

e. To provide emotional support for the parents

i. Allow parents to visit their infant whenever they would like

COMMENTS/TIPS/CAUTIONS

It is important to note the character of the IV site hourly to discourage severe IV infiltration and necrosis of tissues; the site provides an excellent medium for bacterial growth

In renal dysfunction the infant will become edematous, display an abnormal gain in weight, and may require administration of diuretics; certain diuretics, e.g., furosemide (Lasix), can cause hypokalemia

Since hypothermia is an infant's common reaction to infection, special attention is directed toward thermoregulation

When Servo control is used, a steady increase in Isolette temperature indicates the infant's increased need for warmth to maintain normal body temperature and alerts the nurse to hypothermia

To avoid the airborne transmission of an infective agent to other infants, all infants should remain in their Isolettes while an infected infant is removed from the Isolette for a procedure

Silver will reflect radiant heat onto the infant, thus increasing temperature

Much of the infant's heat loss is through the scalp; placement of a skull cap will discourage excessive heat loss by this route

Most neonatal nurseries have 24 hour visiting privileges for parents

	COMMENTS/TIPS/ CAUTIONS
ii. Explain the infant's condition to them	
iii. Describe the equipment and procedures being used to support their infant	First assess the parents' desire for information, level of comprehension, and anxiety; the nurse can then better communicate with them
iv. Emphasize the infant's personal characteristics	It is important that the parents recognize the infant as real and as their own; pointing out special characteristics will assist the parents in bonding
v. Allow the parents to ask questions and answer them promptly	
vi. Encourage the parents to participate in their infant's care	Often the parents of an ill neonate feel helpless; providing them with simple tasks, such as changing a diaper or recording the infant's daily weight, will make them feel more useful
vii. If possible, provide the family with privacy to interact with their infant	
viii. Provide a comfortable environment for interaction and avoid focusing on the barriers of isolation such as masks and gloves	Precautions used in isolation many times are emotional barriers; thus it is the nurse's responsibility to assist the parents to overcome these barriers and relate to their infant
ix. Validate the parents' understanding of their baby's condition and treatment; encourage them to ventilate	

CONCLUSIONS

It is through diligent nursing care and supervision that neonatal infection can be minimized. Many institutions have an infection control nurse. Working closely with the nurse may facilitate the early detection of contaminants and assist in determining the most effective way to control nursery outbreak. Knowledge of microorganisms and their transmission is the most effective means available to combat neonatal infection.

REFERENCES

1. Avery, G.B.: Neonatology: Pathophysiology and Management in the Newborn, 2nd ed. Philadelphia, J.B. Lippincott Co., 1981.
2. Bobitt, R.: The group-B beta-hemolytic streptococcus. Semin. Perinatol., *1*:1 (Jan.), 1977.
3. Goldman, D.A., et al.: Bacterial colonization of neonates admitted to an intensive care environment. J. Pediatr., *93*:2, 1978.
4. Herpes on Delivery. Emerg. Med., *12*(May 30):1980.
5. Hodes: Penicillin prophylaxis and neonatal streptococcal disease. Hosp. Pract., *15*: (March) 1980.

6. Klaus, M.H., and Fanaroff, A.A.: Care of the High Risk Neonate, 2nd ed. Philadelphia, W.B. Saunders Co., 1979.
7. Korones, S.B.: High Risk Newborn Infants. St. Louis, C.V. Mosby Co., 1976.
8. Looking for lethal listeriosis. Emerg. Med., *11:*(Aug. 15), 78, 1979.
9. McCracken, G.H., and Shinefield, H.R.: Changes in the pattern of neonatal septicemia and meningitis. Am. J. Dis. Child., *112*:33, 1966.
10. Oakes, A.R.: Critical Care Nursing of Children and Adolescents. Philadelphia, J.B. Lippincott Co., 1981.
11. Parry, M.F., et al.: Gram Negative Sepsis in Neonates: A Nursery Outbreak Due To Hand Carriage of Citrobacteria Diversus. Pediatrics, *65*:1980.
12. Wallis, S., and Harvey, D.: Disorders in the newborn. Nurs. Times, (Aug. 2), 1972.

SECTION V

THE FUTURE OF HIGH RISK PERINATAL CARE

CHAPTER 21

PREDICTIONS, IMPLICATIONS, AND PLANNING FOR HIGH RISK PERINATAL CARE

*Carole Ann Miller McKenzie, C.N.M., Ph.D.,
and Katherine W. Vestal, R.N., Ph.D.*

OBJECTIVES

Upon completion of this chapter the reader will be able to accomplish the following:

1. Describe the trends in perinatal care for the future
2. List 10 projected components of neonatal regional care in the year 2001
3. Describe the trends in regional perinatal education
4. Describe projected changes in parenting in the future
5. Identify the cost of reproductive risk, both material and human
6. List priorities and interventions for managing the high risk family in the future
7. Discuss the challenges of perinatal care in the future
8. Discuss why planning is so important to the future of perinatal care
9. List the principles and techniques for futuristic planning
10. List the outcomes desired in perinatal care

Future maternal-newborn care will be characterized by sophisticated technology and care delivered by highly specialized professionals and technicians in regional centers. The emphasis on family centered care will continue. With increased sophistication in computer technology, diagnoses will be swift, aided by continuous monitoring. The calculation and reporting of statistical rates of perinatal mortality and morbidity will be continuous and instantaneous, thus facilitating research as well as future treatment.

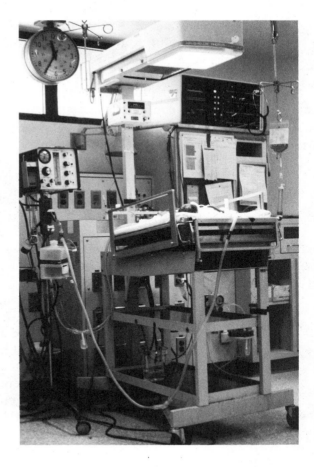

Figure 21-1. Technology in use today will be obsolete by the year 2000. Improved instrumentation will be important, but it cannot replace the humanistic nature of nursing care. (Courtesy of Don Shaeffer, Hermann Hospital, Houston, Texas.)

Problem areas will be rapidly identified and assessed and interventions planned.

The literature indicates that obstetrical care will continue to be more highly technological than ever. One scenario[2] written about childbirth in the year 2000 indicates that even normal births will be engulfed in the "high tech" world that will be a part of our future. The challenge of those involved in the care of perinates will be to provide the high tech care to those who need it, while maintaining a concept of family centered care for all and childbirth options for families with normal pregnancies. The exciting side of high tech is that perinatal mortality and morbidity will decrease, and the sophistication of care will be greater than ever, thus enabling management of perinatal problems to achieve more than ever before.

RISK ASSESSMENT

The potential for risk assessment to begin long before pregnancy will exist and any conditions contributing to the patient's obstetrical risk will be noted throughout the patient's life in computerized medical records. At the time of mate selection, genetic counseling and risk identification could occur. At the time of conception, registration of pregnancy and insertion of continuous cervical monitoring devices could allow a pregnancy with potential risks to be monitored on a 24 hour a day basis.[2]

The fetal assessment tools now in use will be greatly perfected. The possibility of in utero surgical correction of defects, direct fetal blood transfusion, and direct medical management of fetal problems that are being researched at this time, as well as genetic diagnosis, will be part of the perinatal center of the future.[6] Monitoring will no doubt be much more sophisticated, allowing continuous assessment of all maternal and fetal body systems, thus alerting the perinatal team to the need for intervention.

PERINATAL CARE

If disease cures continue to manifest themselves, some of the more common obstetrical problems will likely be curable (e.g., pregnancy induced hypertension and diabetes). Patients with difficulty in conceiving and maintaining pregnancy will be utilizing in vitro fertilization and the artificial uterus. Part of the perinatal center will be devoted to a human "hatchery" facility.

Fetal medicine, reaching incredibly high levels of sophistication, will include not only fetal monitoring, fetal surgery, fetal genetic diagnosis, and fetal transfusion but will also include fetoscopy to allow observation for medical care and for psychological management as well. Fetal drug injection will be part of the medical management.[2]

The highly technological maternal monitor may also allow more active obstetrical intervention than currently exists. Oxytocin induction will be more predictable, as will obstetrical surgical intervention. With cesarean section rates approaching 25 per cent in some areas, and having more than quadrupled (4.8 per cent in 1960)[10] in 30 years, the possibilities are somewhat staggering.

Neonatal care will also be experiencing high tech care, although McCarthy and Butterfield are of the opinion that technology will not change significantly.[7] Since the neonatal area has been somewhat more advanced technologically than the obstetrical area, that does not seem so surprising.

McCarthy and Butterfield further indicate that, based on their projection of trends and population, neonatal regional care in 2001 will be as follows:

1. The trend toward regionalization and consolidation of perinatal services will continue.
2. Maternal utilization patterns will not change.
3. All maternal and newborn referrals will be made to the nearest appropriate perinatal center.
4. All referrals will occur with a uniform frequency distribution.
5. Preventive measures will have no major impact in reducing number of high risk infants.
6. In 2 per cent of all live births neonatal intensive care will be required; 3 per cent of all live births will require neonatal intermediate care.
7. Present technology will not change significantly in the future.
8. Fertility and birth rates will remain the same.
9. Out of state participation in the system will increase.
10. Occupancy rates will remain constant.[7]

On the basis of some of the futuristic literature, the concept of no change in technology and maternal utilization may be challengeable.[2, 12]

However, McCarthy and Butterfield based their predictions on trends in Colorado projected from population figures available there.[7] It appears that the concept of maternal utilization will be more widely accepted, and, it is hoped, maternal transport will be more widely developed. A continuous maternal monitoring device would decrease some of the need, but more overt obstetrical emergencies would still require transport.

With advanced education available in the perinatal area, development of more sophisticated and widely used transport systems appears likely. The educated perinatal team will not only develop the area of transport but also the educational program for all hospitals and health care personnel in each region. With highly developed software, personnel would be able to complete programs on all areas of perinatal interest. With computer television and telephone hookup, instructors could remain at the regional center but be able to render expert assistance to personnel as educational modules were completed and to render on the spot assistance for emergencies at level I and II hospitals.

THE FAMILY

A number of profound changes will occur to affect the family. Familial size will continue to decrease. With this continued decline in birth rate, each child will assume premium importance, thus increasing the need for salvage and positive outcomes in the perinatal area. Family instability will likely continue. With marriage at a later age, however, the possibility of more appropriate choices for mates exists. Societal tolerance of alternative living arrangements, increased life span, lowered cost of divorce, and decreased social, moral, and legal prohibitions will probably contribute to increases in the divorce rate and family instability.[8,9]

Parenting will be changing, also. As the adult population increases to three times that of the child population after the year 2000, parents will be reestablishing their parental authority. The economic constraints will keep both partners in the work force, and extended families will be less readily available because of increased mobility and urbanization. Prospective parents may well have to have their childbearing plans approved by the government and take a computerized parenting test to ensure quality parenting.[8]

IMPLICATIONS

Butanarescu and associates identify the cost of reproductive risk as:

1. Stress associated with increased:
    a. Anxiety concerning the outcome of pregnancy
    b. Distortion and disruption of the nuclear family
    c. Economic cost of health services
2. Reproductive casualty, trauma, and loss
    a. Reproductive trauma
    b. Maternal and neonatal trauma from:
        1) Intrusive procedures
        2) Operative procedures
        3) Infection
        4) Drugs
        5) Procedures and policies
        6) Family reactions

     c.   Damage or death due to disease, disorder or decision
     d.   Failure of maternal-infant attachment
     e.   Family disequilibrium
  3. Material cost
     a.   Personnel
     b.   Service and equipment
     c.   Funding[1]

It is unlikely that these risks will change substantially. While the problems associated with some disorders and procedures may be eliminated, other problems will most assuredly take their place. It also appears unlikely that the cost issue will be completely resolved.

Certainly the issues surrounding family disruption will not disappear. Johnson suggests that the following areas are priorities that should incorporate clinical practice, education, and research for dealing more effectively in the future with the high risk family:

1. Determine the causative factors for the high risk situations
2. Prevent risk situations
3. Prevent family difficulties
4. Identify early signs of family difficulties
5. Develop specific nursing actions
6. Determine effective administration of nursing care
7. Evaluate nursing actions[5]

All of these priorities will continue to have significance for the high risk family in the future. The nurse will continue to have a crucial role in identifying and dealing with the psychosocial problems the high risk family will have.

By providing the family with as much support as possible and by facilitating a more family centered approach, the nurse will continue to be able to diminish the negative outcome. The family difficulties common to high risk families are also identified by Johnson:

1. Multiple crisis
2. Increased separation of family members
3. Inability to express their emotional and physical needs, such as:
     a.   Grief
     b.   Guilt
     c.   Low self-esteem
     d.   Lack of energy due to emotional and physical weariness
4. Family role change related to
     a.   Discipline
     b.   Sibling relationships
5. Finances[5]

Interventions to deal with these problems should be:

1. Determined through assessment
2. Aimed at all family members
3. Individualized to the specific family
4. Encouragement for the family's own problem solving
5. Chosen from a repertoire of possible strategies
6. Part of a team plan
7. Evaluated
8. Refined based on evaluation[5]

The nurse will not only be dealing with family difficulties but will also be responsible for providing humanistic care in a world of high technology; as it is now, it will be very easy to "nurse" the machines rather than the patient. Particularly in an emergency it is easy to forget the patient and deal with the entity that is occurring. While this may be appropriate in a crisis, it is important to provide support, if not during the emergency itself, immediately thereafter. This establishes the importance of the person rather than the crisis or the machines.

The future will occur whether we plan for it or not and will occur with amazing rapidity. The year 2000, with all of its inevitable changes and necessary adaptations, is less than 20 years away. Whether the adaptation to changes is successful and whether nurses have a role in determining what that future will be are contingent upon nursing's willingness to look ahead and plan for what will come.

PLANNING

The planning process is based on the same principles as those underlying the nursing process. Before one plans, one must assess, set priorities, and detail the intervention strategies to accomplish those plans. And finally, one must develop evaluation blueprints to assess whether those plans succeed. There must also be objectives for the direction in which to go, whether it be an individual, a group, a family, a society, or a world. Once those objectives are developed, plans can be made to direct the actions toward the desired outcomes.

If one assumes that the outcomes desired by those involved in perinatal nursing are common goals and can be met, planning can begin. If one believes that these goals should include minimizing perinatal risk, reversing perinatal damage, decreasing perinatal loss, and ensuring positive family adaptations regardless of the outcome, then plans can be made to point care in that direction.

One way to effect planning for positive outcome is to look at what happened in the past. Assessment of what did and did not work and evaluation of trends in past care and how they developed can be useful. Priorities can then be set by utilizing a *crisis intensity chart*. This chart separates problem areas according to a measure of their magnitude and urgency. After these measures have been made, areas can be ranked. This chart allows one to assess the consequences if each crisis is not solved in 1–5 years, 10–20 years, or 20–50 years. One can also estimate crisis intensity and how it will affect the organization times the degree of effect.[13]

Various types of *social forecasting* can be utilized after priorities have been set. Social forecasting "assists an individual or an organization to anticipate social trends by reviewing past trends and forecast where change will occur."[8]

A common method of social forecasting is *trend extrapolation*. One must make an assumption that the future will be like the past and that future changes will occur in the same direction.[3]

Individuals or groups may look from present to future by placing themselves on a continuum utilizing their goals. These are called *linear projections* or *time lines*. Various alternatives can be superimposed on the projections and the impact of each analyzed.[11]

McCarthy and Butterfield projected their plans for perinatal care in the year 2001 in Colorado by projecting population, live birth data, neonatal bed occupancy, and fertility rates of 1976. These were projected by computer for the year 2001, thus allowing them to make suggestions for planning.[7] Many other *computerized techniques,* which are very sophisticated, utilize multivariate analysis.[11]

Probably one of the most widely known futuristic planning tools is the *Delphi Process.* In utilizing the Delphi Process one uses a series of questionnaires. The questionnaires begin with broad questions and lead to more specific ones with each "round." The process stops when consensus is reached or enough information is exchanged by a group of experts in the field. In addition, these experts are anonymously questioned about the likelihood of future developments.[4]

Nominal Group Technique, or NGT, is another practical planning tool for the future or a problem solving tool for any time. A structured group meeting is held. Each individual in the group writes down all of his ideas about a given problem. A sharing of ideas occurs, round robin, and each member is able to clarify his ideas. Ultimately, each member votes on ideas by selecting his top five priorities. The individual votes are mathematically pooled to yield the group decision.[4]

The planning techniques mentioned here are more fully explained in the references for this chapter. Any individual or group desiring more information can consult these.

The various state plans for regionalization of perinatal services are an essential component of planning for future perinatal care. However, more planning is needed and must be an ongoing process. The plans already generated must be implemented and evaluated. The evaluations as well as the successes and failures must lead toward future directions. The future cannot be allowed just to happen. Nurses must influence it in the direction they believe quality perinatal care should go.

The future of perinatal care will be exciting as we, as nurses, assume a greater role in prevention and cure. The challenge, however, will not be in operating the machines but in avoiding any horrors of mechanization, in providing humanistic, family oriented care, and in planning for the brightest future possible for perinates.

REFERENCES

1. Butanarescu, G.F., Tillotson, D.M., and Villarreal, P.P.: Perinatal Nursing: Vol. 2, Reproductive Risk, New York, John Wiley & Sons, 1980.
2. Corea, G.: Childbirth 2000. Omni, *2*:48-50, 1979.
3. Cornish, E.: The Study of the Future. Washington, The World Future Society, 1977.
4. Delbecq, A.L., Van de Ven, A.H., and Gustafson, D.H.: Group Technique for Program Planning: A Guide to Nominal Group and Delphi Processes. Glenview, Ill., Scott, Foresman, and Co., 1975.
5. Johnson, S.H.: High-Risk Parenting. Philadelphia, J.B. Lippincott Co., 1979.
6. Lesse, S.: The preventive psychiatry of the future. The Futurist, 1976, pp. 228-235.
7. McCarthy, J.T., and Butterfield, L.J.: Perinatal care in the year 2001. Perinatal News, 1979, pp. 22-23.
8. McKenzie, C.A.M., and Vestal, K.W.: Outlooks on the future of nurse midwifery. J. Nurse-Midwifery, *25*:13-19, 1980.

9. McKenzie, C.A.M., and Vestal, K.W.: Perinatal crises. In Kinney, M., et al. (eds.): AACN's Clinical Reference for Critical-Care Nurses. New York, McGraw-Hill Book Co., 1981.
10. Pritchard, J.A., and MacDonald, P.C.: Williams' Obstetrics, 16th ed. New York, Appleton-Century-Crofts, 1980.
11. Shane, H.G.: The Educational Significance of the Future, Bloomington, Ind., Phi Delta Kappa, 1973.
12. Stine, G.H.: The Life of Allie. Omni, 2:45–47, 1980.
13. Tugwell, P.: Search for Alternatives: Public Policy and the Study of the Future. New York, Random House, 1974.

MATERNAL PROCEDURES AND DRUGS

Sherry A. Gillespie, R.N., M.S.N.,
Pamela Rodgers, B.S., R.Ph.,
and Meredith J. Cowan, R.N., B.S.N.

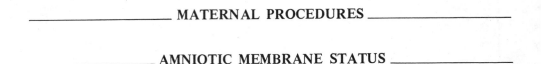

MATERNAL PROCEDURES

AMNIOTIC MEMBRANE STATUS

PURPOSE

Whether the membranes have ruptured is an important factor in obstetrical care. Ruptured membranes predispose both mother and baby to increased risk of intrauterine infection. It is imperative that the status of the membranes be accurately assessed.

EQUIPMENT

Sterile vaginal speculum
Slide
Nitrazine paper
Cotton tip applicators
Sterile gloves

METHOD

ACTION	RATIONALE
Nitrazine Test	
1. Perform sterile speculum examination	Assures more accurate test than placing strip of nitrazine paper into vagina
2. Observe the cervix for escaping amniotic fluid	Rupture is diagnosed when amniotic fluid is seen escaping from os and pooled in the vaginal vault during speculum examination

Adapted from Varney, H.B.: Nurse-Midwifery. Boston, Blackwell Scientific Publications, 1980, pp. 159–162.

ACTION	RATIONALE
3. Place sterile cotton tipped applicator or cotton ball at cervical os	Less chance of an invalid test from touching other structures
4. Touch applicator to nitrazine paper, avoiding all other structures	Avoid contamination of specimen
5. If nitrazine paper turns dark blue, it is strongly suggestive of ruptured membranes; it does not give a definitive diagnosis	Nitrazine paper turns deep blue when moistened by a substance with an alkaline pH—the pH of amniotic fluid is an alkaline 7.0 to 7.5; however, blood, cervical mucus, and other substances are also alkaline and may invalidate the test

Fern Test

1. Perform sterile vaginal examination	To obtain adequate specimen
2. Collect a specimen from the cervix or vaginal pool and place on slide	
3. Allow fluid to dry	To allow development of fern pattern
4. Microscopically examine slide and look for fernlike crystallizations	The sodium chloride in amniotic fluid dries in a fernlike pattern
5. Fern pattern strongly suggests rupture	

DEEP TENDON REFLEXES AND CLONUS

PURPOSE

Hyperactive deep tendon reflexes are indicative of increased central nervous system irritability. All preeclamptic patients should have reflexes checked frequently during labor. Clonus is indicative of disease of the central nervous system.

EQUIPMENT

Reflex hammer

METHOD

ACTION	RATIONALE
1. Reflexes are evaluated on a scale of 0 to 4+ as follows 0 = absent, no response 1+ = decreased; diminished; hypoactive 2+ = normal reflex 3+ = brisk 4+ = very brisk; hyperactive (usually associated with clonus)	
2. General instructions for testing all reflexes:	
a. Compare reflexes on both sides of the body, not just reflexes on one side of body	Different tendons vary considerably in reflex amplitude
b. Limb to be tested should be in a flexed or semi-flexed position	This places slight tension on the muscle that aids in eliciting the reflex
c. Have woman relax as completely as possible	
d. Tap the tendon briskly	Brisk tap produces a sudden additional stretch of the tendon

Knee Jerk Reflex (Quadriceps)

3. Position the patient so that her knees are in a somewhat flexed position	
4. Support her knee by placing one arm beneath it	
5. Feel for the patella and locate the patellar tendon just below	
6. Tap the patellar tendon with the pointed end of the reflex hammer	
7. Observe lower leg extension.	If the patient has had spinal or epidural anesthesia, an accurate response will not be elicited if the knee jerk reflex is tested

Biceps Reflex

8. Feel for the tendon of the biceps brachii muscle in the bend of the elbow	

9. Rest patient's forearm on her trunk

10. Place the thumb of one of your hands on the patient's tendon

11. Tap your thumb briskly with the pointed end of the reflex hammer

12. Observe for movement of biceps muscle and flexion of the lower arm

Clonus (Ankle)

13. Position the woman so her knee is partially flexed

14. Support this position with one hand under her knee

15. Grasp her foot with your other hand and quickly dorsiflex the foot and maintain pressure to keep it in dorsiflexion

16. Observe and feel for beats of clonus (rapid, repetitive, rhythmical contractions)

17. Chart beats of clonus in feet

Adapted from Varney, H.B.: Nurse-Midwifery. Boston, Blackwell Scientific Publications, 1980, pp. 517–521.

DOUBLE SETUP

PURPOSE

This procedure is done to allow manual examination through the internal os for possible visualization of a placenta previa. Since profuse bleeding may occur, everything is at hand to perform immediate cesarean section if complete previa is found.

EQUIPMENT

Instruments and drapes for vaginal delivery
Instruments and drapes for cesarean section

METHOD

ACTION	RATIONALE
1. Prepare patient: explain procedure thoroughly and obtain consent for a cesarean section	To decrease the patient's anxiety Legal consent will be available if needed

ACTION	RATIONALE
2. Obtain type and cross-match, and have blood readily available before procedure begins	
3. Assemble and prepare equipment for vaginal delivery	Sterile vaginal examination will be done; if immediate delivery is required either vaginal delivery or emergency cesarean may be done
4. Set up equipment for cesarean section if needed	
5. Transfer patient to delivery room (or operating room). Bring fetal monitor or Doptone into room	To continuously monitor fetal status
6. Position patient in stirrups, raising both legs at one time	Reduces muscle strain
7. Start IV infusion, if not already started, with a large bore needle. Maintain adequate fluid intake	Large bore needle will insure that blood can be administered rapidly if needed
8. Have scrub nurse readily available	
9. Monitor vital signs and fetal heart rate during procedure	To quickly assess beginning signs of fetal or maternal distress
10. Assist physician during vaginal examination as needed	
11. Depending on findings, treatment will be: a. Rupture of membranes b. Vaginal delivery c. Cesarean section	Method of treatment will depend on presence and degree of placenta previa

ETHANOL (ETHYL ALCOHOL): INTRAVENOUS ADMINISTRATION

PURPOSE

IV administration of ethanol has been used since 1967 to try to arrest premature labor. Ethanol is thought to have a dependent action on the myometrium.*

*Data from Pritchard, J.A., and MacDonald, P.C.: Williams' Obstetrics, 16th ed. New York, Appleton-Century-Crofts, 1980, p. 933.

EQUIPMENT

10 per cent ethanol in D_5W (1000 cc)
Administration set
K-52

METHOD

ACTION	RATIONALE
1. Evaluate patient for the presence of uterine contractions 　a. Attach to external fetal monitor 　b. Palpate uterine fundus for strength of contractions	IV ethanol should be used only if true labor has been established
2. Start IV line with fluid as specified by physician	
3. Administer loading dose of IV ethanol 　a. Infuse 7.5 ml/hour for each kg of body weight 　b. Continue infusion at that rate for 2 hours	To obtain adequate blood levels for suppression of labor
4. Do not give patient anything by mouth	To decrease chances of aspiration
5. When loading dose has infused, decrease rate to 1.5 ml/hour for each kg of body weight	
6. Position patient on her left side in semi-Fowler's position with side rails up	High levels of IV ethanol frequently lead to severe nausea and vomiting; this position may help prevent aspiration of vomitus; the patient becomes heavily sedated and might easily roll out of bed or attempt to get up without assistance
7. Monitor BP, respiration, and state of consciousness every hour	IV ethanol causes mild maternal tachycardia, and extremely high levels are associated with coma
8. Keep oral suction machine at patient's bedside and oxygen readily available	Help prevent aspiration pneumonia
9. Do not leave patient unattended	The patient becomes severely intoxicated during treatment and may unknowingly injure herself because of disorientation

ACTION	RATIONALE
10. Prepare family and patient for usual reactions to therapy: a. Intoxication b. Nausea and vomiting c. Crying jags	Allay patient's and family's anxiety
11. Maintain infusion for 6 hours after contractions stop or maximum of 12 hours	
12. Discontinue ethanol as soon as it is apparent that it has not arrested labor	To permit elimination of as much ethanol as possible from the fetal system before birth
13. Notify pediatrician to be present for delivery	Babies frequently have respiratory distress when mothers have been treated with IV ethanol

EXTERNAL FETAL MONITOR

PURPOSE

The external monitor is used to provide continuous monitoring of fetal heart rate and the frequency and duration of contractions. This is a non-invasive method of monitoring that can be used while the membranes are intact.

EQUIPMENT

Ultrasonic transducer
Tocodynamometer
Abdominal belts
Strip graph paper

METHOD

ACTION	RATIONALE
1. Explain procedure to the patient	Adequate information will help the woman relax and cooperate more fully
2. Ask patient to empty her bladder	A full bladder may cause interference in obtaining a good tracing with the ultrasonic transducer
3. Plug monitor in and turn on power switch	
4. Place two abdominal belts under the patient's back; keep head of bed elevated 45 degrees	Elevating the bed will prevent supine hypotension

ACTION	RATIONALE
5. Plug the ultrasonic transducer into the monitor	
6. Using Leopold's maneuvers, determine fetal position; locate the fetal back and shoulder	FHTs are heard best over the back and shoulder
7. Squeeze ultrasonic transmission gel onto each of the ultrasound crystals and place transducer on patient's abdomen *(do not use ECG paste or alcohol)*	Ultrasonic gel helps the transmission of sound waves
8. Observe the monitor oscilloscope for a uniform wave pattern; move the transducer around until a clear pattern can be seen on oscilloscope	Correct positioning will give the best tracings
9. Secure the transducer with the abdominal belt	
10. Plug the tocodynamometer (toco) into the monitor	
11. Position the toco at the top of the uterine fundus on the woman's abdomen	Fundus is the site where maximum uterine activity can be picked up by the toco
12. Secure the toco with the abdominal belt *(do not make it too snug)*	A belt that is too tight will not allow the toco to register accurate changes in the shape of the fundus
13. Between contractions adjust the pen-set knob on the toco so that the stylet traces between 10 and 25 mm Hg on the strip graph	Baseline tonus cannot be determined with an external monitor; this will prevent the grinding noise the monitor makes if the stylet goes below 0
14. Label the strip graph with: a. Patient's name b. History number c. Date and time d. Gravidity and parity e. Cervical dilatation and status of membranes f. Presence of complications	To insure proper documentation; the strip graph is a permanent part of the mother's medical record
15. Change the position of the toco and ultrasonic transducer as needed during labor to obtain the best tracing	As the baby progresses down the birth canal, the best position for obtaining a good tracing will change

ACTION	RATIONALE
16. To clean the equipment; wipe with a damp soapy cloth	Equipment should be cleaned after every use to prevent the transmission of any potentially infectious agents

PRECAUTIONS

1. Do not make the woman continue to labor on her back just to obtain a good tracing; place her on her side and adjust monitor as needed

2. Do not autoclave the transducer or toco; clean with alcohol

FETAL MONITOR STRIP INTERPRETATION

PURPOSE

Electronic fetal monitoring has become very routine in many labor and delivery units. To obtain the maximum amount of information from the fetal monitor strip, the nurse must systematically appraise the strip.

METHOD

ACTION	RATIONALE
1. Evaluate the uterine activity recording (see Chapter 11) a. Determine frequency of contractions; determine time from beginning of one contraction to beginning of next contraction b. Determine duration of contraction by measuring time from beginning of contraction until end of contraction c. Determine relative strength of contractions i. Palpate uterine fundus during contraction and rate as mild (abdomen indents like a chin); moderate (indents like a nose); and strong (indents like forehead)	To assess adequacy of labor pattern

External monitor does not supply any information about strength of contraction

ACTION	RATIONALE

d. Internal monitor
   i. Baseline tone is the amount of tone in the uterus *between* contractions
  ii. Intensity: Measure the increase in pressure above the baseline tone at the peak of the contraction; record in mm Hg
     mild: 15 to 30 mm Hg
     moderate: 30 to 50 mm Hg/strong: 50 to 70 mm Hg
	All muscles exert some degree of tone

2. Evaluate the fetal heart rate tracing	
a. Determine the baseline heart rate by examining the heart rate between contractions (normal 120 to 160 beats per minute [bpm])	Baseline must be noted so that the presence of acceleration and deceleration can be assessed

b. Assess beat to beat variability which is the normal, irregular, beat to beat changes and fluctuation in the fetal heart rates
   i. Short term variability: beat to beat changes from the fetal heart rate baseline; *may be determined only with scalp electrode*
  ii. Long term variability: rhythmic fluctuations around the fetal heart rate baseline
 iii. Decreased variability, 0 to 5 bpm
     Average variability, 6 to 25 bpm
     Increased variability, over 25 bpm
     Decreased variability is a sign of fetal distress	

ACTION	RATIONALE

c. Identify any periodic changes (transient changes that are associated with antiactions) and classify them

   i. Accelerations: an increase in fetal heart rate associated with fetal movement or contractions
This is a reassuring pattern

   ii. Decelerations: a decrease in fetal heart rate, classified by time in relation to onset of contraction

     (a) Early (due to fetal head compression) — uniform shape; deceleration begins at the onset of the contraction and is finished by the end of the contraction

     (b) Late (due to uteroplacental insufficiency)—uniform shape; deceleration begins after the onset of the contraction and ends after the contraction is finished

     (c) Variable (due to umbilical cord compression) — variable shape (often V or U shaped) and variable onset (may begin at any time)

3. Institute treatment for decelerations and notify physician

ACTION	RATIONALE
4. Record treatments on fetal monitor strip and assess the effect of these measures	Monitor strip is part of the patient's legal record
5. Repeat this sequence every time you reenter patient's room and look at monitor strip	To note any changes from previous observations

FUNDAL HEIGHT MEASUREMENT

PURPOSE

Fundal height is used to estimate gestational age. Between 20 and 36 weeks' gestation, the height of the fundus in centimeters equals the number of weeks' gestation plus or minus 2 cm.

EQUIPMENT

Centimeter tape measure

METHOD

ACTION	RATIONALE
1. Ask the patient to empty her bladder	A full bladder may give a false reading of height
2. Face the patient's head and place your hand on the sides of the uterus	
3. Feel along the sides of the uterus, moving toward the fundus. Hands will meet at the top of the fundus	Improper detection of the top of the fundus will give inaccurate readings
4. Place the zero line of the centimeter tape measure over the symphysis pubis	
5. Stretch the tape measure over the midline of the abdomen to the top of the fundus	
6. Obtain measurement at the lowermost edge of the fundus	

HYDRALAZINE (APRESOLINE) INTRAVENOUS ADMINISTRATION

PURPOSE

Patients with severe preeclampsia (BP more than 160/110) may require additional antihypertensive therapy besides magnesium sulfate. The goal of this therapy is to protect the mother's vital organs from vascular accident without producing hypotension that could compromise the fetus. Hydralazine given IV will decrease BP and may even produce an increase in uterine perfusion.*

EQUIPMENT

Infusion pump
IV solutions

METHOD

ACTION	RATIONALE
1. Prepare 500 ml bag of IV fluid with 40 mg hydralazine	
2. Connect to infusion pump (IMED)	Always give by controlled doses since too rapid administration may cause precipitous drop in BP and lead to fetal distress
3. Begin infusion at rate of 10 ml/hour (hydralazine 0.013 mg/minute) Take BP every 10 to 15 minutes	To assess immediate response to medication
4. Increase dosage by 10 cc every 15 minutes until diastolic pressure is between 90 and 100	Decreasing diastolic pressures below this range decreases placental perfusion
5. Drug should be titrated to keep diastolic pressure between 90 and 100 or as otherwise ordered by physician (i.e., 100 to 110)	
6. Discontinue hydralazine if there is a sudden drop in BP	A sudden drop in maternal BP may cause hypoxia in fetus
7. Maintain accurate intake and output every hour	Assess renal function
8. Observe for the following side effects: a. Headache e. Nausea or vomiting b. Palpitations f. Diarrhea c. Angina g. Sweating d. Tachycardia	To assess intolerance to drug

---

*Data from Kelley, M., and Mongiello, R.: Hypertension in pregnancy: Labor, delivery, and postpartum. Am. J. Nurs., May 1982, pp. 816–817.

PRECAUTIONS

1. Do not give hydralazine to patients with the following conditions:
   a. Hypersensitivity to hydralazine
   b. Rheumatic heart disease
   c. Tachycardia
   d. Lupus erythematosus

2. When mixed with IV solutions containing dextrose, solution may turn yellow, but compatibility has not been altered

3. Do not piggyback this solution with magnesium sulfate or oxytocin (Pitocin) because crystallization may occur; *start a separate IV line*

COMPLICATIONS

1. Rapid fall in BP, which may cause hypoxia in the fetus

_____INTRAUTERINE PRESSURE CATHETER APPLICATION_____

PURPOSE

An intrauterine pressure catheter is inserted when accurate information is needed about the frequency, length, and strength of contractions. It reveals baseline tonus of the uterus between contractions. The information provided assists with IV administration of oxytocin and helps document adequate labor in a patient who fails to progress.

EQUIPMENT

Intrauterine pressure catheter (IUPC)
Syringes filled with sterile water
Sterile drape

METHOD

ACTION	RATIONALE
1. Attach the strain gauge to the holder on the side of the monitor; adjust the holder to the level of the maternal xiphoid	If the strain gauge is not at the correct level inaccurate information will be traced on the strip graph
2. Plug strain gauge into monitor	
3. Position the patient for a vaginal examination; assist with relaxation techniques	Insertion of catheter is often uncomfortable; if patient remains relaxed, discomfort of insertion will be minimized
4. Using sterile technique, hand the physician a sterile drape to be placed between the woman's legs as a sterile field	Decreases the chance of infection

ACTION	RATIONALE
5. Using sterile technique, open the IUPC pack and hold so the physician can obtain the catheter and guide tube	
6. Attach the three way stopcock from the IUPC package to the strain gauge, using the *female* fitting	
7. Using sterile technique, the physician will hand the nurse the end of the catheter with the metal connector	
8. Connect a 20 cc syringe filled with sterile water to the catheter; flush the catheter with sterile water	Flushing the catheter reduces the chance of introducing an air embolus into the uterus
9. Continue to hold the end of the catheter while the physician inserts the catheter; avoid contaminating the tubing below the black dot	This decreases the chance of contamination of the catheter during insertion
10. Assist the patient with relaxation techniques to make the procedure as comfortable as possible	Relaxation makes insertion of the catheter faster and easier
11. After the catheter has been inserted the physician will thread the guide tube out of the vagina toward the metal connector; wipe off blood and amniotic fluid	
12. Remove the syringe and attach catheter to the three way stopcock using the *male* connector	
13. Tape the catheter to the woman's abdomen or thigh	Taping the catheter will reduce the chances of its being pulled out inadvertently
14. Attach the syringe to the remaining fitting on the three way stopcock	
15. Turn the three way stopcock so that the catheter is in the	To remove any air bubbles from the strain gauge

ACTION	RATIONALE
off position; slowly flush the strain gauge	
16. Remove the syringe from the stopcock; uterine activity should fall to 0 on the strip graph	This opens the strain gauge to atmospheric pressure and allows calibration of the monitor
17. If uterine activity does not fall to 0, adjust with zero knob on the side of the monitor (or according to the manufacturer's guidelines)	To assure proper calibration
18. Reattach the syringe and turn stopcock so that the syringe is in the off position; push the test button—uterine activity should register as 50 mm Hg	
19. Turn the stopcock so that strain gauge is in the off position; slowly flush the catheter with 5 to 10 cc sterile water; repeat every 1 to 2 hours	This will flush the tip of the catheter and dislodge any vernix, meconium, or the like; the catheter must be open to obtain accurate data
20. Turn the stopcock to syringe off position; system should begin to record accurate data	
21. Have the patient cough or strain down to test the system; the uterine activity should increase on the strip	An increase in uterine activity demonstrates that the system is registering pressure changes
22. Document on the strip graph that catheter was flushed and calibrated and the time	
23. If the data on the strip graph do not match your subjective interpretation of the contraction pattern: a. Flush and recalibrate b. Check the position of the black dot; it should be visible at vaginal opening; pull out slightly if it is not visible c. If black dot has protruded several inches out of vagina, have catheter replaced	

ACTION	RATIONALE
24. To remove catheter, release tape and gently pull catheter out	
25. Clean strain gauge with a damp, soapy cloth	
26. Replace disposable domes between patients	Decreases chances of infection

PRECAUTIONS

Do not autoclave strain gauge

COMPLICATIONS

1. Risk of uterine infection is increased

2. Uterine perforation may occur

3. Bleeding may occur during insertion

_____ LEOPOLD'S MANEUVERS _____

PURPOSE

The use of Leopold's maneuvers provides a simple approach to palpation of the abdomen. These maneuvers can answer the following questions:
1. Is the lie longitudinal or transverse?
2. What is the presenting part?
3. Where is the fetal back?
4. Where are the small parts and extremities?
5. What is the fundus?
6. On which side is the cephalic prominence?
7. Is baby engaged?
8. How big is the baby?
9. Is there more than one baby?

METHOD: (See Figure A–1)

ACTION	RATIONALE
1. Have patient lie on her back and flex knees slightly	To relax the abdominal wall muscles
2. Stand at patient's side; grasp the lower uterine segment between the thumb and fingers of one hand and feel presenting part	To determine the presenting part

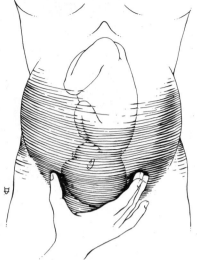

A. First maneuver: What is the Presenting Part?

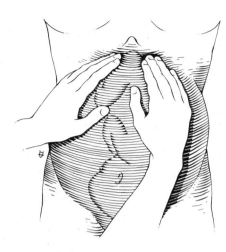

C. Third maneuver: What is the Fundus?

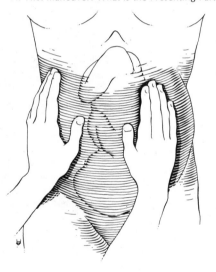

B. Second maneuver: Where is the Back?

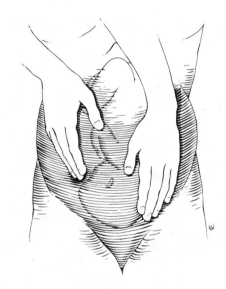

D. Fourth maneuver: Where is the Cephalic Prominence?

Figure A-1. Abdominal palpation. (From Oxorn, H.: Human Labor and Birth, 4th ed. New York: Appleton-Century-Crofts, 1980, pp. 70-71.)

ACTION	RATIONALE
a. Head: harder, smoother, globular, easy to move.	
b. Breech: softer, more irregular, not as mobile	
3. Turn and face the patient; place hands on both sides of the abdomen	To determine on which side the back is lying
4. Use one hand to steady uterus; use the other hand to palpate	

ACTION	RATIONALE
the fetus to determine location of the back and small parts a. Fetal back feels firm and smooth	
5. Move hands up the sides of the uterus and palpate the fundus	To determine what fetal parts are in the fundus
6. Turn and face the patient's feet	To locate cephalic prominence
7. Move the fingers gently down the sides of the uterus toward the pubis	
8. Locate the cephalic prominence on the side where there is greater resistance to the descent of the fingers into the pelvis a. Flexion: Forehead is the cephalic prominence on opposite side from back b. Extension: Occiput is the cephalic prominence on same side as back	
9. Note whether the head is free and floating or fixed and engaged a. Floating: Head lies entirely above the symphysis; examining fingers can be placed between the head and the pubis b. Engaged: Only a small part of the head may be palpable above the symphysis; it cannot be moved laterally c. Dipping: Head is midway between the two locations	To determine engagement

MAGNESIUM SULFATE: INTRAVENOUS ADMINISTRATION

PURPOSE

Magnesium sulfate ($MgSO_4$) is the drug of choice in severe preeclampsia and eclampsia. It is used for its depressant effect on the central nervous system and the peripheral neuromuscular junction. It must be used carefully and in a very controlled fashion since injection leads to depression of the heart and central nervous system, especially the respiratory center. It may also be effective in the treatment of premature labor.

EQUIPMENT

Ampules of magnesium sulfate and calcium gluconate
Soluset
Infusion pump
IV administration set
Needles for piggyback
Oral suction machine

METHOD

ACTION	RATIONALE
Loading Dose	
1. Obtain Soluset and connect to 250 cc bag of D_5 water	
2. Add 4 gm $MgSO_4$ (as ordered by physician) to 75 ml of D_5 water	IV bolus dose is needed to get adequate level of $MgSO_4$ into the blood stream
3. Connect Soluset to IV line and infuse over 20 minute period	Too rapid infusion causes vomiting and severe discomfort
4. Warn patient of hot flush sensation	
Maintenance Dose	
1. Obtain 1000 cc of specified IV solution (D_5–NS or D_5W)	
2. Add 20 to 40 gm of $MgSO_4$ to IV solutions	This keeps fluid intake to a minimum, especially if patient requires oxytocin (Pitocin) induction or augmentation
3. Assemble infusion pump (IMED, IVAC) with $MgSO_4$ solution	Infusion pump is used to deliver accurate, consistent rates
4. Piggyback solution to primary line at connector most proximal to patient	Mainline without medication is needed in the event of hypermagnesemia
5. Set infusion pump to correspond to dosage ordered a. 20 gm = 1000 ml b. 1 gm = 50 ml	

ACTION	RATIONALE
c. 2 gm = 100 ml d. 40 gm = 1000 ml e. 1 gm = 25 ml/hour f. 2 gm = 50 ml/hour	
6. Observe the patient for signs of magnesium intoxication (Early signs) a. Thirst b. Sweating c. Depression of reflexes d. Hypotension e. Flaccidity (Late signs) a. CNS depression b. Respiratory paralysis c. Circulatory collapse	Warning signs of toxicity are easily detected
7. Check deep tendon reflexes hourly	Disappearance of the patellar reflex is one of the most important signs of increasing hypermagnesemia
8. Monitor intake and output carefully; output should be maintained at 30 ml/hour or more; if patient unable to void frequently, insert catheter to straight drainage	Assess renal function and prevent circulatory collapse
9. Monitor vital signs every 30 minutes to 1 hour	Frequent monitoring will document effect or lack of effect of the medication
10. Discontinue MgSO$_4$ if respirations are less than 12 to 14 per minute	To prevent respiratory depression
11. Calcium gluconate should be readily available at the patient's bedside.	Calcium gluconate is the antidote for magnesium toxicity

NON-STRESS TEST

PURPOSE

A non-stress test (NST) is the observance of changes in fetal heart rate associated with spontaneous or evoked fetal movement. Acceleration with fetal movement is indicative of fetal well-being. Mothers experiencing high risk pregnancies are tested periodically (weekly). The NST reflects the influence of the autonomic nervous system on the fetal heart. Fetal activity is correlated with the presence or absence of fetal heart rate accelerations. The presence of accelerations is indicative of fetal well-being.

EQUIPMENT

Fetal monitor
Abdominal belts
Tocodynamometer
Phono/ultrasound transducer

METHOD

ACTION	RATIONALE
1. Explain the procedure to the patient; give patient an estimate of time involved	Decreases anxiety level and allows patient to cooperate more fully
2. Have patient change into hospital gown	
3. Place patient in bed in semi-Fowler's position and in the left lateral position	To prevent supine hypotension
4. Attach patient to external monitor using either a phono-transducer or ultrasound transducer to record fetal heart rate	
5. Ask patient to indicate each time she feels fetal movement by pressing remote event marker or TEST button on monitor	To mark the strip graph at the exact moment of fetal movement
6. Run a 20 minute strip	
7. If there are no fetal movements after 20 minutes, continue tracing for an additional 20 minutes	Fetal sleep cycles may last 20 minutes
8. Interpret test as follows or call physician for interpretation, depending on institutional policy:	
a. Reactive: a minimum of 2 fetal movements over 20 minutes associated with fetal heart rate acceleration of at least 15 bpm lasting at least 15 seconds	
b. Nonreactive: fewer than 2 fetal movements associated with accelerations	

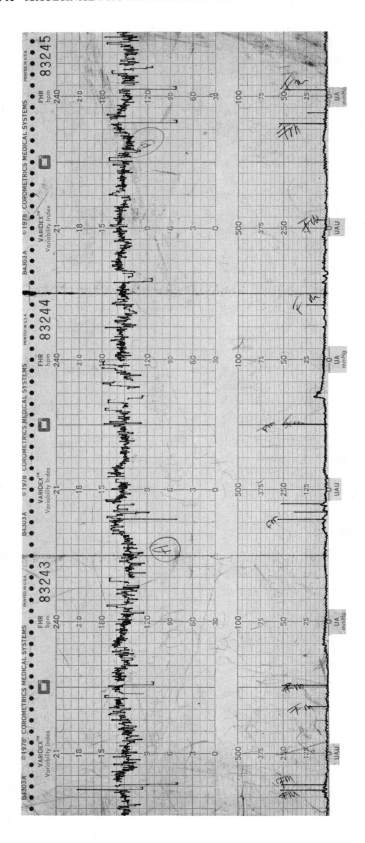

Figure A–2. Non-stress test. *FM*, fetal movement. (Courtesy of Medical University of South Carolina, Charleston, South Carolina.)

_____ OXYTOCIN CHALLENGE TEST _____

PURPOSE

The oxytocin challenge test (OCT) is performed on patients with non-reactive NSTs. The OCT constitutes a measure of determining the respiratory reserve of the uteroplacental unit. It evaluates the capacity of the placenta to transfer O_2 and CO_2. It should be repeated weekly.

EQUIPMENT

> Fetal monitor
> External transducers
> D_5W, 250 cc bag
> Butterfly infusion set
> Oxytocin (Pitocin) solution
> Infusion pump

METHOD

ACTION	RATIONALE
1. Explain procedure to the patient and the time involved (1–3 hours)	A patient who understands what is expected of her is more cooperative
2. Place patient in a semi-Fowler position at a 45 degree angle	To prevent supine hypotension
3. Attach patient to external monitor	
4. Record patient's BP initially and every 15 minutes after test is begun	Baseline for vital signs is necessary to detect deviations from normal
5. Obtain a 10 minute baseline recording of FHR and monitor for spontaneous uterine contractions	A baseline fetal heart rate and uterine activity is needed prior to starting oxytocin administration
6. If there are 3 spontaneous contractions within 10 minutes lasting 40 seconds, call physician to read contraction challenge test	Spontaneous contractions of this frequency and duration are an adequate stress to the placenta
7. If spontaneous contractions are less than 3 in 10 minutes, or no spontaneous contractions are observed, proceed with oxytocin infusion	
8. Prepare oxytocin infusion according to institutional protocol or as specified by physi-	

ACTION	RATIONALE
cian (i.e., 5 units oxytocin in 250 ml D_5W)	
9. Connect oxytocin infusion to an infusion pump (IMED)	By utilizing infusion pump the small dosage of oxytocin will be correctly infused
10. Piggyback oxytocin into primary line at the connector most proximal to the IV site; maintain rate of primary line at 70 to 100 cc/hour	
11. Start oxytocin infusion and increase by 1 milliunit every 15 minutes until 3 contractions in 10 minutes or reach 8 milliunits/minute	
12. When there are 3 contractions in 10 minutes interpret test as follows or call physician for interpretation, depending on institutional policy a. Negative: no late decelerations following contractions b. Positive: late decelerations occurring with 3 contractions c. Unsatisfactory: inadequate uterine contractions or FHR rate pattern d. Equivocal: late decelerations associated with less than 50 per cent of contractions e. Hyperstimulatory: late decelerations associated with hyperstimulatory contractions (90 seconds, every 2 minutes)	
13. If 3 late decelerations occur initiate nursing interventions: a. Repression: discontinue oxytocin administration b. Hydrate c. Correct hypotension if present	Rule out false positive readings and alleviate fetal distress Late decelerations can be caused by supine hypotension, dehydration, hypoglycemia, placental insufficiency

ACTION	RATIONALE
d. Oxygen per rebreathing mask at 8 to 10 liters/minute	
14. Document all treatments on strip graph	Permanent part of mother's medical record
15. Notify physician	Physician must make decision regarding disposition of patient
16. When test has been interpreted, monitor patient until she returns to preoxytocin state or until contractions diminish	Ascertain that labor has not been induced
17. Document results of the test, physician reading test, and disposition at the end of strip graph	
18. Patients with negative OCT should be rescheduled to repeat test in 1 week	Data obtained from OCT are valid for only 1 week

COMPLICATIONS

1. Initiation of labor

OXYTOCIN (PITOCIN) INDUCTION OR AUGMENTATION OF LABOR

PURPOSE

Oxytocin infusion may be utilized for the induction or augmentation of labor. Oxytocin acts directly on uterine muscle to produce clonic contractions. Oxytocin should be administered with caution and under constant medical supervision.

EQUIPMENT

1000 ml bottle of IV fluid as ordered by physician
IV administration set
2 ampules of oxytocin (1 ampule = 10 units)
Infusion pump (IMED, Harvard pump)
IMED cassette

METHOD

ACTION	RATIONALE
1. Obtain 10 minute baseline monitor strip of uterine contractions and fetal heart rate while assembling equipment	To establish baseline fetal heart rate pattern before the stimulation with oxytocin

ACTION	RATIONALE
2. Prepare the oxytocin solution: 20 units in 1000 ml bottle of IV fluids (solution has a concentration of 20 milliunits/ml. Using IMED pump, 3 ml/hour = 1 milliunit/minute)	
3. Take infusion pump to patient's beside	Infusion pump is needed for accurate control of oxytocin administration
4. Assemble infusion pump with oxytocin solution	
5. Set infusion pump to correspond to the oxytocin dosage that was ordered by physician (2 milliunits = 6 cc)	Oxytocin orders should be written by the physician
6. Piggyback oxytocin line (secondary line) into the primary line at the connector most proximal to the patient	IV line without medication is needed in the event that it is necessary to stop infusion of oxytocin immediately
7. Maintain infusion of main line at specified rate (main line 125 cc/hour); total IV fluid rate should not exceed 150 cc/hour	
8. Turn on oxytocin at set rate. Physician must be present on labor and delivery floor while oxytocin is being infused	To treat or respond to adverse reaction to oxytocin
9. Observe contraction pattern and fetal heart rate on the monitor; if no abnormalities are noted, increase oxytocin every 15 to 20 minutes as ordered by physician so that contractions are every 2 to 3 minutes and last approximately 60 seconds—document on nurse's flow sheet	To prevent hyperstimulation of the uterus
10. Once a regular contraction pattern has been established, hold the infusion at that rate and observe	To prevent hyperstimulation of the uterus
11. If at any time there is a question of hyperstimulation (fre-	

ACTION	RATIONALE
quency less than 2 minutes, lasting longer than 90 seconds) or any abnormality in the fetal heart rate pattern, the nurse should immediately: a. Turn off oxytocin infusion b. Turn patient on left side c. Start to administer oxygen by face mask at 6 to 8 liters/minute d. Notify physician	
12. While patient is receiving IV oxytocin, a qualified nursing staff member must remain with her at all times	Constant observation is necessary to detect changes in FHR or uterine activity
13. Continually assess the patient's progress physically and emotionally as well as by monitor tracing	It is important to rely on observation of the patient, not just observation of the monitor
14. Monitor vital signs (TRP) and BP every 15 minutes and record on intrapartum nursing record and monitor strip	To detect deviations from the normal; hypotension may occur because of vasodilating effect of oxytocin
15. Record the frequency, duration, and strength of contractions on intrapartum nursing record	Necessary data to justify how and when oxytocin is increased or decreased
16. Maintain accurate record of intake and output; encourage patient to void frequently	When large amounts are administered, oxytocin has an antidiuretic effect, leading to water intoxication

PRECAUTIONS

1. If there is any doubt about hyperstimulation or fetal distress, stop oxytocin administration and notify physician immediately

COMPLICATIONS

1. Hyperstimulation
2. Fetal distress
3. Rupture of uterus
4. Amniotic fluid embolus
5. Water intoxication

RITODRINE: INTRAVENOUS
ADMINISTRATION IN PREMATURE LABOR

PURPOSE

Premature labor is labor occurring prior to 37 weeks' gestation. Ritodrine is the tocolytic agent recommended by the FDA for treatment of premature labor.

EQUIPMENT

Fetal monitor
Infusion pump
IV solution

METHOD

ACTION	RATIONALE
1. On her admission to labor and delivery, attach patient to external monitor to observe frequency and duration of contractions; draw blood for CBC and SMA-6 (sequential multiple analysis) (glucose, electrolytes, blood urea nitrogen)	To determine if patient is really in premature labor and to obtain baseline laboratory data
2. Place patient on strict bedrest and encourage left lateral position	Provides increased blood flow to uterus
3. Obtain clean catch specimen for urinalysis, culture, and sensitivity test	Urinary tract infections are frequently associated with the onset of premature labor
4. After patient has been attached to external monitor for 15–20 minutes, evaluate contraction pattern	
5. If labor is established, start IV fluids (lactated Ringer's) and infuse 500 ml in 30 minutes.	Adequate hydration will counteract the hypotensive effects of ritodrine
6. Prepare 500 cc bag of D_5W with 3 (50 mg) ampules of ritodrine	
7. Connect ritodrine solution to an infusion pump and piggyback into main line; maintain total IV intake at 100 cc/hour	Overhydration with ritodrine therapy has been associated with pulmonary edema
8. Begin ritodrine infusion by infusion pump at a rate of 100 μg/minute (20 cc/hour)	

ACTION	RATIONALE
9. Once infusion has begun obtain vital signs every 15 minutes until maintenance dose is established	Cardiovascular effects of the drug are the most common side effects; hypotension and tachycardia are common
10. Increase ritodrine by 50 μg (10 cc/hour) every 10 minutes until contractions stop or a maximum is reached of 350 μg/minute (70 cc/hour)	
11. Maintain effective infusion for 1 hour; note time of last contraction on nurse's records	IV infusion is maintained for 12 hours after the last contraction
12. Begin to decrease ritodrine by 50 μg/minute (10 cc/hour) every 30 minutes to achieve lowest effective maintenance dose	Intolerance to high levels of drug is common because of cardiovascular side effects
13. With maintenance dose, monitor BP and pulse every 2 hours; accurate intake and output should be recorded every 4 hours; notify physician of pulse greater than 120 and fall in BP of 15 mm Hg or more	Tachycardia and hypotension may be first signs of body's intolerance of drug
14. Draw blood for hemoglobin and SMA-6 (sequential multiple analysis) determinations 6 hours after starting IV infusion and again when infusion is discontinued	Intravenous infusion of ritodrine is associated with a decrease in hemoglobin and serum potassium; patients may require supplemental IV potassium
15. When contractions have been stopped for 12 hours, start oral administration of ritodrine 10 mg every 2 hours for 24 hours	To maintain adequate blood levels of ritodrine before infusion is discontinued
16. Thirty minutes after first oral dose, discontinue IV administration of ritodrine	
17. Continue to monitor patient for 1 to 2 hours and then transfer her to antepartal unit	To ascertain if oral treatment is going to be effective
18. After 24 hours of oral administration change dosage of ritodrine to 10 mg orally every 4 hours	

PRECAUTIONS

1. If patient begins to complain of palpitations or chest pain *decrease ritodrine and notify physician immediately*

2. Patient may experience the following side effects:
   a. Tachycardia, palpitations, sweating
   b. Headache, nervousness, tremors, restlessness
   c. Nausea, vomiting

3. If patient is given corticosteroids concomitantly with ritodrine watch her closely for signs of pulmonary edema

SPIRAL ELECTRODE APPLICATION

PURPOSE

The spiral electrode is applied directly to the presenting part of the fetus and records a fetal ECG. It gives an accurate tracing of the fetal heart rate. It can be applied only by a skilled examiner after rupture of the membranes and partial dilatation of the cervix.

EQUIPMENT

Spiral electrode (helix)
ECG paste
Leg belt
Leg plate

METHOD

ACTION	RATIONALE
1. Plug monitor in and turn power switch on	
2. Position the woman for a vaginal examination; assist with relaxation techniques	A relaxed patient will make insertion easier for the physician
3. Assist the physician with the vaginal examination, pour povidone-iodine (Betadine) solution as physician introduces fingers into vagina	Efforts should be made to decrease the chances of infection
4. Open the helix package, using sterile technique, and hand to physician	Sterile technique will decrease the chances of infection
5. After application of the helix, attach a leg belt to the woman's thigh closest to the monitor	Allows for increased maternal movement
6. Plug leg plate into monitor	

ACTION	RATIONALE
7. Place small drop of ECG paste on the underside of the leg plate (paste should lightly cover the metal plate)	ECG paste helps provide the best transmission of the electrical signal
8. Secure the leg plate to the anterior aspect of the patient's thigh with the leg belt	Provides the patient with greater freedom of movement
9. Attach the colored wires of the helix to the color coded posts on the leg plate by pushing the posts down and inserting the wire into the slots	
10. Observe the oscilloscope for an ECG tracing	To assure an accurate tracing
11. If fetal heart rate tracing becomes poor, check for dislodgment of the helix by *gently* tugging on the helix; if resistance is felt, helix is still attached	Tracing may become poor if the helix becomes loosened from the presenting part of the fetus
12. Label the strip graph with date and time helix applied	Permanent part of medical records; all treatments should be recorded on strip graph
13. To remove the helix from the fetus, turn the helix counterclockwise	Helix is applied in a clockwise fashion
14. If the helix will not come free, clip helix with a pair of scissors and notify the physician that helix has not been removed	Decreases the chance of trauma to the fetus
15. To clean the leg plate, wipe with a damp, soapy cloth	Equipment should be cleaned after every use to decrease the chances of infection

PRECAUTIONS

1. Clean the electrode site on the baby with a betadine swab at the time of birth

COMPLICATIONS

1. Scalp abscess may develop at the site of attachment
2. Scalp lacerations may occur
3. Risk of maternal infant is slightly increased

_____ STERILE SPECULUM EXAMINATION* _____

PURPOSE

Sterile speculum examinations are done to determine the status of the membranes, to obtain specimens and cultures, and to visualize the cervical os.

EQUIPMENT

Sterile vaginal speculum
Sterile gloves

METHOD

ACTION	RATIONALE
1. Explain procedure to patient	An informed patient is better able to relax during the examination
2. Have patient empty bladder	To make examination more comfortable for the woman
3. Place patient in lithotomy position on the examining table; have her place buttocks slightly beyond the edge of the table	For ease in inserting speculum
4. Drape the woman to provide minimum exposure	To protect patient's modesty and privacy, which will aid in relaxation
5. Put on sterile gloves	
6. Take speculum from package, using sterile technique (if no assistant present, open package before putting on gloves)	
7. Ask the woman to spread her legs	
8. Assist the woman with relaxation techniques	A relaxed patient makes insertion easier
9. Tell the woman that you are going to touch her and gently spread the labia with one hand	To expose vaginal orifice
10. Hold the speculum in the other hand with index finger over the top of the proximal end of the anterior blade and other fingers around the handle	This will assure the blades remaining closed
11. Insert the speculum into the vagina at an oblique angle	Avoids trauma to urethra and periurethral structures

ACTION	RATIONALE
12. Rotate the speculum to a horizontal angle and, while pressing firmly downward, insert the speculum the length of the vaginal canal	Downward pressure avoids trauma to the urethra
13. While maintaining downward pressure, open the speculum by pressing on the thumb piece	
14. Sweep the speculum slowly upward from its posterior position until cervix comes into view	
15. Manipulate the speculum a little further into the vagina until the cervix is well exposed between the blades	Adequate exposure is needed for obtaining specimens
16. Tighten the thumbscrew on the thumb piece	To free hands for handling other equipment
17. Obtain needed specimens	
18. Release the thumbscrew on the thumbpiece; hold blades apart and begin withdrawal until the cervix is released	To avoid pinching or pulling on the cervix during removal of the speculum
19. Release pressure on thumbpiece, allowing blades to close; rotate speculum to oblique angle and remove from vagina	For woman's comfort
20. Deposit speculum in proper container	For sanitary purposes

TERBUTALINE: INTRAVENOUS ADMINISTRATION IN PREMATURE LABOR

PURPOSE

Terbutaline is administered intravenously to suppress uterine contractions in the patient in premature labor whose medical and obstetrical status does not preclude continuation of the pregnancy and in whom betamimetic drugs are not contraindicated. Provision of safe nursing care to the patient receiving terbutaline therapy includes surveillance of electrolytes, fluid balance, cardiovascular status, uterine activity, and fetal well-being.

---

*Data from Varney, H.B.: Nurse-Midwifery. Boston, Blackwell Scientific Publications, 1980. pp. 530–533.

ACTION	RATIONALE

EQUIPMENT

External fetal monitor
IV solutions as ordered
Infusion pump
Tubes for blood collection

METHODS

1. On admission to labor and delivery obtain clean catch urine specimen for urinarlysis, culture, and sensitivity testing	Urinary tract infections are frequently associated with the onset of premature labor
2. Attach patient to external fetal monitor. Obtain blood specimens for CBC, rapid plasma reagin (RPR) test, group types screen, electrolyte profile	To determine frequency and duration of uterine contractions and to establish fetal well-being; to obtain baseline laboratory data
3. Place patient on strict bed rest and encourage left lateral position	Provides maximal blood flow to the uterus and promotes uterine relaxation
4. A pelvic examination is performed to determine cervical dilatation and effacement; fetal presenting part and station must also be identified	Terbutaline therapy is not generally thought to be effective after 3 to 4 cm dilatation; identification of fetal presenting part and station is necessary to decide on mode of delivery should delivery become imminent
5. If labor is diagnosed, start an IV with crystalloid solution ordered; 500 cc to 1 liter is often infused rapidly	Adequate hydration will counteract the hypotensive effects of terbutaline; hydration may also inhibit the oxytocic effect of antidiuretic hormone should a condition of dehydration exist
6. Mix 0.25 terbutaline in 3–5 cc IV solution and inject IV as a bolus over 5 to 10 minutes	Administration of bolus results in effective blood levels of the drug being reached quickly; it is hoped that uterine activity will be inhibited sooner than if the drug were administered gradually
7. Monitor maternal pulse, BP, and fetal heart rate closely while administering the bolus	The most common side effects of terbutaline are cardiovascular; blood pressure is not usually greatly affected, but there may be a widening of pulse pressure with

ACTION	RATIONALE
	increased systolic and decreased diastolic pressures; maternal and fetal tachycardias may be severe
8. Mix 5 mg terbutaline in 500 cc of a dextrose free solution and administer as a constant infusion beginning at 10 μg/minute (60 cc/hour) via a secondary line and infusion pump; total IV intake is usually regulated to 100 to 150 cc/hour	Terbutaline therapy causes an increase in blood glucose as well as depletion of potassium; total intake is carefully monitored because overhydration is associated with maternal pulmonary edema
9. Increase dose rate of terbutaline by 5 mg/minute every 15 to 20 minutes until uterine activity ceases, unacceptable maternal/fetal side effects occur, or a maximum of 60 mg/minute is reached	The dose rate of terbutaline required to successfully inhibit uterine activity varies from patient to patient
10. If higher dose rates of terbutaline are required, the concentration may be doubled to decrease the amount of fluid given	Fluid load and terbutaline may result in pulmonary edema
11. Maintain infusion at effective rate for 1 to 2 hours after uterine activity ceases; then gradually decrease infusion to the slowest effective dose rate and maintain for at least 12 hours*	Cardiovascular effects are more severe at higher dose rates; side effects may be reduced by utilizing the least amount of medication necessary to maintain suppression of labor
12. Check and document vital signs and BP as follows: a. BP, pulse, and respiration every 10 to 15 minutes after first hour or until maintenance dose rate is reached b. Temperature every 4 hours if membranes are intact; every 1 to 2 hours if membranes are ruptured c. FHTs every 30 minutes if	Cardiovascular effects increase the workload of the heart and, if prolonged, may lead to congestive heart failure and pulmonary edema; some institutions advocate continuous maternal cardiac monitoring to identify arrhythmias associated with tachycardia; the presence of infection may disqualify the patient as a candidate for inhibition of labor; the fetus as well as the mother may experi-

*Data from Zuspan, F.P.: Premature labor. *In* Zuspan, F.P., and Quilligan, E.J. (eds.): Practical Manual of Obstetrical Care. St. Louis, C.V. Mosby Co., 1982, pp. 184–191.

ACTION	RATIONALE
clear monitor tracing is not obtainable	ence cardiac failure at prolonged excessive rates; fetal tachycardia may also be an early sign of infection, making differential difficult
d. Notify physician of pulse rate greater than 120, FHT greater than 180, marked maternal hypotension, arrhythmias, or if mother becomes febrile	
13. A record of intake and output should be maintained; notify physician if output is less than 50 cc/hour	Fluid load and terbutaline may result in pulmonary edema and ultimate renal shutdown
14. Fetal monitoring should be continuous with all pertinent data recorded on monitor strips as well as nurse's notes	It is important to document the presence or absence of uterine activity to determine the efficacy of therapy and to establish the presence or absence of fetal well-being
15. Draw blood for electrolyte profile every 4 to 6 hours; if potassium is required, add 20 to 30 mEq KC1, as ordered, to IV of crystalloid solution and mark the IV appropriately	Terbutaline therapy is associated with a decrease in potassium and an increase in glucose; potassium replacement therapy is usually required
16. After uterine activity has ceased, and the decision has been made to stop IV therapy, give 0.25 mg terbutaline subcutaneously and decrease infusion over an hour in four equal parts	Maintaining the suppression of premature labor may depend on maintaining consistent blood levels of terbutaline while infusion is discontinued; terbutaline therapy is usually given subcutaneously every 2 to 4 hours for 24 hours, and oral therapy is started after 24 hours and is given on a variable schedule
17. Continue to monitor the patient for 1 to 2 hours after the first subcutaneous dose, and then transfer her to the antepartum unit	Patient's response to subcutaneous therapy should be established before transfer
18. Provide continuous emotional support and keep patient informed of her status; if patient's condition is stable, allow interaction with family and friends as appropriate	Patient will experience anxiety from drug induced side effects, from fear for physical safety of herself and fetus, and from separation from usual support persons

VAGINAL EXAMINATION DURING LABOR

PURPOSE

A vaginal examination during labor is done to determine cervical effacement, dilatation, fetal presenting part and position, station, and the status of
the membranes.

EQUIPMENT

Sterile gloves
Lubricant

METHOD

ACTION	RATIONALE
1. Have the mother empty her bladder	A full bladder makes the examination more uncomfortable and may interfere with thorough palpation
2. Explain the procedure completely; warn her ahead if something may be particularly uncomfortable	An informed patient can cooperate more fully
3. Drape legs to prevent unnecessary exposure; support person does not have to leave, unless mother so wishes	Aids in relaxation of the mother
4. Wash hands and put on sterile gloves	To prevent introduction of bacteria into the uterus
5. Ask the woman to separate her legs; assist her with relaxation techniques—force should not be used to separate legs	Pelvic examination, particularly in labor, is a very intrusive procedure; the patient should be permitted to proceed at her own speed
6. Lubricate the index and middle fingers of the examining hand: If membranes intact use KY-jelly or sterile benzalkonium (aqueous Zephiran) If membranes ruptured use povidone-iodine (Betadine) solution	To aid with insertion If membranes are intact, the use of povidone-iodine (Betadine) will make it difficult to accurately assess the color of the amniotic fluid and will invalidate the nitrazine test
7. Separate the labia with gloved fingers of the nonexamining hand	To help prevent the examining fingers from touching the labia
8. Gently insert the index and middle fingers of the examining hand into the vagina a. Keep hand turned sideways	To prevent undue pressure on the urethra

ACTION	RATIONALE
9. Move the fingers the full length of the vagina; keep the fourth and fifth fingers bent inward and touching the palm of the hand	To keep these fingers from touching the rectal area
10. Assess the status of the membranes	
a. Palpate for a soft, movable, bulgy sac through the cervix	If the membranes are not ruptured they tend to bulge
b. Watch for fluid running out of the vagina; note color	Amniotic fluid tends to leak from vagina during examination
11. Determine cervical dilatation by outlining the entire perimeter of the cervix and measuring the distance from side to side (1 finger = 1.5 cm)	At complete effacement the cervix is so thin that it may be difficult to obtain an accurate assessment of dilatation without outlining the rim
12. Palpate the thickness of the cervix and determine the degree of cervical effacement (uneffaced cervix is 1 inch thick; cervix 50 per cent effaced is ½ inch thick)	
13. Palpate the presenting part	
a. Cephalic presentation:	
i. Hard skull	
ii. Presence of anterior and posterior fontanelles	
b. Breech: soft, buttocks	
c. Face: irregular knobby parts	
14. Locate the lowest portion of the presenting part; sweep fingers to one side and locate ischial spine; estimate how far above or below spine the presenting part is	
15. Vaginal examination may be begun between contractions but should be continued through a contraction	To determine the fullest extent of effacement, dilatation, and descent with the force of a contraction
16. Gently remove fingers from the vagina and discard the gloves	
17. Explain findings to the woman and her family	Information may provide reassurance and comfort

MATERNAL DRUGS*

Name, Trademark, Source, Preparation	Maternal Dosage and Administration	Uses	Action and Fate	Side Effects and Contraindications	Nursing Implications and Remarks
AMYL NITRITE Amyl Nitrite Aspirols, Amyl Nitrite Vaporoles Synthetic Breakable aromatic ampules	Inhalant: 0.12–0.30 ml	In hypertonicity of uterus	Smooth muscle relaxation Absorbed via mucus membranes Action seen within 10–15 seconds, lasts ≅ 5 minutes Inactivated in liver; significant "first pass effect" Inactive by oral route	Relaxes smooth muscle, including vascular small muscle, and decreases BP Face flushing, headache, throbbing, tachycardia. More rarely causes syncope, nausea and vomiting, restlessness	Appropriate measures for patient protection; rails up, close observation Monitor BP
BETAMETHASONE Celestone Synthetic injection: use "Soluspan" injection Injectable suspension to be used IM in the mother	IM: 12 mg q 24 hr × 2 doses "Soluspan": 6 mg/ml	In patients with premature labor to increase lung maturity in fetus	Action not fully understood; thought to bind with glucocorticoid receptors in alveolar cell to increase production of surfactant Peak effectiveness achieved 48 hr after initial dose Treatment effective for only 7 days	Decreased resistance to infection	Monitor patient closely for signs of infection Should never be given IV since drug is a suspension Drug is not approved by FDA for this use; effects on fetus unknown
BUPIVACAINE Marcaine Synthetic Injection: 0.25%, 0.5%, 0.75% solution (Also available with epinephrine)	Injection: Epidural: 0.25–0.75% solution (10–20 ml) Caudal: 0.25–0.5% solution (15–30 ml) Effect lasts ≅ 4–5 hr (long acting)	Local anesthetic ("amide")	Metabolized in liver and excreted in urine	Allergic symptoms and hypersensitivity Fetal bradycardia Nervousness, dizziness, tremors, headache, nausea and vomiting, drowsiness, hypotension, bradycardia	Observe for allergic reaction Do not use products with preservatives for caudal or epidural blocks Monitor fetal heart rate Supportive care Do not inject intravascularly
BUTORPHANOL Stadol Synthetic Injection: 2 mg/ml	IM or IV: 1–4 mg q 3–4 hr	Non-narcotic analgesic	Stronger than morphine and meperidine Metabolized and excreted in urine Less respiratory depression than with narcotics	Sedation, vertigo, nausea, sweating, lethargy, headache, flushing Because of narcotic antagonist properties, it should not be used in	Monitor cardiac and respiratory status Have supportive facilities available

*Warning: Before administering any drug, check carefully for dosages specific to neonate or mother.

Table continues on following page.

MATERNAL DRUGS* *(Continued)*

Name, Trademark Source, Preparations	Maternal Dosage and Administration	Uses	Action and Fate	Side Effects and Contraindications	Nursing Implications and Remarks
			cotic analgesics	physically dependent patients, since withdrawal symptoms may be precipitated	
CALCIUM GLUCONATE INJECTION Synthetic Injections: 10%	Slow IV: by injection preferably. ≅ 10–15 ml at ≅ 1–3 ml/min; observe for signs of recovery before giving additional amounts (10 ml of 10% solution contains 4.8 mg Ca++ ion)	Magnesium antagonist in hypermagnesemia	Use as antagonist to magnesium intoxication	Rapid IV injection may cause tingling sensations, "calcium taste," or "heat waves"	Close observation with close monitoring of respiratory status and BP IM injections are very painful
CHLOROPROCAINE Nesacaine, Nesacaine-CE Synthetic	Injection: Infiltration and nerve block: 1–2% solution Nesacaine (2–5 ml) Caudal or epidural block: 2–3% solution Nesacaine-CF (no preservative) (15–25 ml) Effects last ≅ 1 hr (short acting)	Local anesthestic ("ester")	Hydrolyzed in the circulation by plasma pseudocholinesterase and excreted in urine	Allergic reactions and hypersensitivity Nervousness, dizziness, tremors, drowsiness, nausea and vomiting, hypotension, bradycardia Fetal bradycardia with paracervical block	Observe for allergy Do not use products with preservatives for caudal or epidural anesthesia Monitor fetal heart rate Supportive care; monitor ventilatory rapidity Do not inject intravascularly
ERGONOVINE MALEATE Ergotrate maleate Semisynthetic Injection: 0.2 mg/ml Oral: 0.2 mg tablets	IM: 0.2 mg q 2–4 hr; usually not necessary to go beyond 24 hr IV: reserved for emergency use; side effects much increased	To hasten involution of postpartum uterus	Decreases uterine bleeding by increasing strength, duration, and frequency of contractions	Nausea and vomiting, dizziness, headache, palpitation, tinnitus, diaphoresis; generally these are not sufficient for discontinuance of therapy Onset of side effects IV: immediate IM: 2–5 min PO: 5–10 min Use with caution in renal disease, liver disease, some vascular diseases	Monitor BP, uterine tone May decrease prolactin levels and interfere with lactation Observe lochia

Drug	Dosage	Action	Side Effects	Nursing Considerations
EPHEDRINE Alkaloid or synthetic Generic preparation Injection: 25 mg/ml 50 mg/ml	IV: 10–25 mg Administer smallest dose to maintain BP at or less than 130/80 mm Hg	Sympathomimetic, relatively long acting; a β-adrenergic agent Very good absorption Excreted essentially unchanged in urine; some liver metabolism Effects seen ≅ 1 hr	hypertension, toxemia, pregnancy, hypersensitivity	Tachyphylaxis may develop Monitor fetal and maternal heart rate Monitor maternal BP
ETHYL ALCOHOL (Ethanol) (5–10% ethanol in D_5W) Grain fermentation	IV drip: usually 10%, calculated according to body weight; begin infusion slowly and increase gradually	Crosses placenta Decreases uterine activity in labor theoretically by inhibiting oxytocin release from pituitary Hepatically metabolized	Giddiness, excitement, headache, nausea and vomiting, sweating, tachycardia, palpitations, tremors, restlessness, weakness, urinary retention Fetal tachycardia	Observations and appropriate measures for patient protection Patient may experience hangover Fetal monitoring
	To prevent premature delivery		Alcohol intoxication if infusion rate exceeds rate of metabolism Vertigo, sedation, flushing, vein irritation Very cautious use in liver impaired patients	
HYDRALAZINE Apresoline Synthetic Injection: 20 mg/ml ampules Oral: 10, 25, 50, 100 mg tablets	IM & IV: 5–20 mg (occasionally up to 40 mg) Use parenterally only when oral route cannot be used or hypotensive effects are urgently needed Oral: 10–100 mg 4 × daily	To reduce activity of uterus; to control premature labor; to raise and/or maintain BP during spinal anesthesia Antihypertensive Exerts its action by peripheral dilating effect on venous capacitance vessels (reduces afterload) Renal flow is often improved Metabolized in liver (extensively removed during first pass)	Hypotension, reflex tachycardia, headache, flushing Cardiac arrhythmias and shock may develop Contraindicated in hypersensitivity	Regular monitoring of BP Observe for orthostatic changes Avoid pressor agents if possible Treat shock with volume expanders
HYDROXYZINE Atarax, Vistaril Oral: 25, 50, 100 mg tablets; 10 mg/5 ml, 25 mg/5 ml syrup Injection: 25, 50 mg/ml	IM: 25–100 mg every 4–6 hr Oral: 25–100 mg 4 × daily	Sedative, antianxiety Antiemetic Enhances action of narcotic agents Rapidly absorbed (metabolic fate unknown)	Hypersensitivity Dry mouth, drowsiness Cautious use in ambulatory patients	Observe for excessive sedation Appropriate measures for patient protection
ISOXSUPRINE Vasodilan Synthetic Injection: 2 mg (5 mg/ml) Oral: 10 and 20 mg tablets	IV infusion: 100 mg/500 cc IV fluid (rarely done because of increased likelihood of side	Uterine relaxant; to control premature labor Metabolized in liver and excreted by kidneys Acts on uterine muscle (relaxation) Very well absorbed β-adrenergic agent	Flushing, hypotension, tachycardia, nausea and vomiting, dizziness, restlessness, nervousness, weakness	Regular monitoring of BP, maternal and fetal Monitor heart rates during and for ≅ 12 hr after control is established If patient is orthostatic,

Table continues on following page.

Page 589

MATERNAL DRUGS* *(Continued)*

Name, Trademark, Source, Preparation	Maternal Dosage and Administration	Uses	Action and Fate	Side Effects and Contraindications	Nursing Implications and Remarks
	effects) Start at 1 ml/min and titrate by response up to 2.5 ml/min (0.2–1 mg/min) then IM: 10 mg q 3 hr × 24 hr then IM: 10 mg q 4–8 hr × 48 hr then Oral: 20–40 mg qid for as long as physician orders			Probably contraindicated in heart disease	caution her about sudden changes in posture
LIDOCAINE Xylocaine, Dilocaine, Ultracaine Synthetic Injection: 0.5%, 1%, 1.5%, 2%, 4%, 5% solution (Also available with dextrose and with epinephrine)	Injection: Spinal: 5% solution Saddleblock: 1.5% solution Epidural and caudal: 1% solution Paracervical: 1% solution	Local anesthetic ("amide")	Metabolized in liver and excreted in urine	Nervousness, dizziness, tremors, drowsiness, nausea and vomiting, bradycardia Allergic reactions and hypersensitivity Fetal bradycardia with paracervical block	Observe for allergy Do not use products with preservatives for caudal or epidural anesthesia Monitor fetal heart rate Supportive care, monitor ventilatory rapidity Do not inject intravascularly
MAGNESIUM SULFATE Injection: 10%, 12.5%, 50% Source: Chemical	IV drip: 10–40 gm/ IV fluid; up to 1–2 gm/hr	To prevent and control seizures in preeclampsia and eclampsia Acts as myometrial relaxant and can counteract uterine tetany that can be caused by use of oxytoxics	Acts immediately and lasts for about 30 min after discontinuance Excreted by kidney	Flushing, thirst, hypotension, loss of reflexes, respiratory depression, hypermagnesemia *Magnesium intoxication* causes drop in BP, respiratory paralysis, and even heart block	Monitor Mg++ blood levels: effective range 2.5–7.5 mg/liter; normal range 1.5–3.0 mg/liter Monitor clinical status, especially additive depressant effects with barbiturates and other sedatives If magnesium intoxica-

Drug	Action/Use	Dosage and Route	Metabolism/Excretion	Side Effects/Contraindications	Nursing Considerations
					artificial respiratory support until IV calcium (usually gluconate salt) can be administered to antagonize Mg++ effects
MEPERIDINE Demerol Synthetic Injection: 25, 50, 75, 100 mg/ml Oral: 50, 100 mg tablets; 50 mg/5 ml oral solution	Narcotic analgesic	IM: 50–100 mg usual dose after regular labor Repeated 1–3 hr intervals May also be given IV	Metabolized by liver and excreted by kidneys Crosses placenta Excreted in breast milk	Hypersensitivity, respiratory depression, constipation, depression of cough reflex, sedation Fetal respiratory depression	Monitor respiratory status Resuscitative facilities should be available
METHYLERGONOVINE MALEATE Methergine Synthetic Injection: 0.2 mg/ml Oral: 0.2 mg tablets	To hasten involution of postpartum uterus	IM: 0.2 mg after delivery of shoulder, after delivery of placenta, or during puerperium. Usually repeated q 2–4 hr for ≅ 24 hr (may be longer if necessary) IV: This route is reserved as a lifesaving measure because it may induce sudden hypertension and stroke. If given IV, give over at least 1–2 min Oral: 0.2 mg during 3rd stage of labor, usually q 4 hr × 24 hr; may go longer prn	Causes rapid, sustained, stronger, longer, and more frequent postpartal uterine contractions, minimizing blood loss and shortening stage 3 of labor	Nausea and vomiting, dizziness, headache, palpitation, tinnitus, diaphoresis; generally not sufficient to discontinue therapy Onset of side effects: IV: immediate IM: 2–5 min Oral: 5–10 min Use with caution in renal disease, liver disease, some vascular diseases Contraindicated in hypertension, toxemia, pregnancy, hypersensitivity	Monitor BP, uterine tone May decrease prolactin levels and interfere with lactation Observe lochia
MORPHINE Alkaloid Injection: 2, 4, 8, 10, 15 mg/ml Oral: 10 mg/5 ml liquid; 10, 15, 30 mg tablets	Narcotic analgesic	IM or IV: 2–15 mg Repeat q 4–6 hr	Metabolized in liver (exquisite first pass effect seen) Excreted in feces and by kidney Crosses placenta	Hypersensitivity Respiratory depression, pupil constriction, muscle relaxation, sedation Fetal respiratory depression	Monitor respiratory status Resuscitative facilities should be available

Table continues on following page.

MATERNAL DRUGS* *(Continued)*

Name, Trademark, Source, Preparation	Maternal Dosage and Administration	Uses	Action and Fate	Side Effects and Contraindications	Nursing Implications and Remarks
OXYTOCIN Pitocin, Syntocinon Synthetic Injection: 10 units/ml	IV drip: 5–40 units/ liter IV fluid IM: usually 10 units Induction: 5–20 units/ liter IV fluid (dosage required to stimulate uterine contractility is usually 1–10 mμ/minute but may occasionally use up to 30 mμ/min, dependent upon institution policy Postpartum: 10–40 units/liter IV fluid (dosage required to control postpartum bleeding is usually 0.5–2.5 units/hour, but may occasionally use up to 5 units/ hour; generally used until lochia is within normal limits)	To induce or stimulate labor To control postpartum bleeding	Oxytocin appears to act on uterine myofibril activity, increasing the effectiveness of contractions; uterine sensitivity increases as gestation progresses, especially immediately prior to parturition Effects disappear rapidly when infusion is stopped Renal and hepatically metabolized	Hypersensitivity Uterine hypertonicity, uterine rupture, spasm Nausea and vomiting, cardiac arrhythmias Pelvic hematoma Afibrinogenemia Water intoxication Fetal bradycardia Neonatal jaundice Contraindicated in significant cephalopelvic disproportion; unfavorable fetal presentations that are not deliverable without conversion; cases in which vaginal delivery contraindicated (e.g., cord presentation or prolapse, placenta previa)	Close observation and accurate flow control essential Infusion pump preferred Frequent monitoring of contraction rate, strength, and fetal heart rate
PHENOBARBITAL Synthetic Injection (various strengths) Oral: tablets, capsules, and liquids (various strengths) Usually used as a sodium salt for increased solubility	Oral or injection: up to 15–60 mg qid (long acting)	To treat preeclampsia and eclampsia Anticonvulsant	Onset of action at about 60 min with peak activity at 10–12 hr Absorbed very well from GI tract Metabolized in liver, may induce enzymes, and excreted by kidney Crosses placental barriers	Respiratory depression, excessive CNS depression bradycardia, syncope, nausea and vomiting, diarrhea, constipation Has been associated with clotting problems in infants	Must have resuscitation facilities for adults and infants Monitor level of consciousness Prophylactic vitamin K is recommended
PROMETHAZINE Phenergan Synthetic	IM, oral, or rectal: 25–50 mg IV: 25 mg May repeat every 4 hr	Enhances action of narcotics Decreases dose of	Crosses placental barrier Sedative and antihis-	Hypersensitivity Headache, dizziness, tinnitus, irritability,	Observe for excessive sedative effects Provide for patient pro-

Drug	Dosage	Use	Action	Side Effects/Contraindications	Nursing Considerations
Phenothiazine derivative Injection: 25, 50 mg/cc ampules Oral: 12.5, 25, 50 mg tablets	(not more than 100 mg/24 hr)	narcotic agents Sedative	taminic agent Absorbed well Metabolized in liver and excreted in urine and feces as inactive metabolites	GI symptoms, nausea and vomiting Cautious use in ambulatory patients	tection May interfere with lactation
PROPIOMAZINE Largon Synthetic (Phenothiazine derivative) Injection: 20 mg/ml	IM or IV: Injection 20–40 mg May repeat at 3 hr intervals	Sedative Enhances action of narcotic agents	Crosses placenta Metabolized in liver Antiemetic	Irritative to vessels hypertension (occasionally hypotension), tachycardia, drowsiness Cautious use in ambulatory patients	Observe patient for excessive sedative effects Provide for patient protection
PROSTAGLANDIN E_2 Dinoprostone, Prestin E_2 Synthetic Vaginal suppository: 20 mg	Insert one (20 mg) suppository high into vagina of supine patient (patient should remain supine for at least 10 min) Additional suppository at 3 to 5 hr intervals until abortion or contractions occur	Abortifacients (in 12th to 20th week); not feticidal To induce or stimulate labor Still experimental	Acts on smooth muscle, causing uterine musculature to contract in a manner similar to that of a term uterus in labor	Nausea and vomiting, pyrexia, diarrhea, headache, rigors, slight hypotension Contraindicated in hypersensitivity	Store in freezer (<20°C); bring to room temperature just prior to use Monitor uterine contractility response Assess tolerance Monitor cardiac status
RITODRINE Yrytopar Synthetic Injection: 50 mg/5 ml Oral: 10 mg tablets	IV drip: 3 ampules (150 mg) per 500 ml IV fluid; (concentration 0.3 mg/ml); start 0.05–0.1 mg/min every 10 min until adequate response attained; usual effective range (0.15–0.35 mg/min) generally continued at least 12 hr Oral: Initiate 10 mg q 2 hr; start 30 min prior to discontinuance of infusion and continue × 24 hr; then decrease 10 to 20 mg every 4 to 6 hr; not more than 120	To prevent premature labor and prolong gestation	Crosses placenta (drug and metabolites) Stimulates sympathetic B_2 receptors, inhibiting contractility of uterine smooth muscle Metabolized in liver; 70–90% of drug and metabolites excreted ir. urine in 10–12 hr	Pulmonary edema (steroids increase this risk), tachycardia, increased BP, sweating, nausea and vomiting, tremor, flushing Occult heart disease may be manifested during ritodrine use Use with caution in preeclampsia, hypertension, or diabetes unless benefits outweigh risks	Closely monitor maternal and fetal heart rates, maternal BP Observe for signs of pulmonary edema; patient should remain supine to avoid hypotension side effects and maternal heart rate should not be allowed to exceed 135/min void concomitant use of β-blocking agents Anesthetics may potentiate hypertensive effects

Table continues on following page.

MATERNAL DRUGS* *(Concluded)*

Name, Trademark, Source, Preparations	Maternal Dosage and Administration	Uses	Action and Fate	Side Effects and Contraindications	Nursing Implications and Remarks
	mg/day orally Continue as long as physician considers it necessary to prolong pregnancy				
TERBUTALINE Brethine, Bricanyl Synthetic Injection: 0.1 mg/ml Oral: 2.5, 5 mg tablets	IV infusion: 5 mg/500 ml; initiate at 10 μg/min and titrate to a maximum of 80 μg/min (1–8 ml/min). Maintain for at least 8–12 hr at minimum effective dose then Subcutaneously: 2.5 mg q 4 hr × 24 hr Oral: 2.5 mg q 4–6 hr prn	To arrest premature labor	β-Adrenergic agent Partial GI absorption Partially metabolized in liver Excreted unchanged by kidneys and fecally	Cardiovascular side effects are more severe than with ritodrine, increasing glucose and depletion of potassium Use with caution in patients with hypertension, cardiovascular disease, diabetes, hyperthyroidism	Monitor BP and maternal and fetal heart rates Monitor electrolyte profiles, hourly intake and output Monitor uterine activity Monitor cardiovascular and respiratory status

_____ REFERENCES _____

1. Facts and Comparisons: Drug Information. 111 West Port Plaza, Suite 423, St. Louis, MO 63141
2. The Extra Pharmacopoeia (Martindale). The Pharmaceutical Press. 1 Lambeth High Street, SE1, London, England
3. American Hospital Formulary Services. American Society of Hospital Pharmacists, 4630 Montgomery Ave., Bethesda, MD 20814

NEONATAL PROCEDURES AND DRUGS

Sheila Southwell, R.N., M.S.N.,
Anita Root, R.N., Ph.D.,
Jane Pohodich, R.N., M.S.,
Alice Illian, R.N., B.S.N.,
and Kathy Hausman, R.N., M.S.N.

NEONATAL PROCEDURES

APGAR SCORING*

PURPOSE

The condition of the neonate must be rapidly and accurately assessed immediately after birth to determine what interventions are needed. The Apgar scoring system, which assesses five characteristics, is the framework for this.

EQUIPMENT

Stethoscope with neonatal-size bell (optional)
Bulb syringe or suction catheter

METHOD

ACTION	RATIONALE
1. To assess heart rate, auscultate or palpate heart through chest wall, or palpate pulsations at the base of the umbilical cord for 15 seconds; multiply by 4.	Entire assessment (five items) must be done at 1 minute; if heart rate is slow or absent, infant obviously needs resuscitation without waiting to count a full minute

*Data from Clark, A.L., and Affonso, D.D.: Childbearing: A Nursing Perspective, 2nd ed. Philadelphia, F.A. Davis Co., 1979.

ACTION	RATIONALE
2. To evaluate respiratory effort, observe quality and loudness of cry and depth of respirations.	Weak or shallow respirations usually can be detected visually and can be heard without a stethoscope, but one may be used for more accurate assessment
3. To assess muscle tone, attempt to extend extremities and evaluate resistance to movement. Evaluate whether extremities return to flexion or remain partially or fully extended	Determination of resistance as well as observation of flexion gives more accurate evaluation of tone
4. To evaluate reflex irritability, gently suction nares or pharynx with bulb or catheter and observe infant's defensive movements	Assess response to noxious stimulus; not a test of specific "reflexes"
5. To evaluate color, simply observe the skin of the infant's head, trunk, and extremities in a good light and with adequate warmth	Cold may produce vasoconstrictive cyanosis, which does not reflect directly upon the infant's immediate cardiorespiratory status; therefore the infant should be dried and warmed as soon as possible

PRECAUTIONS

If one or two items on the scale score zero, particularly heart rate, respiratory effort, or both, abandon further scoring and institute immediate resuscitative measures.

ARTERIAL BLOOD GAS SAMPLING FROM A CENTRAL LINE

PURPOSE

The purpose of arterial blood gas sampling from a central line is to obtain baseline or continuing data to assess the respiratory and metabolic condition of the infant.

EQUIPMENT

3 cc syringe
Heparinized TB syringe or a commercially prepared preheparinized
  syringe
3 cc syringe filled with heparinized flush solution
Cup or bag of ice
Syringe cap or stopper

METHOD

ACTION	RATIONALE
1. Approach the central line at the three way stopcock located between the central catheter and the arterial tubing	
2. Turn the stopcock level clockwise halfway between the flush syringe and the female end of the stopcock connected to the arterial tubing	
3. Place the empty 3 cc syringe into the port (sampling port), which is at right angles to the catheter and the arterial tubing	
4. Turn the stopcock level off to the fluid (arterial tubing) line. Level will be "pointing" to the fluid line	
5. Draw back 2 to 3 cc of blood into the attached empty 3 cc syringe and leave connected to the stopcock. Return the stopcock level to the midway position, then remove the blood filled syringe and cap it off with a sterile needle	
6. Place the heparinized syringe onto the sampling port. Return the stopcock lever to the off to fluid line position. Draw back 0.3 to 0.5 cc blood from the catheter and leave connected to the stopcock	The amount of blood required varies from laboratory to laboratory; remember that an infant's total blood volume is limited, and keep a record of the total amount of "blood out" from various laboratory tests
7. Return the stopcock lever to the midway position, remove the sample, cap the sample, place the sample in ice, and replace the 3 cc syringe filled with blood onto the stopcock	
8. Return the stopcock lever to the off to fluid line position,	Removing air removes the chance of air emboli; flushing slowly

ACTION	RATIONALE
draw back again into the blood filled syringe to remove air bubble, and then push the blood slowly back into the catheter	allows for assessment of vasospasm to the lower extremities and buttocks
9. Return the stopcock lever to midway, remove the empty syringe, and replace the syringe with a new flush filled syringe	
10. Return the stopcock lever to the off to fluid line position, draw back on the flush syringe just enough to clear any air bubbles. Flush the catheter slowly until clear	Avoid using any more flush than is the minimum required to clear the line of blood; frequent laboratory sampling, and therefore frequent flushing, can lead to inadvertent fluid overload; the amount of flush must be recorded and added into the total daily intake figures
11. Rotate the stopcock lever until it once again points toward the flush syringe	
12. Grasp the blood sample, hold vertically, and gently roll it between your hands until all air bubbles have reached the tip of the syringe. You may need to gently tap the syringe. Push the air out of the syringe, cap the syringe, replace it into the ice and send it to the laboratory. Mark the laboratory slip with the time, date, site of acquisition (umbilical artery catheter line), ventilator settings, and the percentage of oxygen the infant is receiving	Bubbles entering the sample and staying there may give falsely higher PO_2 readings than those of the infant, so do not pull the plunger back to try to remove air as room air gas will mix with the sample; this also gives falsely high results

RELATED CARE

1. Be sure the central line is free from air bubbles and that all connections are secure
2. Assess extremities for signs of vasospasm such as cyanosis to toe tips, feet, legs, or any spot area of tissue; if any duskiness is noted, wrap the opposite extremity with a warm cloth until the affected extremity is pink; if it does not "pink up," notify the physician at once and have the line evaluated for removal

3. Observe and check central line connections constantly; tape all connections to central lines

4. Observe for and clear all air from the lines

COMPLICATIONS

1. Exsanguination from disconnected lines
2. Tissue damage or death from vasospasm, air embolus, or dislodged blood clots

CHEST INTUBATION AND MANAGEMENT

PURPOSE

An intrapleural drainage tube is inserted to safely remove air and fluid from the thoracic cavity and to maintain negative pressure in the intrapleural space to facilitate reexpansion of the lung after surgery or trauma.

EQUIPMENT

Chest intubation tray
Suction apparatus, when applicable
Adhesive tape
Water seal bottle, when applicable
Pleur-Evac, when applicable

METHOD FOR PREPARATION OF WATER SEAL BOTTLE

ACTION	RATIONALE
1. Wash hands	
2. Open package containing sterile water seal drainage bottle and tubing	
3. Remove cap from bottle, maintaining sterility of inside of cap; maintain sterility of long tube that extends down into bottle and lip of bottle	
4. Pour sterile water into water seal drainage bottle to 300 cc level as indicated on bottle; end of the long tube must be submerged at least 1 to 2 cm to maintain water seal; when tube is submerged too deeply below water level, higher intrapleural pressure is required to expel air and fluid	

ACTION	RATIONALE
5. Replace cap or stopper in bottle *tightly*	The system must be airtight; inspect every outlet for leaks
6. Tape cap or stopper to bottle	
7. Tape the part of tubing entering drainage bottle to tongue blade	

METHOD FOR PREPARATION OF PLEUR-EVAC

ACTION	RATIONALE
1. Wash hands	
2. Open package containing Pleur-Evac	
3. Pour approximately 100 cc of sterile water into sterile container from irrigation tray	
4. Withdraw a total of 50 cc into Toomey syringe from irrigation tray	
5. Inject this water into water seal chamber of Pleur-Evac via short tubing extending from unit	
6. Repeat steps 3 and 4 using 45 cc of sterile water so that a *total* of 95 cc has been placed in the water seal chamber; this should bring water level in water seal chamber to 2 cm	
7. Pour sterile water into opening of suction control chamber until desired level is reached, as specified by physician; for example, if physician orders 10 cm of negative pressure then suction control chamber is filled to 10 cm level	
8. Place muffler into opening of suction control chamber	

METHOD OF INTUBATION

ACTION	RATIONALE
1. Wash hands	
2. Position infant as specified by physician	
3. Open sterile chest intubation tray, using aseptic technique	
4. Assist physician as indicated	
5. Remove protective cap from end of long tubing extending from water seal bottle or Pleur-Evac	
6. Attach long tubing from water seal bottle or Pleur-Evac to sterile five in one connector on chest catheter	
7. Tape all connections between chest catheters and chest bottles with adhesive tape	The system must be airtight; inspect any outlet for leaks
8. Observe for oscillation of fluid level in long glass tube in water seal bottle	This indicates proper functioning of the drainage system
9. Observe for *constant* bubbling in water seal bottle that would indicate an air leak in the system	Bubbling may normally occur on expiration
10. Stabilize drainage bottle or Pleur-Evac by placing it in wire holder on floor or by hanging Pleur-Evac on side of bed	A precaution to prevent pressure on airtight seal
11. Connect short tube on water seal bottle or Pleur-Evac to suction apparatus when ordered (when suction apparatus is not used, this tube must be uncovered)	
12. Tape two chest tube clamps for each chest catheter to head of bed	Chest tube clamps should be available in case of accidental break in the system
13. Place strip of adhesive tape vertically on outside of water	

ACTION	RATIONALE

seal bottle to allow for marking levels of accumulating drainage

14. Mark water level, time, and date

15. Wash hands

16. Document on medical record

EXCHANGE TRANSFUSION*

PURPOSE

The infant's blood sometimes contains substances that are toxic or harmful. In these cases, blood is removed and replaced with donor blood. The main indications for exchange transfusion are:

1. Hyperviscosity syndrome: to prevent its complications by lowering the hematocrit to 50–55 per cent by replacing part of the blood with 5 per cent albuminated saline
2. Hyperbilirubinemia: to prevent the complications of kernicterus by replacing the blood and its unconjugated bilirubin with donor blood
3. Disseminated intravascular coagulation (DIC): to restore the clotting mechanisms to normal by replacing blood containing toxins and coagulation degradation products with fresh donor blood containing clotting factors

EQUIPMENT FOR PARTIAL EXCHANGE FOR HYPERVISCOSITY

Heat source, restraints
Cardiorespiratory monitor with blood pressure readout
Syringes
IV flush solution
Setup for umbilical artery catheter placement
5 per cent albuminated saline

EQUIPMENT FOR TOTAL EXCHANGE FOR HYPERBILIRUBINEMIA OR DIC

Items 1 to 5 listed under Partial Exchange

Heating coil
Water basin and thermometer
Four way stopcocks
Blood filter
Extension tubing

Discard bag or bottle
Appropriate blood product
Calcium gluconate 10 per cent
Protamine sulfate
Dextrostix

*Data from the following sources:
1. Cloherty, J.P., and Stark, A.R.: Manual of Neonatal Care. Boston, Little, Brown & Co., 1980.
2. Perez, R.H.: Protocols for Perinatal Nursing Practice. St. Louis, C.V. Mosby Co., 1981.
3. University of California at San Francisco: Intensive Care Nursery: Nursing Procedure Manual, 1979–80.

METHOD

ACTION	RATIONALE
1. Restrain infant	Prevents accidental dislodging of catheters
2. Aspirate stomach contents	Prevents regurgitation and aspiration from abdominal manipulation
3. Provide heat source	Hypothermia results in decreased peripheral perfusion and bilirubin-albumin binding
4. Provide continuous cardiorespiratory and BP monitoring	Early recognition of complications
5. Check that medium is appropriate for purpose, properly typed, and cross-matched a. Partial exchange: 20 cc 25 per cent salt poor albumin + 80 cc normal saline	
b. Total exchange: Fresh (<24 hours old) heparinized whole blood, low titer typed, and cross-matched with mother and infant	Preferred medium for total exchange Advantages: no change in glucose, electrolytes, calcium, acid or base Disadvantages: increase in fatty acids (may interfere with bilirubin binding); risk of hemorrhage; must be used within 24 hours
c. Total exchange: Fresh (<24 hours old) ACD or CPD whole blood: low titer typed, and cross-matched with infant and mother	Second choice Advantages: can be returned to storage if not used Disadvantages: binds calcium (citrate preservative); hypoglycemia from hyperinsulinemia (dextrose preservative); acidemia (acid preservative: use blood 24 hours old to decrease acid)
6. Run blood through filter, heating coil immersed in bath of warm (96–97°F, 36–36.5°C) water, four way stopcocks (attach to catheter stopcocks);	Prevention of hypothermia (protect connections from contamination by water); prevention of contamination or air embolus by making a closed system; this system

ACTION	RATIONALE
attach extension tubing to four way stopcock on discard bag	should be set up using aseptic technique as much as possible. Gloves should be worn during procedure for protection of infant and personnel
7. Place catheter(s) if not already in place	Partial exchange usually done through umbilical artery (UA) or umbilical vein (UV) catheter (placement verified by x-ray); total exchange usually done by "push pull" technique; continuous exchange out through UA, in through UV (faster, less stress on cardiovascular system by keeping blood volume stable, decreasing clotting and emboli by keeping flow continuous); total exchange can be done through UA or UV alone if necessary
8. Record all blood removed and replaced, with running total	Usually done in 10 to 20 cc aliquots
	Partial exchange formula: volume of exchange = $$\frac{Kg \times 85\ cc/kg \times (\text{infant crit} - \text{desired crit})}{\text{infant crit}}$$
	Total exchange usually done for 2 × infant's blood volume
9. Gently shake whole blood at frequent intervals	Prevention of settling of RBC and serum
10. ACD or CPD blood: stop after every 100 cc and give calcium gluconate 100 mg by slow IV injection	Prevention of arrhythmias from binding of calcium by citrate
11. Heparinized blood: at end of exchange give protamine sulfate 1 mg IV for every 1 mg of heparin left in infant (87 per cent of blood volume is donor blood; after two volume exchange, donor blood contains heparin 25 mg/500 cc blood) or 1 mg/100 cc exchanged	Prevention of hemorrhage

PRECAUTIONS

1. Two volume exchange should take at least 1 hour to allow for cardio-vascular adaptation
2. Check Dextrostix reading before exchange, immediately after, and every 30 minutes after exchange until stable at 45–130: Hypoglycemia may result from hyperinsulinemia due to dextrose in ACD or CPD blood
3. Check arterial blood gas before, midway in, and after total exchange: hypoxemia and acidemia due to ACD blood, hypothermia, cardiovascular stress

RELATED CARE

1. Continuous cardiovascular monitoring; check vital signs with BP at least before, midway, and after exchange
2. Send first and last aliquot of infant blood for tests
    a. Hyperviscosity: hematocrit, electrolytes, calcium
    b. Hyperbilirubinemia: 1+ bilirubin, albumin, or total protein, arterial blood gas
    c. DIC: 1+ arterial blood gas; PT, PTT, fibrinogen from peripheral vein if possible (heparin in UA and UV lines and heparinized blood will distort tests)
3. Dextrostix reading before, midway during, and after exchange

COMPLICATIONS

Complications include congestive heart failure, cardiac arrest (usually due to hypocalcemia or hyperkalemia), acidosis, sepsis, hemorrhage, embolism (air or clot), transfusion reaction, hypothermia, hypoglycemia

HYPERALIMENTATION:*
Central Venous Line Catheter Care

Many neonates by virtue of gestational age or clinical condition are incapable of achieving adequate nutritional intake orally.

Most likely to benefit from total parenteral nutrition (TPN) are:

1. Infants requiring major surgery such as
    a. Necrotizing enterocolitis
    b. Gastric perforation and resection
    c. Omphalocele or gastroschisis
    d. Tracheoesophageal fistula

---

*Data from the following:

1. Babson, S.G., Pernoll, M.L., and Benda, G.I.: Diagnosis and Management of the Fetus and Neonate at Risk. St. Louis, C.V. Mosby Co., 1980.

2. Brans, Y.W.: Parenteral nutrition in the very low birthweight neonate: a critical view. Clin. Perinatol., 4:367–76, 1977.

3. Filler, R.M., and Eraklis, A.J.: Care of the critically ill child: Intravenous alimentation. Pediatrics, 46:465, 1975.

4. Hall, D.M., and Fhuysen, G.: Percutaneous catheterization of the internal jugular vein in infants and children. J. Pediatr. Surg., 12:719–722, 1977.

5. Kerner, J.A., and Sunshine, P.: Parenteral alimentation. Semin. Perinatol., 3:417–434, 1979.

2. Infants experiencing severe chronic respiratory distress
3. Infants experiencing recurrent complications with oral feeding
    a. Apneic episodes
    b. Abdominal distention
    c. Intractable diarrhea
    d. Chronic vomiting or feeding residuals
4. Very immature infants, that is, those of less than 28 weeks' gestation or weighing less than 900 gm; this category is still controversial, and indiscriminate use of TPN in low birth weight infants is discouraged

TPN can be achieved by two major routes; peripheral and central.

Peripheral sites are preferred when TPN is anticipated to be short term (less than 2 weeks). However, this route has been used many times for as long as 3 months and infants up to 3 kg in weight. Major consideration is related to the actual concentration of the solution for infusion, as a maximum concentration of 12 per cent glucose can be tolerated by a peripheral vein.

A *central vein* can be used to provide higher glucose concentration (up to 25 per cent) and therefore higher caloric intake without increased fluid load than can be tolerated by a peripheral vein. A central vein may also become the site of choice when available peripheral sites have been exhausted.

There are some general considerations and suggested policies regarding central venous catheters.

1. Placement of a central venous catheter in a very small premature infant may be very difficult as the size required may be too large for the vessel
2. Central venous catheters allow direct access to the *right side of the heart;* therefore, special precautions must always be taken to prevent an air embolus when line continuity is disrupted—*do not use three way stopcocks.*
3. All air must be purged from tubing before it is connected to the central venous catheter
4. The amount of flush solution (D_5 in 0.2 N saline with heparin 1 unit/cc) used during dressing and tubing change should be kept to a minimum, since many TPN formulas also contain heparin
5. Dressing changes are best done when IV solution and tubing are changed to reduce risk of contamination with repeated catheter manipulations
6. Tubing and amino acid–glucose solution must be changed at least once every 24 hours; no new TPN solution should ever be attached to old tubing
7. Lipid solutions should not hang longer than 12 hours
8. Dressings should be changed at least every 48 to 72 hours
9. Infusion pumps must be used to regulate flow
10. No housecleaning activities are permitted in the area during dressing change

Components of TPN include protein, carbohydrates, water, electrolytes, trace elements, and fat.

Solutions should be *prepared daily* in the pharmacy department by a trained team. Accuracy of solution content and scrupulous aseptic technique in preparation are essential.

Administration of amino acid–glucose solution should include the following policies

1. Central lines are to be considered inviolate and *are not* to be used to admin-

ister or draw blood, administer medications, or measure central venous pressure

2. In-line filters 0.22 μ size) should be used to filter amono acid–glucose solution

3. *Do not* use filters on lipid administration

4. Simultaneous administration of amino acid–glucose solution and lipids should be done in a manner that allows the lipids to be piggybacked into the main solution line *below* the filter; to avoid a "back-up" of lipids into the TPN solution the lipid line should always be kept *superior* to the amino acid–glucose line

PURPOSE

To provide the fluid and nutritional requirements via a central venous line to the neonate who cannot be supported by alternate oral or peripheral routes

EQUIPMENT

CVP dressing change tray
1 roll each
   3 inch Elastoplast tape
   3 inch and 1 inch Micropore tape
   2 inch cloth adhesive tape
Benzoin
Skin preparation spray or swabs
1 pair sterile gloves
4 packs sterile 4 × 4 pads if dressing tray not available
Antiseptic ointment
3 cc syringe with flushing solution
Extension tubing with one way valve
Amino acid–glucose solution
IV tubing with in line buret
0.22 μ filter
Povidone-iodine swabs or preparation pads
Alcohol preparation pads
½ inch Dermiclear tape
Infusion pump

METHOD

ACTION	RATIONALE
Tubing and Solution Change	
1. Verify solution accuracy with physician's orders: date, time, and signatures should appear on solution containers *and* in medication record	Administration of incorrect solution can be disastrous to infant's metabolic status
2. Prepare bag, tubing, and buret in approved manner	
3. Attach filter	

ACTION	RATIONALE
4. Connect extension tubing with one way valve to filter	
5. Purge entire line of air (check that Y sites are also free of air)	Air can produce embolus if allowed to enter right atrium
6. Remove current IV solution from pump and regulate flow with roller clamp	
7. Prepare catheter hub and tubing connection site with povidone-iodine and allow to dry for minimum of *1 minute*	Requires at least 1 minute of contact to be effective as a bactericidal agent
8. Clamp off catheter and old tubing (when using silicone catheters *always* clamp catheter while there is still an active flow through catheter; otherwise blood back-up can occur)	To prevent air embolus during tubing disconnection and change
9. Disconnect old tubing from catheter hub	
10. Attach new tubing; catheter *must* remain clamped off during tubing change	
11. Unclamp catheter	
12. Start infusion pump at desired infusion rate	
13. Tape all connections using figure of 8 or spiral taping	Prevents accidental disconnection in the line

Dressing Change
1. Prepare all tubing as described in steps 1 to 5 in Tubing and Solution Change

2. Position and restrain infant in bed
Help may be required to immobilize infant's head if the jugular vein has been used for the central line
— Restraints are necessary to prevent infant from moving during procedure

3. Wash hands

4. Carefully lift dressing from bottom, exposing catheter site
— Rapid removal may result in dislodgment or contamination of catheter

ACTION	RATIONALE
5. Note presence of edema, discoloration, drainage, odor, or other unusual findings	Signs of complications
6. Dispose of soiled dressing	
7. Wash hands	
8. Change IV tubing as described in steps 6 to 13 in Tubing and Solution Change	
9. Cleanse catheter site	
a. If kit is available	
i. Open kit, using aseptic technique	
ii. Open extra pair of sterile gloves	
b. If kit is not available	
i. Open all packages, using aseptic technique	
ii. Pour benzoin solution on one 4 × 4 pad, povidone-iodine solution on two 4 × 4 pads, and alcohol on one 4 × 4 pad	
c. Put on sterile gloves	
d. Clean around catheter site and surrounding skin area with defatting agent (acetone, alcohol swabs, or 91 per cent isopropyl alcohol on 4 × 4 pad)	Removes loose skin particles and old tape residue; acetone breaks down cell wall of some bacteria
e. Using iodine based solution on 4 × 4 pad or swabs, carefully cleanse area for *2 full minutes;* begin at catheter insertion site and work in circular fashion from center to periphery; alcohol or Mercresin can be substituted in iodine sensitive patients	Essential in providing the cleanest possible surface for catheter site; extreme care must be taken to avoid dislodging catheter during scrubbing
f. Apply benzoin or skin preparation to areas of	Protects skin and facilitates adherence of tape to skin

ACTION	RATIONALE
skin where tape will be applied	
g. Remove gloves	
h. Open one package sterile 4 × 4 pads and *drop* antiseptic ointment on top	4 × 4 pad will be contaminated if it is allowed to come in contact with outside of ointment container
i. Put on sterile gloves	New gloves are required to provide cleanest possible environment for dressing application
j. Apply antiseptic ointment to catheter insertion site and all suture sites	
k. Apply sterile 4 × 4 pad to site; fold lengthwise to cover insertion site, needle cover (if that type of catheter is used), and catheter tubing connection	
l. Remove gloves	
10. Apply tape; if Op-site occlusive dressing material is available it may be used to secure dressing in place and no further taping is required	Op-Site is a semipermeable occlusive material that will seal dressing site
a. Place 2 inch paper tape over entire dressing area and secure to skin; skin must be completely dry before application of tape	For infant with subclavian catheter abduct arm to give full range of motion without pulling on tape; for internal jugular catheter rotate head as far as possible to opposite side to allow full range of motion without pulling on tape
b. Cover paper tape with 2 inch adhesive tape; *do not* apply adhesive tape directly to infant's skin	Adhesive tape is very irritating to skin and difficult to remove without traumatizing it
c. Seal all edges of adhesive with 1 inch paper tape; dressing does not need to be a large one; however, the adhesive tape *must* be sealed on all edges	Keeps dressing occlusive and as airtight as possible
d. Loop tubing over dressing and secure in place with tape; *do not kink* tubing	Tube for subclavian catheter should exit at clothing neck or infant should be arranged in a manner to keep tube out of infant's reach;

ACTION	RATIONALE
	wet or nonocclusive dressings must be changed immediately

    e. When dressing is in proximity to draining wounds tracheostomy plastic adhesive drape should be used to protect dressing from secretions

    f. Date and initial dressing

11. Check and reregulate IV flow if necessary

12. Chart in nurse's notes
    a. Time of dressing change
    b. By whom
    c. Appearance of site
    d. Catheter potency
    e. Any problems or complications

13. Persons qualified to perform procedure
    a. Hyperalimentation nurse
    b. RN or GN

PRECAUTIONS

1. Amino acid–glucose solutions are perfect growth media for bacteria; strict asepsis in management of line and solution is essential
2. Solutions should be checked prior to administration for cloudiness or particulate matter and, if present, returned to pharmacy
3. Presence of particulate matter or cloudiness in the existing infusion requires an *immediate* change of all solutions and tubing; solution should then be cultured
4. Variance of flow rate ± 10 per cent can result in hypoglycemia or hyperglycemia—therefore infusion pumps should always be used; attempts should never be made to *catch up* slowed infusions
5. A padded hemostat should always be at the bedside to prevent air embolus in event of accidental system break

RELATED NURSING CARE

1. Check flow rate at least every 30 to 60 minutes
2. Do not alter rate more than ± 10 per cent
3. Observe for signs of sepsis and allergic reaction
    a. Sudden febrile reaction
    b. Unexplained glucose intolerance
    c. Hypothermia
    d. Hemodynamic instability

COMPLICATIONS

1. Technical: Most frequently develop at or soon after initial catheter placement
   a. Pneumothorax, hemothorax, hydrothorax
   b. Arterial puncture with transection and hemorrhage
   c. Injury to tracheal plexus
   d. Malposition of catheter
   e. Formation of arteriovenous fistula
   f. Phlebitis or thrombus formation
   g. Air embolus
   h. Pericardial tamponade
2. Mechanical
   a. Clotting
   b. Pump or filter failure
   c. Kinking of catheter tubing
   d. Dislodgment of catheter with extravasation of fluid
   e. Accidental puncture of catheter with suture or scissors during dressing change
3. Septic complications: Incidence of catheter related sepsis is directly correlated with technique employed for proper catheter care
4. Metabolic complications

—————— INTRAVENTRICULAR DRAIN INSERTION*——————

PURPOSE

To treat intraventricular hemorrhage in the newborn a catheter can be inserted into the ventricle and connected to an external drainage device. Although several drainage systems are commercially available, a spinal needle, connector, IV tubing, and an empty sterile vacuum bottle may also be used. The drain may be inserted in the operating room.

In addition to draining bloody fluid from the ventricles, the drain is utilized to prevent or treat increased intracranial pressure.

EQUIPMENT

(If external ventricular drainage set with ventricular catheter is not used)
Spinal needle
T connector or three way connector
IV tubing
Sterile, empty vacuum container
Povidone-iodine
Alcohol
Sterile gloves
Sterile drape
2 X 2 inch gauze pads (4)
Tape
Masks and gowns

*Data from Core Curriculum for Neurosurgical Nursing, Chicago, American Association of Neurosurgical Nurses, 1977.

METHOD

ACTION	RATIONALE
1. Prepare external ventricular drainage set	
a. Remove from package	Needed to measure amount of drainage
b. Hang drainage bag	Whooshing sound will be heard
c. Place or vent	To prevent tubing from kinking and preventing drainage
or	
a. Place tape alongside bottle and mark time and date	Physician uses head landmarks to determine site of catheter insertion; infant's bones, including skull bone, may easily fracture
b. Insert IV tubing into bottle; be sure vacuum is broken	
c. Loop IV tubing as demonstrated	
d. Connect T connector to IV tubing	
2. Prepare insertion tray	
a. Open pack; pour povidone-iodine and alcohol; be sure all equipment is on sterile field	
b. Have gown, mask, and sterile gloves for physician	
c. Have gown and mask for everyone assisting in procedure	
3. Immobilize infant's head	
a. It may be necessary to mummy wrap a larger infant; use extreme caution when immobilizing premature infant	
4. Assist physician with procedure; ensure that strict technique is followed	
a. Head is prepared with povidone-iodine and alcohol	Iodine should dry prior to preparation with alcohol
b. Needle or catheter is inserted into ventricle	If soft catheter is used the skull is first punctured with a needle
c. T connector is attached to end of catheter when bloody CSF returns	Fluid is often sent for culture, cell count, protein determination

ACTION	RATIONALE
d. Position bottle or drainage bag per physician's order	Bottle usually is placed slightly below level of ventricle to facilitate drainage of blood
5. Anchor needle so it cannot move or become dislocated	Movement may cause trauma and increased bleeding; if needle is dislodged or up against ventricle wall, it may not drain
a. Tape and use sterile cotton ball or 2 × 2 inch pads for positioning	
b. When catheter or needle is placed correctly the fluid in the tubing will fluctuate slightly	
6. Care of intraventricular device	
a. Record amount of drainage on each shift	Infant may need fluid replacement
b. Notify physician if amount of drainage increases or fluid indicates increased bleeding or fresh hemorrhage	Fluid will appear bright red if hemorrhage is fresh
c. Change drainage bag or bottle and tubing per institution routine, usually every 24 hours	Prevent development of infection
d. Observe insertion site for signs of infection	Incidence of infection reported to be 1–10 per cent
e. Observe tubing each hour to ensure drainage or proper function	Fluid should fluctuate in tubing
7. Give antibiotic as indicated	
a. Be sure dosage is correct	Methicillin used prophylactically
b. Check cultures as indicated	

PRECAUTIONS

1. Be sure needle or catheter is sufficiently anchored to prevent dislodgment or moving
2. Record drainage amount; infant may become hypovolemic from fluid loss

RELATED CARE

1. Monitor vital and neurological signs
2. Monitor hematocrit and hemoglobin to prevent development of hemorrhagic shock

COMPLICATIONS

1. Infection

_____ INTUBATION _____

PURPOSE

To provide a patent airway to initiate and maintain ventilation.

EQUIPMENT

Laryngoscope
Miller blades size 0 or 1 (curved or straight)
Endotracheal tubes size:
   2.5 mm: up to 1000 gm
   3.0 mm: 1000 to 2500 gm
   3.5 mm: 2500 to 4000 gm
   4.0 mm: greater than 4000 gm
Tincture of benzoin
Q-tips
Adhesive tape
Magill forceps or bayonet forceps
Stylet (optional)
Inflation bag (500 cc) and mask
Oxygen tubing
Suction tubing size:
   6 F (2.5 mm tubes)
   6.5 F (3 to 3.5 mm tubes)
   8 F (3.5 to 4 mm tubes; may fit some 3 mm tubes, depending on brand)
Stethoscope
Personnel needed: at least two
Feeding tubes, size 5 F or 8 F
Sterile K-Y jelly

METHOD

ACTION	RATIONALE
1. Place infant on a radiantly warmed work surface with head at the end of the bed	Prevents cold stress and provides for proper body mechanics of the person doing the procedure
2. Place infant's head in the sniff position by folding a towel and placing it under the shoulders	Places the airway in a linear position and properly positions the head, thus freeing the practitioner's hands
3. Turn on both oxygen and suction	Enables the assistant to place the oxygen source directly to the infant's nose during the procedure
4. Refer to Figure B-1 for a schematic representation	
5. Place the laryngoscope gently into the infant's mouth by in-	Side entry to the mouth will prevent unnecessary blunt trauma to

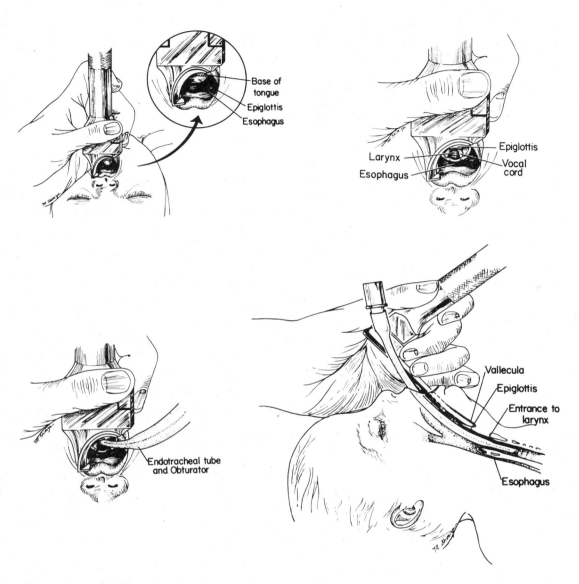

Figure B-1. Technique of endotracheal intubation. The Miller blade should be inserted near the midline and moved to the left side of the mouth, gently deflecting the tongue. As the blade is advanced, the base of the tongue and epiglottis are visualized. The blade should be advanced in the same plane of movement into the vallecula (see *D*); as the blade is gently raised, the epiglottis swings anteriorly, revealing the opening of the larynx. If secretions or meconium is noted, gentle suctioning should be done before insertion of the endotracheal tube. On certain occasions when the epiglottis is not adequately raised, the blade tip may be placed posterior to the epiglottis, which can then be gently raised to expose the vocal cords. The endotracheal tube is advanced from the right corner of the mouth and inserted while direct visualization is maintained. The laryngoscope blade is then carefully withdrawn while the position of the tube is maintained by the right hand on the infant's face. Note the tip of the blade in the vallecula. (From Klaus, M.H., and Fanaroff, A.A.: Care of the High Risk Neonate. Philadelphia, W.B. Saunders, 1979, p. 33.)

ACTION	RATIONALE
troducing the blade into the side of the mouth and over the tongue	the mouth, tongue, or palatal areas
6. Advance the blade forward into the pharyngeal area	
7. Gently lift the entire blade; as the blade is lifted the epiglottis should swing anteriorly	Lifting the entire blade will prevent tension and grooving of the upper gum; it also prevents the distal blade tip from gouging the infant
8. Visualize the upside down V shaped vocal cords	
9. Briefly suction any fluid visualized, especially meconium	If meconium is present it should be removed with direct mouth to tube suctioning until fluid is clear
10. Nasally or orally introduce the tube through the vocal cords and into the trachea	*Caution.* It is not uncommon to pass the tube through the esophagus, especially when the practitioner is unskilled or the infant is struggling; Magill forceps, bayonet forceps, or stylets are sometimes used to assist in intubation because some brands of tubes are soft and flexible, adding extra difficulty to the procedure
	Remember that speed is essential; however, tracheal manipulation stimulates the vagus nerve, causing bradycardia; a common mistake is to prolong attempts at intubation and more severely depress an already compromised infant
	If the heart rate drops below 100, the procedure must be stopped and the infant ventilated with the bag and mask until the heart rate has returned to normal
11. Auscultate and observe the chest while ventilating the infant with the bag	The chest should expand with use of bag, and the breath sounds should be equal bilaterally; if the sounds are louder on the right, the right main stem bronchus has probably been entered; slowly pull the tube back by 0.5 cm measures until the breath sounds are equal on both sides

ACTION	RATIONALE
12. Prepare the nasal area, upper lip, and cheeks with benzoin soaked Q-tips and secure the tube with two strips of ¼ inch adhesive tape	This provides a tacky semicoated surface for the adhesive tape to stick to; some commercial skin preparations, such as those used by ostomy patients, may be employed; tubes need to be retaped many times if the infant is receiving long term respiratory treatment, and these preserve the infant's tender skin
13. Quickly suction the tube with sterile technique to remove any further mucus or secretions	
14. Insert a nasogastric tube and place to gravity drainage	The esophagus is easily entered during intubation, particularly if the infant is struggling; air is introduced into the stomach from use of the bag and causes distention. By pressing against the diaphragm; excess air may also cause the infant to vomit; the NG tube will prevent aspiration of vomitus by providing a relief port
15. Obtain a chest radiograph to assess tube placement	The tube should be midline and 0.5 to 1 cm above the carina

RELATED CARE

1. Monitor the vital signs during and after the procedure until stable
2. Keep the tube clear by suctioning as needed
3. Restrain the active infant to prevent accidental extubation

COMPLICATIONS

1. Inappropriate tube placement
2. Laryngeal spasm or trauma
3. Severe bradycardia
4. Pneumothorax from inappropriate use of the bag

PERIPHERAL CANNULATION*

PURPOSE

The neonate is highly vulnerable to hemodynamic derangements. Placement of a peripheral IV line in the neonate may be indicated:

---

*Data from the following:
1. McIntyre, K.M., and Lewis, A.J. (eds.): Textbook of Advanced Cardiac Life Support. American Heart Association, 1981.
2. Perez, R.H.: Protocols for Perinatal Nursing Practice. St. Louis, C.V. Mosby Co., 1981.

1. When oral intake cannot equal basic fluid requirements
2. When a supplemental nutrient source is required because the gastrointestinal system is compromised
3. As a direct venous route for the administration of pharmacotherapeutic agents
4. As a direct venous route for administration of blood and blood components

The purpose of peripheral cannulation is to provide a safe venous route for administration of special fluid or nutritional requirements of the high risk neonate.

EQUIPMENT

250 to 500 ml container of intravenous fluid
In-line volume buret
Infusion pump
Butterfly needles 23, 25, 27 gauge
Tourniquet
Sterile gauze pads
Povidone-iodine preparation swabs
Tape ½ inch and 1 inch
IV site protector
Transilluminator
2 to 3 cc syringe with flush solution
Small infant arm board or padded tongue blade if extremity is used

METHOD

ACTION	RATIONALE
1. Prepare IV solution a. Insert in-line buret into IV tubing system	In-line buret allows constant monitoring of amount of fluid infused and reduces risk of inadvertent "dumping" of large quantities of fluid into circulatory system Buret should not contain more than 2 hour supply or 20 cc/kg of body weight
b. Insert IV tubing into infusion pump	
2. Select infusion site a. Scalp vein: other major veins available are frontal, temporal, posterior auricular, supraorbital, occipital, and posterior facial (transilluminator may aid in visualization of vein)	Preferred site in the neonate because of ease of visualization and reduced incidence of infiltration due to movement (Fig. B–2)

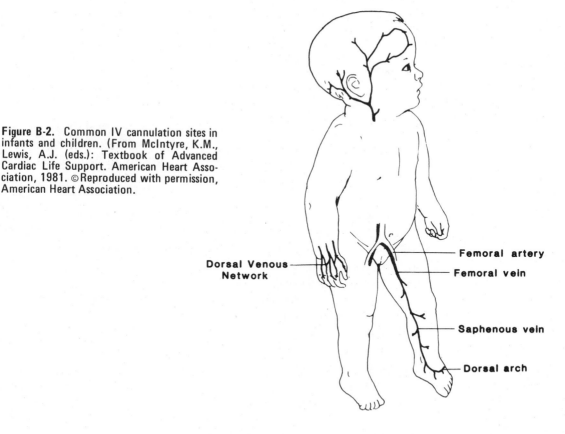

Figure B-2. Common IV cannulation sites in infants and children. (From McIntyre, K.M., Lewis, A.J. (eds.): Textbook of Advanced Cardiac Life Support. American Heart Association, 1981. ©Reproduced with permission, American Heart Association.

Dorsal Venous Network

Femoral artery

Femoral vein

Saphenous vein

Dorsal arch

ACTION	RATIONALE
b. Dorsal venous network of hand and foot	Upper extremity is preferred, as risk of phlebitis is reduced; caution required in use of hand or foot, as infiltration may compromise circulation in hand or foot
3. Scalp vein cannulation a. Restrain infant b. Shave selected site and surrounding area	Good visualization is required Avoid cutting skin, as this will increase risk of infection
c. Apply tourniquet around head	Wide rubber band around head acts as tourniquet; a tape tab on rubber band makes it easier to grasp rubber band to release pressure after cannulation
d. Clean area with povidone-iodine solution and allow to remain on surface for 2 to 3 minutes	Reduces risk of infection; povidone-iodine solution most effective when left on skin for this period

ACTION	RATIONALE
e. Attach syringe to butterfly needle and purge system of air	
f. Stretch skin overlying vein and identify direction of flow	Needle insertion should be in direction of flow
	The filling of a vessel from below and pulsation indicate that it is an artery and should be avoided
g. Grasp butterfly needle with bevel up	
h. Insert needle under skin 0.5 to 1 cm below the actual site at which the vein is to be entered	Angle of entry should be almost parallel to the skin with gradual deepening of angle
i. Check for entry into vein:	
i. Leave 2 to 3 cc syringe attached to butterfly tubing and gently aspirate until blood is returned	Assistance for this technique is generally useful
ii. Remove syringe and advance needle until blood flows back into tubing	
j. Release tourniquet	
k. Inject about 1 to 2 cc of flushing solution and observe infusion site	Inject slowly to observe patency of vein and to determine that an artery has not been entered accidentally (if an artery has been cannulated blanching will usually occur with flushing)
l. Tape needle in place; several methods can be used	Care should be taken not to tape over actual puncture site to protect against infection
i. Place small wedge of cotton under "wings" of butterfly to allow slight elevation and avoid pressure on vessel wall; then tape in "H" fashion to secure	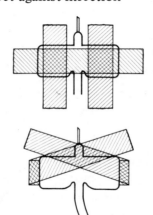
ii. Take approximately 3 inch piece of tape, slide it, adhesive side up, under wings of butterfly and tape it in a crisscross fashion	

ACTION	RATIONALE
m. Connect butterfly tubing to infusion tubing and start infusion pump	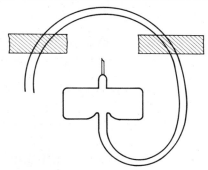
n. Tape butterfly tubing securely in a loop on scalp to avoid accidental dislodgment	
o. Apply antiseptic ointment to puncture site if required by hospital policy	
p. Apply protector to IV site	A 30 cc plastic medicine cup cut in half and with the bottom cut out and edges covered with tape for padding works well, as does a paper souffle cup with the bottom cut out
	When taping IV site protector in place, remember to tape in a fashion that permits untaping, when necessary, at the protector rather than requiring untaping that pulls hair or skin
4. Extremity cannulation	
a. Restrain infant	
b. Select vein	Transilluminator may aid in visualization
i. Hand: tributaries of basilic and cephalic veins or dorsal arch	
ii. Foot and leg: saphenous vein, median marginal and dorsal venous arch of left foot	Caution should be used in lower extremities because of risk of phlebitis
c. Select appropriate needle:	
i. 21 to 25 gauge butterfly preferred	
ii. Over-the-needle plastic cannula	Usually reserved for larger infants
d. Immobilize extremity; when hand is used the wrist should be flexed to stretch and immobilize vessel	Particularly important when an over-the-needle cannula is to be used
e. Follow steps c to m under Scalp vein cannulation	

ACTION	RATIONALE
when butterfly needle is used	
f. Secure hand to arm board	
i. 1 inch tape should be used to immobilize fingers and thumb	
ii. Place small roll of 2 × 2 inch gauze under wrist	
iii. Secure upper arm to arm board by sticking together two pieces of 1 inch tape of unequal length, leaving enough adhesive edge on each end of longer piece to permit securing tape to underside of arm board but preventing tape from adhering to skin	
g. Secure foot to arm board or padded tongue blade but maintain foot in normal position to prevent footdrop	
h. Loop butterfly tubing and secure with tape to prevent accidental dislodgment	
i. Apply antiseptic ointment to IV site if required by hospital policy	
j. Apply protector to IV site	

PRECAUTIONS

1. Assure aseptic technique
2. Exercise caution when using transilluminator or high intensity light, as burns may occur with prolonged exposure
3. Observe carefully for signs of infiltration or cannulation of artery

COMPLICATIONS

1. Infiltration
2. Inadvertent cannulation of artery
3. Infection
4. Phlebitis

SUBDURAL TAP*

PURPOSE

A subdural tap may be used to drain blood or effusions from the subdural space in the treatment of chronic subdural hematoma or subdural effusion that occurs as a complication of many neurological diseases. In unusual circumstances, a subdural tap may be indicated in the treatment of acute subdural hematoma.

EQUIPMENT

Spinal needle
Sterile drapes and towels
Povidone-iodine solution
Alcohol
Sterile gloves
Collection tubes
A standard infant lumbar puncture tray, with substitution of a needle of the correct size, may be used instead

METHOD

ACTION	RATIONALE
1. Check sterile tray to be sure all equipment and supplies are present	Ask physician if additional collection tubes are needed
2. Be sure extra spinal needles are available	Most physicians prefer a particular type of needle; furthermore, it may be necessary to tap both sides of head
3. Pour povidone-iodine and alcohol	
4. Position infant to prevent movement; wrap in blanket or sheet	
5. Place small roll under infant's shoulders	Hyperextension of head assists flow of fluid
6. Head is prepared with povidone-iodine and alcohol	
7. Needle is inserted into subdural space	

*Data from Milhorat, T.H.: Pediatric Neurosurgery. Philadelphia, F.A. Davis Co., 1978.

ACTION	RATIONALE
8. Fluid will flow better if infant is stimulated, e.g., crying	
9. Fluid is collected into tubes and sent for routine studies	First collection sent for culture, Gram stain, cell count, and protein and gluocse measurement. Fluid from subsequent taps is sent for cell count and protein measurement unless otherwise indicated
10. Cover puncture sites: Usually a cotton ball saturated with collodion is placed over puncture site	Prevents fluid leakage

PRECAUTIONS

1. Prevent movement of the infant's head when needle is inserted and during drainage of fluid

RELATED CARE

1. Monitor vital and neurological signs per routine
2. Observe needle insertion site for infection

COMPLICATIONS

1. Increased bleeding
2. Change in neurological status: hemiparesis

SUCTIONING: BULB SYRINGE

PURPOSE

Excess mucus in the nostrils and mouth can obstruct the airway of a neonate and interfere with exchange of oxygen and carbon dioxide. It must be safely removed to facilitate breathing.

EQUIPMENT

Bulb syringe

METHOD

ACTION	RATIONALE
1. Wash hands	
2. Hold infant's head firmly	

ACTION	RATIONALE
3. Squeeze bulb and insert into nostril or mouth as indicated	Steady, gentle suction will prevent damage to the mucosa
4. Release bulb and withdraw from nostril or mouth	
5. Discard mucus between each suctioning to clear bulb	
6. Rinse bulb syringe with hot water and replace near infant's bedside	
7. Wash hands	
8. Document procedure in medical record	

SUCTIONING: DeLEE APPARATUS

PURPOSE

Excess mucus in the nostrils or mouth and stomach can obstruct the airway of a neonate and interfere with exchange of oxygen and carbon dioxide and must be removed.

EQUIPMENT

DeLee suction apparatus

METHOD

ACTION	RATIONALE
1. Wash hands	
2. Insert catheter through infant's nose or mouth to stomach	
3. Insert mouth piece between your own lips	
4. Create mild suction with mouth	
5. Repeat procedure as necessary	
6. Pinch catheter and remove tube gently and quickly	Do not allow fluid to drain from catheter as it is removed

ACTION	RATIONALE
7. Wash hands	
8. Document procedure in medical record	

___ SUCTIONING: STERILE ENDOTRACHEAL OR NASOTRACHEAL ___

PURPOSE

Mucus secretions can obstruct a patent airway and interfere with the exchange of oxygen and carbon dioxide. Suctioning via an endotracheal or nasotracheal tube is utilized to safely remove secretions from the tracheobronchial tree to maintain a patent airway.

EQUIPMENT

Sterile suction catheter 5, 8, or 10
Single sterile glove
Connecting tubing
Source of negative pressure
Normal saline
Sterile water, 120 cc bottle

METHOD

ACTION	RATIONALE
1. Wash hands	
2. Peel open suction catheter package, allowing sterile catheter to remain in package until ready for use	
3. Open sterile water bottle	
4. Turn negative pressure source to on position	Negative pressure source should be regulated for continuous pressure of 60 to 80 mm Hg, depending on size of patient and viscosity of mucus
5. Don sterile glove on dominant hand	Other hand remains ungloved so nonsterile items can be handled
6. Remove suction catheter from package with gloved hand	

ACTION	RATIONALE
7. Grasp connecting tubing with ungloved hand and connect catheter to connecting tubing	
8. Ventilate infant by means of manual resuscitation	Oxygenate infant prior to suctioning of secretions
9. Moisten catheter tip with sterile water	Instill 0.25 cc normal saline into the endotracheal tube to loosen secretions when indicated
10. Turn infant's head to right side	
11. Insert suction catheter into endotracheal tube until resistance is met	Do not apply negative pressure while catheter is being inserted; this would be traumatizing to tissue and deplete the infant's oxygen prior to actual procedure
12. Withdraw catheter approximately 0.5 cm and apply suction by placing thumb over control valve	
13. Withdraw catheter with a rotating motion	Suctioning should last maximum of 5 to 10 seconds
14. Administer oxygen immediately after suctioning	Oxygenate the infant following suctioning procedure
15. Rinse catheter with sterile water	
16. Turn infant's head to left side and repeat procedure	
17. Suction mouth	
18. Turn negative pressure source to off position	
19. Discard catheter and glove	
20. Wash hands	
21. Document procedure in medical record	

SUCTIONING: UNSTERILE ORONASOPHARYNGEAL

PURPOSE

Mucus secretions can obstruct a patent airway and interfere with exchange of oxygen and carbon dioxide. Suctioning is utilized to remove secretions safely from the oronasopharynx to maintain a patent airway.

EQUIPMENT

Sterile suction catheter 8 or 10 F
Connecting tubing
Source of negative pressure
Sterile water

METHOD

ACTION	RATIONALE
1. Open bottle of sterile water	
2. Turn negative pressure source to on position	
3. Peel open suction catheter package, allowing clear catheter to remain in plastic peel-back package until ready for use	
4. Attach suction catheter to connecting tubing	
5. Moisten catheter tip with sterile water	
6. Insert suction catheter into back of mouth	
7. Apply suction intermittently by placing thumb on and off suction control valve	
8. Move catheter gently around back of mouth and throat	
9. Rinse catheter with water	
10. Gently insert catheter upward into right naris, then continue downward, advancing catheter on inspiration only	
11. Withdraw catheter	Suctioning should last 5 to 10 seconds
12. Rinse catheter with water	
13. Repeat procedure, inserting catheter into left naris	
14. Turn negative pressure source to off position	
15. Wash hands	
16. Document on medical record	

THORACOTOMY

PURPOSE

The chest wall is incised so that air or fluid can be evacuated from the pleural space and therefore correct the marked change in respiratory condition.

EQUIPMENT

Thoracotomy tray
12 F chest tubes
4-0 or 5-0 silk suture
Tincture of collodion
Chest drainage device and thoracic suction
Sterile water to fill water chambers
Sterile gown and mask (mask optional)
Sterile gloves
Cardiorespiratory monitor
Personnel needed: two

METHOD

ACTION	RATIONALE
1. Restrain infant properly and prepare the area to be taped with povidone-iodine (Betadine)	
2. Make a small (1 cm) incision to the midaxillary line at the 3rd to 5th intercostal space	Avoid the breast tissue area in female infants, as trauma can cause damage that may affect efforts at lactation later
3. Using a Kelly clamp with the chest tube gripped between the teeth, guide the tip up and over the ribs and puncture the chest wall	The major vessels are located in a groove underneath the ribs; going over the ribs prevents puncture of these vessels
4. Encircle the insertion site with a pursestring suture and then wrap the suture ends around the tube several times; seal the site with collodion	This method (rather than bandaging) allows for direct visualization and cleaning of the site
5. Attach the tube to a drainage device that has been filled with at least 10 to 12 cm of H_2O	Orders for cm of H_2O pressure will vary according to the infant's age, condition, and size of air leak
6. Attach the drainage device to continuous suction of at least 80 cm H_2O pressure	

RELATED CARE

1. Constant observation of vital signs and respiratory management
2. Draw and send blood gases as soon as procedure is over
3. Obtain radiograph to confirm placement and effectiveness of the tube
4. Observe and record the type and amount of drainage obtained at least every 8 hours

COMPLICATIONS

1. Lung damage from trauma
2. Hemorrhage from nicking vessels under the ribs
3. Reaccumulation of leaking air
4. Infection from an invasive procedure

_____TRANSCUTANEOUS MEASUREMENT OF OXYGEN_____

PURPOSE

This method of measuring oxygen is accomplished with the use of a skin electrode heated to 44°C. The electrode produces a reading equal to that observed on a blood sample measured in a blood gas machine at 37°C. The number of blood gas samples necessary has been reduced with the use of this monitor. It has also allowed the physician to have a real time indication of the effect on PO_2 of changes in the respiratory rate, pressures, and FiO_2. The PO_2 can be stabilized rather quickly, and a blood sample can then be drawn for determination of PCO_2 and pH values. It is a means to safely and accurately measure the partial pressure of arterial (PaO_2) and transcutaneous partial pressure of oxygen ($TcPO_2$).

EQUIPMENT

Transcutaneous electrode	3 cc syringe
Contact gel	TB syringe
4 X 4 gauze pad	6 cc syringe
Alcohol swab	Cup of ice

METHOD

ACTION	RATIONALE
1. Wash hands	
2. Prepare skin to apply electrode	Use alcohol to remove oily substances and dried skin; allow to air dry
3. Check electrode membrane for excessive air bubbles	
4. Select site with good capillary circulation for measurement, e.g., chest, abdomen, thighs, back	

ACTION	RATIONALE
5. Remove paper from back of double adhesive paper ring and apply flat side of electrode fixation ring to adhesive ring	
6. Remove remaining adhesive cover and place fixation ring onto selected site	
7. Press firmly to ensure no leakage	
8. Apply thin film of contact gel in middle of electrode	
9. Snap electrode into fixation ring	
10. Observe monitor for evidence of stabilization (approximately 15 to 20 minutes) a. The following will occur: i. Initial decrease in $TcPO_2$ ii. Increase in $TcPO_2$ after skin has warmed	
11. Set desired alarm limits and engage alarms	
12. Position infant off electrode at all times a. Frequency for changing sites: i. Infant under 2 lb every 2 hours ii. Infant 3 to 5 lb every 3 hours iii. Infant over 5 lb every 4 hours b. Method for changing site: i. Snap electrode out of fixation ring ii. Wipe off gel, using dry 4 × 4 gauze pad iii. Follow procedure for initial preparation and placement	Electrodes left at the same site in excess of the hours indicated may cause burns on the skin
13. Monitor patient activity	
14. Obtain FiO_2 measurement from meter on monitor	

ACTION	RATIONALE

15. Draw specimen for arterial blood gases

16. Observe $TcPO_2$ measurement on digital readout

17. Subtract $TcPO_2$ from PaO_2 to give the gradient, when applicable

18. Document on the medical record:
    a. Each change in electrode site on FiO_2
    b. Each time $TcPO_2$ falls below 60 mm Hg or rises above 100 mm Hg
    c. Each time blood is drawn

TUBE FEEDING*

PURPOSE

Infants of less than 32 weeks' gestation lack adequate sucking, swallowing, and gag reflexes to be effectively and safely nipple fed. Other sick infants may be physically too weak to ingest formula by nipple. Nasojejunal feeding may be employed to meet the necessary fluid and caloric intake of the preterm infant or one in whom sucking and gag reflexes are weak or absent, that is, when it may not be in the infant's best interest to receive intermittent bolus feeding by nipple or gavage.

EQUIPMENT

1. Gavage
   15 inch gavage tube 5 or 8 F
   Stethoscope
   20 cc syringe or infant Volufeed container
   Tape
   Sterile water
   Prescribed formula

2. Nasojejunal feeding
   15 inch Silastic or silicon catheter 5 or 8 F (polyvinyl tubes tend to harden during long term placement)

*Data from the following:
1. Cheek, J., and Staub, G.: Nasojejunal alimentation in premature and full-term newborn infants. J. Pediatr., 82:955, 1973.
2. Chen, J., and Wong, P.: Intestinal complication in nasojejunal feeding in low-birthweight infants. J. Pediatr., 85:109, 1974.
3. Klaus, M.H., and Fanaroff, A.A.: Care of the High-Risk Neonate, 2nd ed. Philadelphia, W.B. Saunders Co., 1979.
4. Pierog, S.H., and Ferrara, A.: Medical Care of the Sick Newborn, 2nd ed. St. Louis, C.V. Mosby Co., 1976.

Stethoscope
Infusion pump with burette and IV administration set
Tape

METHOD

ACTION	RATIONALE
1. Gavage	
a. Change infant's diaper and linens as needed to prevent handling after feeding	
b. Wash hands	
c. Place infant on right side with head of bed elevated 15 degrees	Restrain infant if necessary
d. Open gavage tube and formula	
e. Measure tube from bridge of nose to tip of xiphoid cartilage and mark with tape, or measure from tip of nose to ear lobe to xiphoid process and mark with tape	
f. Place tip of feeding tube on anterior surface of tongue; as infant swallows insert tube past oropharynx	Advancing tube as infant swallows may aid in reducing incidence of vagal stimulation and gagging; it also decreases risk of inadvertently entering trachea, as the epiglottis occludes tracheal opening during swallowing
g. Continue to advance feeding tube as infant swallows until measured mark has been reached	
h. Observe infant for gagging, coughing, apnea, bradycardia, and color change during tube placement; if any of these occurs withdraw the tube and allow infant's condition to stabilize before attempting procedure again	Generally a result of 1. Tube entry into trachea 2. Stimulation of gag reflex if tube touches sensitive area of oropharynx 3. Stimulation of vagus nerve
i. Secure tube to chin with small piece of tape	Prevents tubing from slipping when infant moves
j. Attach syringe and gently insert 1 to 2 cc of air while listening with stethoscope over epigastric region; a	Hearing swishing sound upon auscultation after insertion of air confirms tube placement in stomach

ACTION	RATIONALE
swishing sound will be heard as air enters stomach	
k. Aspirate stomach and observe contents	Air injected previously should be aspirated to reduce risk of distention or vomiting during feeding
i. Bile stained or coffee ground appearance of stomach contents should be recorded and feeding withheld until physician notified of findings	Observation of stomach contents and amount is essential for assessing infant's readiness to feed and gastrointestinal status Aspirate can also be checked for pH; pH of 5 or less indicates acid content of stomach
ii. Partially digested formula should be returned to stomach and amount of residual subtracted from amount of formula to be given	If residual is greater than one fifth of previous feeding, consider: 1. Infant may be receiving volume greater than ability to digest in given period 2. Bowel motility may be reduced, delaying gastric emptying (may be an early sign of necrotizing enterocolitis)
iii. Thick mucus should not be replaced, and stomach may be lavaged with 5 to 10 ml of sterile water to reduce risk of vomiting during or after feeding	
l. Pinch off feeding tube and wait a few moments to verify that tube is not causing distress	
m. With tube pinched off pour necessary amount of water or formula into syringe	
n. Release pinched end of feeding tube and allow feeding to flow by gravity	Pressure of syringe plunger may result in sudden stomach distention and vomiting
o. Observe infant behavior during feeding	
i. Sucking on tubing	Pacifier given at this time may aid in the infant's ingestion of formula
ii. Gagging or heaving	Pinch off tubing and allow infant to rest, as feeding may be proceeding too fast or tube may have triggered reflex

ACTION	RATIONALE
iii. Coughing, cyanosis, bradycardia, apnea	Improper tube placement or aspiration, possible vagal stimulation; discontinue feeding
p. When feeding complete, pinch off tubing at syringe and at point where tube enters mouth	
q. Remove tape	
r. Remove pinched tubing quickly	When feeding tube is removed slowly, infant may gag and aspirate formula
s. Burp infant	
t. Place infant on abdomen or right side with head of bed elevated	Right side with head elevated promotes gastric emptying and reduces risk of aspiration if infant vomits

2. Nasojejunal feeding

a. Measure infant for tube placement: from bridge of nose to heel (with leg straight) and mark tubing with tape	Indicates distance tube is to be advanced into stomach
	If nasoduodenal feeding is desired, measurement is same as tube length for gavage plus 2 cm
b. Lubricate tip of tubing with sterile water	Aids passage of tubing through nostril
c. Introduce tubing and check for placement in stomach as for gavage	
d. Position infant on right side with head of bed elevated. *Infant must be kept in this position until tube placement in jejunum is confirmed*	Aids in passage of tubing from stomach through pylorus into small bowel
e. Aspirate tubing every hour and determine pH of aspirate (transpyloric passage usually takes 1 to 4 hours)	pH 5 or less indicates tubing is still in stomach; pH 5 to 7 indicates tubing has passed through pylorus and is in bowel
f. Obtain roentgenogram to confirm tube placement	
g. Start feeding only after tube placement is confirmed	

PRECAUTIONS

1. Use cardiac and respiratory monitors when infant is receiving continuous feeding to warn of vagal induced bradycardia due to tube placement

RELATED CARE IN NASOJEJUNAL FEEDING

1. Change tubing every 8 hours
2. Volume of formula should not exceed 4 hour supply because of risk of bacterial growth
3. Stomach residual should be checked every 4 to 8 hours to assure that infant is not receiving formula faster than it can be utilized
4. Feeding tube should be changed every 3 days if polyvinyl or every 7 to 8 days if Silastic

GENERAL COMPLICATIONS

1. Aspiration
2. Bradycardia
3. Apnea
4. Vagal stimulation

COMPLICATIONS OF NASOJEJUNAL FEEDING

1. Infection
2. Perforation
3. Necrotizing enterocolitis
4. Jejunal intussusception

____ UMBILICAL ARTERIAL OR VENOUS CATHETER PLACEMENT ____

PURPOSE

An umbilical artery catheter (UAC) or umbilical venous catheter (UVC) is placed to provide direct entry to the cardiovascular system for the passage of medications, fluids, blood, or blood products; to obtain blood samples for laboratory tests; and for direct pressure monitoring.

EQUIPMENT

Radiant warmer with Servo control
Cardiac monitor
Povidone-iodine (Betadine) skin preparation
Umbilical catheterization tray
Umbilical catheters sizes 3.5, 5, or 8 F
Stopcock
Adapter (Luer type) for the catheter
Suture (4-0 or 5-0 black silk)
½ inch adhesive tape
Sterile gloves, sterile gown (optional), mask (optional)
Heparinized flush solution
Restraints
Tape measure
Personnel needed: 2

METHOD

ACTION	RATIONALE
1. Place the infant in a supine position on a radiantly heated surface with the Servo control attached	Thermoregulation is a priority; be sure heat reflector patch is not covered by drapes, as that causes ineffective functioning of the warmer and possible overheating or cooling; the thermistor should be moved higher on the chest wall
2. Connect cardiorespiratory monitor	
3. Four point restraint of infant over 1500 gm; in infant less than 1500 gm restrain the lower extremities by wrapping a diaper around the legs, taping the diaper closed, and then securing the legs to the warmer by placing long pieces of tape from side to side across the knees	A circumcision restraint board is helpful, as it provides quick, secure, and atraumatic restraint of the infant

Diapers protect the fragile skin of premature weighing less than 1500 gm |
4. The assistant will hold up the cord stump with an instrument handed over from the practitioner performing the procedure; the cord is then painted by the practitioner with povidone-iodine (Betadine), using a circular motion starting from the base of the cord and progressing at least 5 cm outward	
5. As the assistant continues to hold the painted cord up, the practitioner will place umbilical tape around the cord base and tighten it slightly; the stump is then trimmed to approximately 1 to 2 cm above the base; the assistant will discard the detached portion of the cord	
6. The vessels are then located; two arteries, which appear as tightly close together vessels, and one vein, which is usually flat and dilated, will be present	
7. The catheter to be used (3.5 or 5 F for UAC or 8 F for UVC) is prepared by cutting	It is preferable to prepare the catheter in this way to prevent excess clot formation, which is common

ACTION	RATIONALE
off the large flanged distal end and inserting an 18 gauge blunt needle or Leur adapter; the male end of the three way stopcock is introduced into the hub of the adapter, and the catheter is flushed with the heparinized solution	around the end of a stopcock that has been placed directly into the flanged end of a catheter
	This method also provides a secure connection among the central line, the stopcock, and the fluid line; accidental disconnection is also prevented
8. The artery or vein is now located and dilated as needed with a straight dilator or a special curved arterial vessel dilator	
9. Once the vessel is dilated the catheter may be slowly introduced	Catheters should never be forced in as it is possible to "false track" tissue around the vessel rather than actually to be in the vessel
10. The length of UAC insertion is calculated as 0.75 of the shoulder to umbilical length in centimeters or by doubling the distance from the umbilicus to the midpoint of the inguinal ligament	Proper position of UAC is between the third and fourth lumbar space and is verified by radiography of the chest and abdomen together—a kidney, ureter, and bladder (KUB) film; if the catheter is too high it must be pulled back; length of pullback is measured in centimeters directly on the radiograph itself
	Proper UVC position is just above the diaphragm in the inferior vena cava or atrium; this line provides an excellent source for central venous pressure monitoring which assesses the hydration status of the heart
11. Once in place the catheter may be secured by suturing it in, or by "bridge taping"

To suture in the line a small piece of adhesive tape is placed around its base as the line enters the abdomen; a suture is passed through the tape and then through the umbilical stump | This method's advantage is that the catheter is "marked" at the initial proper length; it also prevents the abdominal wall from exposure to large amounts of tape and provides direct visualization of the entire abdomen and entire cord stump |

ACTION	RATIONALE
12. A KUB film is obtained immediately	Radiograph verifies placement; gonad shields should be used on the infant
13. Final taping or suturing may be completed after verification of placement	If the suture method is used, an additional safety tip could be utilized: Place a length of umbilical tape (2 to 3 cm larger than the circumference of the abdomen) around the abdomen; loop the central line and secure it to the umbilical tape—this will remove tension from the line and prevent accidental removal by inadvertent manipulation (e.g., changing position)

RELATED CARE

1. Observe vital signs closely before, during, and after procedure
2. Tape all central line connections
3. Attach central pressure monitoring devices to all central lines if possible
4. Monitor the status of the arterial line by observing the pressure wave form displayed on the oscilloscope; the proper curve is one in which a slight notch is present immediately after the peak of the wave
5. Observe for damping wave form (one that is becoming progressively flat), which could indicate a clotting line
6. Adequately flush the central line after each blood sampling to prevent clot formation within the catheter
7. Constantly watch for any darkening of the lower extremities, trunk, toes, or toenail beds; notify the physician immediately if this occurs

ARTERIAL COMPLICATIONS

1. Obstruction after the catheter tip is passed 1 to 2 cm into the vessel
2. Obstruction slightly deeper into the abdominal wall because of a tortuous vessel, subendothelial cushions, or possibly a false passage
3. Perforation and hemorrhage
4. Exsanguination from accidental disconnection of the line
5. Vasospasm in the lower extremities, trunk (below the umbilical level), or buttock areas due to air embolus or clots in the vessels
6. Clotted aorta

VENOUS COMPLICATIONS

1. Inappropriate placement into the portal vein or liver
2. Descent of catheter into the inferior vena cava therefore entering the left atrium or pulmonary vein
3. Portal vein or liver exposure to caustic drugs such as alkali, $D_{25}W$, and calcium; all of these can cause necrosis to the area

NEONATAL DRUGS*

Name, Source, Trademarks, Preparations	Neonatal Dosage and Administration	Uses	Action and Fate	Side Effects and Contraindications	Nursing Implications and Remarks
AMINOPHYLLINE (THEOPHYLLINE ETHYLENEDIAMINE) (aminocardol, ammophyllin, cardophyllin, carena, diophyllin, genophyllin, inophylline, metaphyllin, phyllindon, theolamine, theophyldine) Synthetic RECTALAD-AMINOPHYLLINE	Loading dose: 3–5 mg IV, PD Maintenance: 2 mg IV q 8–12 IM or IV: given very slowly; often added to IV infusions	Bronchial asthma, pulmonary emphysema, chronic bronchitis, other pulmonary diseases Adjunct in acute pulmonary edema or paroxysmal nocturnal dyspnea with left-sided heart failure May be helpful in Cheyne-Stokes respiration Reduces neonatal apnea	Relaxes smooth muscle, notably bronchial, stimulates CNS, acts on kidneys to cause diuresis and stimulates cardiac muscle to increase output; on cellular level said to act by inhibiting phosphodiesterases that metabolize cyclic AMP Erratically absorbed orally so determination of theophylline serum levels may help prevent dangerously high blood levels Metabolized by liver; rate differs with individual; unchanged drug and metabolites excreted primarily in urine—small amounts unchanged in feces; secreted in human milk in concentrations of about 70% that in plasma Therapeutic serum levels 10–20 μg/ml; toxic effects above 20 μg/ml	GI irritation, with anorexia, nausea, vomiting, epigastric pain, abdominal pain, rarely diarrhea. CNS stimulation causes headache, irritability, restlessness, nervousness, insomnia, dizziness, convulsions Cardiovascular side effects mild, transient palpitations, sinus tachycardia, increased pulse rate Severe toxic reactions manifested by vomiting, agitation, and sometimes convulsions With IV administration watch for signs of cardiovascular distress IM administration not advised, since drug irritating to tissues Theophylline increases excretion of lithium carbonate; may enhance sensitivity and toxic potential of cardiac glycosides; may exhibit synergistic toxicity with ephedrine and other sympathomimetics	Aminophylline is synthetic theophylline—one of xanthine preparations; all cause varying degrees of CNS stimulation, increased urinary output, smooth muscle relaxation Widely used for so many conditions, could be placed in many categories Oral preparations should be given after meals with full glass of water with antacid to minimize local GI irritation To minimize side effects, IV administration should be slow; rapid injection may produce dizziness, faintness, palpitation, precordial pain, syncope, flushing, bradycardia, severe hypotension, cardiac arrest Theophylline has low therapeutic index; therefore, patients receiving IV therapy should be monitored closely

Drug	Action/Use	Dosage	Pharmacology	Side Effects	Nursing Considerations
CAFFEINE Active principle of *Thea sinensis*, *Coffea arabica*, kola nut, guarana and yerba; other active principles: theobromine, theophylline	General cerebral stimulant and analeptic; Component of many over the counter "pepper uppers" Diuretic general body stimulant Will help relieve certain types of headache	Loading dose: 20 mg/kg IV, PD Maintenance: 5–10 mg/kg once or twice a day × 3 days	A descending central nervous system stimulant; small doses affect cerebrum mainly—larger doses, brain stem, including medulla; large doses increase heart action and cause peripheral vasodilation Absorption of caffeine erratic; salts of caffeine more readily absorbed Rapidly distributed throughout body tissues, readily crossing placenta and blood brain barrier metabolized in liver Excreted by kidneys as 1-methyl uric acid and 1-methylxanthine, about 10% unchanged	Excreted in breast milk, but not readily excreted by newborn; therefore mother taking this drug should probably not nurse baby Rarely severe Mild symptoms include insomnia, restlessness, nervousness, palpitation, nausea, vomiting; functional cardiac symptoms may occur Tolerance may develop to diuretic and cardiovascular and CNS effects	Since most people drink either coffee or tea, they are used to daily dose of caffeine, have tolerance for it and do not usually develop toxic symptoms from using it as drug If functional cardiac symptoms occur, stop drug and give evacuants and sedatives
CAFFEINE CITRATED					
CURARE, SYNTHETIC STRYCHNOS. TUBOCURARINE HYDROCHLORIDE	To produce respiratory paralysis for elimination of resistance to mechanical ventilation; decrease O_2 consumption Pancuronium bromide (Pavulon) now more generally used	IV: first dose 0.2 mg/kg then 0.1 mg/kg prn movement	Smooth muscle relaxant; blocks passage of impulse at myoneural junction	Vasodilation, hypotension, which can be potentiated by aminoglycosides	Monitor vital signs and BP continuously; vasodilation, hypotension can be reversed with combination of neostigmine (Prostigmin) and atropine ABG 10–15 min after dose; changes in ventilation pattern may be necessary

Table continues on following page.

Warning: Before administering any drug, check carefully for dosages specific to neonate or mother.

NEONATAL DRUGS* *(Continued)*

Name, Source, Trademarks, Preparations	Neonatal Dosage and Administration	Uses	Action and Fate	Side Effects and Contraindications	Nursing Implications and Remarks
DIGOXIN Derived from leaves of *Digitalis lanata* Lanoxin Oral: 0.05 mg/cc IM or IV: 0.1 mg/cc	Total digitalizing dose (TDD): Preterm infant 0.03–0.06 mg/kg PO; 0.03–0.05 mg/kg IV Term infant: 0.05 mg/kg; (0.04–0.08 mg/kg PO; 0.03–0.06 mg/kg IV) give ½ TDD, then ¼ TDD, then ¼ TDD at 8 hour intervals Maintenance dose: ¼ TDD divided into two doses 12 hours apart	To increase cardiac output in congestive heart failure	Decreases heart rate and increases strength of contraction by slowing conduction at AV node (increases P-R interval) Excreted by kidneys Absorption and excretion altered in neonate; toxic dose may build up over time	Slow pulse, arrhythmias, especially hypokalemia, if digoxin is given with furosemide (Lasix); precipitates toxicity	Doublecheck calculations and drawn-up medication with another nurse: dose is small and inadvertent overdose is possible Continuous cardiovascular monitoring Check heart rate prior to dose; withhold dose and notify physician if rate < 100 or arrhythmias Check lead II of ECG 2 hr after each dose and show to physician to monitor increased P-R interval Monitor electrolytes KCl supplements often given routinely
DOPAMINE HYDRO-CHLORIDE Synthetic sympathomimetic agent Intropin 200 mg/5cc (200,000 μg)	IV: continuous infusion through central or peripheral vein of diluted solution at 5–10 μg/kg/min to start; double rate if no response Maximum dose in newborns controversial, usually 20–50 μg/kg/min, research in neonates is limited	To maintain systemic blood pressure and increase renal blood flow in shock	Sympathomimetic, beta receptor stimulating effects of low doses, has alpha receptor effects in adults at high doses (vasoconstricting) Intropic effect on myocardium: increases cardiac output and pulse pressure: decreases blood flow to peripheral vascular beds while increasing flow to mesenteric vessels	Ectopic beats, tachycardia, elevated BP, vomiting, decreased urinary output with high doses Inactivated in alkaline solutions Incompatible with amphotericin, ampicillin, gentamicin, penicillin G	Reduce rate of administration until symptoms disappear but therapeutic responses still occur Do not dilute in alkaline solution Control infusion so that bolus is not given inadvertently Monitor vital signs, BP, urine output continuously Correct hypovolemia prior to infusion if possible

Drug	Dosage	Action	Use	Side effects/Toxicity	Nursing considerations
FUROSEMIDE Anthranilic acid derivative Lasix 10 mg/cc	IM, IV, oral: 1-2 mg/kg/dose usually given q 6-12 hr Maintenance: 1-4 mg/kg/day divided in 2-3 doses	Believed to dilate renal vessels, resulting in increased glomerular filtration rate, renal blood flow, sodium excretion Inhibits reabsorption of sodium in proximal and distal tubules and loop of Henle Response usually within 1 hr Metabolized in liver; excreted in urine	Diuresis in infants with CHF	Hypokalemia, hyponatremia, ototoxicity Competes with bilirubin for albumin binding sites	Monitor urine output, specific gravity, urine and serum electrolytes, weight Continuous cardiorespiratory monitoring Should not be given to severely jaundiced infants, especially those with low serum albumin levels Administer slowly (over 5-10 min) to decrease sudden peaks in serum concentration, which increase risk of ototoxicity
HEPARIN SODIUM From intestinal mucosa or lungs of animals Lipo-Hepin, Panheparin 1000 units/cc	IV: Loading dose: 50-100 units/kg Maintenance dose: 600 units/kg/day by continuous infusion or 100 units/kg 4 hours IV To yield PTT 2-3 × control value rate and dose adjusted by screening test results Usually given in conjunction with transfusions of fresh frozen plasma or fresh whole blood to replace clotting factors	Believed to inhibit conversion of prothrombin to thrombin and fibrinogen to fibrin; prevents extension of old clots and formation of new clots Metabolized by liver; excreted by kidneys; should occur within 6 hr but may be delayed in sick infants	DIC with thrombosis or bleeding not controlled by transfusions	Hemorrhage Not compatible with amikacin, gentamicin, tobramycin	Management of hemorrhage: Stop drug; give protamine sulfate 1 mg for each mg of heparin given in last 4 hr (1 mg heparin $\cong$ 100 units) Check coagulation screening tests frequently; observe closely for increased bleeding; monitor vital signs and BP continuously

Table continues on following page.

NEONATAL DRUGS* *(Continued)*

Name, Source, Trademarks, Preparations	Neonatal Dosage and Administration	Uses	Action and Fate	Side Effects and Contraindications	Nursing Implications and Remarks
ISOPROTERENOL HYDROCHLORIDE Synthetic sympathomimetic agent Isuprel 1:5000, 1 mg/5 cc (0.2 mg/cc)	IV: continuous infusion 3 mg diluted in 250 D_5 W yielding 12 µg/cc. Start at 0.2 µg/kg/min (12 µg/kg/hr); double rate if no response; titrate dose with heart rate and BP	To support circulation, increase cardiac output in cases of shock	Beta receptor stimulant, sympathomimetic Inotropic effect on myocardium by increasing rate and strength of contraction	Tachycardia resulting in congestive heart failure; if tachycardia occurs, stop or decrease rate of infusion arrhythmias Not compatible with amphotericin, aminophylline, ampicillin Not effective in pH < 7.10	Monitor vital signs and BP continuously Have defibrillator and emergency antiarrhythmic drugs on hand Acidosis should be corrected prior to infusion Control rate of infusion so bolus is not inadvertently infused
MORPHINE SULFATE Derived from opium 1 mg/cc	IM, SC or IV: 0.1–0.2 mg/kg q 4 hr	Analgesia for pain, pulmonary edema, possible anxiety from use of smooth muscle relaxants Sedation		Respiratory depression, addiction, decreased peristalsis of GI tract, hypotension	Monitor vital signs and BP continuously
PANCURONIUM BROMIDE Pavulon 1 mg/cc	IV: 0.1 mg/kg prn for movement. May have to ↑ dose, as tolerance builds quickly	For respiratory paralysis to eliminate resistance to mechanical ventilation; decreases O_2 consumption	Smooth muscle relaxant Blocks passage of impulse at myoneural junction More potent than curare	Effects last longer than those of curare; not completely reversible by anticholinesterase agents	Monitor vital signs and BP continuously; ABG 10–15 min after dose; change in ventilation pattern may be necessary
PROSTAGLANDIN E_1 PGE_1 Naturally occurring 500 µg/cc (diluted to 50 µg/cc by addition of 9 cc normal saline)	IV: solution of 500 µg/cc diluted with 9 cc normal saline to yield 50 µg/cc; this solution then diluted with IV fluid to yield infusion of 0.05 µg/kg/min at ordered rate; dose may be decreased to 0.025 µg/kg/min after 4–6 hr if therapeutic effects con-	To promote dilation of the ductus arteriosus in infants with congenital heart disease dependant on ductus shunting for oxygenation/perfusion In right ventricular outflow obstruction In transposition of great arteries In left ventricular	Rapidly disappears from circulation; infusion must be continuous Therapeutic effect should occur within 30–45 min	Cardiovascular: vasodilation, edema CNS: hyperthermia, seizures, irritability, lethargy Respiratory: apnea, hypoventilation Infectious disease: interferes with WBC function	This is a controlled drug available only at specific cardiac centers. *It should not be used by persons unfamiliar with its use.* Monitor vital signs and BP continuously; observe skin color and measure ABG q 10 min × 30 min then prn

	Dosage	Use	Action	Side Effects/Precautions	Nursing Considerations
	tinue or serious side effects occur; given through peripheral or central vein (no arterial infusion)	outflow obstruction			Observe CNS for changes Infant should receive prophylactic ampicillin and gentamicin
PROTAMINE SULFATE Synthetic systemic anticoagulant	IV or IM: 1 mg/100 units heparin	Heparin antagonist	Anticoagulant when alone, but when given with heparin attracted to heparin and forms stable salt Rapid action after IV use (5 min)	Reported in adults: hypotension, bradycardia, dyspnea, transitory flushing	Monitor vital signs and BP continuously Observe for bleeding Monitor clotting screening tests Protamine must be refrigerated
SODIUM BICARBONATE (Baking soda)	3 mEq/kg/dose IV over 10 min; do not infuse faster than 1 mEq/kg/minute	Many purposes; to decrease gastric acidity, to reduce acidity systemically, and locally as antipruritic	Alkaline salts that act as antacid because of their basic nature are soluble and widely distributed Excreted by the kidneys and will cause urine to be alkaline	Rare in therapeutic dosage Excessive amounts may cause alkalosis; sodium salts, especially bicarbonates, are more apt to cause alkalosis; sodium bicarbonate may cause acid rebound and increase in CO_2 in stomach	Used IV to combat metabolic acidosis, especially in cardiac arrest When sodium citrate is given to alkalinize urine, patient should receive low calcium diet (no milk or milk products), since calcium will precipitate in alkaline urine In alkalosis due to excessive amounts, stop drug and give mild acids
THAM	Least amount of 0.2 M solution required to bring blood pH to normal levels (equivalent acid buffering to equal mmol of $NaHCO_3$)	Correction of metabolic acidosis during cardiac bypass surgery or that associated with cardiac arrest	Weak base, which, after IV administration, attracts and combines with hydrogen ions and their associated acid anions; there is reduction of PCO_2, a potent respiratory stimulus Also acts as weak osmotic diuretic	Anuria and uremia; use only in life threatening cases during pregnancy; do not use more than one day; use cautiously in patients with renal disease or reduced renal output Local irritation and tissue inflammation at site of injection,	Dosage must be carefully adjusted so blood pH does not increase above normal (7.4); facilities for mechanical ventilation should be available Monitor before, during, and after therapy: blood pH, PCO_2, bicarbonate, glucose, electrolytes

Table continues on following page.

NEONATAL DRUGS* *(Concluded)*

Name, Source, Trademarks, Preparations	Neonatal Dosage and Administration	Uses	Action and Fate	Side Effects and Contraindications	Nursing Implications and Remarks
			Not metabolized appreciably; ionized tromethamine (chiefly as bicarbonate salt) rapidly and preferentially excreted in urine at rate dependent on infusion rate	chemical phlebitis, venospasm, intravenous thrombosis; extravasation may result in inflammation, necrosis, sloughing Hypoglycemia and respiratory depression may occur	
THEOPHYLLINE Active principle of *Thea sinensis*; synthetic Aerolate, Elixophyllin, Slo-Phyllin, Theocin, Theo-Dur	1.5–2 mg/kg PO q 4 hr Oral: 200–300 mg tid or qid	Neonatal apnea	See *Aminophylline*	See *Aminophylline*	Oral preparations: See *Aminophylline*
TOLAZOLINE HYDROCHLORIDE Priscoline hydrochloride 25 mg/cc	Test dose: 1–2 mg/ kg IV over 10 minutes; if response positive (cutaneous flush, increased arterial PO_2), infusion of 1–2 mg/kg/hr through peripheral or central vein, pulmonary artery catheter	Pulmonary vasodilation in persistent fetal circulation	Alpha sympathomimetic blocking agent producing vasodilation of pulmonary and other peripheral arterioles	Hypotension, GI hemorrhage, abdominal distension, oliguria, hematuria, thrombocytopenia	Volume expanders should be on hand before test dose given Vasopressors on hand for continuous IV infusion Monitor vital signs and BP continuously ABG 10–15 minutes after first dose; monitor q h until stable maintenance dose reached, then q 2 h Use in pulmonary hypertension in neonates still experimental; use with extreme caution; should be used only where facilities for cardiovascular and respiratory monitoring, immediate volume expansion, and cardiovascular support are

INDEX

Numbers in *italics* refer to illustrations; numbers followed by (t) refer to tables.

Abdomen
  assessment of, in gastrointestinal obstruction, 504
    in high risk neonate, 285(t)
    in necrotizing enterocolitis, 498
  palpation of, Leopold's maneuvers in, 564–566, **565**
  wrapping of, in omphalocele and gastroschisis, 501–502, 503
Abdominal pain, in high risk pregnancy, 135
Abdominal wall, neonatal, defects of, and neonatal renal failure, 444(t)
Abortion, spontaneous, 157–159
  classification of, 157
  nursing management in, 158–159
Abruptio placentae, 166–168, 238–242, **238, 239**
  assessment of, 167–168, 240
  classification of, 239–240
  hypovolemia from, 378
  nursing management in, 168, 241–242
  vs. placenta previa, 245(t)
Abscess, breast, 269
Acceptance, as stage of grief, 87
Achalasia, 504
Acid-base balance, and acute renal failure, 448
Acidosis, fetal, 147–148
  assessment of, 147
    nursing management in, 147–148
  hyperalichloremic metabolic, in parenteral hyperalimentation, 496(t)
  in neonatal hypoglycemic shock, 309
  in neonatal hypovolemic shock, 307
  in respiratory distress syndrome, 327, 330
Acute pulmonary vasoconstriction, neonatal, 356
Acute pyelonephritis, 174–175
  assessment of, 174
  nursing management in, 175
  postpartal, 269
Acute renal failure, 443, 446–451, 444–445(t)
  assessment of, 446–447
  nursing management in, 447–449
  postrenal, 446
  prerenal, 443
  renal, 446
Acute tubular necrosis, in hypovolemia, management of, 379–380
Admission, of perinatal transport patient, to high risk perinatal center, 48
Admission assessment, of patient in labor, 192–193, 194–195(t)

Adolescent parents, as factor in inhibition of bonding, 70(t), 71
Aganglionic megacolon, 504
Age
  fetal, estimation of, in assessment of well-being, 12(t)
  gestational, assessment of, 281
    small or large for, common problems of, 290(t)
  of father, in criteria for high risk pregnancy, 10(t)
  of mother, in criteria for high risk pregnancy, 10(t)
Agenesis, renal, causing acute renal failure, 443
Air block
  neonatal, 317–319
    assessment of, 317–318
    nursing management of, 318–319
Air transport
  of perinatal high risk patient, 28, **29**
    advantages and disadvantages of, 30(t)
    fixed-winged, 30(t), 32
    rotary-winged, 30(t), 32
    vs. ground transport, 28
Alcohol
  ethyl, as maternal drug, 589(t)
    intravenous administration of, 552–554
  maternal ingestion of, effect on infant, 361
Alkaline phosphatase
  in neonate, normal blood values, 462(t)
  serum, in parenteral hyperalimentation, 497(t)
Alkalosis, causing neonatal hypocalcemia, 436
Ambivalence, parental, toward high risk pregnancy, 102
Ambulance, in transport of perinatal high risk patient, 30(t), 32
Amikacin, dosage schedule, in newborn, 522(t)
Amino acid-glucose solution, in total parenteral nutrition, administration of, 607–608
Amino acids, in neonate, 461–462(t)
  metabolism of, in parenteral hyperalimentation, 496(t)
Amino acid solutions, in parenteral therapy, 486(t)
Aminophylline, in neonates, 642(t)
Amniocentesis, in assessment of fetal well-being, 12(t)
Amniography, in assessment of fetal well-being, 12(t)
Amnioscopy, in assessment of fetal well-being, 12(t)
Amniotic fluid embolism, 213–215
Amniotic fluid
  in assessment of fetal well-being, 12(t)
  meconium in, 332
    fetal distress due to, 230

Amniotic membrane, status of, tests for, 548–549
Ampicillin, dosage schedule, in newborn, 522(t)
Amyl nitrite, as maternal drug, 587(t)
Analgesia, obstetrical, causing intrapartum crisis, 254
Anemia(s), as pregnancy risk factor, 130
  hemolytic, hyperbilirubinemia in, 391
    as sign of cytomegalovirus infection, 527
  in criteria for high risk pregnancy, 11(t)
  in parenteral hyperalimentation, 497(t)
  in pregnancy, 188–190
  in toxoplasmosis, 523
Anesthesia
  obstetrical, causing intrapartum crisis, 254
    general, 255
    regional, 255
Anger, as stage of grief, 87
Ankle, clonus in, testing of, 551
  dorsiflexion of, in assessment of high risk neonate, 288, 289
Antepartal assessment, 154–157
Antepartum bleeding, as indication for high risk maternal/fetal transport, 39(t)
Antepartum risk scoring index, 128–129(t)
Antibiotics
  commonly prescribed, dosage schedule in newborn, 522(t)
  in herpes simplex infection, 533
  in sepsis due to group B beta hemolytic streptococcus and Listeria monocytogenes, 519, 520
Anticipatory grief, 88
Anticipatory guidance, by nurse, of childbearing family in crisis, 93
Anus, in assessment of high risk neonate, 285(t)
  imperforate, 504, 505(t)
Anxiety, level of, in crisis situations, 91–93
  relieving of, in nursing role for perinatal transport, 47, 54(t)
Aorta, coarctation of, 365
Aortic arch interruption, 365
Aortic stenosis, 365, 365
Apgar score, hypovolemia and, 378
  neonatal asphyxia and, 297, 297(t)
Apgar scoring
  method of, 596–597
  of high risk neonate, in assessment, 280, 280(t)
  precautions in, 597
Apnea, neonatal, common causes of, 338(t)
  in central nervous system failure, 327(t)
  in sepsis due to group B beta hemolytic streptococcus and Listeria monocytogenes, 518
  in pneumothorax, 342
Apneic episodes, neonatal, 337–341
  assessment of, 337–339
  nursing management in, 339–341
"Apple peel" small bowel, 507(t)
Apresoline, as maternal drug, 589(t)
  intravenous administration of, 559–561
Arizona, maternal/fetal transport in, 25
Arizona Regional Perinatal Program, maternal transport equipment list, 36(t)
Arm, recoil of, in assessment of high risk neonate, 288, 289
Arnold-Chiari type 2 malformation, with congenital hydrocephalus, 407
  with myelomeningocele, 404
Arterial blood gases
  in congenital heart defects, 369
  in persistent fetal circulation, 358, 359

Arterial blood gases (Continued)
  sampling of, from central line, 597–600
    related care, 599
  testing of, in neonatal resuscitation, 300
Asphyxia, 419–422
  causing hypovolemia, 377–378
  assessment of, 420–421
  nursing management of, 421–422
  neonatal, 295–303
    and Apgar score, 297, 297(t)
    fetal factors in, 296
    maternal factors in, 296
    nursing management of, 297–303
  perinatal, as indication for high risk maternal/fetal transport, 40(t)
Aspiration, in neonatal air block, 318–319
  meconium, 331–335
Aspiration pneumonia, 331–335
Aspiration syndromes, in persistent fetal circulation, 356
Assessment
  admission, of patient in labor, 192–193, 194–195(t)
  antepartal, 154–157
  in crisis situations, 90–93
  of family-infant bonding, 67, 67(t)
  of fetal well-being, methods of, 11, 12(t)
  of high risk maternal-fetal unit, 124–130, 128–129(t)
  of high risk neonate, 279–292
    equipment for, 290(t)
  of high risk perinatal patient,
    by transport team, 31
    in pre-transport process, 46
    nursing role in transport, 52(t)
  of maternal well-being, methods of, 11, 12(t)
  of perinatal risk factors, 7, 8
    vs. ground transport, 28
  of postpartal psychological risk, 273–274
  of risk, in perinatal care, future of, 541–542
  postpartum, 259
Atarax, 589(t)
Atony, gastric, 505(t)
  uterine, postpartum hemorrhage due to, 261
Atresia
  choanal, 349–351
    assessment of, 349
    nursing management of, 350–351
  duodenal, 506(t)
  esophageal, 506(t)
    with tracheoesophageal fistula, neonatal, 319–322
  gastrointestinal, 504
  jejunal and ileal, 506–507(t)
  pulmonary valve, 362
  tricuspid valve, 362
Atrial septal defect, 362
Atropine, in neonatal resuscitation, 301(t)
Attachment, parent-infant, enhancement of, in nursing role for perinatal transport, 54(t)
  vs. bonding, 66, 66(t)
Auscultation, in congenital heart defects, 368
  in congestive heart failure, 375

Back, in assessment of high risk neonate, 286(t)
Bacteremia, postpartal, 268–269
Bacterial meningitis, neonatal, 415–419
Bargaining, as stage of grief, 87
Barrel chest, in diaphragmatic hernia, 345

Basal metabolic rate, in normal neonate, 455(t)
Baseline data, of perinatal patient, in nursing role for perinatal transport, 52(t)
Beds, neonatal intensive care, system to locate, 19
Betamethasone, 587(t)
Bicarbonate, in neonatal resuscitation, 300, 301(t)
Biceps reflex, testing of, 550–551
Bilirubin, conjugation and excretion of, 390–391
Bimanual compression of uterus, 143, **143**
Biochemical testing, in assessment of fetal well-being, 12(t)
Biologic factors, influence of, on pregnancy and outcome, 9(t)
Biopsy, rectal, in Hirschsprung's disease, 508(t)
Biventricular mixing lesions, 365–367
Bleeding. See also *Hemorrhage*.
  in high risk pregnancy, 135
  in neonatal coagulopathies, 384
  in toxoplasmosis, 523
Blood, neonatal, hyperviscosity of, in persistent fetal circulation, 356
  whole, in parenteral therapy, 487(t)
Blood circulation
  fetal, 355
  fetal to neonatal, normal, 354–355
  neonatal, **355**
Blood clotting
  in normal newborn, 384
    deficiencies of, 384
    protein system in, **385**
Blood gases
  arterial, in congenital heart defects, 369
    in persistent fetal circulation, 358, 359
  sampling of, from central line, 597–600
  testing of, in neonatal resuscitation, 300
  in necrotizing enterocolitis, 498
Blood group, of father, in criteria for high risk pregnancy, 10(t)
Blood pressure, abnormal, in high risk pregnancy, 135
  in assessment of high risk neonate, 282(t)
Blood products, causing neonatal hypocalcemia, 436
Blood transfusion. See *Transfusion*.
Blood transfusion reaction, 487(t)
"Blues," postpartal, 273
Blurred vision, in high risk pregnancy, 135
Body movement, in family-infant bonding, 66(t)
Body proportions, in assessment of high risk neonate, 283(t)
Bonding
  family-infant, 64–79
    adaptive tasks of pregnancy for, 70(t)
    infant response in, 66
    inhibiting factors in, 70(t)
    nursing interventions to facilitate, 71–73
    nursing objectives in, 64
    nurse and, 67–71
    principles of, 65–66
    real or threatened loss and, 66
  in death or imminent death of newborn, 77–79
    nursing interventions in, 75–76
  parent-congenitally deformed infant, nursing interventions in, 76–77
  parent-high risk infant, nursing interventions to facilitate, 73–75
  parent-transported infant, nursing interventions in, 75–76
  vs. attachment, 66, 66(t)
Bowel
  decompression of, in gastrointestinal obstruction, 509

Bowel *(Continued)*
  large, obstruction of, 505(t)
    malrotation of, 507(t)
  small, obstruction of, 505(t)
Bradycardia, fetal, 232
Brain scan, in asphyxia, **420**
Breast(s)
  abscess of, 269
  engorgement of, postpartal, 269
  in assessment of high risk neonate, 285(t), 287(t)
  infections of, postpartal, 269
  postpartum educational needs related to, 260(t)
Breast feeding, in assessment of family-infant bonding, 67(t)
  of high risk infant, in bonding process, 75
Breast milk
  in management of acute renal failure, 448
  suggested regimens for feeding, 476–477(t)
  trace elements in, 472(t)
Breathing, onset of, in neonate, 326
Breech presentation, 222–223, **224**
Brethine, as maternal drug, 594(t)
Bricanyl, as maternal drug, 594(t)
Brow presentation, 221–222
Bulb syringe, in suctioning, 626–627
Bullae, in scalded skin syndrome, 532
BUN, in neonate, normal blood values, 462(t)
  serum, in neonatal acute renal failure, 446
Bupivacaine, as maternal drug, 587(t)
Burning urination, in high risk pregnancy, 135
Burnout, of intensive care nurse, reduction of, 115
Butorphanol, as maternal drug, 587(t)
Butterfly needles, in peripheral cannulation, 622, 623

Caffeine, as neonatal drug, 643(t)
Calcitonin, in neonatal hypercalcemia, 439
Calcium
  in neonate, assessment of, 464
    normal blood values, 464(t)
  intestinal malabsorption of, causing neonatal hypocalcemia, 436
  metabolism of, 435
    in parenteral hyperalimentation, 496(t)
  neonatal requirements, 457(t)
  oral, in treatment of serum calcium imbalances, 438
  serum. See *Serum calcium*.
Calcium chloride, in neonatal resuscitation, 300, 301(t)
Calcium gluconate, causing neonatal hypercalcemia, 436
  in treatment of neonatal acute renal failure, 448
Calcium gluconate injection, as maternal drug, 588(t)
Calorie intake, neonatal, assessment of, 457
Calorie requirements, of normal neonate, 455(t)
  factors increasing, 458
Calories, in neonatal reading, assessment record of, **483**
Cannulation, peripheral, 619–624
Caput succedaneum, in assessment of high risk neonate, 283(t)
Carbenicillin, dosage schedule, in newborn, 522(t)
Carbohydrate(s)
  in neonate, assessment of, 460(t)
    normal blood values, 460(t)
    requirements, 457(t)
Carbohydrate malabsorption, formula for feeding in, 481(t)
Cardiac arrest, maternal, 138–140

Cardiac arrest, maternal *(Continued)*
    assessment of, 138
    nursing management of, 138–140
Cardiac catheterization, in congenital heart defects, 370
Cardiac compression, in maternal cardiac arrest, 139–140
Cardiogenic shock, neonatal, 314–316
    assessment of, 315
    nursing management of, 315–316
Cardiopulmonary resuscitation, quick reference guide to, **323**
Cardiorespiratory monitor, in exchange transfusion, 603, 604
Cardiovascular disorders, as pregnancy risk factor, 128(t)
Care givers, high risk, 16
    education of, **16**, 17
Catheter
    central venous line, care of, 606–613
    intrauterine pressure, application of, 561–564
    umbilical, in neonatal resuscitation, 300
    arterial or venous, placement of, 638–641
Catheterization, cardiac, in congenital heart defects, 370
    in hyperalimentation, guidelines for, 490(t)
Celestone, as maternal drug, 587(t)
Central nervous system failure, 326, 327(t)
Central vein, in hyperalimentation, 607
Central venous line, arterial blood gas sampling from, 597–600
    catheter care in, 606–613
Cerebrospinal fluid, circulation of, **407**
Cervix, lacerations of, postpartum hemorrhage due to, 261–262
    postpartal infections of, 267
Cesarean section, as pregnancy risk factor, 130
    impending, 145–146
        assessment of, 145
        nursing management in, 145–146
    previous, in criteria for high risk pregnancy, 10(t)
Chart, crisis intensity, 545
Chest, barrel, in diaphragmatic hernia, 345
    space occupying lesions of, 356, 357
Chest intubation, 600–603
Chest lag, in neonatal peripheral respiratory difficulty, 327(t)
Chest tube, placement of, in neonatal air block, 319
Chest x-ray
    in congenital heart defects, 364, 369–370
    in congestive heart failure, 375
    in neonatal air block, 318
    in persistent fetal circulation, 358
Childbearing family
    assessment of, for perinatal risk factors, 7, 8
    in crisis, coping resources of, 85–86
        evaluation of, 82
        importance of professional assistance to, 82
        importance of quality of relationships in, 82
        meaning of crisis situation for, 82
        nursing management of, 93–94
    of infant in intensive care, impact on, 110–111
        nursing care of, 111–113
    response to crisis, 88–90
Childbirth. See also under specific topics.
    anesthesia in, 254–256
    trauma of, and neonatal asphyxia, 296
Chin tug, in neonatal peripheral respiratory difficulty, 327(t)
Chloramphenicol, dosage schedule, in newborn, 522(t)
Chloride, in neonate, assessment of, 470(t)

Chloride *(Continued)*
    neonatal requirements, 457(t)
Chloroprocaine, as maternal drug, 588(t)
Choanal atresia, 349–351
    assessment of, 349
    nursing management of, 350–351
Cho-Free, 480(t)
Cholesterol, in neonate, normal blood values, 462(t)
Chromosomal defects, in congenital heart defects, 361
Chronic disease, of parents, in criteria for high risk pregnancy, 10–11(t)
Chronic intrauterine hypoxia, 357
    causing hyperviscosity syndrome, 381
Chvostek sign, in neonatal hypocalcemia, 436, 437
Citrobacter, in neonatal meningitis, 416
Clinical decision making, by high risk perinatal transport team, 31
Clinistix, in assessment of neonatal hyperglycemia, 432, 434
Clinitest, 491(t)
    in assessment of neonatal hyperglycemia, 432, 434
Clonus, testing of, 551
Clotting factors, **384**
Coach, in transport of perinatal high risk patient, 30(t), 32
Coagulopathies, neonatal, 383–390
    assessment of, 387–388
    in sick infant, etiology of, 386–387
    in well infant, etiology of, 385–386
    nursing management in, 388–390
    predisposing factors, in sick infant, 384
        in well infant, 383
    screening tests for, 388(t)
Coarctation of aorta, congestive heart failure from, 374
Communication
    pre-transport, 40–46
    post-transport, 48–49
    with perinatal family, in nursing role for perinatal transport, 54(t)
    with primary care nurse, in nursing role for perinatal transport, 50(t)
    within childbearing family in crisis, 82, 88–89
Community-based transport, to regional perinatal care center, 18
Community hospitals
    as part of regionalized perinatal intensive care program, 19
    definition of, 19
    high risk services and, 19
Computerized techniques, in perinatal care planning, 546
Computerized tomogram
    in intracranial hemorrhage, **424**
    in myelomeningocele, 403, **403, 404**
    in neonatal meningitis, **417**
Congenital heart defects, 360–372
    assessment of, 362–369
    etiology of, 361–362
    nursing management in, at hospital of birth, 370–371
        at perinatal center, 371–372
    predisposing factors in, 361
    surgical treatment of, 371–372
Congenital heart disease, 357
    and gastrointestinal atresia, 506(t)
Congenital malformations, as indication for high risk maternal/fetal transport, 40(t)
Congenitally deformed infant, bonding of, nursing interventions in, 76–77
Congestive heart failure, neonatal, 372–376

Congestive heart failure, neonatal *(Continued)*
    assessment of, 374–375
    etiology of, 373–374
    nursing management in, 375–376
Conjunctivitis, in ophthalmia, 530
Continuous positive airway pressure, 330
Contractions
    monitoring of, 554–556
        interpretation in, 556–557
        by intrauterine pressure catheter, 561–564
    tetanic, 146–147
        nursing management in, 146–147
Coombs' test, in hyperbilirubinemia, 392, 393
Coordination of resources, by nurse, of childbearing
    family in crisis, 93
Coordinator, in pre-transport communication process,
    46
Cord
    in assessment of high risk neonate, 285(t)
    milking of, hyperviscosity syndrome from, 380
    prolapse of, 205–208, **206**
        as pregnancy risk factor, 131
        assessment of, 206–207
        nursing management of, 207–208
Cord clamping, early, hypovolemia from, 378
    late, hyperviscosity syndrome from, 380
Cow's milk, whole, causing neonatal hypocalcemia,
    436
CPAP, 330
Creases, plantar, in assessment of high risk neonate,
    286(t), 287(t)
Creatinine, in neonate, normal blood values, 462(t)
Crisis
    general principles of, 98
    response of childbearing family to, criteria for
        evaluation of, 82
    situational, high risk pregnancy as, 101–103, 101(t)
Crisis intensity chart, 545
Crisis theory, 85–86
Cry, in assessment of high risk neonate, 282(t)
    in neonatal meningitis, 521
Cultural belief systems, and childbearing family in
    crisis, 84–85
Cultural factors, in criteria for high risk pregnancy,
    10(t)
Cultural needs, community, in regionalization process,
    14
Curare, in neonates, 643(t)
Cutaneous infections, 532(t)
CVM infection, 526–527
Cyanosis
    caused by overhydration in parenteral therapy,
        488(t)
    central, in persistent fetal circulation, 357, 362
    in congenital heart defects, 362
    in hyperviscosity syndrome, 380
    in neonatal hypovolemic shock, 307
    in neonatal urinary tract infection, 530
    in respiratory distress syndrome, 329
    in transposition of great arteries, 364
Cystitis, postpartal, 269
Cysts, lung, in persistent fetal circulation, 357
    neonatal, 327(t)
Cytomegalovirus infection, 526–527
    assessment of, 526
    problems and complications of, 527
    transmission of, 526

Data retrieval system, as part of regional dispatch
    system in neonatal intensive care, 19
Death, intrauterine fetal, 236–238
    of newborn, and parents, 77–79
Deceleration, early, of fetal heart rate, 232, **232**
    nursing management of, 232
    late, of fetal heart rate, 234–235, **234**
Decision making, clinical, by high risk perinatal
    transport team, 31
    in stabilization of patient in pre-transport process,
        46
Decreased peripheral perfusion, in congestive heart
    failure, 375
Decreased variability, fetal heart rate, 235–236
Deep tendon reflexes, testing of, 549–551
Deformed infant, bonding of, nursing interventions
    in, 76–77
Dehydration, neonatal, causing hypercalcemia, 435
DeLee apparatus, in suctioning, 627–628
    method for, 627–628
DeLee trap, in neonatal asphyxia, 299
Delivery, cesarean. See *Cesarean section.*
    emergency, 149–152
        assessment of, 149
        nursing management in, 149–152
    stresses of, 105–106
Delphi process, in perinatal care planning, 546
Demerol, as maternal drug, 591(t)
Denial, as stage of grief, 86
Depression
    as pregnancy risk factor, 131
    as stage of grief, 87
    of neonatal respiratory center, 326
    postpartal, 272–275
Dextrose, in treatment of neonatal hyperglycemia,
    435
Dextrose solutions, in parenteral therapy, 486(t)
Dextrostix
    in congenital heart defects, 369
    in neonatal hyperglycemia, 432
    in neonatal hypoglycemia, 310, 432, 433–434
    testing by, in neonatal resuscitation, 303
Diabetes mellitus, as indication for high risk maternal/
    fetal transport, 39
    as pregnancy risk factor, 125, 128(t), 130
    in pregnancy, 181–184
        assessment of, 182–183
    White's classification of, 182
Diabetic mother, infant of. See *Infant of diabetic
    mother.*
Diagnosis, pregnancy, high risk categories in, 122
Diagnostic testing, of perinatal patient, in nursing
    role for perinatal transport, 52(t)
Dialysis, peritoneal, in management of acute renal
    failure, 448
Diaphoresis, in neonatal hypoglycemic shock, 310
Diaphragmatic hernia
    neonatal, 327(t), 344–348
        assessment of, 345
        in persistent fetal circulation, 357
        nursing management of, 345–348
Diarrhea, in necrotizing enterocolitis, 499, 500
Diarrheal disease, 531–532
DIC. See *Disseminated intravascular coagulopathy.*
Digoxin
    in congestive heart failure, 375
    in neonatal cardiogenic shock, 316
    in neonates, 644(t)
Dilocaine, as maternal drug, 590(t)
Dinoprostone, as maternal drug, 593(t)
Disseminated herpes simplex infection, 528

Disseminated intravascular coagulopathy
  antepartal, 170–172
    assessment of, 170–171
    nursing management in, 172
  intrapartal, 247–249
    assessment of, 248
    nursing management of, 248–249
  neonatal, exchange transfusion in, 603
    trigger events for, 386, 386(t)
  postpartum, as pregnancy risk factor, 131
Diving seal reflex, and necrotizing enterocolitis, 489
Divorce, in childbearing family in crisis, 82
Documentation, of transport process, in nursing role
    for perinatal transport, 57(t)
Dopamine hydrochloride, in neonates, 644(t)
Double setup, 551–552
  method for, 551–552
Down's syndrome
  congenital heart defects in, 361
  duodenal atresia in, 506(t)
  hyperviscosity syndrome in, 381
Drain(s), in intracranial hemorrhage, 426
  intraventricular, insertion of, 613, 615
Dressings, in hyperalimentation, change of, 609–612
Drugs, maternal. See names of specific drugs.
  neonatal. See under Neonatal drugs.
Dubowitz system, in assessment of gestational age, 281
  in assessment of high risk neonate, 287(t), 288
Duodenal atresia, 506(t)
Duodenal stenosis, 507(t)
Duplication, gastrointestinal, 504
Dysfunctional labor, 208–213
  assessment of, 209–211
  nursing management in, 211–213
  patterns of, comparison of, 209, 209(t)
Dysplasia, renal, associated with neonatal renal failure,
    444(t)
Dyspnea, caused by overhydration in parenteral
    therapy, 488(t)
Dystocia, as pregnancy risk factor, 130

Early deceleration, of fetal heart rate, 232, **232**
  nursing management of, 232
Ears, in assessment of high risk neonate, 284(t), 287(t)
Ecchymoses, in neonatal coagulopathies, 384
ECG. See Electrocardiogram.
Echocardiogram, in congenital heart defects, 370
Eclampsia
  as intrapartum crisis, 198–199
  classification of, 178
  causing neonatal hypocalcemia, 435, 436
  causing neonatal hypoglycemia, 432, 433
  magnesium sulfate in, intravenous administration of,
    556–568
Eclamptic seizure, 143–144
  assessment of, 144
  nursing management in, 144, 181
Economic factors, influence of, on pregnancy and
    outcome, 9(t)
Ectopic pregnancy, 159–161
  assessment of, 160
  implantation sites of, **160**
  nursing management in, 161
  previous, as risk factor in pregnancy, 130
Edema
  in assessment of high risk neonate, 287(t)
  maternal, in high risk pregnancy, 135
  neonatal, in acute renal failure, 446

EDTA, in neonatal hypercalcemia, 439
Education, of new mother, postpartum needs, 260(t)
  of transport personnel, 27, 41
Elective procedures, in stabilization of perinatal
    patient for transport, 47
Electrocardiogram
  fetal, spiral electrode application in, 578–579
  neonatal, in acute renal failure, 448
    in congenital heart defects, 370
    in congestive heart failure, 375
    in hypercalcemia, 437
Electrode, spiral, application of, 578–579
  transcutaneous, in measurement of oxygen, 632, 633
Electrolytes, basic, in neonate, assessment of,
    464–471(t)
Electrolyte imbalance, in parenteral therapy,
    488–489(t)
Embolism, amniotic fluid, 213–215
    assessment of, 213–214
    nursing management of, 214–215
Emotional factors, influence of, on pregnancy and
    outcome, 9(t)
Emotional immaturity, parental, as factor in inhibition
    of bonding, 70(t), 71
Emotional needs, of high risk perinatal families,
    importance of, 17
Emotional state, of mother, in criteria for high risk
    pregnancy, 10(t)
    postpartum educational needs related to, 260(t)
Emotional support systems, lack of, as factor in
    inhibition of bonding, 70(t), 71
Emphysema, lobar, neonatal, 327(t)
Encephalitis, as sign of herpes simplex infection, 528
Endocardial cushion defect, 366, 367
Endotracheal intubation, 616–619
Endotracheal tube, displacement of, in infant in
    ventilator, 346(t)
  sterile, in suctioning, 628–629
Enfamil, 478(t)
Engle-Barrett syndrome, associated with neonatal
    renal failure, 444(t)
Engorgement, of breasts, postpartal, 269
Enterocolitis, necrotizing, hyperviscosity syndrome
    causing, 380
  in hypovolemia, management of, 379
Environmental factors, influence of, on pregnancy
    and outcome, 9(t)
Environmental toxins, causing congenital heart
    defects, 361
Ephedrine, as maternal drug, 589(t)
Epidural block, in obstetrical anesthesia, 255
Epigastric pain, in high risk pregnancy, 135
Epinephrine, in neonatal resuscitation, 300, 301(t)
Equipment
  checking of, in nursing role for perinatal transport,
    50(t)
  for maternal/fetal transport, 35, 36(t)
  for neonatal transport, 35, 37, 38(t)
  for perinatal transport, monitoring of, 48
  restocking of, in nursing role for perinatal transport,
    58(t)
Ergonovine maleate, as maternal drug, 588(t)
Ergotrate maleate, as maternal drug, 588(t)
Escherichia coli, in neonatal infection, 516
  in neonatal meningitis, 415, 416
Esophageal atresia, 506(t)
  with tracheoesophageal fistula, neonatal, 319–322
Esophageal fistula, 506(t)
Esophageal sphincter, lower, and neonatal ability and
    readiness to feed, 456

Esophagus, neonatal, malformations of, **320**
Ethanol, as maternal drug, 589(t)
  intravenous administration of, 552–554
Ethyl alcohol, as maternal drug, 589(t)
  intravenous administration of, 552–554
Examination, of perinatal patient, in nursing role
  for perinatal transport, 52(t)
Exchange transfusion, 603–606
  method of, 604–605
  precautions in, 606
Expiratory grunt, in neonatal peripheral respiratory
  difficulty, 327(t)
External fetal monitor, 554–556
  precautions in, 556
  strip interpretation in, 556–559
Extrauterine pregnancy, previous, as pregnancy risk
  factor, 130
Extremity(ies), cannulation in, method of, 623–624
  in assessment of high risk neonate, 286(t)
Eye(s), in assessment of high risk neonate, 284(t)
  infection of, 530(t)
Eye contact, in family-infant bonding, 66(t)

Face presentation, 220–221, **220**
Failure, parental feelings of, at unsuccessful pregnancy,
  102, 107
Fallot, tetralogy of, 362, 363
Family, childbearing. See also *Childbearing family.*
  future of, 543
  of high risk perinate, 4
    and nurse, 4
  perinatal, contact with, in nursing role for transport,
    51(t), 58(t)
Family centered care
  concept of, in regionalized perinatal care centers, 17
  in high risk delivery setting, **3**
  reconciled with regionalized high risk perinatal care,
    18
Family history, in criteria for high risk pregnancy,
  10(t)
Family life, disruption of, in crisis, 89–90
Family physician, importance of, to high risk perinatal
  families, 17
Father
  as bonding figure, 71–72
  characteristics of, in criteria for high risk pregnancy,
    10(t)
  contact with, in nursing role for perinatal transport,
    51(t)
Fat(s)
  in neonate, assessment of, 462(t)
    malabsorption of, formula for feeding in, 481(t)
    requirements, 457(t)
Fatty acids, essential, metabolism of, in parenteral
  hyperalimentation, 497(t)
  free, in neonate, normal blood values, 463(t)
Feeding regimens, suggested, based on weight and
  age at birth, 476–477(t)
Feet, in assessment of high risk neonate, 286(t)
Female genitals, in assessment of high risk neonate,
  285(t)
Femoral pulse, in assessment of high risk neonate,
  285(t)
Fern test, of amniotic membrane, 549
Fetal acidosis, 147–148
  assessment of, 147
  nursing management in, 147–148

Fetal alcohol syndrome, congenital heart defects in,
  361
Fetal circulation, **355**
Fetal death, intrauterine, 236–238
Fetal distress, 229–236
Fetal growth, serial measurements of, in assessment of
  fetal well-being, 12(t)
Fetal heart rate
  abnormalities of, 231–236
  accelerations of, 558
  baseline, 231, **231**
  decelerations of, 558
    early, 232–233, **232**
    late, 234–235, **234**
    variable, 233–234, **233**
  decreased variability of, 235–236
  external monitoring of, 554–556
    interpretation of, 556–559
  in assessment of well-being, 12(t)
  in neonatal asphyxia, 229
  non-stress test and, 568–569
Fetal heart tones, in assessment of high risk fetal/
  maternal unit, 130
Fetal hypoxemia, 147–148
  assessment of, 147
  nursing management in, 147–148
Fetal medicine, future of, 542
Fetal monitor
  external, 554–556
    precautions in, 556
    strip interpretation in, 556–559
Fetal scalp sampling, in hypoxemia and acidosis, 147,
  148
Fetal weight, in assessment of well-being, 12(t)
Fetus
  age of, estimation of, in assessment of well-being,
    12(t)
  high risk, identification of, 122–124
    in maternal/fetal transport, 24–28
  malposition of, 215–218
    in criteria for high risk pregnancy, 11(t)
    nursing management of, 218
  malpresentation of, 218–225
    nursing management of, 219
  movements of, in assessment of well-being, 12(t)
  non-stress test of, 568–570
  well-being of, assessment of, 11, 12(t)
Fever, in high risk pregnancy, 135
  in neonatal herpes simplex, 528
  in neonatal meningitis, 417
  in neonatal toxoplasmosis, 523
Fistula
  esophageal, 506(t)
  tracheoesophageal, nursing management in, 321–322
    with esophageal atresia, neonatal, 319–322
Fixed-winged air transport, of perinatal high risk
  patient, 30(t), 32
Flaring, of nares, in choanal atresia, 349
  in respiratory distress syndrome, 329
Flow rate, in hyperalimentation, 491(t)
  of IV fluids, 484(t)
Fluid and electrolyte balance, maintenance of, in
  gastrointestinal obstruction, 510
  in herpes simplex infection, 535–536
  in neonatal diarrhea, 531
Fluid(s), intravenous, nurse's role in administering,
  484(t)
Fluid intake, neonatal, assessment of, 457, **483**
  increased, in parenteral therapy, 488(t)

Fluid requirements, neonatal, 455
    factors increasing, 458
Follow-up, in nursing role for perinatal transport,
    58(t), 59(t)
Fontanel(s), in assessment of high risk neonate, 283(t)
    in neonatal herpes simplex, 528
    in neonatal meningitis, 521
Foramen ovale, 362, 364
Form(s), crisis intensity chart, 545
    for neonatal resuscitation medication, **302, 304–305**
    for neonatal transport, **42–45**
Formula(s), components, effects, and indications for,
    478–482(t)
    milk-based, 478(t)
    modular, 482(t)
    suggested regimens in, 476–477(t)
Frothing, at lips, in neonatal peripheral respiratory
    difficulty, 327(t)
Fundus, height of, measurement of, 559
Furosemide, in neonates, 645(t)
    in cardiogenic shock, 316
    in congestive heart failure, 375
Furuncles, in neonatal cutaneous infections, 532

Gases, blood. See *Blood gases.*
    trapped, in perinatal patient in transport, 48
        monitoring for, in nursing role for perinatal
            transport, 56(t)
Gasping, in neonatal central nervous system failure,
    327(t)
Gastric atony, 505(t)
Gastric capacity, neonatal, 456
Gastric distention, in infant in ventilator, 347(t)
Gastric emptying, neonatal, 456–457
Gastrointestinal obstruction, 504–512
    assessment of, 504–509
    classification of, 504
    locations of, 505(t)
    nursing management in, 509–511
Gastrointestinal tract, infection of, 531–532
Gastroschisis, and omphalocele, 500–503
    assessment of, 501
    nursing management in, 501–503
Gavage, method of, 635–637
General obstetrical anesthesia, 255
Genetic diagnosis, antenatal, in assessment of fetal
    well-being, 12(t)
Genital herpes, 527–529, 533–537
Genital herpes simplex viral infection, 177
    nursing management in, 177
Genitals, in assessment of high risk neonate, 285(t),
    287(t)
Genitourinary anomalies, and gastrointestinal atresia,
    506(t)
Gentamicin, dosage schedule, in newborn, 522(t)
Gestational age
    estimation of, by fundal height, 559
    of high risk neonate, assessment of, 281
    reading of, 291
    small or large for, common problems of, 290(t)
Glucagon, in treatment of neonatal hypoglycemia, 434
Glucose
    in neonatal resuscitation, 300, 301(t)
    in treatment of neonatal hypoglycemia, 310, 434
    metabolism of, in parenteral hyperalimentation,
        496(t)
    serum. See *Serum glucose.*
Glucose water, suggested regimens for feeding, 476(t)

Glycosuria, in hyperalimentation, 491(t)
    in parenteral therapy, 485(t)
Grades, of heart murmurs, 369
Great arteries, transposition of, 362, 364–365, **364**
    congestive heart failure from, 375
Grief
    anticipatory, 88
    as emotional response, 87–88
    process of, in intrauterine fetal death, 237–238
        in parents of congenitally deformed infant, 77
        in parents of high risk infant, 74
    stages of, in childbearing family in crisis, 86–87
Ground transport, of perinatal high risk patient, 28, **29**
    advantages and disadvantages of, 30(t)
    vs. air transport, 28
Group B beta hemolytic streptococcus, in neonatal
    septic shock, 312
    sepsis due to, 518–520
Group B streptococcus, in neonatal meningitis, 415,
    416
Growth, of fetus, in assessment of well-being, 12(t)
Growth retardation, in cytomegalovirus infection, 527
Grunt, expiratory, in neonatal peripheral respiratory
    difficulty, 327(t)
    in pneumothorax, 342
Guidance, anticipatory, by nurse, of childbearing
    family in crisis, 93

Halothane, in obstetrical anesthesia, 255
Hands, in assessment of high risk neonate, 286(t), 288,
    289
Head, in assessment of high risk neonate, 283–284(t)
Head lag, in assessment of high risk neonate, **288,** 289
Headache, severe, in high risk pregnancy, 135
Health care institution, in perinatal transport,
    definition of, 23
Heart, in assessment of high risk neonate, 282(t)
Heart defects
    congenital, 360–372
        etiology of, 361–362
        nursing management in, at hospital of birth,
            370–271
        surgical treatment of, 371–372
Heart disease
    classification of, 185(t)
    congenital, 357
        and gastrointestinal atresia, 506(t)
    in pregnancy, 184–187
        assessment of, 185–186
        nursing management in, 186
Heart rate, fetal. See *Fetal heart rate.*
    neonatal, in hypovolemia, 378
Heart sounds, normal, 368–369
Heel to ear maneuver, in assessment of high risk
    neonate, **288,** 289
Heel stick, in assessment of hyperviscosity syndrome,
    382
Helicopter, in transport of perinatal high risk patient,
    29, 30(t), 32
Hematocrit
    determination of, in neonatal resuscitation, 303
    in hyperviscosity syndrome, 382
    in neonatal hypovolemic shock, 306
    in persistent fetal circulation, 358
    in respiratory distress syndrome, 330
Hematological data, in necrotizing enterocolitis, 498
Hematoma
    postpartum hemorrhage due to, 262–263

Hematoma *(Continued)*
  nursing management in, 262–263
  subdural, 423
Hemolytic anemia, as sign of cytomegalovirus
    infection, 527
  hyperbilirubinemia in, 391
Hemolytic incompatibility, 169–170
Hemophilia A and B, 386
Hemorrhage
  antepartum, as indication for high risk maternal/
    fetal transport, 39(t)
  in high risk pregnancy, 135
  intracranial, 423–427
    assessment of, 424–425
    classification of, 423
    nursing management in, 425–427
  hypovolemia from, 378
  maternal, 140–143
    assessment of, 141
    nursing management of, 141–143
  postpartum, 259–263
    as pregnancy risk factor, 131
    conditions that predispose to, 261(t)
Hemorrhagic disease of newborn, 385–386
Heparin sodium, in neonates, 645(t)
Hepatitis, as sign of syphilis, 525
Hepatomegaly, in congestive heart failure, 374
Hepatosplenomegaly, in toxoplasmosis, 523
Hernia, diaphragmatic. See *Diaphragmatic hernia.*
Herpes simplex infection, 527–529, 533–537
  assessment of, 528
  disseminated, 528
  genital, 175–177
    assessment of, 176
    nursing management in, 177
  nursing management in, 529, 533–537
  problems and complications in, 528–529
  transmission of, 527–528
High risk fetus, identification of, 122–124
High risk infant, bonding and, 73–75
  transported, bonding and, 75–76
High risk maternal-fetal unit, assessment of, 121–130,
    121
High risk perinatal care, regionalized, definition of, 14
High risk perinatal center
  and referring hospital, pre-transport communication
    between, 41
  post-transport communication within, 48
  pre-transport communication within, 46
High risk pregnancy
  as situational crisis, 101–103, 101(t)
  assessment of, 121–130, **121**
  criteria for, 8, 10–11(t)
  identification of, 8, 9–11(t)
Hirschsprung's disease, 505(t), 508(t)
History
  as pregnancy risk factor, 128(t)
  medical/surgical, influence of, on pregnancy and
    outcome, 9(t)
  obstetric/gynecologic, influence of, on pregnancy
    and outcome, 9(t)
  pregnancy, high risk categories in, 121–122
Holosystolic murmur, 369
Hospital(s), community. See also *Community hospitals.*
  referring, post-transport communication in, 41
    pre-transport communication in, 41
Hostility, as reaction to high risk pregnancy, 102
  as stage of grief, 87
Hot line, to high risk perinatal center, in pre-transport
    communication process, 46

Hyaline membrane disease, 326–331. See also
    Respiratory distress syndrome.
  in air block, 317
Hydatidiform mole, 162–163
Hydralazine, as maternal drug, 589(t)
  intravenous administration of, 559–561
Hydrating solutions, in parenteral therapy, 486(t)
Hydrocephalus, 406–411
  assessment of, 408–409
  nursing management in, 409–411
  with myelomeningocele, 404, 405
Hydrocortisone, in neonatal hypoglycemia, 434–435
  in neonatal hypoglycemic shock, 311
Hydroxyzine, as maternal drug, 589(t)
Hyperalimentation
  neonatal, 461–462(t)
    central venous line care in, 606–613
    complications in, 613
    guidelines for, 490–494
    precautions in, 612
    related nursing care in, 612–613
  parenteral, metabolic problems in, 496–497(t)
Hyperammonemia, in parenteral hyperalimentation,
    496(t)
Hyperbilirubinemia, 390–395
  assessment of, 391–392
  common causes of, 391
  exchange transfusion in, 603
  nursing management in, 393–395
Hypercalcemia
  definition of, 435
  in parenteral hyperalimentation, 497(t)
  intravenous fluids in, 439
  kidney insult in, 437
  predisposing factors, 435–436
Hyperchloremia, causes of, in infant at risk, 471(t)
Hyperchloremic metabolic acidosis, in parenteral
    hyperalimentation, 496(t)
Hyperemesis gravidarum, 172–174
  as pregnancy risk factor, 130
  assessment of, 172–173
  nursing management in, 172–174
Hyperglycemia
  neonatal, 461(t)
    definition of, 430
    predisposing factors, 430–431
    in parenteral hyperalimentation, 496(t)
Hyperkalemia
  causes of, in infants at risk, 466(t)
  in neonatal acute renal failure, 448
  in parenteral hyperalimentation, 497(t)
  in parenteral therapy, 489(t)
Hypermagnesemia
  causes of, in infant at risk, 470(t)
  neonatal, assessment of, 441
    nursing management in, 442–443
    predisposing factors in, 440
Hypernatremia, causes of, in infant at risk, 468–469(t)
Hyperosmolar solutions, in parenteral therapy,
    486–487(t)
Hyperparathyroidism, maternal, causing neonatal
    hypocalcemia, 435, 436
Hyperreflexia, in high risk pregnancy, 135
Hypertension
  as indication for high risk maternal/fetal transport,
    39
  pregnancy induced, as antepartal crisis, 177–181
    assessment of, 179
    nursing management of, 180–181
    complications of, as intrapartal crisis, 193, 196–199

Hyperventilation, from respirators, causing neonatal hypocalcemia, 436
in persistent fetal circulation, 359
Hyperviscosity, of neonatal blood, in persistent fetal circulation, 356
Hyperviscosity syndrome, 380–383
assessment of, 381–382
exchange transfusion in, 603
nursing management in, 382–383
Hypervitaminosis A, in parenteral hyperalimentation, 497(t)
Hypervitaminosis D, in parenteral hyperalimentation, 497(t)
Hypocalcemia
definition of, 435
in parenteral hyperalimentation, 497(t)
neonatal, assessment of, 436–437
calcium therapy in, 438
predisposing factors, 435
Hypochloremia, causes of, in infant at risk, 470(t)
Hypoglycemia
neonatal, 460(t)
assessment of, 431–432
definition of, 430
glucose replacement in, 434
nursing management in, 433–435
predisposing factors, 430
postinfusion, in parenteral hyperalimentation, 496(t)
symptomatic, therapy in, 460–461(t)
Hypoglycemic shock, neonatal, 308–311
Hypokalemia
causes of, in infants at risk, 465(t)
in parenteral hyperalimentation, 497(t)
in parenteral therapy, 488–489(t)
Hypomagnesemia
definition of, 439
in parenteral hyperalimentation, 497(t)
neonatal, assessment of, 441
causes of, in infant at risk, 469(t)
nursing management in, 442
Hyponatremia, causes of, in infant at risk, 467–468(t)
Hypoparathyroidism, maternal, causing fetal hypercalcemia, 436
Hypoperfusion, renal, neonatal, causing acute renal failure, 443
Hypophosphatemia, in parenteral hyperalimentation, 496(t)
Hypoplasia, lung, in persistent fetal circulation, 357
Hypoplastic left heart syndrome, 365
Hypotension, in infant in ventilator, 346(t)
in neonatal hypovolemic shock, 307
Hypothermia, in gastrointestinal obstruction, prevention of, 510
in omphalocele and gastroschisis, 501
Hypovolemia
neonatal, 306–308
assessment of, 378–379
etiology of, 377–378
nursing management in, 379–380
predisposing factors, 377
Hypovolemic shock, neonatal, 306–308
Hypoxemia
birth, as risk factor, 123
fetal, 147–148
assessment of, 147
nursing management in, 147–148
in perinatal patient, in transport, 48
nursing role in, 56(t)

Hypoxemia (Continued)
in treatment of neonatal septic shock, 312
intrauterine, chronic, 357
causing hyperviscosity syndrome, 381
resulting from apnea, 337
Hypoxic ischemic encephalopathy, caused by asphyxia, 419

Idiopathic respiratory distress, neonatal, 327(t)
IgA, and newborn, 514
IgC, fetal, 514
IMED casette, in administration of oxytocin, 573, 574
Imminent death, of newborn, and parents, 77–79
Immune thrombocytopenia, 385
Immunoglobulins, and newborn, 514–515
Imperforate anus, 504, 505(t), 508(t)
Incubator, transport, in high risk neonatal transport, 37
Infant. See also Neonate.
ability and readiness to feed of, 456–457
emergency delivery of, 148–152
high risk, bonding and, 73–75
transported, bonding and, 75–76
in intensive care, as postpartal crisis, 109–113
nutritional requirements of, 453, 454, 457(t)
factors increasing, 455–456
multiple gestational, in family-infant bonding, 65
premature, nutritional deprivation in, 454
small or large for gestational age, common problems of, 290(t)
vitamin requirements of, 457(t)
Infant of diabetic mother
congenital heart defects in, 361
hyperviscosity syndrome in, 381
hypocalcemia in, 435, 436
hypoglycemia in, 432, 433
hypomagnesemia in, 440
Infant formulas, components, effects, and indications for, 478–482(t)
Infant warmers. See Radiant warmers.
Infections
as indication for high risk maternal/fetal transport, 40(t)
as pregnancy risk factor, 131
genital, herpes simplex viral, 175–177
neonatal, 516–517
common local, 530–532(t)
necrotizing enterocolitis and, 489
predisposing factors in, 516
postpartal, 266–272
puerperal, 266–272
Infiltration, in parenteral therapy, 484(t)
Injection site, in parenteral therapy, 484(t)
Intensive care, infant in, as postpartal crisis, 109–113
Intercostal retractions, in neonatal peripheral respiratory difficulty, 327(t)
Intestine. See Bowel.
Intracath, in parenteral therapy, 485(t)
Intracranial hemorrhage, 423–427
assessment of, 424–425
classification of, 423
nursing management in, 425–427
Intracranial pressure, increased, signs and symptoms of, 409, 409(t)
Intralipid, 493(t)
Intrauterine fetal death, 236–238
Intrauterine hypoxia, chronic, 357

Intrauterine pressure catheter, application of, 561–564
Intravenous equipment, in high risk maternal/fetal transport, 36(t)
Intravenous fluids, in herpes simplex infection, 536
    nurse's role in administering, 484(t)
    suggested feeding regimens, 476(t)
Intravenous needles, in parenteral therpay, 485(t)
Intravenous nutritional support, 475(t)
Intravenous pressure catheter, application of, method of, 561–564
Intravenous tubing, and bags, in parenteral therapy, 487(t)
    guidelines for use of, 491–492(t)
Intraventricular drain, insertion of, 613–615
Intropin, in neonates, 644(t)
Intubation
    chest, 600–603
    endotracheal, 616–619
    in stabilization of perinatal patient for transport, 47
Isolation precautions, in herpes simplex infection, 529, 533
    in neonatal infection, **515**
Isolette, transport, in high risk neonatal transport, 37
    use of, in herpes simplex infection, 529
Isomil, 478(t)
Isoproterenol, in neonatal cardiogenic shock, 316
    in neonatal resuscitation, 301(t)
Isoproterenol hydrochloride, in neonates, 646(t)
Isoxsuprine, as maternal drug, 589(t)
IUD, and ectopic pregnancy, 161

Jaundice
    in neonatal septic shock, 312
    in cytomegalovirus infection, 526
    in hyperbilirubinemia, 391
    in toxoplasmosis, 523
    physiological, 391
Jejunal and ileal atresia, 506–507(t)

Kanamycin, dosage schedule, in newborn, 522(t)
Kernicterus, 393
Ketoacidosis, in parenteral hyperalimentation, 496(t)
Kidneys. See also under *Renal.*
    multicystic, childhood type, associated with neonatal renal failure, 444(t)

Labor
    dysfunctional, 208–213
        nursing management in, 211–213
        patterns of, comparison of, 209, 209(t)
    monitoring of, in nursing role for perinatal transport, 56(t), 57(t)
    oxytocin in, 573–575
    phases of, normal lengths of, 210(t)
    premature, 199–202
        as indication for high risk maternal/fetal transport, 39
        assessment of, 200
        nursing management of, 201–202
        ritodrine in, 576–578
        terbutaline in, 581–584
    risk factors in, 123
    stresses of, 105–106

Labor length, in criteria for high risk pregnancy, 10(t)
Laboratory parameters, in assessment of fetal and maternal well-being, 12(t)
Lacerations, intrapartum, postpartum hemorrhage due to, 261–262
Lactose intolerance, formula for feeding in, 478–479(t)
Lanoxin, in neonates, 644(t)
Lanugo, in assessment of high risk neonate, 283(t), 287(t)
Large bowel, obstruction of, 505(t)
Large for gestational age infants, common problems of, 290(t)
Largon, as maternal drug, 593(t)
Lasix, in neonates, 645(t)
Late deceleration, of fetal heart rate, 234–235, **234**
Lecithin, in pulmonary surfactant deficiency, 327
Left heart syndrome, hypoplastic, 365
Left to right shunts, 365–367
Left ventricular outflow obstruction, 362, 365–367, **365**
Leg, recoil of, in assessment of high risk neonate, **288**, 289
Leopold's maneuvers
    method of, 564–565, **565**
    to detect malpresentation, 219
    to detect multiple pregnancy, 228
Lethargy
    in congenital heart defects, 362
    in hyperviscosity syndrome, 381
    in neonatal herpes simplex infection, 528
    in neonatal meningitis, 521
Level I facilities, for obstetrical and newborn care, definition of, 15
Level II facilities, for obstetrical and newborn care, definition of, 15
Level III facilities, for obstetrical and newborn care, definition of, 15
    transport as responsibility of, 27
Lidocaine, as maternal drugs, 590(t)
Lie, transverse, of fetus, 223–225, **225**
Linear projections, in perinatal care planning, 545
Lipids, total, in neonate, normal blood values, 463(t)
Liposyn, 493(t)
Listeria monocytogenes, in neonatal meningitis, 416
    sepsis due to, 518–520
Liver disease, formula for, feeding in, 480(t)
Lobar emphysema, neonatal, 327(t)
Lochia, in postpartal uterine infections, 268
    postpartum educational needs relating to, 260(t)
Lofenalac, 478(t)
Logistics, of transport, importance of, 40–41
Lonalac, 478(t)
Low spinal block, in obstetrical anesthesia, 255
Lower esophageal sphincter, and neonatal ability and readiness to feed, 456
Lung(s). See also *Pulmonary.*
    in assessment of high risk neonate, 282(t)
Lung cysts, in persistent fetal circulation, 357
    neonatal, 327(t)
Lung hypoplasia, in persistent fetal circulation, 357

Magnesium
    neonatal, assessment of, 469–470(t)
        intestinal malabsorption of, causing hypocalcemia, 436
    requirements, 457(t)
    serum. See *Serum magnesium.*

Magnesium deficiency, maternal, causing neonatal hypocalcemia, 436
  causing neonatal hypomagnesemia, 440
Magnesium sulfate, 590(t)
  in preeclampsia, causing neonatal hypermagnesemia, 440
  intravenous administration of, 566–568
    loading dose, 567
    maintenance dose, 567–568
    method of, 567–568
Male genitals, in assessment of high risk neonate, 285(t)
Malposition, of fetus, 215–218
Malpresentation, of fetus, 218–225
Malrotation, of bowel, 507(t)
Marcaine, as maternal drug, 587(t)
Mastitis, 269
  as pregnancy risk factor, 131
Maternal drugs. See names of specific drugs.
Maternal/fetal transport, 24–28
  advantages of, over newborn transport, 26
  equipment for, 35
  indications for, 39, 39(t)
  stabilization of patient for, 46–47
Maternal/fetal unit, as perinatal patient, 3
Maternal monitor, future of, 542
Maternal touch progression, in bonding, 72
Meconium, in fetal digestive system, 453
Meconium aspiration, 331–335
  assessment of, 332–333
  in neonatal air block, 317
  nursing management of, 333–334
Meconium ileus, 504, 507(t)
Meconium plug, 504
Meconium staining, of amniotic fluid, fetal distress due to, 230
Medical/surgical history, in criteria for high risk pregnancy, 10–11(t)
  influence of, on pregnancy and outcome, 9(t)
Medication(s)
  for neonatal resuscitation, 301(t), **302**
  in maternal transport equipment, 36(t)
  in neonatal transport equipment, 38(t)
  maternal and neonatal. See under specific names of medications.
Megacolon, aganglionic, 504
Membrane(s), amniotic, premature rupture of. See *Premature rupture of membranes.*
  status of, tests for, 548–549
Men, pregnancy as maturational milestone in, 99(t)
  stresses of pregnancy affecting, 100
Meningitis, neonatal, 415–419, 520–522
  as sign of herpes simplex infection, 528
  assessment of, 416–417, 521
  bacterial and viral causes of, 520–521
  nursing management in, 418–419
  problems and complications in, 521
  treatment of, 522
Meningocele, vs. myelomeningocele, 401
Mental state, of pregnant woman, 99–100
Meperidine, as maternal drug, 591(t)
Metabolic demands, of perinatal patient in transport, 47
Metabolic disorders, as pregnancy risk factor, 128(t)
Methergine, as maternal drug, 591(t)
Methicillin, dosage schedule, in newborn, 522(t)
Methylergonovine maleate, as maternal drug, 591(t)
Milia, neonatal, 283
Milk-based formulas, 478(t)

Milk
  breast, in management of acute renal failure, 448
    suggested regimens for feeding, 476–477(t)
    trace elements in, 472(t)
  cow's, whole, causing neonatal hypocalcemia, 436
Milk leg, 263–266
Milk protein hypersensitivity, formula for feeding in, 479(t)
Mineral requirements, neonatal, 455–456
Modular formula, 482(t)
Mole, hydatidiform, 162–163
Monitor, fetal, external, 554–556
    precautions in, 556
  maternal, future of, 542
Monitoring, of patient condition, in nursing role for perinatal transport, 56(t)
Morphine, as maternal drug, 591(t)
Morphine sulfate, in neonates, 646(t)
Mortality, perinatal, 2
Mother
  age of, in criteria for high risk pregnancy, 10(t)
  cardiac arrest in, 138–140
  characteristics of, in criteria for high risk pregnancy, 10(t)
  diabetes mellitus in. See *Infant of diabetic mother.*
  disease in, as indication of high maternal/fetal transport, 39(t)
  hemorrhage in, 140–143
  history in, in criteria for high risk pregnancy, 9–11(t)
  postpartum educational needs of, 260(t)
  shock in, 140–143
  transport of, in high risk perinatal care, 18, 24–28
  well-being of, assessment of, 11, 12(t)
Motion, and vibration, causing changes in patient conditon during transport, 47
Motion sickness, in transported maternal/fetal patient, 47
Mouth, in assessment of high risk neonate, 284(t)
Mouth-to-mouth resuscitation, in maternal cardiac arrest, 139
Multicystic kidneys, childhood type, associated with neonatal renal failure, 444(t)
Multiple gestational infants, in family-infant bonding, 65
Multiple pregnancy, as antepartal crisis, 187–188
  as indication for high risk maternal/fetal transport, 39(t)
  as intrapartum crisis, 227–229
Murmurs
  in congenital heart defects, 362
    contour of, 369
    grades of, 369
    holosystolic, 369
    radiation of, 369
  systolic, in persistent fetal circulation, 357
    systolic ejection, 369
Muscle tone, in neonatal hypovolemic shock, 307
Myelomeningocele, 400–406, **402**
  assessment of, 402–403
  neurological dysfunction and level of lesion in, 401(t)
  nursing management in, 404–406
  surgical repair of, 405
  vs. meningocele, 401
Myocarditis, congestive heart failure from, 374

Naloxone, in neonatal resuscitation, 301(t)
Naming, of high risk infant, in bonding process, 75
Narcosis, neonatal, 327(t)
Nares, flaring of, in choanal atresia, 349
    in respiratory distress syndrome, 329
Nasogastric intubation, in omphalocele and
    gastroschisis, 502
Nasogastric nutritional support, 474(t)
Nasogastric tube, in neonatal diaphragmatic hernia,
    345
    in neonatal septic shock, 313
Nasojejunal feeding, 634–638
Nasojejunal nutritional support, 575(t)
Nasotracheal tube, sterile, in suctioning, 628–629
Neck, in assessment of high risk neonate, 283–284(t)
Necrotizing enterocolitis, 459, 489, 495, 498–500
    assessment of, 498
    hyperviscosity syndrome causing, 380
    in hypovolemia, management of, 379
    nursing management in, 499–500
    possible causes of, 489, **495**
    predisposing factors in, 489
Needles
    butterfly, in peripheral cannulation, 622, 623
    intravenous, in parenteral therapy, 485(t)
    spinal, in intraventricular drain insertion, 613, 614
        in subdural tap, 625
Neo-Mull-Soy, 478(t)
Neonatal care, regional, future of, 542–543
Neonatal circulation, **355**
Neonatal coagulopathies, 383–390
    assessment of, 387–388
    in sick infant, etiology of, 386–387
        predisposing factors, 384
    in well infant, etiology of, 385–386
        predisposing factors, 383
    nursing management in, 388–390
    screening tests for, 388, 388(t)
Neonatal heart rate, in hypovolemia, 378
Neonatal intensive care, crisis of, 109–113
Neonatal intensive care units, stress of nurses in,
        113–114, **114**
    care for, 115–116
Neonatal meningitis, 415–419
Neonatal transport, 24–26. See also *Newborn
        transport.*
    equipment for, 35, 37, 38(t)
    history of, 25
    in regionalized perinatal care, 18
    indications for, 40, 40(t)
    stabilization of patient for, 47
Neonate. See also *Infant.*
    asphyxia in, 395–303
    drugs in. See names of specific drugs.
    hypovolemic shock in, 306–308
    infection in, 516–517
    normal, basic caloric requirements of, 455(t)
    septic shock in, 311–314
    transport of. See *Neonatal transport.*
Nervous breakdown, postpartal, 272–275
Nesacaine, as maternal drug, 588(t)
Neurobehavioral responses, in assessment of high risk
    neonate, 286–287(t)
Neurological assessment, of high risk neonate, **288,**
    289
Neurological problems, as indication for high risk
    maternal/fetal transport, 40(t)
Newborn transport, advantages of maternal/fetal
    transport over, 26

Newborn transport worksheet, **42–45**
Nipples, in assessment of high risk neonate, 285(t),
    287(t)
Nitrazine test, of amniotic membrane, 548–549
Nitrous oxide, in obstetrical anesthesia, 255
Nominal group technique, in perinatal care planning,
    546
Nonimmune thrombocytopenia, 385
Non-stress test (NST), 568–569, **570**
    method of, 569
    interpretation of, 569
Nurse, and high risk pregnancy family, 104–105
    as transport team leader, 32
    bonding process and, 67–71
    emotional response of, to childbearing family in
        crisis, 94
    in neonatal intensive care unit, stress on, 113–114,
        114
Nursery, factors predisposing to infection in, 516
Nursing interventions
    in stillbirth and early infant death, 108, 109(t)
    to facilitate bonding, 71–73
        of congenitally deformed infant, 76–77
        of high risk infant, 73–75
        of transported infant, 75–76
Nursing role, in perinatal transport, 49, 50–59(t)
Nursoy, 478(t)
Nutramigen, 480(t)
Nutrition, of mother, in criteria for high risk
    pregnancy, 11(t)
Nutritional requirements, neonatal, 453, 454, 457(t)
    factors increasing, 455–456
Nutritional support, sources of, 475–475(t)

Objectives, for reader. See *Reader objectives.*
Obstetrical history, abnormal, as indication for high
        risk maternal/fetal transport, 39(t)
    influence of, on pregnancy and outcome, 9(t)
Obstetrical loss, unresolved parental grief from, 70(t),
    71
Occiput posterior, 125
    right, 216–217, **216**
Occiput transverse, 215
    left, 217, **217**
OCT, 571–573
Oliguria, neonatal, 443, 446
Oliohydramnios, 357
Omphalitis, 532(t)
Omphalocele, 361
    and gastroschisis, 500–503
One-way perinatal transport, in maternal/fetal
        transport situations, 27, **27,** 28
    nursing role in, 50–59(t)
    problems of, 27–28
Opacity of skin,
    in assessment of high risk neonate, 287(t)
Ophthalmia, neonatal, 530(t)
Op-site occlusive dressing, in hyperalimentation, 611
Oral feedings, suggested regimens, 476(t)
Oral nutritional support, 474(t)
Orogastric intubation, in omphalocele and
    gastroschisis, 502
Orogastric nutritional support, 474(t)
Oronasopharynx, unsterile, suctioning of, 629–630
Overhydration, by parenteral therapy, 488(t)
Over-reaction, as characteristic of pregnant women,
    99–100

Oxygen
in herpes simplex infection treatment, 534–535
in persistent fetal circulation, 359
transcutaneous measurement of, 632–634
Oxygenation, adequate, in infant in ventilator, 346(t)
Oxytocin, 592(t)
administration of, intrauterine pressure catheter use with, 561
induction or augmentation of labor with, 573–575
Oxytocin challenge test (OCT), 571–573
method of, 571–573

Packed cells, in parenteral therapy, 487(t)
Pain, abdominal, in high risk pregnancy, 135
epigastric, in high risk pregnancy, 135
Pallor, in hypovolemia, 378
Palpation, in congenital heart defects, 368
in congestive heart failures, 375
Pancreatic disease, formula for feeding in, 480(t)
Pancuronium bromide, in neonates, 646(t)
Parathormone, causing neonatal hypercalcemia, 436
Parenteral hyperalimentation, metabolic problems in, 496–497(t)
Parenteral therapy. See also *Hyperalimentation* and *Nutritional support.*
nutritional monitoring of, 459(t)
physical actions in administering, 484–485(t)
side effects in, 486–489(t)
Parenthood, as maturational crisis, 98–100
Parents, of transported infant, conflict between, 76
Paresis, in high risk pregnancy, 135
Parity, in criteria for high risk pregnancy, 10(t)
Partial thromboplastin time (PTT), in neonatal coagulopathies, 388, 388(t)
Patent ductus arteriosus, 366
congestive heart failure from, 375
Paternal influences, on pregnancy and outcome, 9(t)
Patient, perinatal, definition of, 3
Patient focus, in perinatal transport, 24–26
PEEP, 330
Penicillin G, dosage schedule, in newborn, 522(t)
Perfusion, peripheral, decreased, in congestive heart failure, 375
poor, in congenital heart defects, 362
Perinatal asphyxia, as indication for high risk maternal/fetal transport, 40(t)
Perinatal care
future of, 542–543
high risk, regionalization of, 13
implications for, 543–545
planning in, 545–546
Perinatal care center
and referring hospital, pre-transport communication between, 41
post-transport communication within, 48
pre-transport communication within, 46
regionalization of, 13–14
Perinatal family, contact with, in nursing role for perinatal transport, 51(t), 58(t)
Perinatal nursing care, high risk, nature of, 2–6
Perinatal outcome, in United States, 13
Perinatal patient, definition of, 3
safety of, during transport, 47
Perinatal transport, equipment in, 34–37, 36(t)
vehicle selection in, 32–34
Perinatal team, 5
stress and, 5

Perinatal team (Continued)
support of, by institution administration, 5
Perinatal transport
concept of, 23
equipment in, 34–37, 36(t)
one-way, 27, 27, 28
nursing role in, 50–59(t)
system for, 23–24
two-way, 27, 27
nursing role in, 50–59(t)
types of, 24–28
vehicle selection in, 32–34
Perinatology
nurse and, 5
nursing research in, 5
risk factors in, 7–12
Perineum
maternal, lacerations of, postpartum hemorrhage due to, 261–262
postpartal educational needs related to, 260(t)
postpartal infections of, 267
Peripheral cannulation, 619–624
common intravenous sites in infants and children, 621
Peripheral perfusion, decreased, in congestive heart failure, 375
Peripheral respiratory difficulty, 326, 327(t)
Peripheral sites, in hyperalimentation, 607
Peritonitis, postpartal, 268
Persistent fetal circulation, 354–360
assessment of, 357–358
nursing management in, at hospital of birth, 358–359
at perinatal center, 359–360
Petechiae, in neonatal coagulopathies, 384
in neonatal septic shock, 312
Phenergan, as maternal drug, 592(t)
Phenobarbital, as maternal drug, 592(t)
Phenylketonuria, formula for feeding in, 479(t)
Phlebitis, in injection site, in parenteral therapy, 484(t)
Phosphates, dietary, high, causing neonatal hypocalcemia, 436
Phosphorus, metabolism of, in parenteral hyperalimentation, 496(t)
neonatal requirements, 457(t)
Photographs, of transported infant, in bonding process, 76
Phototherapy, fluid requirements in, 455
in hyperbilirubinemia, 394–396
Physician, family, importance of, to high risk perinatal families, 17
Pitocin, 592(t)
administration of, intrauterine pressure catheter use with, 561
induction or augmentation of labor with, 573–575
Placenta, abnormal adherence of, 246–247
Placenta previa, as antepartal crisis, 163–166
as intrapartum crisis, 242–245
as pregnancy risk factor, 130
double setup procedure in, 551–552
hypovolemia from, 378
vs. abruptio placentae, 245(t)
Placental transfusion, hyperviscosity syndrome in, 381
Plantar creases, in assessment of high risk neonate, 286(t), 287(t)
Platelet count, in neonatal coagulopathies, 388, 388(t)
Pleur-Evac, in chest intubation, 601
Pneumonia, aspiration, 331–335

Pneumonia, aspiration *(Continued)*
  in persistent fetal circulation, 356
  neonatal, 327(t)
    in sepsis due to group B beta hemolytic
      streptococcus and *Listeria monocytogenes,*
      518
Pneumothorax, neonatal, 327(t), 341–344
  tension, in infant in ventilator, 346(t)
    neonatal, 317–319
Polycythemia, associated with hyperviscosity
  syndrome, 380
Polyethylene tubing, in parenteral therapy, 485(t)
Popliteal angle, in assessment of high risk neonate,
  288, 289
Portagen, 480(t)
Positioning, of nurse, in transport vehicle, 55(t)
Positive end expiratory pressure (PEEP), 330
Postinfusion hypoglycemia, in parenteral
  hyperalimentation, 496(t)
Postmaturity, as risk factor, 123
Postpartal adjustment, vs. dysfunctional bonding,
  72–73
Postpartal crisis, infant in intensive care, 109–113
Postrenal acute renal failure, 446
Post-term birth, as risk factor, 123
Post-transport communication, 48–49
Posture, in assessment of high risk neonate, **288,**
  289
Potassium
  deficit of, in parenteral therapy, 488–489(t)
  excess of, in parenteral therapy, 489(t)
  in neonate, assessment of, 456–466
  neonatal requirements, 457(t)
Potassium salts, concentrated, "safe" range for,
  489(t)
Potter's syndrome, 357, 443, 444(t)
Prednisone, in neonatal coagulopathies, 389
Preeclampsia
  as indication for high risk maternal/fetal transport,
    39
  assessment of, 196
  classification of, 178
  hydralazine in, 559–560
  magnesium sulfate in, causing neonatal
    hypermagnesemia, 440
    intravenous administration of, 566–568
  severe, assessment of, 196–197
    nursing management of, 197–198
  testing of deep tendon reflexes and clonus in,
    549–551
Preeclampsia-eclampsia, as pregnancy risk factor,
  122, 128(t), 130
Pregestimil, 480(t)
Pregnancy
  adaptive tasks of, for successful bonding, 70(t)
  as maturational crisis, 98–100, 99(t)
  concerns and stresses of, 98–100, 99(t)
  ectopic, 159–161
  high risk. See *High risk pregnancy.*
    implantation sites of, **160**
    nursing management in, 161
  maladaptation to, identification of, 103–104, 104(t)
  multiple, as antepartal crisis, 187–188
    as indication for high risk maternal/fetal transport,
      39(t)
    as intrapartum crisis, 227–229
  potential influences on, 8, 9(t)
  previous, in criteria for high risk pregnancy, 10(t)
  risk characteristics of, 101(t)

Pregnancy *(Continued)*
  unplanned, as factor in inhibition of bonding, 70(t),
    71
  unwanted, as factor in inhibition of bonding, 70(t),
    71
Pregnancy induced hypertension, as antepartal crisis,
  177–181
  assessment of, 179
  nursing management of, 180–181
  complications of, as intrapartal crisis, 193, 196–199
Pregnancy outcome, potential influences on, 8, 9(t)
  previous, in criteria for high risk pregnancy, 10(t)
Premature infant, nutritional deprivation in, 454
Premature labor, 199–202
  as indication for high risk maternal/fetal transport,
    39
  assessment of, 200
  nursing management of, 201–202
  ritodrine in, 576–578
  terbutaline in, 581–584
Premature rupture of membranes, 202–205
  as indication for high risk maternal/fetal transport,
    39
  assessment of, 203
  in high risk pregnancy, 131, 136
  nursing management in, 204–205, **205**
Prematurity
  as indication for high risk maternal/fetal transport,
    40
  as risk factor, 123
  as sign of rubella, 524
  as sign of syphilis, 525
Prerenal acute renal failure, 443
Prerenal azotemia, in parenteral hyperalimentation,
  496(t)
Presentation
  breech, 222–223, **224**
  brow, 221–222
  face, 220–221, **220**
  shoulder, 223–225, **225**
Prestin E_2, as maternal drug, 593(t)
Pre-transport communication, 40–46
  within referring hospital, 41
Primary facilities, for obstetrical and newborn care,
  definition of, 15
Problem solving, by childbearing family in crisis, 90
Programming, in regionalization of high risk perinatal
  care, 14
Progression, pregnancy, in criteria for high risk
  pregnancy, 11(t)
Prolapse, of cord, 205–208, **206**
  as pregnancy risk factor, 131
  assessment of, 206–207
  nursing management of, 207–208
Promethazine, as maternal drug, 592(t)
Propiomazine, as maternal drug, 593(t)
ProSobee, 478(t)
Prostaglandin E_1, in neonates, 646(t)
Prostaglandin E_2, as maternal drug, 593(t)
Protamine sulfate, in neonates, 647(t)
Protein, in neonate, assessment of, 461(t)
  neonatal requirements, 457(t)
  total, in neonate, normal blood values, 462(t)
Protein hypersensitivity, formula for feeding in, 480(t)
Protein solutions, in parenteral therapy, 486(t)
Prothrombin time (PT), in neonatal coagulopathies,
  388, 388(t)
Prune belly syndrome, associated with neonatal renal
  failure, 444(t)

Psychological factors, influences of, on pregnancy and outcome, 9(t)
Psychological risk, postpartal, 272–275
Psychological support, of perinatal patient or family in transport, 47
Psychosis, as pregnancy risk factor, 131
Pudendal block, in obstetrical anesthesia, 255
Puerperal infection, 266–272
Pulmonary hypoperfusion, neonatal, 328
Pulmonary stenosis, severe, 362
Pulmonary surfactant deficiency, 327–328
Pulmonary valve atresia, 362
Pulmonary valvular stenosis, 362
Pulmonary vascular bed, decreased cross-sectional area of, 357
Pulmonary vascular development, increased, 356–357
    normal, 356
Pulmonary vasoconstriction, acute, neonatal, 356
Pulmonary venous return, total anomalous, 367–368, **367**
    congestive heart failure from, 375
Pulse(s)
    femoral, in assessment of high risk neonate, 285(t)
    in congenital heart defects, 368
    in congestive heart failure, 374
    in hypovolemia, 378
Pustules, in neonatal cutaneous infections, 532
Pyelonephritis, acute, 174–175
    assessment of, 174
    nursing management in, 175
    postpartal, 269
Pyloric stenosis, 504, 507(t)

Race, in criteria for high risk pregnancy, 10(t)
Radiant warmers, fluid requirements of infant treated in, 455
    in esophageal malformations, 321
    in hypovolemic shock, 307
    in omphalocele and gastroschisis, 502
    in septic shock, 313
Radiography, in assessment of fetal well-being, 12(t)
Rales, in congestive heart failure, 374
Rapport, importance of, in transport, 40
Rash, in assessment of high risk neonate, 283(t)
RBC. See Packed cells.
Reader objectives
    in antepartal crises, 153
    in assessment and classification of high risk maternal-fetal unit, 120
    in cardiovascular and hematological crises in neonates, 353
    in future of high risk perinatal care, 540
    in gastrointestinal crises and nutritional support, 452
    in intrapartum crises, 191
    in neonatal emergencies, 294
    in neonatal infections, 514
    in neurological crises, 399
    in obstetrical emergencies, 137
    in postpartal crises, 258
    in renal and metabolic crises, 429
    in respiratory crises, 325
    in stress, 97
Readjustment, to nonpregnant state, in women following childbirth, 100
Reality testing, in crisis situations, 90–91
Record, of newborn transport, **42–45**
Record keeping process, in nursing role for perinatal transport, 52(t)

Rectal biopsy, in Hirschsprung's disease, 508(t)
Referral
    as part of regional dispatch system in neonatal intensive care, 19
    as synonym for perinatal transport, 23
    by hospital, pre-transport communication for, 41
    follow-up, in nursing role for perinatal transport, 59(t)
Referring hospital, post-transport communication in, 41
    pre-transport communication in, 41
Reflex(es)
    biceps, testing of, 550–551
    deep tendon, testing of, 549–551
    diving seal, necrotizing enterocolitis and, 489
    knee jerk, testing of, 550
Reflex activity, influencing neonatal ability and readiness to feed, 456
Regional dispatch systems, in high risk perinatal care, 19
Regional obstetrical anesthesia, 255
Regionalization, of high risk perinatal care, nature of, 14
    program for, 14
Regionalized high risk perinatal care, 18, 20
Regionalized perinatal care centers
    conceptual model of, 15, **16**
    cost of, 17
    personnel for, 16–17
Regionalized transport systems, 18
Renal acute renal failure, 446
Renal agenesis, causing acute renal failure, 443
Renal disorders, as pregnancy risk factor, 128(t)
Renal dysplasia, associated with neonatal renal failure, 444(t)
Renal excretion, impaired, causing neonatal hypocalcemia, 436
Renal hypoperfusion, neonatal, causing acute renal failure, 443
Renal vein, thrombosis of, associated with neonatal renal failure, 444(t)
Renovascular accidents, associated with neonatal renal failure, 444(t)
Replogle tube, in neonatal septic shock, 313
Resentment, as characteristic of pregnant women, 99–100
    parental, of high risk pregnancy, 102
Resignation, as stage of grief, 87
Respirations, in assessment of high risk neonate, 282(t)
    rapid, in neonatal peripheral respiratory difficulty, 327(t)
Respiratory difficulty, peripheral, 326, 327(t)
Respiratory distress
    as indication for high risk maternal/fetus transport, 40(t)
    causes of, 328(t)
    effects of, 328(t)
    fluid requirements in, 455
    in congenital heart defects, 362
    in congestive heart failure, 374
    in diaphragmatic hernia, 345
    in high risk pregnancy, 135
    in omphalocele and gastroschisis, 501
    in persistent fetal circulation, 356, 367
Respiratory distress syndrome, 326–331
Respiratory failure, neonatal, 326, 327(t)
Resuscitation
    mouth-to-mouth, in maternal cardiac arrest, 139
    neonatal, **298**

Resuscitation *(Continued)*
   equipment for, 295(t)
Retractions
   in pneumothorax, 342
   intercostal, in neonatal peripheral respiratory
      difficulty, 327(t)
   subcostal, in neonatal peripheral respiratory
      difficulty, 327(t)
   substernal, in respiratory distress syndrome, 328
Rh sensitization, 169
Right ventricular outflow obstruction, 362, **363**
Risk assessment, in perinatal care, future of, 541–542
Risk identification, in candidate for maternal
   transport, 25
Risk scoring index, antepartum, 128–129(t)
Ritodrine, 593–594(t)
   intravenous administration of, in premature labor,
      576–578
Role therapy, and childbearing family in crisis, 83–84
Rotary-winged air transport, of perinatal high risk
   patient, 30(t), 32
Rubella, maternal, effect on infant, 361
   neonatal, 524–525
"Runaway IV," 490(t)

Sabin-Feldman dye test, in toxoplasmosis, 523
Saddle block, in obstetrical anesthesia, 255
Saran wrap, in gastrointestinal obstruction, 510
   in omphalocele and gastroschisis, 502
Safety, of perinatal patient, during transport, 47
   responsibility for, of high risk perinatal transport
      team, 31
Scalded skin syndrome, 532(t)
Scalp, as site of intravenous nutritional support,
   475(t)
   fetal, sampling from, in hypoxemia and acidosis,
      147, 148
Scalp vein, cannulation in, 620–623
Scarf sign, in assessment of high risk neonate, **288,**
   289
Schizophrenia, postpartal, 272–275
Secondary facilities, for obstetrical and newborn
   care, definition of, 15
Sedatives, avoidance of, in mother of congenitally
   deformed infant, 77
Seizure(s), eclamptic, 143–144
   nursing management in, 144, 181
   assessment of, 413–414
   classification of, 412–413
   etiology of, 412–413, 412(t)
   in neonatal hypocalcemia, 436
   in neonatal hypoglycemia, 433
   in neonatal hypoglycemic shock, 310
   in neonatal hypomagnesemia, 442
   nursing management in, 414–415
   recording of, 414(t)
Sensitive period, in family-infant bonding, 65–66
Separation, in childbearing family in crisis, 82
   of sick infant from parents, 17
Sepsis
   as pregnancy risk factor, 131
   due to group B beta hemolytic streptococcus,
      assessment of, 518
   due to *Listeria monocytogenes,* 518–520
   in omphalocele and gastroschisis, 501, 502
Sepsis neonatorum, 517–518
Septic shock, neonatal, 311–314
Septicemia, 517–518

Serum albumin, in neonate, normal blood values,
   462(t)
Serum BUN, in neonatal acute renal failure, 446
Serum calcium
   imbalances of, 435–439
      assessment of, 436–437
      nursing management in, 437–439
   in congenital heart defects, 369
   in persistent fetal circulation, 358, 359
Serum glucose
   imbalances of, 430–435
      assessment of, 431–432
      nursing management in, 433
   in congenital heart defects, 369
   in persistent fetal circulation, 358, 359
Serum magnesium
   imbalances of, 439–443
      assessment of, 441
      nursing management in, 442–443
   in persistent fetal circulation, 358, 359
Setting sun sign, in assessment of high risk neonate,
   284(t)
Sexual desire, change in, in pregnant woman, 100
SGOT, elevations of, in parenteral hyperalimentation,
   497(t)
   in neonate, normal blood values, 461(t)
SGPT, elevations of, in parenteral hyperalimentation,
   497(t)
   in neonate, normal blood values, 462(t)
Shame, parental, at unsuccessful pregnancy, 106
Shock
   as pregnancy risk factor, 131
   cardiogenic, 314–316
   hypoglycemic, 308–311
   hypovolemic, 306–308
   maternal, 140–143
   neonatal, 303–306
   septic, 311–314
   symptoms of, 171(t)
Shoulder dystocia, 225–227
Shoulder presentation, 223–225, **225**
Shunt(s), in treatment of hydrocephalus, 410, **411**
   left to right, as congenital heart defects, 365–367
Siblings, responses of, to family crisis, 89
Sickle cell disease, in pregnancy, 188
Sickle cell hemoglobin C, 189
Sickle cell trait, 189
Silastic mesh, in omphalocele and gastroschisis, 503
Silver nitrate, in herpes simplex infection prevention,
   533
Similac, 478(t)
Similac PM 60/40, 478(t)
Situational crisis, high risk pregnancy as, 101–103,
   101(t)
Skin, in assessment of high risk neonate, 283(t)
   infection of, 532(t)
Skin eruptions,
   in sepsis due to group B beta hemolytic
      streptococcus and *Listeria monocytogenes,* 518
SMA, 478(t)
Small bowel, obstruction of, 505(t)
Small for gestational age infants, common problems
   of, 290(t)
Smooth muscle relaxants, in persistent fetal
   circulation, 359
Social factors, influences of, on pregnancy and
   outcome, 9(t)
Social forecasting, in perinatal care, 545
Sodium
   in neonate, assessment of, 467–469(t)

Sodium *(Continued)*
  neonatal requirements, 457(t)
  retention of, in parenteral therapy, 488(t)
Sodium bicarbonate, in neonates, 647(t)
Solutions
  amino acid, in parenteral therapy, 486(t)
  dextrose, in parenteral therapy, 486(t)
  hydrating, in parenteral therapy, 486(t)
  hyperosmolar, in parenteral therapy, 486–487(t)
  in total parenteral nutrition, change of, 608–609
  protein, in parenteral therapy, 486(t)
Soy-based formulas, 478–479(t)
Space occupying lesions, of chest, 356, 357
Species-specific responses, in family-infant bonding, 65
Speculum, sterile, examination with, 580–581
Spiral electrode, application of, 578–579
Spinal block, low, in obstetrical anesthesia, 255
Spinal needle, in intraventricular drain insertion, 613, 614
  in subdural tap, 625
Spontaneous abortion, 157–159
Stabilization, of patient, in pre-transport process, 46–47
  nursing role in, 52(t)
Stadol, as maternal drug, 587(t)
Status epilepticus, 415
Stenosis
  aortic, 365, **365**
  duodenal, 507(t)
  gastrointestinal, 504
  pulmonary, severe, 362
  pulmonary valvular, 362
  pyloric, 507(t)
Sterile speculum examination, 580–581
Stillbirth, unresolved parental grief from, 70(t), 71
Stomach. See *Gastric.*
Stools, in necrotizing enterocolitis, 498
  in neonatal diarrhea, 531
Streptococcus(i)
  causing neonatal infection, 516
  group B beta hemolytic, in neonatal septic shock, 312
  sepsis due to, 518–520
Stomach, obstruction of, 505(t)
Stress
  general principles and effects, 97–98
  to family of high risk perinate, 4
  to family of infant in intensive care, 109–113
  to nurse, in care of childbearing family in crisis, 113–115
  to perinatal team, 5
Stress testing, in assessment of fetal well-being, 12(t)
Stridor, inspiratory, in choanal atresia, 349
Strip graph, in fetal monitoring, interpretation of, 556–559
Strychnos, synthetic, in neonate, 643(t)
Stump, umbilical, in omphalitis, 532
Subcostal retraction, in neonatal peripheral respiratory difficulty, 327(t)
  in respiratory distress syndrome, 327(t)
Subdural hematoma, 423
Subdural tap, 625–626
Substernal retractions
  in pneumothorax, 342
  in respiratory distress syndrome, 328
Suck-swallow pattern, 456
Suctioning
  bulb syringe in, 626–627
  DeLee apparatus in, 627–628
  of unsterile oronasopharynx, 629–630

Supervision, in perinatal transport, definition of, 23
Support systems, emotional, lack of, as factor in inhibition of bonding, 70(t), 71
Surgery, in congenital heart defects, 317–372
  in myelomeningocele, 405
Surgical delivery. See also *Cesarean section.*
  previous, in criteria for high risk pregnancy, 10(t)
Syntocinon, as maternal drug, 592(t)
Syphilis, 525–526
Syringe, bulb, in suctioning, 626–627
Systems theory, and childbearing family in crisis, 84
Systolic ejection murmur, 369
Systolic murmur, in persistent fetal circulation, 357

Tachycardia
  fetal, 231
  in neonatal hypoglycemic shock, 309
  in neonatal hypovolemic shock, 307
Tachypnea
  in neonatal acute renal failure, 448, 450
  in neonatal hypoglycemic shock, 309
  in pneumothorax, 342
  in respiratory distress syndrome, 328
  transient, of newborn, 335–337
Taking hold phase, in postpartal adjustment, 73
Taking in phase, in postpartal adjustment, 73
Tap, subdural, 625–626
TE fistula. See *Tracheoesophageal fistula.*
Team, in transport of perinatal high risk patient, 28–32
Teflon mesh, in omphalocele and gastroschisis, 503
Temperature, neonatal, instability of, as cause of apnea, 338(t)
Tension pneumothorax, in infant in ventilator, 346(t)
Teratogens, causing congenital heart defects, 361
Terbutaline, 594(t)
  intravenous administration of, in premature labor, 581–584
Tertiary facilities, for obstetrical and newborn care, definition of, 15
Tes-Tape, 491(t)
Testing, biochemical, in assessment of fetal well-being, 12(t)
  stress, in assessment of fetal well-being, 12(t)
Test(s), non-stress, 568–570
  of amniotic membrane status, 548–549
  oxytocin challenge, 571–573
Tetanic contractions, 146–147
Tetralogy of Fallot, 362, **363**
Texture, of skin
  in assessment of high risk neonate, 287(t)
THAM, in neonates, 648(t)
Theophylline, in neonates, 647(t)
Thiopental sodium, in obstetrical anesthesia, 255
Thoracotomy, 631–632
  in neonatal air block, 319
Thrill, in congenital heart defects, 368
Thrombocytopenia
  as sign of cytomegalovirus infection, 527
  as sign of rubella, 524
  immune, 385
  nonimmune, 385
Thrombophlebitis, postpartal, 263–266
Thrombosis, renal vein, associated with neonatal renal failure, 444(t)
Ticarcillin, dosage schedule, in newborn, 522(t)

Time lines, in perinatal care planning, 545
Tobramycin, dosage schedule, in newborn, 522(t)
Tocodynamometer, 554, 555
Tolazoline hydrochloride, in neonates, 697(t)
  in persistent fetal circulation, 359
Tone, muscle, in neonatal hypovolemic shock, 307
TORCH infections, 522
  causes of, 517
Total anomalous pulmonary venous return, 367–368, **367**
  congestive heart failure from, 375
Total parenteral nutrition (TPN)
  central vein sites in, 607
  components of, 607
  dressing change in, 609–612
  peripheral sites for, 607
  solutions for, 607
    change of, 608–609
Touch, maternal, progression of, in bonding, 72
Toxins, environmental, causing heart defects, 361
Toxoplasmosis, 522–524
Trace elements
  effects of deficiencies of, 472(t)
  in breast milk, 472(t)
  minimum level recommended, 472(t)
  neonatal requirements of, 455–456
Tracheoesophageal fistula, and gastrointestinal atresia, 506(t)
  with esophageal atresia, neonatal, 319–322
Transcutaneous electrode, in measurement of oxygen, 623, 633
Transfer
  as synonym for perinatal transport, 23
  of patient, in nursing role for perinatal transport, 55(t), 57(t)
  of responsibilities, in nursing role for perinatal transport, 50(t)
Transfusion
  blood, reaction to, 487(t)
  exchange, 603–606
  in management of hypovolemia, 379
  in neonatal coagulopathies, 388–389
  partial exchange, in hyperviscosity syndrome, 383
  placental, hyperviscosity syndrome in, 381
  twin to twin, hypovolemia in, 378
Transient tachypnea of newborn, 335–337
Transillumination, of hydrocephalus, 408, **408**
Transport
  air, of perinatal high risk patient, 28, **29**, 30(t)
  changes in patient condition due to, 47
  ground, of perinatal high risk patient, 28, **29**
  high risk perinatal, indications for, 37, 39–40
  maternal, in regionalized perinatal care, 18
  maternal/fetal. See *Maternal/Fetal transport.*
  neonatal. See *Neonatal transport.*
  one-way, 27, **27**, 28
    nursing role in, 50–59(t)
  perinatal. See *Perinatal transport.*
  process of, 40–49
  two-way, 27, **27**
    nursing role in, 50–59(t)
Transport incubator, in high risk neonatal transport, 37
Transport isolette, in high risk neonatal transport, 37
Transport systems, community based, 18
  regionalized, 18–19
Transport team
  composition of, 28, 31
  preparation of, 31–32
  roles of members of, 32
  size of, 31

Transported infants, bonding and, 75–76
Transposition of great arteries, 362, 364–365, **364**
  congestive heart failure from, 375
Transverse lie, 223–225, **225**
Trend extrapolation, in perinatal care planning, 545
Tricuspid valve atresia, 362
Triple dye, in herpes simplex infection prevention, 533
Trisomy 13, congenital heart defects in, 361
Trisomy 18, congenital heart defects in, 361
Trisomy 21, congenital heart defects in, 361
Trousseau sign, in neonatal hypocalcemia, 437
Truncus arteriosus, 366, **366**
  congestive heart failure from, 374
Tubes
  endotrachael, 616
  endotracheal or nasotracheal, in suctioning, 628–629
  Replogle, in neonatal septic shock, 313
Tube feeding, 634–638
Tubing
  in hyperalimentation, change of, 608–609
  intravenous, and bags, in parenteral therapy, 487(t)
    guidelines for use of, 491–492(t)
  polyethylene, in parenteral therapy, 485(t)
Tubocurarine hydrochloride, in neonates, 643(t)
Tubular necrosis, acute, in hypovolemia, management of, 379–380
Tubular/cortical necrosis, associated with neonatal renal failure, 444(t)
Turner's syndrome, congenital heart defects in, 361
Twin to twin transfusion, hypovolemia in, 378
Twins
  diamnionic, hyperviscosity syndrome in, 380
  hypervolemia in, 377
  in family-infant bonding, 65
Two-way perinatal transport, 27, **27**
  nursing role in, 50–59(t)

Ultrasound, in assessment of fetal well-being, 12(t)
Ultracaine, as maternal drug, 590(t)
Umbilical arterial catheter, placement of, 638–641
Umbilical stump, in omphalitis, 532
United States, perinatal outcome in, 13
University Hospital, San Diego, neonatal transport equipment list, 38(t)
University of Colorado Medical Center classification of newborns, **291**
Unplanned pregnancy, as factor in inhibition of bonding, 70(t), 71
Unwanted pregnancy, as factor in inhibition of bonding, 70(t), 71
Urinalysis, in neonatal acute renal failure, 447
Urinary output
  in hypovolemia, 378
  inadequate, in parenteral therapy, 488(t)
  monitoring of, in maternal hemorrhage, 142
Urinary tract
  defects of, and neonatal renal failure, 444(t)
  infection of, 530(t)
  obstructive lesions of, and neonatal renal failure, 444(t)
Urination, burning, in high risk pregnancy, 135
Urine
  dark or blood-tinged, in acute renal failure, 450
  in assessment of high risk neonate, 282(t)
  specific gravity of, in assessment of neonatal fluid and calorie intake, 457
Uterine size, in assessment of fetal and maternal well-being, 12(t)

Uterus
  atony of, postpartum hemorrhage due to, 261
  bimanual compression of, 143, **143**
  inversion of, 252–254
  postpartal infections of, 267–268
  rupture of, 249–252

Vagina, lacerations of, postpartum hemorrhage due to,
    261–262
  postpartal infections of, 267
Vaginal examination, during labor, 585–586
Valsalva's maneuver, in catheterization, 492(t)
Valvular stenosis, pulmonary, 362
Van, in transport of perinatal high risk patient, 30(t),
    32
Vancomycin, dosage schedule, in newborn, 522(t)
Variability, decreased, of fetal heart rate, 235–236
Variable deceleration, of fetal heart rate, 233–234,
    233
Vasodilan, 589(t)
VATER association, 361
  neonatal renal failure and, 444(t)
VDRL test, in syphilis, 526
Vehicle selection, in perinatal high risk transport,
    33–34
Ventilation
  in herpes simplex infection treatment, 535
  in neonatal asphyxia, 299
  in stabilization of perinatal patient for transport, 47
Ventilator
  infant in, safety of, 347(t)
    standards of care for, 346–347(t)
  malfunctions of, 347(t)
Ventral septal defect, 362
Ventral suspension, in assessment of high risk neonate,
    288, 289
Ventricular outflow obstruction, right, 362, **363**
Ventricular septal defect, 366, **366**
  congestive heart failure from, 374
Vernix caseosa, in assessment of high risk neonate,
    283(t)
Vibration, and motion, causing changes in patient
    condition during transport, 47
Vision, blurred, in high risk pregnancy, 135
Vistaril, 589(t)
Vital signs, in parenteral therapy, 485(t)
  monitoring of, in nursing role for perinatal
    transport, 56(t), 57(t)
Vitamin D, deficiency of, in parenteral
    hyperalimentation, 497(t)

Vitamin D (Continued)
  high maternal intake of, causing neonatal
    hypercalcemia, 436
Vitamin requirements, neonatal, 455, 457(t)
Vitamin K deficiency, 385–386
  in parenteral hyperalimentation, 497(t)
Vitamins
  effects of deficiencies of, 473(t)
  effects of excesses of, 473(t)
  normal blood levels of, 473(t)
Volvulus, 507(t)
Vomiting, in necrotizing enterocolitis, 498
von Willebrand's disease, 386
Vulva, postpartal infections of, 267

Warmers, infant. See *Radiant warmers.*
Water, glucose, suggested regimens for feeding, 476(t)
Water seal bottle, in chest intubation, 600–601
Weight, gain of, in assessment of neonatal fluid and
    calorie intake, 457
  loss of, in neonatal urinary tract infection, 530
  of fetus, in assessment of well-being, 12(t)
  of mother, in criteria for high risk pregnancy, 10(t)
Wheezing, in acute renal failure, 450
White's classification, of diabetes mellitus, 182
Whole blood, in parenteral therapy, 487(t)
Withdrawal, as stage of grief, 87
Women, pregnancy as maturational milestone in,
    99(t)
Worksheet, for neonatal resuscitation medications,
    302, 304–305
  newborn transport, 42–45

Xiphoid retraction, in neonatal peripheral respiratory
    difficulty, 327(t)
X-ray
  chest, in congenital heart defects, 364
    in congestive heart failure, 375
    in neonatal air block, 318
    in persistent fetal circulation, 358
  in gastrointestinal obstruction, 506, 507(t)
  in necrotizing enterocolitis, 498
Xylocaine, 590(t)

Yrytopar, as maternal drug, 593–594(t)